Myofascial Pain
and Fibromyalgia

Trigger Point
Management

Myofascial Pain and Fibromyalgia

Trigger Point Management

Second Edition

Edward S. Rachlin, MD
Assistant Clinical Professor of Orthopedic Surgery
UMDNJ–Robert Wood Johnson School of Medicine
New Brunswick, New Jersey

Instructor in Clinical Orthopedics
New York University School of Medicine

Assistant Adjunct
Department of Orthopedics
Lenox Hill Hospital
New York, New York

Isabel S. Rachlin, PT
Specialized Physical Therapy
Ithaca, New York

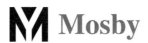 Mosby

An Imprint of Elsevier Science

St. Louis   London   Philadelphia   Sydney   Toronto

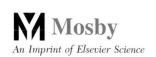
Mosby
An Imprint of Elsevier Science

Acquisitions Editor: Natasha Andjelkovic
Developmental Editor: Kimberley Cox
Production Editor: Edna Dick
Production Manager: Guy Barber
Illustration Specialist: Robert Quinn
Book Designer: Andrew Johnson

Copyright © 2002, 1994 by Mosby, Inc.

NOTICE

Orthopedics is an ever-changing field. Standard safety precautions must be followed, but as new research and clinical experience broaden our knowledge, changes in treatment and drug therapy may become necessary or appropriate. Readers are advised to check the most current product information provided by the manufacturer of each drug to be administered to verify the recommended dose, the method and duration of administration, and contraindications. It is the responsibility of the licensed prescriber, relying on experience and knowledge of the patient, to determine dosages and the best treatment for each individual patient. Neither the publisher nor the editor assumes any liability for any injury and/or damage to persons or property arising from this publication.

Mosby, Inc.
An Imprint of Elsevier Science
11830 Westline Industrial Drive
St. Louis, Missouri 63146

Printed in the United States of America

International Standard Book Number 0–323–01155–1

01 02 03 04 code/code 9 8 7 6 5 4 3 2 1

We dedicate this book to our family in appreciation of their encouragement and support.

Contributors

Elsayed Abdel-Moty, PhD
Research Associate Professor, University of Miami, Coral Gables. Administrator of Clinical Services/Systems and Supervisor of Ergonomics, University of Miami Comprehensive Pain and Rehabilitation Center, Miami Beach, Florida.
The Role of Ergonomics in the Prevention and Management of Myofascial Pain

Louis F. Amorosa, MD
Professor of Clinical Medicine, University of Medicine and Dentistry of New Jersey–Robert Wood Johnson Medical School. Chief of Endocrinology (St. Peter's University Hospital) and Attending Physician (Robert Wood Johnson University Hospital), New Brunswick, New Jersey.
Metabolic and Endocrine Causes of Muscle Syndromes

Shihab S. Asfour, PhD
Industrial Engineering Department, University of Miami, Coral Gables, Florida.
The Role of Ergonomics in the Prevention and Treatment of Myofascial Pain

Mary F. Bezkor, MD
Clinical Associate Professor of Rehabilitation, New York University School of Medicine. Staff, New York University Medical Center; Rusk Institute of Rehabilitation Medicine, New York, New York.
Trigger Point Management

Harold V. Cohen, DDS
Professor, Division of Oral Medicine, University of Medicine and Dentistry of New Jersey–New Jersey Dental School, Newark. Robert Wood Johnson University Hospital, New Brunswick, New Jersey.
Diagnosis and Management of Orofacial Pain

Andrew A. Fischer, MD, PhD
Associate Clinical Professor, Department of Rehabilitation Medicine, Mount Sinai School of Medicine, New York. Attending Physician, Mount Sinai Hospital, Elmhurst Hospital, and St. Francis Hospital, Roslyn, New York.
Functional Diagnosis of Musculoskeletal Pain and Evaluation of Treatment Results by Quantitative and Objective Techniques; New Injection Techniques for Treatment of Musculoskeletal Pain

Joan T. Gold, MD
Clinical Associate Professor of Rehabilitation Medicine, New York University School of Medicine. Clinical Director of Children's Rehabilitation Services, Howard A. Rusk Institute of Rehabilitation Medicine, New York University Medical Center, New York, New York.
Diagnostic Challenges in the Pediatric Patient with Musculoskeletal Pain

Roy C. Grzesiak, PhD

Clinical Associate Professor of Psychiatry, University of Medicine and Dentistry of New Jersey–New Jersey Medical School, Newark. Consulting Psychologist, New Jersey Pain Institute, University of Medicine and Dentistry of New Jersey–Robert Wood Johnson Medical School, New Brunswick, New Jersey.
Psychological Considerations in Myofascial Pain, Fibromyalgia, and Related Musculoskeletal Pain

Fatma İnanici, MD

Assistant Professor in Physical Medicine and Rehabilitation, Department of Physical Medicine and Rehabilitation, Hacettepe University Medical School. Attending Physician, Department of PMR, Hacettepe University Hospital, Ankara, Turkey.
Fibromyalgia Syndrome: Clinical Features, Diagnosis, and Biopathophysiologic Mechanisms; Management of Fibromyalgia Syndrome

Joseph Kahn, PhD, PT

Clinical Assistant Professor Emeritus, SUNY Stony Brook, New York. Chief, Physical Therapy (Retired), East Nassau Medical Group/HMO, Syossett, New York. Private Practice (Retired).
Electrical Modalities in the Treatment of Myofascial Conditions

Tarek M. Khalil, PhD, PE

Industrial Engineering Department, University of Miami, Coral Gables, Florida.
The Role of Ergonomics in the Prevention and Treatment of Myofascial Pain

Paul J. Kiell, MD

Far Hills, New Jersey
Trigger Point Management

Hans Kraus, MD†

Former Associate Professor, Department of Rehabilitation Medicine, New York University, New York, New York.
Muscle Deficiency

Mathew H.M. Lee, MD

Chairman, Department of Rehabilitation Medicine, New York University School of Medicine. Medical Director, Rusk Institute of Rehabilitation Medicine, New York, New York.
Trigger Point Management

Brian Miller, PT, OCS

Owner, Miller Physical Therapy, Marquette, Michigan.
Manual Therapy for Myofascial Pain and Dysfunction

Matthew Monsein, MD, MBA

Clinical Instructor, Department of Dentistry, University of Minnesota. Medical Director, Chronic Pain and Rehabilitation, Abbot-Northwestern Hospital and Sister Kenny Institute, Minneapolis, Minnesota.
Disability Evaluation and Management of Myofascial Pain

Beth Paris, PT, LMT

Director, Hands On Physical Therapy, Ithaca, New York.
The Practical Application of Trigger Point Work in Physical Therapy

---

†Deceased.

Winston C.V. Parris, MD
Clinical Professor of Anesthesiology, University of South Florida School of Medicine. CEO, Universal Anesthesia Company, Tampa, Florida.
Nerve Block Therapy for Myofascial Pain Management

Richard A. Pertes, DDS
Clinical Professor and Director, Fellowship Program in Orofacial Pain, Division of Oral Medicine, University of Medicine and Dentistry of New Jersey–New Jersey Dental School, Newark, New Jersey.
Diagnosis and Management of Orofacial Pain

Edward S. Rachlin, MD
Assistant Clinical Professor of Orthopedic Surgery, University of Medicine and Dentistry of New Jersey–Robert Wood Johnson School of Medicine, New Brunswick, New Jersey. Instructor in Clinical Orthopedics, New York University Hospital for Joint Diseases. Assistant Adjunct, Department of Orthopedics, Lenox Hill Hospital, New York, New York.
Trigger Points; History and Physical Examination for Myofascial Pain; Trigger Point Management; Injection of Specific Trigger Points

Isabel S. Rachlin, PT
Specialized Physical Therapy, Ithaca, New York.
Trigger Point Management; Physical Therapy Treatment Approaches for Myofascial Pain Syndromes and Fibromyalgia

Hubert L. Rosomoff, MD
Comprehensive Pain and Rehabilitation Center, University of Miami, Miami Beach, Florida.
The Role of Ergonomics in the Prevention and Treatment of Myofascial Pain

Renee Steele-Rosomoff, BSN, MBA
Comprehensive Pain and Rehabilitation Center, University of Miami, Miami, Florida.
The Role of Ergonomics in the Prevention and Treatment of Myofascial Pain

Muhammad B. Yunus, MD
Professor of Medicine, Section of Rheumatology, University of Illinois College of Medicine at Peoria. Attending Physician, OSF St. Francis Medical Center, Peoria, Illinois.
Fibromyalgia Syndrome: Clinical Features, Diagnosis, and Biopathophysiologic Mechanisms; Management of Fibromyalgia Syndrome

Foreword

The vast majority of patients seen in pain management programs have myofascial pain. Yet to most physicians and other health care providers, this is a very confusing area in which they have received little training. This instructional text explores new concepts in the etiology, pathophysiology, clinical presentations, laboratory evaluation, diagnosis, and treatment of myofascial pain syndromes, fibromyalgia, and trigger points. It stresses theory as well as technique. It emphasizes a comprehensive, interdisciplinary approach to the subject by drawing upon experts in physiatry, orthopedic surgery, anesthesiology, psychology, physical therapy, rheumatology, endocrinology, dentistry, and industrial engineering. Each of the chapter authors is a well-known expert who has published extensively in the area of pain management. For this new edition, nine new contributing authors have been added.

The scope of this second edition has been extensively revised and broadened and includes the following new material:

- A new chapter on the metabolic causes of muscle pain
- Discussion of muscle pain in the pediatric population
- Facts on new methods in myofascial pain and trigger point diagnosis
- Analysis of new injection techniques for the treatment of muscular/skeletal pain
- A new chapter on nerve block therapy for myofascial pain management
- A new chapter detailing manual trigger point examination and treatment in physical therapy
- An expanded chapter on orofacial pain
- Additional information on regulatory efforts to address workplace ergonomics
- Chapters on the diagnosis and treatment of fibromyalgia that have been rewritten and updated
- New approaches to treatment involving alternative and integrative medicine in acute and chronic pain, and new approaches to prevention and wellness

All of the chapters have been updated to incorporate new information, new references, and many new photographs and illustrations. The book is organized into three parts: Part I, General Considerations, presents background material on the pathophysiologic mechanisms, the clinical features, the pertinent laboratory tests, and the pharmacologic, nonpharmacologic, and psychological treatment approaches to muscle pain.

Part II, Trigger Point Management, is an important section including theory, background information, and technique. This section is designed to be used in the treatment room. Each skeletal muscle is discussed sequentially, with subheadings outlining the corresponding symptoms and referral pain pattern findings, differential diagnosis, anatomy and trigger point location, noninvasive therapy, injection technique of the trigger point, precautions, post-injection physical therapy program, exercise and home program, and corrective and preventive measures. The descriptive illustrations of the typical trigger point injection technique, augmented by the detailed illustrations showing the precise injection of the specific trigger point location in individual skeletal muscles, should aid the reader in correct performance of these procedures.

Part III covers physical therapy and rehabilitation including exercise, electric modalities, therapeutic massage techniques, manual therapy techniques, body mechanics, and ergonomics.

This second edition will be a very valuable reference and a practical laboratory guide for physicians and other health care professionals who treat patients suffering from the various types of muscle pathology. It also emphasizes the need for further research to clarify our understanding of the interrelationship among fibromyalgia, myofascial pain syndromes, referred pain, and trigger points. The better we understand this type of skeletal muscle pain, the more rationally we can plan our treatment approach. Dr. Edward Rachlin is to be congratulated again for conceptualizing, editing, and rewriting this useful text. His dedication to the subject matter and to the care of patients suffering from these conditions is obvious, as is that of his equally knowledgeable and dedicated coauthors.

Joel A. DeLisa, M.D., M.S.
Professor and Chair
Department of Physical Medicine and
 Rehabilitation
UMDNJ–New Jersey Medical School
Newark, New Jersey
President & CEO
Kessler Medical Rehabilitation Research and
 Education Corporation
West Orange, New Jersey

Acknowledgments

We wish to express our gratitude to the following:

Dr. Katherine Rachlin for her valuable organizational assistance. Jo Anne Caporaso and Susan Miarmi for all of the time and energy they devoted to this project; the librarian, Lana Strazhnik, for her valiant efforts in researching the numerous and often difficult to obtain references necessary for the preparation of the Second Edition of this text; Sarah Rubenstein-Gillis for her helpful suggestions and photographic contributions; Stacy Snyder, LAc, Dipl Ac, for her expertise in Chinese Medicine; and to Anna Winkvist, PhD, for her help in obtaining Swedish research articles.

Preface

There has been a great increase in the awareness of muscle pain as a cause and/or major contributing factor in acute and chronic pain conditions. Since the publication of our First Edition, new concepts in pain mechanisms, theory of etiology, and treatment have evolved in the fields of both myofascial pain and fibromyalgia. The goal of the Second Edition is to fill the growing need for an instructional text that provides state-of-the-art technique as well as theory and research in these fields. This text is designed to be used in the treatment room as well as for reference.

We have maintained our original format, consisting of three parts: General Considerations, Trigger Point Management, and Physical Therapy and Rehabilitation. In addition to new chapters, all previous chapters in the text have been updated and many completely revised. References have been extensively expanded to include the latest sources. The text remains a practical text, with additional illustrations, to enable the physician and therapist to incorporate new techniques in managing muscle pain. Concise and detailed presentation for the comprehensive management of single muscle pain syndromes, a hallmark of the text, continues to be one of its most important and practical features. New concepts in diagnosis of muscle pain and trigger point injection technique are clearly described, with extensive illustrations. Every attempt has been made to maintain a "how to do it" approach, without losing sight of the importance of the multifaceted nature of muscle pain. We have added nine new contributing authors, emphasizing the comprehensive interdisciplinary approach that is required in treating myofascial pain and fibromyalgia. The scope of the Second Edition has been broadened to include several new chapters. New insights are described in detail by Dr. Andrew A. Fischer in his chapters on new concepts in myofascial pain, in addition to diagnosis and new injection techniques. Nerve block therapy for myofascial pain management by Dr. Winston C.V. Parris has contributed an anesthesiologist's perspective to our treatment armamentarium.

We have placed equal emphasis on noninvasive approaches in the management of muscle pain. The physical therapy and rehabilitation chapters have been updated and expanded to include manual techniques, movement therapies, exercise, electrical modalities, ergonomics, and important clinical observations and information. Beth N. Paris, P.T. has expanded the scope of physical therapy in her chapter entitled The Practical Application of Trigger Point Work in Physical Therapy, in which she gives detailed instruction on performing manual trigger point examination and treatment of commonly found "patterns" of muscle involvement.

A unique chapter has been contributed by Dr. Joan Gold dealing with unusual aspects of musculoskeletal pain in the pediatric population. Another new chapter, Metabolic and Endocrine Causes of Muscle Syndromes, was contributed by Dr. Louis F. Amorosa. Chapters on the diagnosis and treatment of fibromyalgia have been rewritten and updated by Drs. Muhammad B. Yunus and Fatma İnanici. Drs. Harold V.

Cohen and Richard A. Pertes have extensively revised the chapter on the diagnosis and management of facial pain. Drs. Mathew H.M. Lee and Mary F. Bezkor have contributed to the comprehensive approach in treating myofascial pain and fibromyalgia by including alternative medicine (integrative approaches in acute and chronic pain), as well as focusing on prevention and wellness, in the chapter discussing management of muscle pain and trigger points. The importance of exercise and endorphin production has been emphasized by Dr. Paul Kiell.

We wish to thank our contributing authors for continuing to share their expertise and their enthusiasm. Their contributions have enabled the text to incorporate all of the most current and effective methods in management of myofascial pain syndromes, fibromyalgia, and trigger points.

We mourn the passing of Dr. Hans Kraus, who has been the inspiration for this text. Time has proven his methods on muscle deficiency and exercise to be so valuable that only slight revisions have been made to his chapter. We recommend that all practitioners involved in treating patients with muscle pain take the time to read his chapter. This whole book expounds on Dr. Kraus' comprehensive approach and his commitment to recognition of the whole person in evaluating and treating muscle pain.

Edward S. Rachlin, M.D.
Isabel S. Rachlin, P.T.

Contents

Part I

General Considerations

Fibromyalgia Syndrome: Clinical Features, Diagnosis, and Biopathophysiologic Mechanisms

Muhammad B. Yunus, MD ▪ Fatma İnanici, MD

Definition and Classification of Fibromyalgia

Fibromyalgia, also described as fibromyalgia syndrome (FMS), is characterized by chronic widespread musculoskeletal aching, pain, and stiffness, as well as tenderness on palpation at multiple sites, called tender points.[18, 72, 174, 205, 226, 234] Fibromyalgia and FMS will be used synonymously in this chapter. FMS may be classified as primary and concomitant. When unqualified, the term *fibromyalgia* is currently used to include both primary and concomitant varieties.

The term *primary fibromyalgia* is used when a significant underlying or concomitant condition that may contribute to pain is absent. FMS may be classified as *concomitant* when another condition, such as rheumatoid arthritis (RA), osteoarthritis, or hypothyroidism, is present and contributes to pain or fatigue of fibromyalgia. No significant differences in clinical characteristics exist between primary and concomitant fibromyalgia.[206] However, concomitant conditions should be treated appropriately,[99] and for research purposes should be described if they are relevant to the results. The term *secondary fibromyalgia* should not be used for concomitant fibromyalgia because satisfactory treatment of a concurrent disease such as RA or hypothyroidism does not significantly ameliorate fibromyalgia features, e.g., pain, fatigue, and number of tender points.

Myofascial pain syndrome (MPS) causes regional soft tissue pain (in contrast to widespread pain in FMS), but there is evidence that MPS (or regional soft tissue pain) and FMS are overlapping syndromes, both clinically[100] and biophysiologically.[14, 214] In our follow-up study of regional soft tissue pain, 40% of patients developed widespread musculoskeletal pain after a mean period of 6 years.[102] Lapossy and associates also reported that 25% of their 53 patients who had initially presented with low back pain developed fibromyalgia.[114]

Brief History of Fibromyalgia

Aches and pains in the muscles and joints were described as muscular rheumatism in the European literature since the 17th century.[162] In 1904, Gowers coined the term *fibrositis* in an article on lumbago, a localized condition.[75] However, in 1968, Traut used the nomenclature *fibrositis* to describe *generalized* musculoskeletal aching, fatigue, poor sleep, and tender points at multiple sites.[182] Moldofsky and his associates published the findings of a sleep electroencephalogram (EEG) study in "fibrositis" in 1975.[137] The validity of the concept of fibromyalgia, however, remained in doubt until 1981, when the first controlled study of the clinical characteristics of this syndrome by a formal protocol was published by Yunus and his colleagues.[234] This study showed that multiple symptoms, including pain, fatigue, poor sleep, a subjective swelling of tissues, paresthesia, irritable bowel syndrome (IBS), and headaches, as well as multiple tender points, were significantly more common in fibromyalgia patients than in age-, sex- and race-matched, normal controls, thus raising fibromyalgia to a recognizable *syndrome* level. A large number of controlled studies have since been published to confirm these associated features of fibromyalgia.[18, 40, 202, 204, 206] The blinded, multicenter criteria study incorporating control groups of patients with various types of chronic pain[206] has been very helpful in further validation of the syndrome of fibromyalgia.

Epidemiology and Clinical Features of Fibromyalgia Syndrome

Sex, Age, Race, and Prevalence

FMS occurs most commonly among women in the 40- to 60-year-old age group; 85% to 90% of the patients are women.[18, 201, 206, 230, 234] However, fibromyalgia has been described among juveniles[163, 229] as well as in the elderly.[222] Most fibromyalgia patients described in the literature are of European origin, probably because of clinic and referral biases. FMS has been described among the Japanese,[145] South African blacks,[123] and among a population in the Indian subcontinent.[45]

By American College of Rheumatology (ACR) criteria, prevalence of fibromyalgia in a community was found to be 2% in Wichita, Kansas, USA,[205] and 3.3% in London, Ontario, Canada.[195] The peak prevalence was in the 60- to 79-year-old age group in the Wichita community and in the 55- to 64-year-old age category in the Ontario population. As in the clinic population, FMS is more common in women than men in population studies. The prevalence was 3.4% among women vs. 0.5% in men in the Wichita study[205] and 4.9% among women vs. 1.6% in men in the London, Ontario, study.[195] In population studies, fibromyalgia is associated with lower levels of education.[195, 205]

Age, sex, and race distribution, as well as duration of symptoms, in FMS are shown in Table 1–1. Fibromyalgia is a chronic disease with an average symptom duration of 6 to 7 years at the time of presentation in a rheumatology clinic.[230]

Symptoms

The most common and characteristic symptoms of fibromyalgia are generalized pain, stiffness, fatigue, and poor sleep. Other symptoms include a swollen feeling in soft tissues and paresthesia. The onset of fibromyalgia symptoms often follows infection (particularly viral infection) or trauma as well as mental stress.[39, 78, 158, 198]

Several associated illnesses, e.g., irritable bowel syndrome, headaches, and restless legs syndrome (RLS), have been well described in fibromyalgia and are shown in Table 1–2. These disorders are more common in fibromyalgia patients than in normal controls as well as in those with other chronic pain conditions, such as RA.[18, 202, 206, 214, 231] A knowledge of these associated conditions is important for avoiding unnecessary investigations and for proper management of a patient.

Pain is the integral and most common presenting symptom of fibromyalgia. It is usually present in all four limbs, as well as the upper or lower back. About two thirds

Table 1–1.
Age, Sex, Race, and Symptom Duration in Fibromyalgia in Several Selected Series

	Yunus et al.[231] (n = 113)	Goldenberg[72] (n = 118)	Wolfe et al.[206] (n = 293)	Combined° (n = 524)
Mean age (yr)	40	43	49	44
Females (%)	94	87	89	90
Caucasian (%)	98	92	93	94
Duration of symptoms (yr)	7	5	NR†	6

°Results are based on the mean values of the three series.
†NR, not reported.
Modified from Yunus MB, Masi AT: Fibromyalgia, restless legs syndrome, periodic limb movement disorder and psychogenic pain. In McCarty DJ Jr, Koopman WJ (eds): Arthritis and Allied Conditions: A Textbook of Rheumatology, 12th ed. Philadelphia, Lea & Febiger, 1993, pp 1383–1405. Reproduced by permission.

Table 1–2.
Symptoms in Fibromyalgia Syndrome Based on Several Large Series

	Frequency (%)	
Symptoms[*]	Mean[†]	Range
Musculoskeletal		
Pain at multiple sites	100	100
Stiffness	78	76–84
"Hurt all over"	64	60–69
Swollen feeling in tissues	47	32–64
Nonmusculoskeletal		
General fatigue	86	75–92
Morning fatigue	78	75–80
Poor sleep[‡]	65	56–75
Paresthesia	54	26–74
Associated Symptoms		
Headaches	53	44–56
Dysmenorrhea	43	40–45
Irritable bowel syndrome	40	30–53
Restless legs syndrome	31	31
Sicca symptoms	15	12–18
Raynaud's phenomenon[§]	13	12–18
Female urethral syndrome	12	9–17

[*]See ref. 230 for individual references pertaining to various symptoms.
[†]Mean values derived from percentage figures reported in several studies.[230]
[‡]Based on the question, "Do you sleep well?" or a similar question.
[§]Definition specified as "dead white pallor on exposure to cold."
Modified from Yunus MB, Masi AT: Fibromyalgia, restless legs syndrome, periodic limb movement disorder and psychogenic pain. In McCarty DJ Jr, Koopman WJ (eds): Arthritis and Allied Conditions: A Textbook of Rheumatology, 12th ed. Philadelphia, Lea & Febiger, 1993, pp 1383–1405. Reproduced by permission.

of the patients state that they "hurt all over," and this symptom has been found to be useful in differentiating fibromyalgia from other conditions.[206, 231, 232] Pain is spontaneously described as aches, soreness, hurting, and burning. Leavitt and associates compared the pain characteristics in 50 patients with FMS and 50 patients with RA, using an adapted McGill Pain Questionnaire, and found that pain in fibromyalgia had a greater spatial distribution and involved a greater number of pain descriptors.[118] Commonly used words used for description of pain by the FMS patients were aching, exhausting, nagging, hurting, sore, annoying, shooting, miserable, radiating, unbearable, and throbbing.[47] Several words, e.g., radiating, steady, spasm, spreading, and gnawing, were significantly more common in description of FMS than of RA.[118]

Common sites of pain or stiffness are low back, neck, shoulder region, arms, hands, knees, hips, thighs, legs, and feet.[118, 231] However, many other areas, including the anterior chest,[104, 150] may be affected. Chest pain in fibromyalgia is sometimes a prominent symptom and may cause confusion with cardiopulmonary disease.[104, 150] The presence of prominent tender points on palpation in the chest wall and other parts of the body (see the following section, "Physical Examination") suggests fibromyalgia but does not help to rule out concomitant cardiopulmonary diseases because such diseases are not uncommon in FMS. Metacarpophalangeal and proximal interphalangeal joint areas may also be painful[222] and may lead to misdiagnosis of arthritis, particularly if patients also complain of swelling in these areas. Pain in a subgroup of patients is, indeed, predominantly articular rather than muscular.[161]

Although uncommon, some patients may have predominantly or exclusively one-sided pain.[234] These patients may not fulfill the currently proposed ACR criteria for fibromyalgia,[206] but they should be diagnosed as having this disorder and treated as such if other features of this illness, e.g., fatigue, poor sleep, paresthesia, and multiple tender points, are present.

Pain or stiffness is often aggravated by cold or humid weather, anxiety or stress, overuse or inactivity, poor sleep,[40, 119, 206, 231, 234] and noise.[158, 206] Psychological distress is associated with severity of pain.[21, 216] Moderate physical activity, local heat, massage, rest and relaxation, and stretching exercises are reported to be beneficial by many patients.[40, 231, 234] Most patients state that their pain and stiffness are worse in the morning and the evening.[234] In studies of chronobiologic influences on FMS, Moldofsky reported that the worst times for a fibromyalgia patient are in the morning, latter half of the afternoon, and evening.[134] During these periods, patients feel more achy, stiff, and lethargic, and experience more emotional distress and decreased cognitive performance.[134] Unlike most normal controls, the FMS patients feel their best between 10 AM and 2 PM, the peak time being around noon. A physician should inquire about such diurnal variation of symptoms in a patient and advise her or him to utilize this narrow window of relative comfort in accomplishing important daily activities, if such variation is present in a given patient. Moldofsky also reported seasonal effects on fibromyalgia symptoms.[134] By self-report, patients experience worse mood, pain, and lower energy levels during the months of November and March. This finding is consistent with our earlier report that 44% of our patients felt better during summer or summer and spring; only one of our 50 patients had preferred the winter months.[234] However, Hawley and Wolfe analyzed pain, depression, global severity, and depression recorded longitudinally and found no influence of seasons on these variables among fibromyalgia patients.[87] Thus, patient-reported seasonal influence on FMS symptoms may be a subjective perception and needs further studies.

Stiffness, usually worse in the morning and the evening, is common, but unlike in RA, morning stiffness does not correlate with severity of fibromyalgia as determined by degree of pain, number of tender points, or level of fatigue.[231] Most (about 85%) but not all patients have stiffness.[234] Pain and stiffness sites correlate with each other (our unpublished data).

Fatigue is quite common in fibromyalgia; moderate or severe fatigue occurs in about 75% to 90% of patients.[18, 198, 206, 234] A typical patient describes it by saying that "I am always tired." It is variously described as exhaustion, tiredness, lack of energy, fatigue, and sometimes as a global feeling of general weakness. It is aggravated by physical activity and may cause significant dysfunctions in daily living. Fatigue, rather than pain or stiffness, may be the presenting feature in some patients. Fatigue, like pain, seems to be primarily of central origin, as is the case with chronic fatigue syndrome (CFS).[108] The neuromuscular responses recorded during and after a fatiguing load were similar between fibromyalgia patients and healthy controls.[83] Fatigue may be contributed to, or associated with, poor sleep, excessive physical activity, and physical deconditioning, as well as psychological factors.[226, 234] Fatigue is also associated with pain, global severity, and functional disability.[226]

Nonrestorative sleep is common in fibromyalgia.[18, 40, 72, 206, 231, 234] About 75% of the patients describe sleep difficulties. Morning fatigue, which may be a better indicator of the quality of sleep, is present in about 75% to 90%. Poor sleep may be indicated by difficulty in falling asleep, frequent awakening, light sleep, and morning fatigue. Restless legs syndrome and periodic limb movement disorder may also contribute to disturbed sleep. In our studies,[226, 234] poor sleep was correlated with fatigue as well as psychological distress. Poor sleep may aggravate pain[4, 206, 226, 234] and may contribute to its pathophysiologic mechanisms (see "Biopathophysiologic Mechanisms," discussed later). There is a relationship between poor sleep and pain as well as attention to pain. Affleck and coworkers[4] demonstrated that poor sleep the previous night predicts pain the next day, which is then followed by a poor night's sleep.

Swollen feeling and paresthesia are present, overall, in about half the patients.[18, 40, 72, 206, 231, 234] Both symptoms are predominantly present in the extremities, although other anatomic regions may be involved. In some patients, these symptoms can be quite severe, but no objective joint swelling or sensory deficits are present on physical examination (discussed in "Physical Examination," the following section). Paresthesias often diffusely involve all the fingers or an extremity and are described as "tingling," "pins and needles," or "numb." However, paresthesia, like pain, may have a radiating quality, simulating radiculopathy. This symptom is reported by about 40% to 60% of patients overall, but has been reported to be as high as 84%.[172] Paresthesia, with or without radiating distribution, along with other neurologic symptoms such as headaches, weakness, and fatigue, may mimic a neurologic disorder, and some patients may consult a neurologist before a diagnosis of FMS is made. A concomitant neurologic problem in these patients should be ruled out by proper neurologic examination and investigations, if necessary.

The mechanisms of paresthesia and subjective swelling are unknown, but they do not correlate with the psychological status of the patients.[216, 231] However, both paresthesia and swollen feeling may be related to pain and perhaps represent an abnormal sensory processing, as will be discussed under "Biopathophysiologic Mechanisms." Total number of numbness and swollen feeling sites correlated with the number of pain sites,[231] and about 40% of patients describe their pain as either numb or pins and needles.[118] Autonomic dysfunction may also play a role. Electromyographic (EMG) and nerve conduction velocity studies are normal in patients with fibromyalgia per se, unless another concomitant neurologic condition is present.[172]

Several *associated symptoms and conditions* have been described in fibromyalgia (see Table 1–2 and Fig. 1–3). More than one study has shown these to be significantly more common in fibromyalgia patients than in pain-free normal controls, as well as those with other chronic pain conditions, such as RA, as mentioned earlier. Apart from chronic headaches, IBS, primary dysmenorrhea, RLS, and female urethral syndrome, several other similar syndromes including fibromyalgia are now considered to form a spectrum of illnesses with central sensitivity as a common biopathophysiologic mechanism and have been collectively called *central sensitivity syndromes* (CSS).[214] CSS will be discussed later in this chapter.

Sicca symptoms are also found to be significantly more common in fibromyalgia patients than in controls.[206, 223] The cause of dry mouth in fibromyalgia is not known. This symptom was not related to drugs (such as an antidepressant medication) or to psychological symptoms of anxiety, stress, or depression among our patients.[223] None of our patients with dry mouth had Sjögren's syndrome or other connective tissue disease, either at presentation or on follow-up.[223] Sicca symptoms may possibly be related to autonomic dysfunction or an abnormal sensory perception. However, one should be aware that several connective tissue diseases have been reported to be associated with fibromyalgia. These include RA,[201] systemic lupus erythematosus,[133] and Sjögren's syndrome.[28]

Physical Examination

Physical examination in primary fibromyalgia shows no joint swelling, muscle weakness, or neurologic abnormalities. Range of motion may sometimes be mildly limited because of pain, and peripheral joints may be tender because of the diffuse nature of tenderness in some fibromyalgia patients. The most significant finding related to FMS is the presence of *multiple tender points*.[17, 40, 72, 174, 206, 231, 234] Tender points are best elicited by manual palpation by digital pressure using an approximate force of 4 kg. To learn this amount of force, an examiner should first apply a steady digital pressure on a hard or firm surface, such as a patient's forehead, and watch for blanching of the examining fingernail. The pressure required to fully blanch the fingernail is usually about 4 kg, although this guide is rough. A reliable method for an estimation of 4-kg force is to use a dolorimeter. After applying a dolorimetric force of 4 kg on one side first, the examiner should manually palpate the opposite site, asking the patient if the digital pressure applied is roughly equivalent to the pressure that the patient had felt by the dolorimeter. Digital pressure may be applied by either of the first three fingers, depending on the site palpated and the natural comfort of the examiner. A regular use of a dolorimeter is not necessary for clinical practice, although it is often used in research settings.

For tender point examination, the examiner should first apply only gentle pressure and increase the pressure gradually, so that the patient then feels pain, being able to discriminate between pain and pressure. For a definition of tender point, a subject must feel pain. Once pain is verbalized by the patient, the pain may be further graded as mild, moderate, or severe. Mild or greater pain will qualify for the definition of a

Table 1–3.
Physical Signs in Fibromyalgia Syndrome

Positive Findings	Negative Findings°
Multiple tender points†	Absent joint swelling
Skinfold tenderness	Normal range of motion of the joints
Cutaneous hyperemia	Normal muscle strength‡
Reticular skin discoloration	Normal sensory functions
Diffuse puffiness of fingers (rare)	Normal reflexes

°The findings may be abnormal due to concomitant disease, e.g., arthritis or neuropathy.
†Diagnostic of FMS.
‡Reduced maximum voluntary muscle strength by isokinetic dynamometer has been reported.

tender point.[206] For a pain response to be graded greater than mild, a visible physical sign such as flinching, grimacing, or withdrawal needs to be present.[206]

Although there are 18 sites to be palpated for tender points in the ACR criteria (see Fig. 1–1), many more sites are tender in fibromyalgia,[199, 206, 232, 234] including the joints.[101, 206] In fact, a small subgroup of patients is diffusely tender all over, but this does not necessarily denote a psychological disturbance.[109] Some FMS patients may feel pain on touch or massage (called allodynia), which is normally nonpainful. Allodynia most likely represents the severity of an underlying chemical and sensory abnormality rather than a psychological disturbance. Tenderness in the so-called control points does not exclude a diagnosis of FMS, nor are they associated with psychological distress, as mentioned earlier.[109]

Tender points are consistent among the patients when examined by the same, as well as by different, observers on more than one occasion,[51, 183, 233] and reliably discriminate fibromyalgia patients from normal controls,[234] as well as those with other forms of chronic pain.[206]

Other physical signs in fibromyalgia, which are not necessary to make a diagnosis of this condition, include skinfold tenderness and cutaneous hyperemia.[206, 232] *Skinfold tenderness* is elicited by pinching a fold of skin and subcutaneous tissue by moderate pressure in the tender point examination sites, although such tenderness may be globally present in many fibromyalgia patients. *Cutaneous hyperemia* is seen at the tender point examination sites following such an examination.[232] Skinfold tenderness correlates with tender point examination[232] and has been shown to have a sensitivity of 60% and specificity of 83% in the multicenter ACR criteria study.[206] Hyperemia had limited sensitivity (50%) and specificity (31%).[206]

Reticular discoloration of skin, first described by Caro,[43] as a "net-like," mottled, blue or purple discoloration of the skin in the extremities, was present in only 15% of patients, but had a high specificity (95%) in the multicenter criteria study.[206] Physical findings in FMS are shown in Table 1–3.

Clinical features of fibromyalgia among men were compared with those in women in a recent study.[226] A number of features were significantly less frequent among men, e.g., fatigue, morning fatigue, irritable bowel syndrome, and "hurting all over." The number of tender points as well as number of total symptoms was also significantly fewer among men. Stepwise logistical regression showed significant differences in number of tender points between men and women. However, pain severity, global severity of illness, and functional disabilities were similar between the two groups. Although global anxiety, stress, and depression were less frequent in men,[226] assessments of the psychological disturbance by validated questionnaires were found to be similar between men and women.[101]

Laboratory Tests

Results of the usual, routine laboratory tests, e.g., complete blood count, erythrocyte sedimentation rate (ESR), chemistry profile (including muscle enzymes), and rheumatoid factor, are normal in FMS.[72, 226, 231, 234] Antinuclear antibodies (ANA) are present

Table 1–4.
Laboratory Tests in Fibromyalgia Syndrome

Abnormal Tests°	Normal Tests†
Sleep EEG studies‡	Complete blood count
Neuroendocrine tests§	Erythrocyte sedimentation rate
	Muscle enzymes
	Thyroid function tests
	Rheumatoid factor
	Antinuclear antibodies
	Radiographs; bone scan
	Electromyography
	Muscle biopsy

°No laboratory tests having a satisfactory sensitivity and specificity are currently available in fibromyalgia.
†Several tests listed as normal may be abnormal if a concomitant disease is present, e.g., rheumatoid arthritis or hypothyroidism.
‡Sleep EEG studies may show such treatable conditions as restless legs syndrome, periodic limb movement disorder, REM sleep behavioral disorder, and sleep apnea. Sleep EEG studies should be requested only if clinically indicated.
§See text and Tables 1–7 through 1–9.

in about 10% of patients, similar to the frequency found in a healthy, normal control group with similar distribution of age, sex, and race.[17, 223] Other tests reported to be normal in FMS include multiphase skeletal scintigraphy[218] and electromyography[130, 172, 235] (Table 1–4). Although sleep electroencephalography (EEG) should not be done as a routine, this test may be performed in a suspected case of periodic limb movement disorder or rapid eye movement (REM) behavior disorder. Restless legs syndrome can also be diagnosed by sleep EEG studies, but it can be easily diagnosed in most cases by a typical history of an unpleasant, difficult to describe sensation (such as worms writhing) in the legs while at rest (such as sitting for a prolonged period) and at night (usually before falling asleep).[113, 141] The sufferers of RLS have a compulsive feeling of moving about their legs to get some relief. The diagnosis is important because it is treatable by medications such as benzodiazepines (clonazepam, temazepam), dopaminergic drugs (carbidopa-levodopa, pergolide, pramipexole), and opiates (codeine, tramadol, propoxyphene, hydrocodone).[113, 141] However, not all of the above medications have been evaluated by double-blind control studies, and their long-term efficacy or adverse reactions are unknown.

Although a large number of neuroendocrine studies are abnormal in FMS (see "Biopathophysiologic Mechanisms"), none of these studies is sensitive and specific enough to be used for diagnosis of FMS.

Diagnosis and Differential Diagnosis

Fibromyalgia can be easily and reliably diagnosed in virtually all cases by its characteristic symptoms and multiple tender points,[206, 230, 231, 232] provided that the examiner is proficient in proper examination of tender points. The ACR criteria for the classification of fibromyalgia include widespread musculoskeletal pain and the presence of mild or greater tenderness in 11 of 18 possible sites (Table 1–5 and Fig. 1–1). The criteria specifically state that other diseases need not be excluded for making a diagnosis of fibromyalgia.[206] In clinical practice, not all patients will have 11 tender points or widespread pain as defined in Table 1–5 but otherwise may have characteristic fibromyalgia features. These patients may be diagnosed as having "incomplete fibromyalgia,"[225] and should be diagnosed as having fibromyalgia for the practical purpose of case management. In our observation, the number of tender points found by inexperienced hands tends to be fewer than the number found by examiners who are appropriately trained.

Because FMS has a protean clinical manifestation, it may be confused with a variety of other conditions, including different forms of arthritis, polymyalgia rheumatica (PMR) among the elderly patients, neurologic disease, cardiopulmonary disease,

Table 1–5.
American College of Rheumatology Criteria for Classification of Fibromyalgia*

1. History of widespread pain.

Definition: Pain is considered widespread when all of the following are present: pain in the left side of the body, pain in the right side of the body, pain above the waist, pain below the waist. In addition, axial skeletal pain (cervical spine or anterior chest or thoracic spine or low back) must be present. In this definition, shoulder and buttock pain are considered as pain for each involved side. "Low back" pain is considered lower segment pain. Thus, pain at three widespread sites (e.g., right arm, low back, and left leg) will satisfy the criterion of widespread pain.

2. Pain in 11 of 18 tender point sites on digital palpation (see also Fig. 1–1).

Definition: Pain (mild or greater) on digital palpation must be present in at least 11 of the following 18 tender point sites:

Occiput: bilateral, at the suboccipital muscle insertions.
Low cervical: bilateral, at the anterior aspects of the intertransverse spaces at C5–7.
Trapezius: bilateral, at the midpoint of the upper border.
Supraspinatus: bilateral, at origins above the scapula spine near the medial border.
Second rib: bilateral, at the second costochondral junctions, just lateral to the junctions on upper surfaces.
Lateral epicondyle: bilateral, 2 cm distal to the epicondyles.
Gluteal: bilateral, in upper outer quadrants of buttocks in anterior fold of muscle.
Greater trochanter: bilateral, posterior to the trochanteric prominence.
Knee: bilateral, at the medial fat pad proximal to the joint line.

*For classification purposes, patients will be said to have fibromyalgia if both criteria (1 and 2) are satisfied. Widespread pain must have been present for at least 3 months. The presence of a second clinical disorder does not exclude the diagnosis of fibromyalgia.
From Wolfe F, Smythe HA, Yunus MB, et al: The American College of Rheumatology 1990 Criteria for the Classification of Fibromyalgia. Report of the Multicenter Criteria Committee. Arthritis Rheum 33:160–172, 1990. Used by permission.

and hypothyroidism (Table 1–6). Careful history taking, physical examination, and appropriate laboratory tests will clarify the confusion in most cases. Like any other disease in the similar age group as FMS, coexisting presence of diseases is not uncommon in FMS and should always be considered. For example, some fibromyalgia patients may have or will develop arthritis, spinal stenosis, hypothyroidism, PMR, disc herniation, and peripheral neuritis.

As discussed earlier, fibromyalgia should be diagnosed by its own clinical characteristics. None of the concurrent diseases *causes* fibromyalgia in the sense that a satisfactory treatment of the accompanying disease, e.g., RA and hypothyroidism, does not

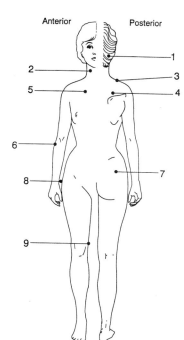

Figure 1–1. Locations of 9 bilateral tender point sites to be palpated for testing American College of Rheumatology criteria for classification of fibromyalgia syndrome (FMS) (see Table 1–5 for description). 1, occiput; 2, low cervical; 3, trapezius; 4, supraspinatus; 5, second rib; 6, lateral epicondyle; 7, gluteal; 8, greater trochanter; 9, knee. (From Yunus MB, Masi AT: Fibromyalgia, restless legs syndrome, periodic limb movement disorder and psychogenic pain. In McCarty DJ Jr, Koopman WJ [eds]: Arthritis and Allied Conditions: A Textbook of Rheumatology, 12th ed. Philadelphia Lea & Febiger, pp 1383–1405, with permission.)

Table 1–6.
Presenting Features of Fibromyalgia with Confounding Diagnosis and Key Points of Differentiation

Presenting Features	Confounding Diagnosis	Present in Confounding Disease
Joint pain and subjective swelling	Arthritis	Objective joint swelling
Diffuse muscular aching and stiffness	Polymyalgia rheumatica	↑ ESR, ↓ Hb, constitutional features
Muscle fatigue, weakness	Myopathy	Objective weakness, ↑ muscle enzymes
Fatigue, sensitivity to cold, muscle pain	Hypothyroidism	↓ T_4, ↑ TSH
Back pain/stiffness	Ankylosing spondylitis	Sacroiliitis
Sciatica-type pain	Disc herniation	Neurologic and radiologic findings
Chest pain	Cardiac or pleural pain	Typical history of cardiac pain, pleural rub; ECG, chest film, or laboratory findings of intrathoracic disease

ESR, erythrocyte sedimentation rate; Hb, hemoglobin; T_4, thyroxin; TSH, thyroid-stimulating hormone; ECG, electrocardiogram; ↑, elevated; ↓, decreased.

Modified from Yunus MB, Masi AT: Fibromyalgia, restless legs syndrome, periodic limb movement disorder, and psychogenic pain. In McCarty DJ, Koopman WJ (eds): Arthritis and Allied Conditions: A Textbook of Rheumatology, 12th ed. Philadelphia, Lea and Febiger, 1993, pp 1383–1405, with permission.

satisfactorily help FMS symptoms, nor does it decrease the number of tender points. However, comorbid conditions should be appropriately diagnosed and managed. It is now known that FMS is much more common in RA than expected.[201] Thus, RA and fibromyalgia may be present in the same patient. In most cases, RA is only mildly or moderately active but the patient has more pain of widespread distribution and more fatigue than can be explained by RA activity alone. Again, a large number of tender points will provide the evidence for the concomitant presence of FMS. Some of these patients are inappropriately treated with a larger dose of nonsteroidal anti-inflammatory drugs, disease-modifying drugs, or corticosteroids at the risk of serious side effects. These patients need reassurance, a centrally acting drug, such as a low-dose antidepressant, and other measures for proper management of fibromyalgia (see Chapter 2, Management of Fibromyalgia Syndrome). Polymyalgia rheumatica may pose a difficult problem. We have encountered patients with typical PMR with much elevated ESR who responded satisfactorily to a low-dose corticosteroid preparation, only to develop features of FMS at a later date with much pain, stiffness, and multiple tender points. Fatigue disproportional to disease activity of PMR, a large number of tender points, a lack of satisfactory response to an increased dose of the corticosteroid preparation, and a normal (or modestly increased) ESR are indicative of a diagnosis of FMS while the PMR is inactive. Sometimes, however, both conditions may coexist, and again, the features described above, including multiple tender points, will be helpful to make a proper diagnosis.

Biopathophysiologic Mechanisms

Although the pathogenesis of FMS is not completely understood, remarkable progress has been made since the first controlled clinical study of this syndrome in 1981.[234] It is clear that FMS is not a psychiatric disorder, but is based on neurochemical abnormalities that are generally different from those reported in psychiatric illnesses such as depression. Despite muscle pain, no histologic or biochemical abnormalities in the muscles have been demonstrated in FMS by appropriately designed studies. FMS has multifactorial etiology, of which neuroendocrine aberration,[52, 164, 210] particularly central sensitization or sensitivity, seems most important.[23, 214, 224] Several other factors interact with these aberrations and further amplify pain; they include nonrestorative sleep, trauma, infection or inflammation, psychological distress, genetics, physical deconditioning, and environmental factors, such as weather and noise (Fig. 1–2).

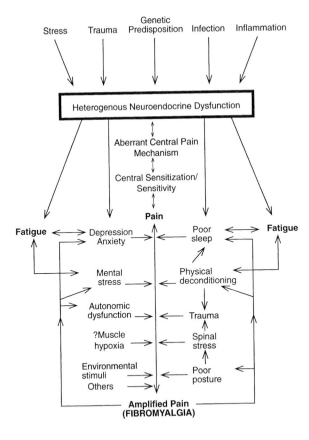

Figure 1–2. A schematic representation of the proposed model for biopathophysiologic mechanisms of FMS showing multiple factors that interact to amplify pain. The primary problem is currently believed to be in the "box," i.e., a heterogeneous neuroendocrine dysfunction, leading to central sensitization or sensitivity. (Adapted from Yunus MB: Psychological aspects of fibromyalgia syndrome: A component of the dysfunctional spectrum syndrome. Baillieres Clin Rheumatol 8:811–837, 1994, with permission.)

Muscle Studies

Because of pain and tenderness in muscles, initial investigations were directed toward muscle pathology. A controlled but unblinded study by Bengtsson and colleagues[20] showed no significant differences between patients and controls by histopathologic or histochemical study, with the possible exception of ragged red fiber, which was present in the trapezius muscles of 15 (37%) of 41 patients and in none of the 10 controls. Drewes and associates, however, found no ragged red fibers in 50 quadriceps muscle biopsies from 20 fibromyalgia patients or in 15 biopsies of 10 normal controls, all blindly assessed.[58a]

We had reported an absence of inflammation, atrophy of type II fiber, and motheaten appearance of type I fiber by histochemistry, and myofibrillar lysis with deposition of glycogen and mitochondria by electron microscopy (EM) in an uncontrolled study.[106] However, our subsequent blinded and controlled study of muscle biopsy by EM was found to be normal.[227]

Bengtsson and her colleagues reported a significant decrease in adenosine triphosphate (ATP), adenosine diphosphate (ADP), adenosine monophosphate (AMP), and phosphocreatine (Pcr) in trapezius muscles by open biopsy,[19] but similar changes were not significantly different between patients and controls by P-31 nuclear magnetic resonance spectroscopy (NMR), when controls were appropriately matched for physical deconditioning, as measured by maximal oxygen uptake ($\dot{V}O_2max$).[171, 173] Using P-31 magnetic resonance spectroscopy, Park and associates reported significantly decreased Pcr and ATP in fibromyalgia muscles,[149] but it is not known if patients and controls had similar muscle conditioning. Muscle oxygenation was found to be significantly low by multipoint oxygen electrode as compared with normal controls in one study,[122] but this finding might have resulted from muscle deconditioning, which is common in fibromyalgia. In conclusion, no definite, ongoing source of pathology was found in the peripheral tissues in fibromyalgia that might account for pain.

Immunochemical and molecular studies of substance P in the muscles of FMS have also been reported to be normal.[178]

Given an absence of generalized nociceptive stimulus at the periphery to account for the widespread pain of fibromyalgia, attention focused on central mechanisms.[210] It became increasingly clear that the major problem is one of neurohormonal aberrations, which have been recently reviewed.[52, 164, 214, 224] It now seems that central sensitization and sensitivity are the key elements to the neurohormonal abnormalities in FMS.[23, 214] Because of its important contribution to the biopathophysiologic mechanisms of FMS, the concept of central sensitization and the evidence for its presence in FMS will be discussed first.

The Concept of Central Sensitization

Central sensitization is defined by an exaggerated response of the central nervous system (CNS) to a peripheral stimulus that is normally painful (hyperalgesia) or non-nociceptive, such as touch (allodynia), denoting hyperexcitability and hypersensitivity of the CNS neurons. Another characteristic of central sensitization is the prolongation or persistence of pain.

A better understanding of central sensitization has evolved in recent years through animal experiments.[49, 56, 62] A nociceptive stimulus, such as inflammation[49] or direct nerve injury[56, 207] at the periphery, sends a bombardment of afferent impulses to the spinal cord dorsal horn via the C fibers, resulting in remarkable chemical, synaptic, molecular, and, in some cases, anatomic changes in the neurons, both at the spinal and supraspinal levels. An increased synaptic efficacy allows "cross-talk" between neurons, modulating their response. Such a "cross-talk" between nociceptive and non-nociceptive neurons may explain the phenomenon of allodynia in FMS. The ability of the CNS to undergo the aforementioned changes has been called CNS neuroplasticity, implying that the CNS function is not fixed but is capable of alterations, depending on various peripheral or environmental factors.

Following a nociceptive stimulation at the periphery, substance P is released at the synapse in the dorsal horn and removes the magnesium block of N-methyl-D-aspartate (NMDA), allowing excitatory amino acids (EAA), e.g., glutamate and aspartate, to activate postsynaptic NMDA receptors. Such activation now permits several intramembranous and intracellular changes, e.g., alteration of cell membrane permeability, influx of calcium, excitement of secondary neurons, and expression of *c-fos*. Besides substance P, other C-fiber neuropeptides are also involved in causing the aforementioned intramembranous and intracellular changes; these neuropeptides include neurokinin A, calcitonin gene-related peptide (CGRP), somatostatin, cholecystokinin, galanine, and vasoactive intestinal polypeptide (VIP), as shown in animal studies.[27, 49] NMDA receptor activation seems very important for induction and maintenance of central sensitivity.[208] Interactions between various neuropeptides as well as EAA[58] orchestrate a magnified stimulus at the dorsal horn and subsequent events, leading to striking functional changes in the secondary neurons with sustained hyperexcitability and sensitivity, amplification of the peripheral stimulus, enlargement of the receptive field, and "wind-up" phenomenon. There is evidence that spinal and supraspinal neurons interact constantly in the complex phenomenon of sensory processing.[120]

Wind-up phenomenon, as described in animal models, is defined by a *progressively* increased response of the secondary neurons following repeated and brief stimulus of the C fibers at the periphery, so that with each successive stimulus the response of these neurons increases and is stronger than the previous one.[208] Wind-up is mediated by NMDA receptor and inhibited by NMDA receptor antagonists. Similar to wind-up in animals, "temporal summation" has been documented in humans.[157] In fact, NMDA may play an important role in the pathogenesis of fibromyalgia, considering that ketamine, an NMDA receptor antagonist, has been shown in placebo-controlled studies to reduce muscle pain[77, 175] as well as temporal summation.[77]

Central Sensitivity/Central Sensitization in Fibromyalgia Syndrome

Although animal studies have clearly demonstrated a state of hyperexcitability in the CNS following a peripheral stimulus of inflammatory nature (central sensitization), leading to central sensitivity, such source of peripheral nociception is not always obvious in FMS. Although a peripheral trauma (such as an automobile accident[39]), inflammation (e.g., RA[201]), a degenerative disease of the joints, or possibly the mechanical stress of poor posture may provide a peripheral source of nociceptive stimulus in FMS, such a concept needs to be proven by appropriate studies. FMS often follows RA, but the other way around has also been observed in our clinic. The association between RA and FMS[201] may be due to other factors besides noxious input from the inflamed joints, such as genetic and endocrine. Animal studies suggest that the peripheral source of inflammation need not continue for sustained neuroplastic changes in the CNS.[49] It is also possible that there is an intrinsic and tonic hyperexcitability and hypersensitivity of the central neurons modulating pain in FMS, probably genetically determined in the absence of a noxious peripheral source.[214]

Irrespective of exact mechanisms involved—which are currently unknown—evidence has accumulated in recent years that central sensitivity is operative in FMS, as has been recently reviewed.[23] Arroyo and Cohen demonstrated that, following a nonnoxious electrocutaneous stimulation, fibromyalgia patients demonstrated significantly decreased pain tolerance as compared with normals. Moreover, the pain in FMS patients was accompanied by a spread to other locations and a persistent dysesthesia, suggesting centralization of pain.[10] Such central mechanisms in FMS were suggested by another study in which it was found that fibromyalgia patients were not only more tender in their muscles following a pressure stimulus, but the pain was qualitatively different from that in controls.[16] Granges and Littlejohn reported widespread pain in fibromyalgia by application of pressure measured by an algometer among 18 tender point and 4 "control" sites, as compared with normal controls as well as regional soft tissue pain, with a correlation between tender and control point sites among the study subjects.[76] Such a diffuse and widespread nature of tenderness among FMS patients would suggest central sensitivity in this disease. As mentioned earlier, NMDA is likely to play an important role in the aberrant central pain mechanism in FMS.

Kosek and Hansson had demonstrated an increased sensitivity to heat and nonpainful cold stimuli, apart from pressure, among FMS patients as compared with normal controls.[111] They also demonstrated that there is an abnormal central inhibitory control in FMS. Increased sensitivity to heat with hyperalgesia was also demonstrated in other studies.[69, 121] Taken together, the foregoing evidence suggests that there is an abnormal sensory processing at the CNS level in fibromyalgia.

Abnormal central sensory processing has also been documented in FMS by somatosensory evoked potential studies in the brain, by analyzing electroencephalographic waveforms following a peripheral stimulus.[69, 121] There is an increased activation of the CNS, including the somatosensory cortex, and as shown by Lorenz and coworkers,[121] the nociceptive response of the brain is widespread beyond the stimulated area in fibromyalgia patients as compared to controls—again suggesting the important role of the CNS in pain modulation in this syndrome.

Brain functions in FMS have been studied by magnetic brain stimulation (MBS) and by imaging techniques. MBS was developed by Barker and colleagues[13] to study human motor cortex functions. MBS involves placing a coil on the skull that corresponds to the cortical representation of a peripheral muscle, and recordings are made through cutaneous electrodes placed at the target peripheral muscle. Using the technology of MBS, Salerno and associates evaluated motor cortical function with recordings from the first dorsal interosseous and anterior tibial muscles in 13 patients with FMS and 13 matched healthy controls, and demonstrated motor cortical dysfunction in FMS that involved both excitatory and inhibitory mechanisms, indicating an aberrant central pain mechanism.[169] Single photon emission computed tomography (SPECT) demonstrated a decreased regional cerebral blood flow in the thalamus and

---

Table 1–7.

Neurosensory and Neuroimaging Abnormalities in Fibromyalgia Syndrome

---

Greater and more diffuse pain on mechanical pressure as compared with pain-free healthy controls.
Marked reduction of pain tolerance by a non-noxious electrocutaneous stimulation, accompanied by spread and persistence of dysesthesia.
Qualitatively different pain in muscles by stimulus-response function for pressure vs. pain.
Temporal summation and hyperexcitability.
Abnormal central endogenous inhibitory control by noxious stimuli.
Abnormal cerebral somatosensory evoked potentials following a painful peripheral stimulus, suggesting increased central nociceptive activation.
Motor cortical dysfunction by magnetic brain stimulation.
Decreased regional cerebral blood flow in the thalamus and caudate nucleus (which modulate pain) by single photon emission computed tomography (SPECT).
Deranged sympathetic function by power spectral analysis of heart rate variability with exaggerated sympathetic activity at resting state.
Exaggerated nocturnal sympathetic activity by spectral analysis of heart rate variability.
Decreased sympathetic activity on various stressful stimulus.
Exaggerated response of norepinephrine to interleukin-6.

Adapted from Yunus MB, Inanici F: Clinical characteristics and biopathophysiological mechanisms of fibromyalgia syndrome. In Baldry P (ed): Myofascial Pain and Fibromyalgia Syndromes: A Clinical Guide to Diagnosis and Management. London, Churchill Livingstone, 2001, pp 351–377, with permission.

caudate nucleus in FMS, as compared with controls, indicating an abnormality in pain perception in FMS.[139] Neurosensory and imaging abnormalities in FMS are shown in Table 1–7.

Autonomic Dysfunction

Autonomic disturbance has long been suspected in FMS.[209] Autonomic functions have been evaluated in recent years in FMS by assessing heart rate variability using a high-resolution electrocardiogram in supine and standing positions, and over 24 hours. A beat-to-beat quantitative assessment of the cardiovascular functioning can be investigated by power spectral analysis (PSA), which evaluates heart rate fluctuation. Three components can be identified in the spectrum, i.e., very low frequency, low frequency, and high frequency. Whereas the high frequency represents efferent vagal activity, the low frequency is most likely contributed by sympathetic function when expressed in normalized units. An increased ratio of low-frequency/high-frequency band values reflects sympathetic hyperactivity.[180] A study of autonomic nervous system function using the aforementioned methodology by Martinez-Lavin and associates showed significant differences between patients and controls in the low-frequency band of power analysis following an upright position, suggesting an abnormal sympathetic function with an impairment of the expected sympathetic surge after an orthostatic stress (standing up), whereas the sympathetic component was markedly increased while the subject was in the supine position.[127] The same group of investigators recorded 24-hour heartbeat variability in a subsequent study and found an increased nocturnal predominance of low-frequency component in the spectral band as compared with healthy controls, suggesting an excessive sympathetic activity modulating the sinus node.[128] An increased nocturnal sympathetic activity has been found to correlate with sleep arousal[30] and may thus contribute to poor sleep and morning fatigue in FMS.

In another study of heart rate variability by PSA employing 22 patients with FMS and 22 healthy controls, electrocardiogram recordings were obtained for 20 minutes in a supine position.[50] FMS patients showed a significantly decreased heart rate variability, a significantly higher heart rate, higher low-frequency (LF) and lower high-frequency (HF) components of PSA as compared with controls, suggesting exaggerated sympathetic and decreased parasympathetic tones at a resting state. However, unlike quality of life, anxiety, stress, and depression, which correlated with the findings of LF/HF, no association was found in FMS symptoms and muscle tenderness. Thus the role of psychiatric distress in the previously discussed findings of excessive sympathetic tone in FMS needs further evaluation. It is possible that there is an intrinsic chronic hyperstimulation of the sympathetic nervous system that contributes to symptoms of FMS as well as anxiety. Martinez-Lavin and Hermosillo suggest that other symptoms of FMS, such as pain, poor sleep, fatigue, sicca symptoms, and Raynaud's-like symptoms can also be explained by a dysfunctional autonomic nervous system.[126] Our view is that symptoms of FMS are too complex to be explained by an abnormality of a single system even if this system interacts with others. Although an autonomic dysfunction may contribute to some symptoms of FMS, these symptoms ensue from a host of complex interactions among many other factors, such as neurohormonal, environmental, psychological, and genetic, which may vary among several subgroups.

Several studies have shown decreased sympathetic tone following a host of stressful stimulations, e.g., cold water and acoustic stimulation,[190, 159] orthostatic stress,[127] isometric muscle contraction,[63] and exercise.[191] Basal plasma neuropeptide Y (NPY) level was decreased in another study, implying a diminished sympathetic output.[53] These incongruent results between NPY level and sympathetic overactivity need further examination and explanation. It is possible that plasma NPY reflects a sustained chronic stress status among a subgroup of fibromyalgia patients. Another recent study has shown an exaggerated response of norepinephrine to interleukin-6, suggesting a dysfunction of the sympathetic nervous system in FMS.[181] Plasma and urinary catecholamines were found to be normal in FMS.[219] These findings are compatible with the view that static blood measurement of autonomic neurotransmitters or measurement of their urine metabolites does not reflect the dynamic, constantly variable autonomic functions.[126]

Neurotransmitter/Neurochemical Dysfunctions

Pain is transmitted by A-delta and C fibers; C fibers utilize substance P (SP) as an important neurotransmitter for pain transmission, although other neurotransmitters as well as excitatory amino acids are also involved,[27, 49, 197] as mentioned earlier. The neurotransmitters involved in pain inhibition include serotonin, norepinephrine, γ-aminobutyric acid (GABA), enkephalin, and other less studied neurochemicals.[27, 49] An increased activity of the excitatory neurotransmitter SP or a deficiency of the inhibitory ones such as serotonin may, therefore, cause amplified pain, as in FMS.

A significantly increased level of SP in the cerebrospinal fluid (CSF) of fibromyalgia patients has been consistently demonstrated as compared with normal controls in several studies.[31, 167, 188, 193] There was no correlation between CSF SP and depression.[167] A related finding is the fact that nerve growth factor, which is known to promote the growth of SP, has also been reported to be elevated in the CSF.[70]

Serotonin deficiency in fibromyalgia is suggested by low levels of plasma or serum tryptophan (a precursor of serotonin[165, 220]), a decreased transport ratio of plasma tryptophan (an indicator of the brain entry of tryptophan[220]), decreased serum serotonin,[94, 166] and a decreased level of CSF 5-hydroxyindoleacetic acid (5HIAA, a metabolite of serotonin).[93, 168] Urinary 5HIAA levels have also been reported to be low in fibromyalgia.[107] The results of imipramine binding on platelets in FMS are conflicting, with both low[112] and high[166] binding, probably due to differences in methodology as well as small number of subjects studied. The role of peripheral serotonin in the pathogenesis of FMS was supported by two recent studies, recognizing the algogenic property of serotonin at the peripheral tissues.[64, 65] Ernberg and colleagues found that provocation by needle injection in the superficial masseter muscle releases more serotonin in FMS than in healthy controls, which was associated with pain, allodynia, and hyperalgesia.[64] However, unlike normal controls, injection of serotonin in the messeter muscle did not provoke pain and hyperalgesia in fibromyalgia patients, probably because of already high serotonin level in this muscle.[65]

Significantly decreased levels of 3-methoxy-4-hydroxyphenethylene glycol (a metabolite of norepinephrine) and homovanillic acid (a metabolite of dopamine) in the CSF of fibromyalgia patients, as compared with normal, pain-free controls, have also been reported.[168] However, the numbers in this study were small, and further studies are indicated.

So far, investigations of opioid peptides in FMS have not provided fruitful results. Both serum[221] and CSF[187] β-endorphin levels have been reported to be normal. In addition, the markers for pro-enkephalin and pro-dynorphin, the other opioid peptides, were elevated rather than decreased.[189] A lack of a significant role of the opioids in FMS is further supported by the fact that neither pain intensity nor tender points improved by intravenous infusion of morphine, which was administered in a double-blind placebo-controlled study.[175]

Yunus and associates showed that a combination of several amino acids and urinary dopamine would better classify FMS than either of them alone, with a sensitivity of 86% and specificity of 77% against normal controls.[217] This observation supports the concept that FMS is caused by a complex interaction between a number of chemicals. Neurochemical findings in FMS are shown in Table 1–8.

Endocrine Factors

Several controlled studies have demonstrated hypothalamic-pituitary-adrenal (HPA) axis abnormalities in FMS, which include decreased 24-hour urinary free cortisol,[52, 53, 81] loss of diurnal cortisol fluctuation and elevated evening cortisol level,[53, 131] and an exaggerated adrenocorticotropin hormone (ACTH) response to corticotropin-releasing hormone (CRH) with similar cortisol level between the FMS patients and controls,[79, 81] suggesting a relative hypocortisolemia to elevated ACTH. This hypocortisolemia is not, however, due to a primary hypofunction of the adrenal cortex, inasmuch as the cortisol response to ACTH stimulation is normal in FMS.[81] A central mechanism is the most likely explanation for hypocortisolemia in FMS.[52, 79, 81] A central deficiency of CRH has been suggested.[52] Also, a recent study showed delayed release of ACTH following IL-6 stimulation, which may suggest a dysfunction of the hypothalamic CRH neurons.[181]

Using a different method in which hypoglycemia was titrated by using clamps, Adler and coworkers found that ACTH response to hypoglycemia was decreased with normal cortisol production and decreased epinephrine level among 15 premenopausal patients with FMS, compared with 13 healthy controls.[3] Given a different approach, the results of this study are not directly comparable to other HPA axis studies already mentioned.

Growth hormone (GH) status has been found to be low in FMS in several studies. Insulin-like growth factor (IGF-1), which represents an integrated secretion of GH, is decreased,[25, 26, 68] as is the directly measured GH.[11, 26, 81, 117] Another study, employing a small number of patients, found the IGF-1 level to be comparable to that of normal controls.[103] However, stimulation studies have shown discordant results. GH secretion was increased following hypoglycemic[81] as well as GH-releasing hormone (GHRH)[117]

Table 1–8.
Neurochemical Findings in Fibromyalgia Syndrome

Elevated substance P in the cerebrospinal fluid (CSF)
Decreased serum serotonin level
Decreased 5-hydroxyindoleacetic acid in the CSF
Decreased 5-hydroxyindoleacetic acid in 24-hour urine
Low serum tryptophan and low transport ratio of tryptophan
^{3}H-imipramine binding on platelets: both normal and increased by two different studies
Low MHPG (metabolite of norepinephrine) in CSF
Low HVA (metabolite of dopamine) in CSF
Decreased plasma neuropeptide Y
Normal pro-enkephalin and pro-dynorphin markers in CSF

MHPG, 3-methoxy-4-hydroxyphenethylene glycol; HVA, homovanillic acid.
From Yunus MB, Inanici F: Clinical characteristics and biopathophysiological mechanisms of fibromyalgia syndrome. In Baldry P (ed): Myofascial Pain and Fibromyalgia Syndromes: A Clinical Guide to Diagnosis and Management. London, Churchill Livingstone, 2001, pp 351–377, with permission.

challenge, but not following administration of clonidine and L-dopa (which increases GH secretion by inhibiting hypothalamic somatostatin via α_2-adrenergic and dopamine receptors, respectively).[26] These differences may be explained by different stimulation tests and the fact that GH release involves a complex mechanism. A deficiency of GH may partly explain several features of FMS, e.g., decreased exercise tolerance and a generalized feeling of muscle weakness and fatigue, although such relationships between GH deficiency and FMS symptoms have not been demonstrated. Interestingly, however, a double-blind controlled study of GH injected subcutaneously showed an improvement in functional capacities, general well-being, and number of tender points.[26] The cause of decreased GH secretion is not known in fibromyalgia. Much of the GH is secreted during stage 3 and 4 sleep, which is disrupted in FMS.[137] It may also be due to a low adrenergic stimulation of the GH axis.[154]

Basal thyroid hormone levels are normal in FMS,[142] but a blunted response of thyrotropin (TSH) and an exaggerated response of prolactin to thyrotropin-releasing hormone (TRH) have been reported.[67, 142] A controlled study of gonadal functions in 57 female FMS patients and 114 controls has shown significantly decreased dehydro-epiandrosterone sulphate (DHEAS) as well as free testosterone levels.[55] There was a significant negative correlation between pain and DHEAS level, and free testosterone level correlated with physical functioning.

Nocturnal secretion of melatonin was reported to be normal,[156] increased,[110] or decreased.[196] Methodologic differences may account for such discrepancy. Given the balance of evidence, it seems at this time that the nocturnal melatonin secretion is normal in FMS. Abnormalities of endocrine functions in fibromyalgia are shown in Table 1–9.

Sleep Studies

Clinically, most patients with FMS complain of nonrestorative sleep, as described under clinical features. The first objective documentation of a sleep anomaly was described by Moldofsky and his colleagues,[137] who studied 10 fibromyalgia patients (7 women, 3 men; mean age of 51.9 years) by sleep EEG. Seven patients demonstrated an intrusion of alpha rhythm in their non–rapid eye movement (non-REM) sleep, whereas the other three patients showed an absence of stage 4, as well as stage 3, sleep. In the same study, six healthy volunteers, all men (aged 19–24 years), were deprived of their stage 4 sleep by auditory stimuli. Following deprivation of their stage 4 sleep, the healthy subjects developed musculoskeletal pain and increased tenderness as measured by dolorimetry. Thus, it would appear that nonrestorative sleep may contribute to fibromyalgia features. In subsequent studies, the same group of investiga-

---

Table 1–9.
Endocrine Findings in Fibromyalgia Syndrome

Decreased 24-hour urine free cortisol
Loss of normal diurnal fluctuation of cortisol
Exaggerated ACTH response to both CRH and hypoglycemia
Low total basal plasma cortisol with normal basal free cortisol
Normal cortisol response to ACTH challenge
Delayed ACTH release after interleukin-6 administration
Decreased response of thyroid hormones and TSH to TRH
Decreased insulin-like growth factor–1 (IGF-1)
Decreased growth hormone (GH)
GH response to stimulation studies: both normal and increased in several studies
    using different agents for stimulation
Normal nocturnal secretion of melatonin in 2 of 3 studies

ACTH, adrenocorticotropin hormone; CRH, corticotropin-releasing hormone; TSH, thyroid-stimulating hormone, TRH, thyrotropin-releasing hormone.
From Yunus MB, Inanici F: Clinical characteristics and biopathophysiological mechanisms of fibromyalgia syndrome. In Baldry P (ed): Myofascial Pain and Fibromyalgia Syndromes: A Clinical Guide to Diagnosis and Management. London, Churchill Livingstone, 2001, pp 351–377, with permission.

tors confirmed the alpha anomaly during non-REM sleep in patients with FMS compared with dysthymic disorder[82] and with RA.[136]

Several other investigators have shown abnormalities in FMS by controlled sleep EEG studies, including increased alpha waves in stage 1 (indicating arousal), intrusion of alpha waves into delta waves (alpha-delta anomaly), decreased delta waves in stage 3 and 4 (indicating nonrestorative sleep), higher number of arousals and awakenings, and decreased sleep time.[32, 59, 60, 138, 152]

However, sleep EEG abnormalities have not been found by all investigators. Some studies were reported to be normal,[91, 105] and others found that alpha-delta sleep abnormality was found in about a third of patients without having any correlation with clinical severity of symptoms.[42] Two independent groups of investigators failed to demonstrate decreased pain threshold by pressure or pain symptoms among healthy subjects following delta wave sleep interruption or deprivation for three consecutive nights.[60, 148] Sleep studies have been recently reviewed by Harding.[84]

The differences between results of various reports may be explained by a lack of standardized sleep EEG methods and their interpretations, as well as a small number of patients investigated in most studies. It should also be remembered that sleep EEG findings are not specific for FMS.[82, 136] Poor sleep does not seem essential for causing FMS among all patients. It is possible that poor sleep alone may not produce this disorder, but would play a permissible role in the presence of other factors, such as genetic, neurohormonal, environmental, and psychological.[60] In a study of 108 consecutive patients who had attended a sleep disorder clinic, only 3 (2.7%) had fibromyalgia,[57] a frequency similar to the normal population. In another study, Alvarez Lario and colleagues found that 1 (3%) of 30 patients with sleep apnea met the criteria for fibromyalgia.[115] A subgroup of patients reported no sleep difficulties in clinical practice. With regard to the role of sleep in FMS, it may be concluded that although sleep seems an important factor in the biopathogenesis of FMS and poor sleep should always be managed in the treatment of FMS (see Chapter 2, Management of Fibromyalgia Syndrome), there is a lack of general consensus among the investigators regarding the sleep EEG findings and their relationship to pathogenesis or symptoms of FMS. It is of interest that zolpidem, a hypnotic agent, helped sleep, but not pain, in FMS.[135]

Psychological Factors in Fibromyalgia Syndrome

Psychological status in FMS has been reviewed elsewhere.[73, 211] Psychological factors are an important determinant of any pain—particularly chronic pain—irrespective of the cause, and FMS is no exception. Psychological distress perpetuates pain in a vicious cycle. Chronic pain may cause psychological disturbance, which in turn may aggravate pain.

It is now clear that psychiatric diseases are not necessary for development of FMS. A good number of studies (but not all) have shown that the frequencies of psychiatric diseases, e.g., anxiety and depression, in FMS are similar to other chronic diseases, e.g., RA.[5, 6, 46, 109] An important insight has been gained by studying nonpatients, i.e., those who have fibromyalgia by ACR criteria in a community survey but do not seek medical help. In such a study, Aaron and associates compared the frequency of psychiatric diagnoses in FMS nonpatients with those of FMS patients seen in a clinic as well as pain-free healthy controls from the community.[1] It was found that although clinic patients had a significantly higher lifetime diagnosis of psychiatric illnesses (anxiety and mood disorders) than community controls, the psychiatric diagnoses were similar between nonpatients and controls. The authors concluded that psychiatric disorders determine a patient's consultation with a health care provider but are not intrinsic to fibromyalgia.[1]

Utilizing the Diagnostic and Statistical Manual of Mental Disorders III (DSM-III) criteria, our group studied, in a blinded way, 35 patients with fibromyalgia, 33 patients with RA, and 31 pain-free normal controls, and found no significant difference between FMS and RA in major depression (34% vs. 39%), panic disorder (14% vs.

6%), obsessive compulsive disorder (6% vs. 3%), or any psychiatric diagnosis (49% vs. 57%). Although the frequency of these diagnoses in FMS and RA was higher than those in normal controls, the difference did not reach statistical significance.[7] Kirmayer and associates also did not find a significant difference between FMS and RA in any psychiatric diagnosis using the DSM-III criteria.[109] However, Hudson and coworkers found a significantly higher current as well as lifetime diagnosis of depression in their study of 31 patients with FMS and only 14 RA patients.[95] An important criticism of this study is that the number of RA patients included in this investigation was small. Alfici and colleagues also found significantly increased depression in FMS compared with RA.[8] Significantly more common anxiety was found by Alfici and colleagues[8] as well as by Hudson and coworkers[95] as compared with control groups. It may be noted that among the studies by DSM criteria,[5, 8, 95, 109] only the study by Ahles and associates[5] was properly blinded.

Several studies utilized validated questionnaires for psychological symptoms and stress and found no difference in anxiety and depression between FMS patients and controls.[6, 46, 54] Uveges and colleagues found greater psychological distress, including depression, among FMS patients as compared with RA patients, but daily stress was a significant covariate.[186] Using the Arthritis Impact Measurement Scales (AIMS) subscale of depression, Hawley and Wolfe found significantly higher depression scores in FMS than in other rheumatology clinic patients.[56] However, using the AIMS subscales of depression and anxiety, Dailey and associates found no difference between FMS and RA.[54]

Virtually all studies have shown a greater degree of lifetime or daily stress in FMS as compared with normal controls as well as RA.[7, 54, 186] It seems that stress is an important factor in FMS, although a relationship between symptoms and stress has not been adequately addressed. In our study of psychological status by Minnesota Multiphasic Personality Inventory (MMPI) in FMS, we found no correlation between psychological status and several important features of FMS, e.g., tender points, fatigue, poor sleep, swollen feeling, paresthesia, irritable bowel symptoms, and headaches; however, pain severity was influenced by psychological factors.

It has been suggested that FMS is a spectrum of depressive illnesses.[95–97] However, elsewhere we have argued that depression and FMS are different diseases, based on psychological, biophysiologic, and therapeutic studies.[211, 224] As discussed earlier, the occurrence of psychiatric diagnoses in FMS is not greater than in other chronic diseases, e.g., RA in a majority of studies. The HPA axis functions and sleep EEG findings are different in FMS than in depression.[119, 211, 224] For example, the HPA axis is hyperactive in depression,[12, 143, 160, 170] with a blunted response of ACTH to CRH.[9, 71] Also, 24-hour urinary cortisol was found to be significantly increased in depression, but not in FMS.[124] As already discussed, the HPA axis functions in FMS are opposite of what has been found in depression. Moreover, the glucocorticoid receptors in the lymphocytes are normal in FMS,[119] in contrast to low values found in depression.[74, 194] Additionally, a recent study found that patients with depression have significantly fewer tender points than those with FMS (1.3 vs. 16.5).[66] Okifuji and associates have shown that current depressive disorders are independent of the core features of FMS; depressed patients were not different from nondepressed ones in pain severity, number of tender points at ACR criteria sites, or control points for tenderness.[147] These results are similar to our previous observations.[216] Therapeutically, FMS responds to a much lower dose of antidepressant medications than is required for treatment of depression, and several medications effective in FMS, e.g., cyclobenzaprine and tramadol (as shown by double-blind controlled studies) do not have significant antidepressant properties.

The psychological status in FMS may be summarized by stating that a minority subgroup of patients (30%–40%) has a significant psychological disturbance, but most studies suggest that the frequency of such distress is similar to that in other chronic diseases, such as RA. Because FMS is a heterogeneous disease with regard to psychological subgrouping,[184, 185, 216] such subgroups should be recognized in the proper management of FMS (see Chapter 2, Management of Fibromyalgia Syndrome). It is known that psychological status is influenced by many factors, such as referral bias, education, and social status.[153, 155]

Genetic Factors

Familial aggregation has been described in several reports.[37, 38, 150] No consistent association of FMS with HLA has been described.[32, 36, 92, 228] However, linkage studies of HLA are more reliable in demonstrating true genetic contribution in a disease. A study of multicase families by our group has shown a weak but significant linkage of HLA with FMS.[228] A recent study has shown a possible association of a polymorphism in the serotonin transporter (5-HTT) gene regulatory region with FMS.[146] The frequency of the genotype S/S of 5-HTT was significantly higher in FMS than healthy controls. However, this difference was found to be insignificant when the subgroup of patients with psychological disturbance was excluded. Thus, there is no true association of S/S genotype with "pure" FMS. Bondy and associates found an association of the silent T102C polymorphism of the 5-HTA-receptor gene among 168 patients with FMS and 115 normal controls and found a significant increase of the T/C and C/C genotypes, and a significant decrease of the T/T genotype in FMS.[29] No correlation was found between these genotypes and psychological distress as measured by validated questionnaires. Thus, a dysfunction of serotonin may be genetically involved in FMS. Gene mapping studies in FMS by a collaborative group, including our own, are currently in progress. Genetic aspects of FMS have recently been reviewed.[215]

An Integrative Hypothesis for Biophysiologic Mechanisms

It is clear that FMS is a heterogeneous disease or illness. Various contributing factors, e.g., genetic, neurohormonal, psychological, nonrestorative sleep, and environmental are important, but not equally so in an individual case. The major biophysiologic aberration in FMS is a neurohormonal one, with resulting central sensitivity (see Fig. 1–2). As shown in the "box" in Figure 1–2, such neurohormonal dysfunctions are heterogeneous, implying that they are different in FMS from psychiatric illnesses, and they are likely to be different between patient subgroups. A host of factors may trigger such dysfunctions, including genetic, infection, trauma, inflammation, and mental or physical stress. Once present, the biophysiologic elements then interact, most likely in a bidirectional manner, with other factors such as poor sleep, psychological distress, physical deconditioning, overuse, trauma, and various socioeconomic and environmental contributions to amplify the pain and other symptoms of fibromyalgia. The contributions of various etiopathogenetic elements previously mentioned in causing fibromyalgia are likely to vary from patient to patient, causing the heterogeneity in this illness, requiring different and individualized approaches in management of patients.

Disability and Quality of Life in Fibromyalgia Syndrome

Disability in FMS is comparable to that in other chronic diseases.[35, 85, 44] In a six-center study involving 1604 patients, disability, as evaluated by the Health Assessment Questionnaire (HAQ), was found to be high in FMS.[200] More than 16% reported receiving U.S. social security disability as compared with 2.2% in the general population and 29% among RA patients in one center; the highest disability rate was present in San Antonio, Texas (36%) and the lowest in Peoria, Illinois (6%). Such discrepancy in the rate of disability at various sites is most likely explicable on the basis of referral bias and socioeconomic and psychological factors. In this study,[200] 64% of patients reported being able to work most days. Disability as evaluated by HAQ and work simulating standardized tasks was found to be similar between by FMS and RA in one study.[44]

Assessment of disability in FMS is a complex issue. While a large majority of patients can work most days,[200] some patients are truly disabled. Disability is often influenced by education, occupation, psychological distress, and other sociopsychological factors, such as spousal support. In the absence of an objective marker in FMS at this time, it is important to evaluate the patient on several visits, carefully documenting symptoms, job description and difficulties, patient attitude, and the number as well as locations of tender points. Repeated documentation is very useful in establishing the reliability of a patient's history and tender points. Some patients have allodynia and are tender to touch everywhere. As mentioned earlier, this does not necessarily imply malingering or severe psychological disturbance. Concomitant diseases or conditions such as arthritis, sleep disorders (to be documented by polysomnography), and severe mood disorders add to morbidity and should be documented and appropriately treated. An inquiry about job history is also useful. Many fibromyalgia patients were efficient and responsible workers and physically fit, doing regular exercises, before the onset of their disease. Thus, evaluation of disability should include an assessment of all the factors, remembering that psychiatric illnesses or psychological distress has a biophysiologic basis also. As eloquently put by Martinez-Lavin,[126] "They [fibromyalgia patients] are not censurable for their suffering."

Self-assessed questionnaires, such as HAQ and fibromyalgia HAQ (FHAQ),[203] and Fibromyalgia Impact Questionnaire,[34] may be used. It has been argued that FHAQ is more sensitive and appropriate for FMS.[203] Such a questionnaire should be administered on more than one occasion. The issue of disability dilemma in FMS has been discussed by Bennett.[22]

Quality of life (QOL) is markedly impaired in FMS.[35, 89, 125] Burckhardt and associates found that QOL in FMS was among the poorest as compared with other chronic conditions, such as osteoarthritis, RA, chronic obstructive pulmonary disease, permanent ostomies, and insulin-dependent diabetes.[35] Henriksson reported that FMS had adversely affected jobs in 75% of patients and their relationships with other family members were affected in more than 70%.[89] Patients with FMS took much longer to complete a task and needed to take frequent rests because of their distressing symptoms.[89]

Central Sensitivity Syndromes

Following the initial descriptions,[209, 211, 231] FMS is now well recognized to be a band in the spectrum of many other similar syndromes,[2, 47] which have recently been named CSS.[213, 214, 224] The members (types) of CSS include fibromyalgia, chronic fatigue syndrome (CFS), irritable bowel syndrome (IBS), female urethral syndrome, myofascial pain syndrome, temporomandibular pain and dysfunction syndrome, restless legs syndrome, periodic limb movement disorder, multiple chemical sensitivity, tension type headaches, migraine, and primary dysmenorrhea (Fig. 1–3). Gulf war syndrome is similar to FMS,[48] except that it is described mostly among men and the stress factors to trigger the illness are uniquely a combination of physical and psychological, as involved in a war. These syndromes are most likely associated with each other, although data are not available for all of them.[211, 214] In controlled studies, FMS has been shown to be associated with many other CSS conditions, e.g., irritable bowel syndrome, tension-type headaches, chronic fatigue syndrome, primary dysmenorrhea, restless legs syndrome, and female urethral syndrome, as discussed elsewhere.[211, 214] Conversely, FMS has been reported to be more frequent in irritable bowel syndrome and CFS compared with a control group, as has been reviewed.[211, 214]

The types of CSS share many clinical characteristics, such as gender (mostly women), age distribution, and symptoms (pain, fatigue, poor sleep, paresthesia, and a state of global hyperalgesia).[211, 214] Moreover, no structural tissue pathology (such as inflammation or degeneration) is present in these conditions by usual laboratory tests

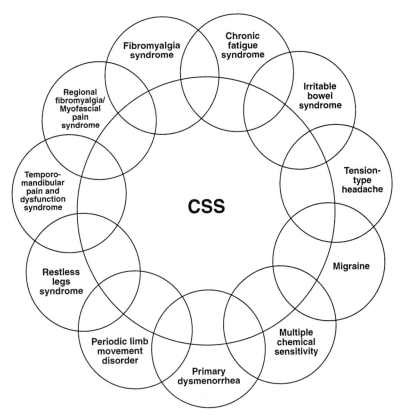

Figure 1–3. The members of the central sensitivity syndromes (CSS) share overlapping features and a common biopathophysiologic mechanism of neuroendocrine dysfunction/centralsensitivity. (Adapted from Yunus MB: Psychological aspects of fibromyalgia syndrome: A component of the dysfunctional spectrum syndrome. Baillieres Clin Rheumatol 8:811–837, 1994, and Yunus MB: Central sensitivity syndromes: A unified concept for fibromyalgia and other similar maladies. J Indian Rheumatism Assoc 8:27–33, 2000, with permission.)

and x-rays. Although psychological factors play a role in a minority subgroup of patients with CSS, the types of CSS cannot be classified as psychiatric illnesses. Thus, CSS cannot be explained by either of the two classical models, i.e., pathology (with structural tissue damage) and psychiatry, but by a new concept of "third paradigm," as suggested by Yunus.[212, 214, 224] These third paradigm illnesses are characterized by neurohormonal aberrations leading to central sensitivity that are generally different from those in psychiatric illnesses.[214, 224] Although there is no structural tissue damage in CSS, a functional abnormality of the neuroendocrine functions can be clearly demonstrated and an abnormality in brain functions can be visualized by neuroimaging techniques, as discussed earlier in this chapter, using FMS as an example. Thus, the distinction between illness ("functional") and disease ("organic," having structural pathology) is blurred. Unlike Jennings,[104] we therefore do not differentiate between the terms *illness* and *disease*. Disease, by definition, simply means "opposite of ease,"[179] meaning suffering, which occurs in all three paradigms, e.g., classic pathology, psychiatry/psychology, and the new third paradigm. Because our role as physicians and other health care providers is to alleviate human suffering, any distinction between illness and disease becomes meaningless and making it does a disservice to our patients.

Central sensitivity may well be the common binding glue of pathogenesis between the various types of the CSS. Evidence for central sensitivity in FMS has been described; it has also been reported in several other members of the CSS family, e.g., myofascial pain syndrome,[14] irritable bowel syndrome,[132] chronic tension type headaches,[15] migraine,[144] and multiple chemical sensitivity.[177] With future investigations, the numbers of illnesses or diseases belonging to the CSS category are likely to increase with further studies on central sensitivity.

It is vital to understand that the boundaries between the three paradigms of disease discussed previously are not rigid. In any chronic disease with structural damage, such as RA, contribution of psychological factors is common. FMS is often associated with a connective tissue disease, such as RA,[201] systemic lupus erythematosus,[133] and Sjögren's syndrome,[28] and the presence of psychological factors is likely to worsen functional disability and overall morbidity in any chronic disease, including those in the CSS family. Chronic diseases, irrespective of cause, should indeed be viewed in a broad biopsychosocial context, and a proper management of these conditions should include a global or holistic approach incorporating proper attention to the pathologic and physiologic as well as psychosocial elements.[129]

CSS is an important and useful concept for more than one reason. It is a newly described paradigm that needs better understanding and a fresh, unbiased approach. CSS syndromes are not synonymous with psychiatric illness, as the old thinking dictated. Multiple symptoms are present in a given patient because of associations with other members of the CSS family, leading to a confusion with somatization. Although a small minority of patients with these syndromes may satisfy the criteria for somatization disorder by virtue of their mutual associations, it may be noted that such a diagnosis is not a valid one, because unlike true somatization disorder, the CSS diseases often have an onset after the age of 30 years and the symptoms can be explained by a defined biophysiologic mechanism. The knowledge that many of the CSS conditions are mutually associated helps their proper diagnosis without extensive investigations. A new biophysiologic mechanism or a form of treatment demonstrated in one may be applicable to others. And finally, CSS as a group is most likely the commonest cause for which patients seek medical help. As a group, they cause immense suffering and disability with great financial burden on a society. A better understanding of and proper research on these conditions are therefore important priorities for the medical community.

Summary

Fibromyalgia syndrome is characterized by *widespread* musculoskeletal pain and *tender points* on palpation at multiple sites, which is based on well-studied biophysiologic mechanisms. Although the biopathophysiologic mechanisms of FMS are not fully understood (like many other chronic diseases, such as RA), it has become clear that the major problem in this condition is a neuroendocrine aberration with central sensitivity as a very important element. FMS is a common condition that causes much suffering and disability. It is part of a spectrum of many other similar syndromes, e.g., irritable bowel syndrome, chronic fatigue syndrome, headaches, and restless legs syndrome, which are now collectively called *central sensitivity syndromes* or CSS. The CSS group of diseases is based on a biopathophysiologic mechanism that is different from both "organic" diseases with structural pathology and psychiatric illnesses. A greater clinical and research interest is warranted for FMS and other similar conditions for better understanding and management of these common and disabling maladies.

References

1. Aaron LA, Bradley LA, Alarcon GS, et al: Psychiatric diagnoses in patients with fibromyalgia are related to health care-seeking behavior rather than to illness. Arthritis Rheum 39:436–445, 1996.
2. Aaron LA, Burke MM, Buchwald D: Overlapping conditions among patients with chronic fatigue syndrome, fibromyalgia, and temporomandibular disorder. Arch Intern Med 160:221–227, 2000.
3. Adler GK, Kinsley BT, Hurwitz S, et al: Reduced hypothalamic-pituitary and sympathoadrenal responses to hypoglycemia in women with fibromyalgia syndrome. Am J Med 106:534–543, 1999.
4. Affleck G, Urrows S, Tennen H, et al: Sequential daily relations of sleep, pain intensity, and attention to pain among women with fibromyalgia. Pain 68:363–368, 1996.

5. Ahles TA, Khan SA, Yunus MB, et al: Psychiatric status of patients with primary fibromyalgia, patients with rheumatoid arthritis, and subjects without pain: A blind comparison of DSM-III diagnoses. Am J Psychiatry 148:1721–1726, 1991.
6. Ahles TA, Yunus MB, Masi AT: Is chronic pain a variant of depressive disease? The case of primary fibromyalgia syndrome. Pain 29:105–111, 1987.
7. Ahles TA, Yunus MB, Riley SD, et al: Psychological factors associated with primary fibromyalgia syndrome. Arthritis Rheum 27:1101–1106, 1984.
8. Alfici S, Sigal M, Landau M: Primary fibromyalgia syndrome—a variant of depressive disorder? Psychotherapy and Psychosomatics 51:156–161, 1989.
9. Amsterdam JD, Maislin G, Winokur A, et al: Pituitary and adrenocortical responses to the ovine corticotropin releasing hormone in depressed patients and healthy volunteers. Arch Gen Psychiatry 44:775–781, 1987.
10. Arroyo JF, Cohen ML: Abnormal responses to electrocutaneous stimulation in fibromyalgia. J Rheumatol 20:1925–1931, 1993.
11. Bagge E, Bengtsson BA, Carlsson L, Carlsson J: Low growth hormone secretion in patients with fibromyalgia—a preliminary report on 10 patients and 10 controls. J Rheumatol 25:145–148, 1998.
12. Banki CM, Bissette G, Arato M, et al: CSF corticotropin-releasing factor-like immunoreactivity in depression and schizophrenia. Am J Psychiatry 144:873–877, 1987.
13. Barker AT, Jalinous R, Prestoni L: Non-invasive magnetic stimulation of the human motor cortex. Lancet 1:1106–1107, 1985.
14. Bendtsen L, Jensen R, Olesen J: Qualitatively altered nociception in chronic myofascial pain. Pain 65:259–264, 1996.
15. Bendtsen L, Jensen R, Olesen J: Decreased pain detection and tolerance thresholds in chronic tension-type headache. Arch Neurol 53:373–376, 1996.
16. Bendtsen L, Norregaard J, Jensen R, Olesen J: Evidence of qualitatively altered nociception in patients with fibromyalgia. Arthritis Rheum 40:98–102, 1997.
17. Bengtsson A, Ernerudh J, Vrethem M, et al: Absence of auto-antibodies in primary fibromyalgia. J Rheumatol 16:1466–1469, 1989.
18. Bengtsson A, Henriksson KG, Jorfeldt L, et al: Primary fibromyalgia. A clinical and laboratory study of 55 patients. Scand J Rheumatol 15:340–347, 1986.
19. Bengtsson A, Henriksson KG, Larsson J: Reduced high-energy phosphate levels in the painful muscles of patients with primary fibromyalgia. Arthritis Rheum 29:817–821, 1986.
20. Bengtsson A, Henriksson KG, Larsson J: Muscle biopsy in primary fibromyalgia: Light microscopical and histochemical findings. Scand J Rheumatol 15:106, 1986.
21. Benjamin S, Morris S, McBeth J, et al: The association between chronic widespread pain and mental disorder. Arthritis Rheum 43:561–567, 2000.
22. Bennett RM: Fibromyalgia and the disability dilemma. A new era in understanding a complex, multidimensional pain syndrome. Arthritis Rheum 39:1627–1634, 1996.
23. Bennett RM: Emerging concepts in the neurobiology of chronic pain: evidence of abnormal sensory processing in fibromyalgia. Mayo Clin Proc 74:385–398, 1999.
24. Bennett RM, Clark SC, Walczyk J: A randomized, double-blind, placebo-controlled study of growth hormone in the treatment of fibromyalgia. Am J Med 104:227–231, 1998.
25. Bennett RM, Clark SR, Campbell SM, Burckhardt CS: Low levels of somatomedin C in patients with the fibromyalgia syndrome. A possible link between sleep and muscle pain. Arthritis Rheum 35:1113–1116, 1992.
26. Bennett RM, Cook DM, Clark SR, et al: Hypothalamic-pituitary-insulin-like growth factor-I axis dysfunction in patients with fibromyalgia. J Rheumatol 24:1384–1389, 1997.
27. Besson JM: The neurobiology of pain. Lancet 35:1610–1615, 1999.
28. Bonafede RP, Downey DC, Bennett RM: An association of fibromyalgia with primary Sjögren's syndrome: A prospective study of 72 patients. J Rheumatol 22:133–136, 1995.
29. Bondy B, Spaeth M, Offenbaecher M, et al: The T102c polymorphism of the 5-HT2A-receptor gene in fibromyalgia. Neurobiol Dis 6:433–439, 1999.
30. Bonnet MH, Arand DL: Heart rate variability: Sleep stage, time of night, and arousal influences. Electroencephalogr Clin Neurophysiol 102:390–396, 1997.
31. Bradley LA, Alberts KR, Alarcon GS, et al: Abnormal brain regional cerebral blood flow (rCBF) and cerebrospinal fluid (CSF) levels of substance P (SP) in patients and non-patients with fibromyalgia (FM). Arthritis Rheum 39(Suppl. 19):S212, 1996.
32. Branco J, Atalaia A, Paiva T: Sleep cycles and alpha-delta sleep in fibromyalgia syndrome. J Rheumatol 21:1113–1117, 1994.
33. Branco JC, Taveres V, Abreu I, et al: HLA studies in fibromyalgia. J Musculoskeletal Pain 4:21–27, 1996.
34. Burckhardt CS, Clark SR, Bennett RM: The fibromyalgia impact questionnaire: Development and validation. J Rheumatol 18:728–733, 1991.
35. Burckhardt CS, Clark SR, Bennett RM: Fibromyalgia and quality of life: A comparative analysis. J Rheumatol 20:475–479, 1993.
36. Burda CD, Cox FR, Osborne P: Histocompatibility antigens in the fibrositis (fibromyalgia) syndrome. Clin Exp Rheumatol 4:355–358, 1986.
37. Buskila D, Neumann L: Fibromyalgia syndrome (FM) and nonarticular tenderness in relatives of patients with FM. J Rheumatol 24:941–944, 1997.

38. Buskila D, Neumann L, Hazanov I, Carmi R: Familial aggregation in the fibromyalgia syndrome. Semin Arthritis Rheum 26:605–611, 1996.
39. Buskila D, Neumann L, Vaisberg G, et al: Increased rates of fibromyalgia following cervical spine injury. Arthritis Rheum 40:446–452, 1997.
40. Campbell SM, Clark S, Tindall EA, et al: Clinical characteristics of fibrositis: I. A "blinded" controlled study of symptoms and tender points. Arthritis Rheum 26:817–824, 1983.
41. Carette S, McCain GA, Bell DA, Fam AG: Evaluation of amitriptyline in primary fibrositis. A double-blind, placebo-controlled study. Arthritis Rheum 29:655–659, 1986.
42. Carette S, Oakson G, Guimont C, Steriade M: Sleep electroencephalography and the clinical response to amitriptyline in patients with fibromyalgia. Arthritis Rheum 38:1211–1217, 1995.
43. Caro XJ: Immunofluorescent detection of IgG at the dermal-epidermal junction in patients with apparent primary fibrositis syndrome. Arthritis Rheum 27:1174–1179, 1984.
44. Cathey MA, Wolfe F, Kleinheksel SM: Functional ability and work status in patients with fibromyalgia. Arthritis Care and Research 1:85–98, 1988.
45. Choudhury AK, Yunus MB, Haq SA, et al: Clinical features of fibromyalgia in a Bangladeshi population. J Musculoskeletal Pain 9:25–33, 2001.
46. Clark S, Campbell SM, Forehand ME, et al: Clinical characteristics of fibrositis. II. A "blinded," controlled study using standard psychological tests. Arthritis Rheum 28:132–137, 1985.
47. Clauw DJ: Fibromyalgia: More than just a musculoskeletal disease. Am Fam Physician 52:843–848, 1995.
48. Clauw DJ: The "Gulf War Syndrome": implications for rheumatologists. J Clin Rheumatol 4:173–174, 1998.
49. Coderre TJ, Katz J, Vaccarino AL, Melzack R: Contribution of central neuroplasticity to pathological pain: Review of clinical and experimental evidence. Pain 52:259–285, 1993.
50. Cohen H, Neumann L, Shore M, et al: Autonomic dysfunction in patients with fibromyalgia: Application of power spectral analysis of heart rate variability. Semin Arthritis Rheum 29:217–227, 2000.
51. Cott A, Parkinson W, Bell MJ, et al: Interrater reliability of the tender point criterion for fibromyalgia. J Rheumatol 19:1955–1959, 1992.
52. Crofford LJ, Demitrack MA: Evidence that abnormalities of central neurohormonal systems are key to understanding fibromyalgia and chronic fatigue syndrome. Rheum Dis Clin North Am 22:267–284, 1996.
53. Crofford LJ, Pillemer SR, Kalogeras KT, et al: Hypothalamic-pituitary-adrenal axis perturbations in patients with fibromyalgia. Arthritis Rheum 37:1583–1592, 1994.
54. Dailey PA, Bishop GD, Russell IJ, Fletcher EM: Psychological stress and the fibrositis/fibromyalgia syndrome. J Rheumatol 17:1380–1385, 1990.
55. Dessein PH, Shipton EA, Joffee BI, et al: Hyposecretion of adrenal androgens and the relation of serum adrenal steroids, serotonin and insulin-like growth factor-1 to clinical features in women with fibromyalgia. Pain 83:313–319, 1999.
56. Devor M: Central changes mediating neuropathic pain. In Proceedings of the Vth World Congress on Pain. Amsterdam, Elsevier Science Publishers BV, 1988, pp 114–128.
57. Donald F, Esdaile JM, Kimoff JR, Fitzcharles MA: Musculoskeletal complaints and fibromyalgia in patients attending a respiratory sleep disorders clinic. J Rheumatol 23:1612–1616, 1996.
58. Dougherty PM, Willis WD: Enhancement of spinothalamic neuron responses to chemical and mechanical stimuli following combined micro-iontophoretic application of n-methyl-d-aspartic acid and substance P. Pain 47:85–93, 1991.
58a. Drewes AM, Andreasen A, Schroder HD, et al: Muscle biopsy in fibromyalgia. Scand J Rheumatol 94(Suppl.):20, 1992.
59. Drewes AM, Gade J, Nielsen KD, et al: Clustering of sleep electroencephalopathic patterns in patients with the fibromyalgia syndrome. Br J Rheumatol 34:1151–1156, 1995.
60. Drewes AM, Nielsen KD, Rasmussen C, et al: The effects of controlled delta sleep deprivation on experimental pain in healthy subjects. J Musculoskeletal Pain 8(3):49–67, 2000.
61. Drewes AM, Nielsen KD, Taagholt SJ, et al: Sleep intensity in fibromyalgia: Focus on the microstructure of the sleep process. Br J Rheumatol 34:629–635, 1995.
62. Dubner R, Ruda MA: Activity-dependent neuronal plasticity following tissue injury and inflammation. Trends in Neurosciences 15:96–103, 1992.
63. Elam M, Johansson G, Wallin G: Do patients with primary fibromyalgia have an altered muscle sympathetic nerve activity? Pain 48:371–375, 1992.
64. Ernberg M, Hedenberg-Magnusson B, Alstergren P, Kopp S: The level of serotonin in the superficial masseter muscle in relation to local pain and allodynia. Life Science 65:313–325, 1999.
65. Ernberg M, Lundeberg T, Kopp S: Pain and allodynia/hyperalgesia induced by intramuscular injection of serotonin in patients with fibromyalgia and healthy individuals. Pain 85:31–39, 2000.
66. Fassbender K, Samborsky W, Kellner M, et al: Tender points, depressive and functional symptoms: Comparison between fibromyalgia and major depression. Clin Rheumatol 16:76–79, 1997.
67. Ferraccioli G, Cavalieri F, Salaffi F, et al: Neuroendocrinologic findings in primary fibromyalgia (soft tissue chronic pain syndrome) and in other chronic rheumatic conditions (rheumatoid arthritis, low back pain). J Rheumatol 17:869–873, 1990.
68. Ferraccioli G, Guerra P, Rizzi V, et al: Somatomedin C (insulin-like growth factor 1) levels decrease during acute changes of stress related hormones. Relevance for fibromyalgia. J Rheumatol 21:1332–1334, 1994.
69. Gibson SJ, Littlejohn GO, Gorman MM, et al: Altered heat pain thresholds and cerebral event-

related potentials following painful CO_2 laser stimulation in subjects with fibromyalgia syndrome. Pain 58:185–193, 1994.

70. Giovengo SL, Russell IJ, Larson AA: Increased concentrations of nerve growth factor in cerebrospinal fluid of patients with fibromyalgia. J Rheumatol 26:1564–1569, 1999.

71. Gold PW, Loriaux DL, Roy A, et al: Responses to corticotropin-releasing hormone in the hypercortisolism of depression and Cushing's disease. Pathophysiologic and diagnostic implications. N Engl J Med 314:1329–1335, 1986.

72. Goldenberg DL: Fibromyalgia syndrome: An emerging but controversial condition. JAMA 257:2782–2787, 1987.

73. Goldenberg DL: Psychological symptoms and psychiatric diagnosis in patients with fibromyalgia. J Rheumatol 16(Suppl. 19):127–130, 1989.

74. Gormley GJ, Lowy MT, Reder AT, et al: Glucocorticoid receptors in depression: Relationship to the dexamethasone suppression test. Am J Psychiatry 42:1278–1284, 1985.

75. Gowers WR: Lumbago: Its lessons and analogues. BMJ 1:117–121, 1904.

76. Granges G, Littlejohn G: Pressure pain threshold in pain-free subjects, in patients with chronic regional pain syndromes, and in patients with fibromyalgia syndrome. Arthritis Rheum 36:642–646, 1993.

77. Graven-Nielsen T, Kendall SA, Henriksson KG, et al: Ketamine reduces muscle pain, temporal summation, and referred pain in fibromyalgia patients. Pain 85:483–491, 2000.

78. Greenfield S, Fitzcharles MA, Esdaile JM: Reactive fibromyalgia syndrome. Arthritis Rheum 35:678–681, 1992.

79. Griep EN, Boersma JW, de Kloet ER: Altered reactivity of the hypothalamic-pituitary-adrenal axis in the primary fibromyalgia syndrome. J Rheumatol 20:469–474, 1993.

80. Griep EN, Boersma JW, de Kloet ER: Pituitary release of growth hormone and prolactin in the primary fibromyalgia syndrome. J Rheumatol 21:2125–2130, 1994.

81. Griep EN, Boersma JW, Lentjes EG, et al: Function of the hypothalamic-pituitary-adrenal axis in patients with fibromyalgia and low back pain. J Rheumatol 25:1374–381, 1998.

82. Gupta MA, Moldofsky H: Dysthymic disorders and rheumatic pain modulation disorder (fibrositis syndrome): A comparison of symptoms and sleep physiology. Can J Psychiatry 31:608–616, 1986.

83. Hakkinen A, Hakkinen K, Hannonen P, Alen M: Force production capacity and acute neuromuscular responses in fatiguing loading in women with fibromyalgia are not different from those of healthy women. J Rheumatol 27:1277–1282, 2000.

84. Harding SM: Sleep in fibromyalgia patients: Subjective and objective findings. Am J Med Sci 315:367–376, 1998.

85. Hawley DJ, Wolfe F: Pain, disability, and pain/disability relationships in seven rheumatic disorders: A study of 1,522 patients. J Rheumatol 18:1552–1557, 1991.

86. Hawley DJ, Wolfe F: Depression is not more common in rheumatoid arthritis: A 10-year longitudinal study of 6,153 patients with rheumatic disease. J Rheumatol 20:2025–2031, 1993.

87. Hawley DJ, Wolfe F: Effect of light and season on pain and depression in subjects with rheumatic disorders. Pain 59:227–234, 1994.

88. Hawley DJ, Wolfe F, Cathey MA: Pain, functional disability, and psychological status: A 12-month study of severity in fibromyalgia. J Rheumatol 15:1551–1556, 1988.

89. Henriksson CM: Longterm effects of fibromyalgia on everyday life. A study of 56 patients. Scand J Rheumatol 23:36–41, 1994.

90. Holsboer F, Von Bardeleben U, Gerken A, et al: Blunted corticotropin and normal cortisol response to human corticotropin-releasing factor in depression. N Engl J Med 311:1127, 1984.

91. Horne JA, Shackell BS: Alpha-like EEG activity in non-REM sleep and the fibromyalgia (fibrositis) syndrome. Electroencephalogr Clin Neurophysiol 79:271–276, 1991.

92. Horven S, Stiles TC, Holst A, Moen T: HLA antigens in primary fibromyalgia syndrome. J Rheumatol 19:1269–1270, 1992.

93. Houvenagel E, Forzy G, Leloire O, et al: Cerebrospinal fluid monoamines in primary fibromyalgia. Revue du Rhumatisme et des Maladies Osteo-Articulaires 57:21–23, 1990.

94. Hrycaj P, Stratz T, Muller W: Platelet 3H-imipramine uptake receptor density and serum serotonin levels in patients with fibromyalgia/fibrositis syndrome. J Rheumatol 20:1986–1988, 1993.

95. Hudson JI, Hudson MS, Pliner LF, et al: Fibromyalgia and major affective disorder: A controlled phenomenology and family history study. Am J Psychiatry 142:441–446, 1985.

96. Hudson JI, Pope HG: Fibromyalgia and psychopathology: Is fibromyalgia a form of "affective spectrum disorder"? J Rheumatol 19(Suppl.):15–22, 1989.

97. Hudson JI, Pope HG: Affective spectrum disorder: Does antidepressant response identify a family of disorders with a common pathophysiology? Am J Psychiatry 147:552–564, 1990.

98. Hyyppa MT, Kronholm E: Nocturnal motor activity in fibromyalgia patients with poor sleep quality. J Psychosom Res 39(1):85–91, 1995.

99. İnanici F, Yunus MB: Management of fibromyalgia syndrome. In Baldry P (ed): Myofascial Pain and Fibromyalgia Syndromes: A Clinical Guide to Diagnosis and Management. London, Churchill Livingstone (in press).

100. İnanici F, Yunus MB, Aldag JC: Clinical features and psychologic factors in regional soft tissue pain: Comparison with fibromyalgia syndrome. J Musculoskeletal Pain 7(1/2):293–301, 1999.

101. İnanici F, Yunus MB, Aldag JC: Psychological features in men with fibromyalgia syndrome: Comparison with women. Ann Rheum Dis 59(Suppl. 1):62, 2000.

102. İnanici F, Yunus MB, Castillo LD, Aldag JC: Prognosis of regional fibromyalgia: Comparison within fibromyalgia syndrome. J Musculoskeletal Pain 6(Suppl. 2):97, 1998.

103. Jacobsen S, Main K, Danneskiold-Samsoe B, Skakkebaek NE: A controlled study on serum insulin-like growth factor-I and urinary excretion of growth hormone in fibromyalgia. J Rheumatol 22:1138–1140, 1995.

104. Jennings D: The confusion between disease and illness in clinical medicine. Can Med Assoc J 135:865–870, 1986.

105. Jennum P, Drewes AM, Andreasen A, Nielsen KD: Sleep and other symptoms in primary fibromyalgia and in healthy controls. J Rheumatol 20:1756–1759, 1993.

106. Kalyan-Raman UP, Kalyan-Raman K, Yunus MB, et al: Muscle pathology in primary fibromyalgia syndrome: Light microscopic, histochemical and ultrastructural study. J Rheumatol 11:808–813, 1984.

107. Kang Y-K, Russell IJ, Vipraio GA, et al: Low urinary 5-hydroxyindole acetic acid in fibromyalgia syndrome: Evidence in support of a serotonin-deficiency pathogenesis. Myalgia 1:14–21, 1998.

108. Kent-Braun JA, Sharma KR, Weiner MW, et al: Central basis of muscle fatigue in chronic fatigue syndrome. Neurology 43:125–131, 1993.

109. Kirmayer LJ, Robbins JM, Kapusta MA: Somatization and depression in fibromyalgia syndrome. Am J Psychiatry 145:950–954, 1988.

110. Korszun A, Sackett-Lundeen L, Papadopoulos E, et al: Melatonin levels in women with fibromyalgia and chronic fatigue syndrome. J Rheumatol 26:2675–2680, 1999.

111. Kosek E, Hansson P: Modulatory influence on somatosensory perception from vibration and hetero-topic noxious conditioning stimulation (HNCS) in fibromyalgia patients and healthy subjects. Pain 70:41–51, 1997.

112. Kravitz HM, Katz R, Kot E, et al: Biochemical clues to a fibromyalgia-depression link: imipramine binding in patients with fibromyalgia or depression and in healthy controls. J Rheumatol 19:1428–1432, 1992.

113. Krueger BR: Restless legs syndrome and periodic movements of sleep. Mayo Clin Proc 65:999–1006, 1990.

114. Lapossy E, Maleitzke R, Hrycaj P, et al: The frequency of transition of chronic low back pain to fibromyalgia. Scand J Rheumatol 24:29–33, 1995.

115. Alvarez Lario B, Teran J, Alonso JL, et al: Lack of association between fibromyalgia and sleep apnea syndrome. Ann Rheum Dis 51:108–111, 1992.

116. Lautenbacher S, Roscher S, Strian D, et al: Pain perception in depression: Relationships to symptomatology and naloxone-sensitive mechanisms. Psychosom Med 56:345–352, 1994.

117. Leal-Cerro A, Povedano J, Astorga R, et al: The growth hormone (GH)-releasing hormone-GH-insulin-like growth factor-1 axis in patients with fibromyalgia syndrome. J Clin Endocrin Metabol 84:3378–3381, 1999.

118. Leavitt F, Katz RS, Golden HE, et al: Comparison of pain properties in fibromyalgia patients and rheumatoid arthritis patients. Arthritis Rheum 29:775–781, 1986.

119. Lentjes EG, Griep EN, Boersma JW, et al: Glucocorticoid receptors, fibromyalgia and low back pain. Psychoneuroendocrinology 22:603–614, 1997.

120. Lima D: Anatomical basis for the dynamic processing of nociceptive input. European J Pain 2:195–202, 1998.

121. Lorenz J, Grasedyck K, Bromm B: Middle and long latency somatosensory evoked potentials after painful laser stimulation in patients with fibromyalgia syndrome. Electroencephalogr Clin Neurophysiol 100:165–168, 1996.

122. Lund N, Bengtsson A, Thorborg P: Muscle tissue oxygen pressure in primary fibromyalgia. Scand J Rheumatol 15:165–173, 1986.

123. Lyddell C, Meyers OL: The prevalence of fibromyalgia in a South African community. Scand J Rheumatol 94(Suppl.):8, 1992.

124. Maes M, Lin A, Bonaccorso S, et al: Increased 24-hour urinary cortisol excretion in patients with post-traumatic stress disorder and patients with major depression, but not in patients with fibromyalgia. Acta Psychiat Scand 98:328–335, 1998.

125. Martinez JE, Ferraz MB, Sato EI, Atra E: Fibromyalgia versus rheumatoid arthritis: A longitudinal comparison of the quality of life. J Rheumatol 22:270–274, 1995.

126. Martinez-Lavin M, Hermosillo AG: Autonomic nervous system dysfunction may explain the multi-system features of fibromyalgia. Semin Arthritis Rheum 29:197–199, 2000.

127. Martinez-Lavin M, Hermosillo AG, Mendoza C, et al: Orthostatic sympathetic derangement in subjects with fibromyalgia. J Rheumatol 24:714–718, 1997.

128. Martinez-Lavin M, Hermosillo AG, Rosas M, Soto ME: Circadian studies of autonomic nervous balance in patients with fibromyalgia: A heart rate variability analysis. Arthritis Rheum 41:1966–1971, 1998.

129. Masi AT: An intuitive person-centered perspective on fibromyalgia syndrome and its management. Baillieres Clin Rheumatol 8:957–993, 1994.

130. McBroom P, Walsh NE, Dumitro D: Electromyography in primary fibromyalgia syndrome. Clin J Pain 4:117–119, 1988.

131. McCain GA, Tilbe KS: Diurnal hormone variation in fibromyalgia syndrome: A comparison with rheumatoid arthritis. J Rheumatol 19(Suppl.):154–157, 1989.

132. Mertz H, Naliboff B, Munakata J, et al: Altered rectal perception is a biological marker of patients with irritable bowel syndrome. Gastroenterology 109:40–52, 1995.

133. Middleton GD, McFarlin JE, Lipsky PE: The prevalence and clinical impact of fibromyalgia in systemic lupus erythematosus. Arthritis Rheum 37:1181–1188, 1994.

134. Moldofsky H: Chronobiological influences on fibromyalgia syndrome: Theoretical and therapeutic implications. Baillieres Clin Rheumatol 8:801–810, 1994.

135. Moldofsky H, Lue FA, Mously C, et al: The effect of zolpidem in patients with fibromyalgia: A dose ranging, double blind, placebo controlled, modified crossover study. J Rheumatol 23:529–533, 1996.
136. Moldofsky H, Lue FA, Smythe HA: Alpha EEG sleep and morning symptoms in rheumatoid arthritis. J Rheumatol 10:373–379, 1983.
137. Moldofsky H, Scarisbrick P, England R, et al: Musculoskeletal symptoms and non-REM sleep disturbance in patients with "fibrositis" syndrome and healthy subjects. Psychosom Med 37:341–351, 1975.
138. Molony RR, MacPeek DM, Schiffman PL, et al: Sleep, sleep apnea and the fibromyalgia syndrome. J Rheumatol 13:797–800, 1986.
139. Mountz JM, Bradley LA, Modell JG, et al: Fibromyalgia in women. Abnormalities of regional cerebral blood flow in the thalamus and the caudate nucleus are associated with low pain threshold levels. Arthritis Rheum 38:926–938, 1995.
140. Mukerji B, Mukerji V, Alpert MA, Selukar R: The prevalence of rheumatologic disorders in patients with chest pain and angiographically normal coronary arteries. Angiology 46:425–430, 1995.
141. National Heart, Lung and Blood Institute Working Group on Restless Legs Syndrome: Restless legs syndrome detection and management in primary care. Am Fam Physician 62:108–114, 2000.
142. Neeck G, Riedel W: Thyroid function in patients with fibromyalgia syndrome. J Rheumatol 19:1120–1122, 1992.
143. Nemeroff CB, Widerlov E, Bissette G, et al: Elevated concentrations of CSF corticotropin-releasing factor-like immunoreactivity in depressed patients. Science 226:1342–1344, 1984.
144. Nicolodi M, Volpe AR, Sicuteri F: Fibromyalgia and headache. Failure of serotonergic analgesia and N-methyl-D-aspartate-mediated neuronal plasticity: Their common clues. Cephalalgia 18(Suppl. 21):41–44, 1998.
145. Nishikai M: Fibromyalgia in Japanese. J Rheumatol 19:110–114, 1991.
146. Offenbaecher M, Bondy B, de Jonge S, et al: Possible association of fibromyalgia with a polymorphism in the serotonin transporter gene regulatory region. Arthritis Rheum 42:2482–2488, 1999.
147. Okifuji A, Turk DC, Sherman JJ: Evaluation of the relationship between depression and fibromyalgia syndrome: Why aren't all patients depressed? J Rheumatol 27:212–219, 2000.
148. Older SA, Battafarano DF, Danning CL, et al: The effects of delta wave sleep interruption on pain thresholds and fibromyalgia-like symptoms in healthy subjects; correlations with insulin-like growth factor I. J Rheumatol 25:1180–1186, 1998.
149. Park JH, Kari S, King LE, Olsen NJ: Analysis of 31P MR spectroscopy data using artificial neural networks for longitudinal evaluation of muscle diseases; dermatomyositis. NMR Biomed 11:245–256, 1998.
150. Pellegrino MJ: Atypical chest pain as an initial presentation of primary fibromyalgia. Arch Phys Med Rehabil 71:526–528, 1990.
151. Pellegrino MJ, Waylonis GW, Sommer A: Familial occurrence of primary fibromyalgia. Arch Phys Med Rehabil 70:61–63, 1989.
152. Perlis ML, Giles DE, Bootzin RR, et al: Alpha sleep and information processing, perception of sleep, pain, and arousability in fibromyalgia. Int J Neurosci 89:265–280, 1997.
153. Pillay AL, Sargent CA: Relationship of age and education with anxiety, depression, and hopelessness in a South African community sample. Percept Mot Skills 89:881–884, 1999.
154. Pillemer SR, Bradley LA, Crofford LJ, et al: The neuroscience and endocrinology of fibromyalgia. Arthritis Rheum 40:1928–1939, 1997.
155. Pincus T, Callahan LF: What explains the association between socioeconomic status and health: Primarily access to medical care or mind-body variables? J Mind-Body Health 11:4–36, 1995.
156. Press J, Phillip M, Neumann L, et al: Normal melatonin levels in patients with fibromyalgia syndrome. J Rheumatol 25:551–555, 1998.
157. Price DD, Mao J, Frenk H, Mayer DJ: The N-methyl-D-aspartate receptor antagonist dextromethorphan selectively reduces temporal summation of second pain in man. Pain 59:165–174, 1994.
158. Prince A, Bernard AL, Edsal PA: A descriptive analysis of fibromyalgia from the patients' perspective. J Musculoskeletal Pain 8:35–47, 2000.
159. Qiao Z, Vaeroy H, Morkrid L: Electrodermal and microcirculatory activity in patients with fibromyalgia during baseline, acoustic stimulation and cold pressor tests. J Rheumatol 18:1383–1389, 1991.
160. Raadsheer FC: Increased Activity of Hypothalamic Corticotropin-Releasing Neurons on Aging, Alzheimer Disease ond Depression [dissertation]. Amsterdam, University of Amsterdam, 1994.
161. Reilly PA, Littlejohn GO: Peripheral arthralgic presentation of fibrositis/fibromyalgia syndrome. J Rheumatol 19:281–283, 1992.
162. Reynolds MD: The development of the concept of fibrositis. J Hist Med Allied Sci 38:5–35, 1983.
163. Roizenblatt S, Tufik S, Goldenberg J, et al: Juvenile fibromyalgia: Clinical and polysomnographic aspects. J Rheumatol 24:579–585, 1997.
164. Russell IJ: Advances in fibromyalgia: Possible role for central neurochemicals. Am J Med Sci 315:377–384, 1998.
165. Russell IJ, Michalek JE, Vipraio GA, et al: Serum amino acids in fibrositis/fibromyalgia syndrome. J Rheumatol 19(Suppl.):158–163, 1989.
166. Russell IJ, Michalek JE, Vipraio GA, et al: Platelet 3H-imipramine uptake receptor density and serum serotonin levels in patients with fibromyalgia/fibrositis syndrome. J Rheumatol 19:104–109, 1992.
167. Russell IJ, Orr MD, Littman B, et al: Elevated cerebrospinal fluid levels of substance P in patients with the fibromyalgia syndrome. Arthritis Rheum 1994. 37:1593–1601.
168. Russell IJ, Vaeroy H, Javors M, Nyberg F: Cerebrospinal fluid biogenic amine metabolites in fibromyalgia/fibrositis syndrome and rheumatoid arthritis. Arthritis Rheum 35:550–556, 1992.

169. Salerno A, Thomas E, Olive P, et al: Motor cortical dysfunction disclosed by single and double magnetic stimulation in patients with fibromyalgia. Clin Neurophysiol 111:994–1001, 2000.

170. Schatzberg AF, Rothschild AJ, Stahl JB, et al: The dexamethasone suppression test: Identification of subtypes of depression. Am J Psychiatry 140:88–91, 1983.

171. Simms RW: Fibromyalgia is not a muscle disorder. Am J Med Sci 315:346–350, 1998.

172. Simms RW, Goldenberg DL: Symptoms mimicking neurologic disorders in fibromyalgia syndrome. J Rheumatol 15:1271–1273, 1988.

173. Simms RW, Roy SH, Hrovat M, et al: Lack of association between fibromyalgia syndrome and abnormalities in muscle energy metabolism. Arthritis Rheum 37:794–800, 1994.

174. Smythe HA: Non-articular rheumatism and psychogenic musculoskeletal syndromes. In McCarty DJ (ed): Arthritis and Allied Conditions: A Textbook of Rheumatology. Philadelphia, Lea & Febiger, 1979, pp 881–891.

175. Sorensen J, Bengtsson A, Backman E, et al: Pain analysis in patients with fibromyalgia. Effects of intravenous morphine, lidocaine, and ketamine. Scand J Rheumatol 24:360–365, 1995.

176. Sorensen J, Graven-Nielsen T, Henriksson KG, et al: Hyperexcitability in fibromyalgia. J Rheumatol 25:152–155, 1998.

177. Sorg B: Multiple chemical sensitivity: Potential role for neural sensitization. Crit Rev Neurobiol 13:283–316, 1999.

178. Sprott H, Bradley LA, Oh SJ, et al: Immunohistochemical and molecular studies of serotonin, substance P, galanin, pituitary adenylyl cyclase-activating polypeptide, and secretoneurin in fibromyalgic muscle tissue. Arthritis Rheum 41:1689–1694, 1998.

179. Stedman's Medical Dictionary. Baltimore, Williams & Wilkins, 1995.

180. Task Force of the European Society of Cardiology and the North American Society of Pacing and Electrophysiology: Heart rate variability standards of measurement, physiological interpretation, and clinical use. Circulation 93:1043–1065, 1996.

181. Torpy DJ, Papanicolaou DA, Lotsikas AJ, et al: Responses of the sympathetic nervous system and the hypothalamic-pituitary-adrenal axis to interleukin-6: A pilot study in fibromyalgia. Arthritis Rheum 43:872–880, 2000.

182. Traut EF: Fibrositis. J Am Geriatr Soc 16:531–538, 1968.

183. Tunks E, McCain GA, Hart LE, et al: The reliability of examination for tenderness in patients with myofascial pain, chronic fibromyalgia and controls. J Rheumatol 22:944–952, 1995.

184. Turk DC, Okifuji A, Sinclair JD, Starz TW: Pain, disability, and physical functioning in subgroups of patients with fibromyalgia. J Rheumatol 23:1255–1262, 1996.

185. Turk DC, Okifuji A, Sinclair JD, Starz TW: Interdisciplinary treatment for fibromyalgia syndrome: Clinical and statistical significance. Arthritis Care Research 11:186–195, 1998.

186. Uveges JM, Parker JC, Smarr KL, et al: Psychological symptoms in primary fibromyalgia syndrome: Relationship to pain, life stress, and sleep disturbance. Arthritis Rheum 33:1279–1283, 1990.

187. Vaeroy H, Helle R, Forre O, et al: Cerebrospinal fluid levels of β-endorphin in patients with fibromyalgia (fibrositis syndrome). J Rheumatol 15:1804–1806, 1988.

188. Vaeroy H, Helle R, Forre O, et al: Elevated CSF levels of substance P and high incidence of Raynaud phenomenon in patients with fibromyalgia: New features for diagnosis. Pain 32:21–26, 1988.

189. Vaeroy H, Nyberg F, Terenius L: No evidence for endorphin deficiency in fibromyalgia following investigation of cerebrospinal fluid (CSF) dynorphin A and met-enkephalin-Arg6-Phe7. Pain 46:139–143, 1991.

190. Vaeroy H, Qiao ZG, Morkrid L, Forre O: Altered sympathetic nervous system response in patients with fibromyalgia (fibrositis syndrome). J Rheumatol 16:1460–1465, 1989.

191. van Denderen JC, Boersma JW, Zeinstra P, et al: Physiological effects of exhaustive physical exercise in primary fibromyalgia syndrome (PFS): Is PFS a disorder of neuroendocrine reactivity? Scand J Rheumatol 21:35–37, 1992.

192. Watson R, Libmann KO, Jenson J: Alpha-delta sleep: EEG characteristics, incidence, treatment, psychological correlates in personality. Sleep Research 14:226, 1985.

193. Welin M, Bragee B, Nyberg F, Kristiansson M: Elevated substance P levels are contrasted by a decrease in met-enkephalin-arg-phe levels in CSF from fibromyalgia patients. J Musculoskeletal Pain 3(Suppl. 1):4, 1995.

194. Whalley LJ, Borthwick N, Copolov D, et al: Glucocorticoid receptors and depression. BMJ (Clinical Research Edition) 292:859–861, 1986.

195. White KP, Speechley M, Harth M, Ostbye T. The London Fibromyalgia Epidemiology Study: The prevalence of fibromyalgia syndrome in London, Ontario. J Rheumatol 26:1570–1576, 1999.

196. Wikner J, Hirsch U, Wetterberg L, Rojdmark S: Fibromyalgia—a syndrome associated with decreased nocturnal melatonin secretion. Clinical Endocrinology (Oxford) 49:179–183, 1998.

197. Willis WD, Westlund KN: Neuroanatomy of the pain system and of the pathways that modulate pain. J Clin Neurophysiol 14:2–31, 1997.

198. Wolfe F: Fibromyalgia. Rheum Dis Clin North Am 16:681–698, 1990.

199. Wolfe F: What use are fibromyalgia control points. J Rheumatol 25:546–550, 1998.

200. Wolfe F, Anderson J, Harkness D, et al: Work and disability status of persons with fibromyalgia. J Rheumatol 24:1171–1178, 1997.

201. Wolfe F, Cathey MA, Kleinheksel SM: Fibrositis (fibromyalgia) in rheumatoid arthritis. J Rheumatol 11:814–818, 1984.

202. Wolfe F, Hawley DJ, Cathey MA, et al: Fibrositis: Symptom frequency and criteria for diagnosis. J Rheumatol 1985. 12:1159–1163.

203. Wolfe F, Hawley DJ, Goldenberg DL, et al: The assessment of functional impairment in fibromyalgia (FM): Rasch analyses of 5 functional scales and the development of the FM health assessment questionnaire. J Rheumatol 27:1989–1999, 2000.
204. Wolfe F, Ross K, Anderson J, Russell IJ: Aspects of fibromyalgia in the general population: Sex, pain threshold, and fibromyalgia symptoms. J Rheumatol 22:151–156, 1995.
205. Wolfe F, Ross K, Anderson J, et al: The prevalence and characteristics of fibromyalgia in the general population. Arthritis Rheum 38:19–28, 1995.
206. Wolfe F, Smythe HA, Yunus MB, et al: The American College of Rheumatology 1990 Criteria for the Classification of Fibromyalgia. Report of the Multicenter Criteria Committee. Arthritis Rheum 33:160–172, 1990.
207. Woolf CJ: Evidence for a central component of post-injury pain hypersensitivity. Nature 306:686–688, 1983.
208. Woolf CJ, Thompson SW: The induction and maintenance of central sensitization is dependent on N-methyl-D-aspartic acid receptor activation; implications for the treatment of post-injury pain hypersensitivity states. Pain 44:293–299, 1991.
209. Yunus MB: Primary fibromyalgia syndrome: Current concepts. Compr Ther 10:21–28, 1984.
210. Yunus MB: Towards a model of pathophysiology of fibromyalgia: Aberrant central pain mechanisms with peripheral modulation. J Rheumatol 1992;19:846–850.
211. Yunus MB: Psychological aspects of fibromyalgia syndrome: A component of the dysfunctional spectrum syndrome. Baillieres Clin Rheumatol 8:811–837, 1994.
212. Yunus MB: Dysregulation spectrum syndrome: A unified new concept for many common maladies. In Multidisciplinary Approaches to Fibromyalgia, FMS Resources Group, LTD. Columbus, Ohio, Anadem Publishing, 1998, pp 243–251.
213. Yunus MB: Fibromyalgia and related syndromes. Current Practice of Medicine On line serial 2000. Available at http://praxis.md/index.cfm?page=cpmref&article=CPM02%2DRH393
214. Yunus MB: Central sensitivity syndromes: A unified concept for fibromyalgia and other similar maladies. J Indian Rheumatism Assoc 8:27–33, 2000.
215. Yunus MB: Genetic aspects of fibromyalgia syndrome. J Rheumatol Med Rehabil 11:143–145, 2000.
216. Yunus MB, Ahles TA, Aldag JC, Masi AT: Relationship of clinical features with psychological status in primary fibromyalgia. Arthritis Rheum 34:15–21, 1991.
217. Yunus MB, Aldag JC, Dailey JW, Jobe PC: Interrelationships of biochemical parameters in classification of fibromyalgia syndrome and healthy normal controls. J Musculoskeletal Pain 3(4):15–24, 1995.
218. Yunus MB, Berg BC, Masi AT: Multiphase skeletal scintigraphy in primary fibromyalgia syndrome: A blinded study. J Rheumatol 16:1466–1468, 1989.
219. Yunus MB, Dailey JW, Aldag JC, et al: Plasma and urinary catecholamines in primary fibromyalgia: A controlled study. J Rheumatol 19:95–97, 1992.
220. Yunus MB, Dailey JW, Aldag JC, et al: Plasma tryptophan and other amino acids in primary fibromyalgia: A controlled study. J Rheumatol 19:90–94, 1992.
221. Yunus MB, Denko CW, Masi AT: Serum beta-endorphin in primary fibromyalgia syndrome: A controlled study. J Rheumatol 13:183–186, 1986.
222. Yunus MB, Holt GS, Masi AT, et al: Fibromyalgia syndrome among the elderly: Comparison with younger patients. J Am Geriatr Soc 35:987–995, 1988.
223. Yunus MB, Hussey FX, Aldag JC: Antinuclear antibodies and "connective tissue disease features" in fibromyalgia syndrome: A controlled study. J Rheumatol 20:1557–1560, 1993.
224. Yunus MB, Inanici F: Clinical characteristics and biopathophysiological mechanisms of fibromyalgia syndrome. In Baldry P (ed): Myofascial Pain and Fibromyalgia Syndromes: A Clinical Guide to Diagnosis and Management. London, Churchill Livingstone, 2001, pp 351–377.
225. Yunus MB, Inanici F, Aldag JC: Incomplete fibromyalgia syndrome: Clinical and psychological comparison with fibromyalgia syndrome. Arthritis Rheum 41(Suppl. 9):S258, 1998.
226. Yunus MB, Inanici F, Aldag JC, Mangold RF: Fibromyalgia in men: Comparison of clinical features with women. J Rheumatol 27:485–490, 2000.
227. Yunus MB, Kalyan-Raman UP, Masi AT, Aldag JC: Electron microscopic studies of muscle biopsy in primary fibromyalgia syndrome: A controlled and blinded study. J Rheumatol 16:97–101, 1989.
228. Yunus MB, Khan MA, Rawlings KK, et al: Genetic linkage analysis of multicase families with fibromyalgia syndrome. J Rheumatol 26:408–412, 1999.
229. Yunus MB, Masi AT: Juvenile primary fibromyalgia syndrome. Arthritis Rheum 28:138–144, 1985.
230. Yunus MB, Masi AT: Fibromyalgia, restless legs syndrome, periodic limb movement disorder, and psychogenic pain. In McCarty DJ, Koopman WJ (eds): Arthritis and Allied Conditions: A Textbook of Rheumatology, 12th ed. Philadelphia, Lea and Febiger, 1993, pp 1383–1405.
231. Yunus MB, Masi AT, Aldag JC: A controlled study of primary fibromyalgia syndrome: Clinical features and association with other functional syndromes. J Rheumatol 19(Suppl.):62–71, 1989.
232. Yunus MB, Masi AT, Aldag JC: Preliminary criteria for primary fibromyalgia syndrome (PFS): Multivariate analysis of a consecutive series of PFS, other pain patients, and normal subjects. Clin Exp Rheumatol 7:63–69, 1989.
233. Yunus MB, Masi AT, Aldag JC: Short-term effects of ibuprofen in primary fibromyalgia syndrome: A double blind, placebo controlled trial. J Rheumatol 16:527–532, 1989.
234. Yunus MB, Masi AT, Calabro JJ, et al: Primary fibromyalgia (fibrositis): Clinical study of 50 patients with matched normal controls. Semin Arthritis Rheum 11:151–171, 1981.
235. Zidar J, Backman E, Bengtsson A, et al. Quantitative EMG and muscle tension in painful muscles in fibromyalgia. Pain 40:249–254, 1990.

Chapter 2

Management of Fibromyalgia Syndrome

Fatma İnanici, MD ▪ Muhammad B. Yunus, MD

Although biopathophysiologic mechanisms of fibromyalgia syndrome (FMS) have not been fully elucidated, significant progress has been made in this area in recent years. Many different factors interact to cause symptoms, and their relative importance varies from patient to patient. Current management, although it remains less than satisfactory, can nevertheless be helpful to most patients.

A substantial number of randomized, controlled clinical trials have demonstrated efficacy of both pharmacologic and nonpharmacologic interventions. Available treatment approaches range from pharmacologic therapy with psychotropic agents to nonconventional interventions, such as acupuncture and hypnotherapy. The optimal management of patients with FMS includes patient education and reassurance, elimination of aggravating factors, utilization of both pharmacologic and nonpharmacologic means, and multidimensional approach. Most effective management can be achieved when it is tailored to the individual patient. Principles of management are summarized in Table 2–1.

Positive and Empathetic Attitude of the Physician

The successful management of FMS begins with a positive and empathetic attitude of the physician. It is particularly important to reassure the patient that the physician understands his or her suffering and is willing to help.

Firm Diagnosis

A firm diagnosis is essential. Unnecessary investigations should be avoided while making a diagnosis (see Chapter 1, Fibromyalgia Syndrome: Clinical Features, Diagnosis, and Biopathophysiologic Mechanisms). Most patients with FMS have had symptoms for 5 to 7 years before their consultation with a physician.[57] Granges and associates[62] suggest that earlier diagnosis and treatment lead to better outcomes.

Table 2–1.
Principles of Management in Fibromyalgia Syndrome

- Positive and empathetic attitude of the physician
- Firm diagnosis
- Diagnosis and management of comorbid conditions
- Patient education and reassurance
- Addressing aggravating factors
- Individualization of management
- Improvement of sleep quality
- Gradual increase of physical activities
- Pharmacologic treatment
- Nonpharmacologic interventions, including cognitive behavioral therapy
- Multidisciplinary approach

Diagnosis and Management of Comorbid Conditions

Recognizing comorbid musculoskeletal conditions is also important. Concomitant pain problems such as osteoarthritis, rheumatoid arthritis, and spinal stenosis are not unusual in patients with FMS. Failure to recognize and treat these concurrent disorders appropriately may cause poor treatment outcomes.[41, 151]

Patient Education and Reassurance

As with any chronic condition, education of the patient is fundamental in FMS.[29] Educational material in the form of an information sheet or booklet is frequently helpful. Patients should be reassured that although the disorder is a very painful one, it does not cause tissue damage, reduced life expectancy, deformity, or crippling.[12, 58] Experience suggests that calling it a "benign condition" is often resented by patients suffering from severe, ceaseless pain. Discussing the diagnosis and explaining the currently known biophysiologic mechanisms and the noninflammatory, nonmalignant nature of the illness can lessen anxiety and can help the patient develop successful coping strategies. Patients should be advised to accept that although fibromyalgia is a chronic condition and there is no cure, effective therapy is available to make them more functional,[121] to reduce pain, and improve quality of life.[158] Patients should be encouraged to take an active, self-help–oriented approach to treatment. Burckhardt and associates[30] evaluated the effectiveness of education and physical training in decreasing FMS symptoms and concluded that they are useful, especially in increasing patients' self-esteem.

Addressing Aggravating Factors

Symptoms of FMS are commonly exacerbated by various factors (Table 2–2). The existence and importance of these aggravating factors differ from patient to patient. Common aggravating factors in FMS are addressed in the following paragraphs.

Sleep Disturbances. In different series, about 75% of the patients with FMS

Table 2–2.
Factors That May Aggravate the Symptoms of Fibromyalgia Syndrome

Neurohormonal/muscular factors	Occupational factors
Nonrestorative sleep	Repetitive trauma
Physical deconditioning	Ergonomic factors
Poor posture	Prolonged sitting/standing/walking
Muscle overload	Weight lifting/bending
Hypothyroidism	Mental/physical stress
Medication side effects	Poor sleep (shift workers)
Psychological factors	Comorbid conditions
Stress	Headache
Anxiety	Irritable bowel syndrome
Depression	Restless legs syndrome
Poor coping skills	Periodic limb movement disorder
Environmental factors	Chronic fatigue syndrome
Hot or cold temperature	Arthritis
Chilling	Hyperlaxity
Humidity	Neuropathy
Weather change	Family/social factors
Excess air conditioning	Lack of social and family support
Noise	Excess family demands
	Lack of hobbies and recreation

Adapted from Yunus MB: Fibromyalgia syndrome: Is there any effective therapy? Consultant 36:1279–1285, 1996, with permission.

complain of sleep problems, including difficulties in falling asleep, frequent awakening, and waking up unrefreshed (nonrestorative sleep) (see Chapter 1, Fibromyalgia Syndrome: Clinical Features, Diagnosis, and Biopathophysiologic Mechanisms). Primary sleep disturbances such as sleep apnea, restless legs syndrome, and periodic limb movement disorder are also associated with FMS.[97] It is uncertain whether disturbed sleep is an antecedent or a consequence of FMS. Poor sleep contributes to pain, fatigue, and impaired physical and mental performance.[69, 100]

Physical Deconditioning. Physical fitness, muscle strength, and endurance of patients with FMS are lower than those of age and sex-matched controls.[16, 95] Physical deconditioning, pain, and fatigue worsen symptoms in a vicious cycle, i.e., widespread pain and fatigue contribute to inactivity; deconditioned muscles use excess energy for a given task and may therefore contribute to fatigue; and weak muscles are also susceptible to microtrauma-induced damage, which then aggravates pain.[12, 15]

Psychological Factors. Most patients with FMS do not have a current psychiatric illness. Ahles and coworkers[2] reported that the prevalence of major depression was not greater in FMS than in rheumatoid arthritis or in healthy controls. However, significant psychological distress has been observed in about 30% to 40% of patients with FMS.[157] Pain, irrespective of its cause, is significantly influenced by psychological factors and accentuated by stress, anxiety, and depression. Proper management of psychological distress helps but does not completely alleviate symptoms in many patients. Psychological management includes emotional support, psychotherapy (including cognitive behavioral therapy [CBT]), and use of antidepressant and anxiolytic drugs. Only a minority of patients, who have severe psychiatric problems, need referral to a psychiatrist.

Environmental and Occupational Factors. Patients frequently believe that their symptoms vary with changes in weather. Some patients are sensitive to high or low temperatures and some report worsening of their symptoms with barometric pressure changes.[66] Thus, patients should be advised to avoid the aggravating weather factors as much as possible.

Waylonis and colleagues[147] described various occupational activities that are associated with increased pain. Job or workplace modifications are often beneficial in the management of FMS.[111, 158] Every attempt should be made to keep FMS patients employed because employment gives them less time to focus on their pain and it also provides them with a sense of self-worth, which is particularly important in chronic illness.[158]

Management of Comorbid Conditions. The presence of concurrent diseases, such as arthritis, hypothyroidism, neurologic diseases, restless legs syndrome, bowel problems, and migraine, often adds to the global distress of a patient and should be appropriately managed.

Individualization of Management

Besides a variety of aggravating factors, different pain processing mechanisms have been shown among FMS patients.[138] Furthermore, individual behavioral and cognitive responses play an important role in pain perpetuation and chronicity.[120] Thus, treatment of FMS needs to be individualized.

Improvement of Sleep Quality

Improving sleep quality is a significant component of FMS management. Important elements of improving sleep quality are summarized in Table 2–3.

Drugs that are used to alleviate poor sleep include tricyclic antidepressants,[18, 27, 33, 56] alprazolam,[125] zolpidem,[99] and zopiclone.[44, 63] In sleep apnea, sleep disruption is caused by either obstruction of the upper airways or decreased respiratory signaling from the central nervous system. Patients with sleep apnea usually require treatment with

Table 2–3.
Important Elements for Improving Sleep Quality

A complete history of patient's sleeping habits
    Sleep/wake time cycle
    Caffeine intake, alcohol, smoking
    Exercising habits
    Sleep environment, noise
Addressing sleep difficulties/disorders
    Nonrestorative sleep (awakening feeling tired or unrefreshed)
    Difficulty falling asleep
    Frequent awakening during sleep
    Early morning awakenings
    Sleep apnea
    Restless legs syndrome
    Periodic limb movements of sleep
Addressing psychological factors
    Stress
    Anxiety
    Depression
Restoring sleep hygiene
    A regular sleep/wake schedule
    Adequate sleep time (i.e., at least 7 or 8 hours/night)
    Daily exercise
    Avoiding heavy meals before bedtime
    Avoiding caffeine, smoking, and alcohol within several hours of bedtime
    Treating rhinitis, acid reflux
    Eliminating environmental disturbances (e.g., noise, light)
    Relaxation
Pain management
Avoiding pharmacologic agents that may disrupt sleep
Medications that facilitate sleep

From Inanici F, Yunus MB: Management of fibromyalgia syndrome. In Baldry P (ed): Myofascial Pain and Fibromyalgia Syndromes: A Clinical Guide to Diagnosis and Management. London, Churchill Livingstone, 2001, pp 379–398, with permission.

continuous positive airway pressure or surgery.[12] Restless legs syndrome and periodic limb movements during sleep can be treated with dopaminergic drugs, e.g., L-dopa 100 to 200 mg/day; benzodiazepines, e.g., clonazepam 0.5 to 1.5 mg/day; or opioids, such as codeine and hydrocodone.[25, 86, 101, 102]

Gradual Increase of Physical Activities

Patients with FMS should be encouraged to exercise progressively and regularly, beginning at a low level, e.g., for just a few minutes initially. Stretching exercises provide short-term help. Aerobic exercises are the most beneficial. Eccentric (contracting and lengthening a muscle) and high-intensity exercises should be avoided in order to prevent postexercise pain and patient compliance problems.[40] Types of exercise should be individualized according to the patient's choice and pain severity. The key is to start exercising at a low level for 5 to 10 minutes, or even less, and to increase it gradually—for example, by 2 minutes every week to 30 to 40 minutes daily.[158] Aerobic exercises should be done three to four times a week at about 70% of maximum heart rate.[40] Patients also benefit from brisk walking, swimming in a warm pool, and bicycling. Treadmill exercise is helpful, particularly in the winter months with low outside temperature.

Pharmacologic Treatment

Because FMS is currently thought to be based on aberrant central pain mechanisms (see Chapter 1, Fibromyalgia Syndrome: Clinical Features, Diagnosis, and Biopathophysiologic Mechanisms), a number of centrally acting drugs have been studied in FMS. Some of them have been found to be beneficial in short-term, randomized, blinded, placebo-controlled trials (Table 2–4). Significant improvement with drug therapy has been found in 25% to 50% of patients,[57] and overall degree of efficacy has been modest in most studies.[5] Buskila[31] has emphasized the necessity of developing new drugs and the importance of long-term comparative trials to evaluate both efficacy and toxicity.

Antidepressant Agents

FMS was initially thought to be a disorder of sleep and pain.[100] Because serotonin modulates both of these, serotonergic antidepressant agents have been evaluated in the management of FMS. Most of them increase the time spent in stage 4 sleep.[151] These drugs are widely used to provide analgesia in FMS and other chronic pain conditions.[5, 55]

Tricyclic Antidepressants

Amitriptyline is the most widely prescribed pharmacologic agent for the treatment of FMS.[88] Wolfe and associates[152] reported a 7-year study at six rheumatology centers showing that 40% of the fibromyalgia patients at these centers used amitriptyline during the course of the investigation. Its beneficial effects on FMS symptoms have been demonstrated in randomized controlled trials.[33–35, 58, 79, 133]

Carette and coworkers[34] studied the efficacy of amitriptyline in a 9-week, double-blind, placebo-controlled trial of 70 patients. Patients received an incremented dose of amitriptyline from 10 mg/day to 50 mg/day at bedtime or placebo. They reported that duration of morning stiffness, pain, sleep quality, and patient and physician overall assessments were improved in the amitriptyline group, but not in the placebo group. No significant changes were noted in tender point scores measured with a dolorimeter in either of the groups.

Goldenberg and colleagues[58] randomized 62 patients into 4 groups to receive 25 mg of amitriptyline at night, 500 mg of naproxen twice daily, both amitriptyline and naproxen, or placebo, in a 6-week, double-blind trial. They reported significant improvement in pain, sleep difficulties, morning fatigue, global assessment, and tender point score in groups receiving amitriptyline. Naproxen was ineffective, with minor synergistic effect with amitriptyline. Scudds and associates[133] reported similar benefits of amitriptyline in a randomized double-blind, crossover trial of 36 patients with FMS.

Jaeschke and coworkers[79] conducted 23 N-of-1 randomized controlled trials of amitriptyline. They noted rapid improvement, generally within 1 week, in 25% of the patients. They found that 10 mg at bedtime is effective in some patients and such low-dose therapy avoids anticholinergic side effects of this drug. Adverse effects such as dry mouth, daytime sedation, weight gain, constipation, orthostatic hypotension, fluid retention, nightmares, and paradoxical insomnia were reported in up to 20% of patients but frequently subsided with continued treatment.[146] The recommended starting dose of amitriptyline was 10 mg at bedtime. If there was no response to the initial dose and side effects were tolerable, the dose could be gradually increased to 50 to 75 mg/day in 10-mg increments on a weekly basis. Some patients may be late responders; hence this drug should be tried for 4 to 6 weeks. If there is no benefit, the drug can be gradually withdrawn and another tricyclic agent, such as cyclobenzaprine, can be given.[41] Inasmuch as tachyphylaxis may occur after 2 to 3 months of continued treatment, a 2- to 4-week amitriptyline-free period may restore the efficacy of amitriptyline.[88] During this time, Russell[123] suggests employing alprazolam; however, another centrally acting analgesic may also be prescribed.

Cyclobenzaprine, another tricyclic antidepressant (TCA), has a similar chemical structure to amitriptyline. It has been marketed as a muscle relaxant because of its ability to reduce brainstem noradrenergic function and motor neuron efferent activity.[8] Several clinical trials have utilized this agent in FMS and reported a modest, short-

Table 2–4.
Pharmacologic Agents That Were Found To Be Effective by Placebo-controlled, Blinded Trials in Fibromyalgia Syndrome

Agent	Ref. No.	Study Design	Trial Duration (weeks)	No. of Pts.	Dose (mg/day)	Better Than Placebo in Improving							Adverse Effects
						Pain	TPs	Sleep	Fatigue	Psych. Status	Func. Status	Global Well-being	
Antidepressants													
Amitriptyline	34	P	9	70	10–50	Yes	No	Yes	—	—	—	Yes	Drowsiness, xerostomia, agitation, gastrointestinal symptoms
Amitriptyline	58	P	6	62	25	Yes	Yes	Yes	Yes	—	—	Yes	Dry mouth, dyspepsia, diarrhea
Amitriptyline	133	C	10	36	50	Yes	Yes	—	—	—	—	Yes	Not reported
Amitriptyline	79	N-of-1	2 × 2°	23	5–50	Yes	Yes	Yes	Yes	—	—	Yes	Not reported
Cyclobenzaprine	18	P	12	120	10–40	Yes	Yes	Yes	No	—	—	Yes	Dry mouth, drowsiness, constipation, dizziness, palpitation, tachycardia, tiredness, headache, nausea
Cyclobenzaprine	119	C	8	12	30	No	No	Yes	Yes	No	—	—	Dry mouth, nausea, weakness
Cyclobenzaprine	33	P	24	208	10	No	No	Yes	Yes	Yes	Yes	Yes	Somnolence, dizziness, abdominal pain, rash, headache, weight gain
Dothiepin	36	P	8	60	75	Yes	Yes	—	—	—	—	Yes	Drowsiness, dry mouth, weakness, abdominal pain, hypertension, headache
Clomipramine	23	C	3	37	75	Yes	Yes	—	—	—	—	Yes	Not reported
Fluoxetine	60	C	4 × 6†	19	20	Yes	No	Yes	Yes	Yes	—	Yes	Not specified
Fluoxetine + AMI	60	C	4 × 6†	19	20 + 10	Yes	No	Yes	Yes	Yes	Yes	Yes	Not specified
Sertraline	3	P	10	14	—	No	Yes	—	—	No	No	—	Not reported
Citalopram	4	P	16	40	20–40	No	—	—	—	Yes	—	Yes	Not reported
Trazadone	27	C	8	13	—	No	No	Yes	No	No	No	No	Not reported
Pirlindole	54	P	4	100	150	Yes	Yes	No	No	No	—	Yes	Dizziness, dry mouth, headache, insomnia, nausea/vomiting, sleep during day, palpitation, vertigo
SAMe	140	C	3	17	200	—	Yes	—	—	Yes	—	—	None documented
SAMe	141	P	2	30	400	Yes	Yes	—	—	Yes	—	—	No major side effects

Benzodiazepines

Alprazolam	125	P	6	78	0.5–3	Yes	Yes	—	—	No	No	Yes	Blurred vision, rash, adenopathy, headaches, swelling
Temazepam	72	C	12	10	15–30	Yes	No	Yes	—	—	—	Yes	Not reported
Hypnotics													
Zopiclone	44	P	12	41	7.5	No	No	Yes	No	—	—	—	Taste alteration, sleepwalking
Zopiclone	63	P	8	33	7.5	No	No	Yes	—	—	—	Yes	Nightmares, headache, diarrhea, nausea, daytime tiredness
Zolpidem	99	C	2	19	5–10–15	No	No	Yes	No	—	—	—	Headache, influenza-like symptoms, diarrhea, abnormal dreaming, anxiety, hallucination
Analgesics													
Tramadol	22	C	Single dose	12	100	No	Yes	—	—	—	—	—	Nausea, dizziness, hypotension, hypertension, tremor, epigastric pain, somnolence
Tramadol	124	P	6	69	50–400	—	Yes	—	—	—	—	—	Not documented
Others													
Growth hormone	17	P	36	50	0.0125/kg	Yes	—	—	—	—	—	Yes	Carpal tunnel syndrome
5-OH tryptophan	37	P	4	50	300	Yes	Yes	Yes	Yes	Yes	—	Yes	Gastric pain, diarrhea, headache, somnolence
Human IFN-α	128	P	6	120	50 IU/day	No	No	No	No	Yes	Yes	—	No adverse effects observed

°2 × 2: 2 weeks treatment period for active drug and 2 weeks for placebo.
†4 × 6: 6-week trials with each of four treatments (i.e., fluoxetine, amitriptyline, a combination of both drugs or placebo).
P, parallel; C, crossover; TP, tender points; SAMe, S-adenosylmethionine; AMI, Amitriptyline; —, not measured.

39

term efficacy.[18, 119] Bennett and colleagues[18] conducted a 12-week double-blind, randomized, controlled study of 120 patients with FMS and found cyclobenzaprine to decrease the severity of pain significantly and improve the quality of sleep after 2 to 12 weeks. Fatigue improved somewhat during weeks 2 to 4. Reynolds and associates[119] evaluated cyclobenzaprine in a 4-week randomized, double-blind, crossover design study of 12 FMS patients. They reported improvement in evening fatigue and total sleep time, but there was no effect on pain, tender points, mood ratings, and sleep parameters.

Santandrea and colleagues[130] evaluated the efficacy and tolerability of two different doses of cyclobenzaprine in a double-blind crossover study. Patients received either a single dose of 10 mg/day cyclobenzaprine at bedtime or 30 mg/day cyclobenzaprine in three equal doses daily for 15 days. After a 15-day washout period, the groups were crossed over to the other regimen. The authors noted that both regimens resulted in a significant improvement in the number of tender points, quality of sleep, anxiety, fatigue, irritable bowel syndrome, and stiffness. The higher dose, however, did not have a better therapeutic effect but did have an increased incidence of side effects.

Long-term efficacy of amitriptyline and cyclobenzaprine vs. placebo was compared in a 6-month, double-blind, randomized, placebo-controlled trial in 208 patients with FMS.[33] It was found that 21%, 12%, and 0% of the amitriptyline, cyclobenzaprine, and placebo patients had significant clinical improvement after 1 month (amitriptyline vs. placebo $P = 0.002$, cyclobenzaprine vs. placebo $P = 0.02$, amitriptyline vs. cyclobenzaprine P not significant). At 3 months and 6 months, however, tolerance to these drugs developed and there was no difference between the three groups. Authors noted that normal Minnesota Multiphasic Personality Inventory (MMPI) profile at baseline was predictive of clinical improvement at 1 month.[33]

Efficacy of several other TCAs has been studied.[23, 36, 156] Seventy-five mg/day dothiepin at bedtime was found superior to placebo in pain relief and tender point score improvement in a double-blind, controlled study of 60 patients.[36] Clomipramine, 75 mg/day, and maprotiline, 75 mg/day, were compared with placebo in a triple-crossover, randomized study of 37 patients over a 3-week period.[23] Clomipramine, which is preferentially serotonergic, significantly reduced the number of tender points, and maprotiline, which has more effect on noradrenaline (norepinephrine), improved psychological scores. An open label trial of imipramine showed that only 2 of 20 patients responded favorably, whereas 14 patients stopped therapy during the initial 3-month period due to lack of response.[156] Nortriptyline, which is an active metabolite of amitriptyline, was also ineffective in a 8-week, double-blind, randomized, placebo-controlled trial of 120 patients.[71]

Selective Serotonin Reuptake Inhibitors

Fluoxetine, a selective serotonin reuptake inhibitor (SSRI) has been studied in FMS. Case reports, as well as open-label and controlled studies with fluoxetine, reported improvements in sleep disturbances and depression, but only one study[60] found a positive effect on pain relief or TP score.[51, 53, 60] Wolfe and associates[154] reported in a controlled study that fluoxetine, 20 mg/day, showed no effect on pain at 6 weeks, although a high dropout rate makes it difficult to interpret these results. Goldenberg and associates[60] evaluated the efficacy of fluoxetine and amitriptyline (AMI). Nineteen patients received 20 mg fluoxetine, 25 mg AMI, a combination of fluoxetine and amitriptyline, or placebo, each over a 6-week period, in a double-blind, randomized, crossover design. Both fluoxetine and amitriptyline were effective and the combination worked better than either drug alone. Small sample, short follow-up, and high dropout rate are the major concerns about this study.

Sertraline was evaluated by Alberts and coworkers[3] in a double-blind, placebo-controlled trial in 14 patients with FMS. Patients treated with this drug showed significantly increased pain thresholds at both tender and control points. Furthermore, compared with baseline, there was a significantly increased blood flow in both left and right frontal cortical regions, a finding that led the authors to suggest that sertraline may act by enhancing activation of the pain inhibition network.

Norregaard et al[108] reported no symptom improvement with citalopram in a randomized, double-blind, placebo-controlled study. In a recent double-blind study of 40 patients, citalopram was found to be effective in improving pain at the end of 2 months.[4] After 4 months, however, this effect diminished. Montgomery Asberg Depression Rating Scale and the Fibromyalgia Impact Questionnaire scores were improved progressively until the end of 4-month trial.[4]

Other Antidepressant Agents

According to their clinical experience, Wilke[151] and Yunus[158] noted the beneficial effects of 50 to 100 mg trazodone taken at bedtime. However, there is only one controlled study with this heterocyclic antidepressant agent.[27] The clinical and polysomnographic effects of trazodone were evaluated by Branco and colleagues[27] in a double-blind, crossover, placebo-controlled, 2-month trial of 12 patients with FMS. The authors concluded that trazodone normalized rapid eye movement (REM) latency and the alpha-delta pattern by sleep studies, but it was not superior to placebo in improving the psychological profile, symptoms, and functional parameters.

Venlafaxine, another heterocyclic antidepressant, which inhibits both serotonin and noradrenaline (norepinephrine) reuptake, has been reported to be beneficial in a case report and in an open-label clinical trial of 11 patients.[45, 46] Double-blind, placebo-controlled studies with larger sample sizes are needed.

The efficacy of two monoamine oxidase A (MAO-A) inhibitors, moclobemide and pirlindole, which inhibit the deamination of serotonin, noradrenaline, and dopamine, was evaluated in the treatment of FMS. The results of randomized, double-blind, placebo-controlled study of moclobemide showed no beneficial effect.[68] On the other hand, pirlindole was found to be superior to placebo in alleviating pain, reducing tender point score, and improving patient and physician global assessment of severity in a 4-week double-blind study of 100 cases of FMS.[54] However, MAO-A inhibitors should be used with caution in the treatment of this disorder and should never be prescribed in combination with other serotonergic and noradrenergic drugs because of potentially serious side effects.

Conflicting results on the efficacy and tolerability of S-adenosylmethionine (SAMe), an anti-inflammatory drug with analgesic and antidepressant effects, has been reported in several clinical trials.[78, 140, 141, 144] Tavoni and associates,[141] in a 3-week, double-blind, placebo-controlled crossover trial of 17 patients with FMS, found that the number of tender points and painful sites decreased and depression scores improved after intramuscular administration of SAMe, but not after placebo treatment. The efficacy of 800 mg orally administered SAMe daily versus placebo for 6 weeks was investigated in 44 patients with FMS in a double-blind trial carried out by Jacobsen and coworkers.[78] Significant improvements were noted in clinical disease activity, pain, fatigue, morning stiffness, and mood evaluated by Face Scale ($P < 0.05$). Authors suggested that SAMe has some beneficial effects on fibromyalgia and could be an important option in the treatment of this condition. Tavoni and colleagues[140] used 400 mg/day intravenous SAMe for 15 days in 30 fibromyalgia patients with connective tissue disease (Sjögren's syndrome in 8, systemic lupus erythematosus in 7, rheumatoid arthritis in 4, systemic sclerosis in 3, mixed connective tissue disease in 3, mixed cryoglobulinemia in 2, and Raynaud's disease in 2 patients) in a randomized double-blind trial. They reported a significant decrease in pain. In contrast to this finding, Volkmann and associates[144] reported no beneficial effect of this drug when administered intravenously at a dose of 600 mg/day or placebo for 10 days in 34 patients with fibromyalgia in a crossover trial. Overall, SAMe seems to be useful in FMS.

Benzodiazepines

Anxiolytic agents may be beneficial in a subgroup of patients. Several clinical trials have assessed the efficacy of benzodiazepines in FMS. Russell and associates[125] randomized 78 patients with FMS to receive ibuprofen and/or alprazolam in a double-blind, placebo-controlled trial. They reported that clinical improvement in patient rating of disease severity and severity of tenderness upon palpation was most apparent, but not significant, in patients who were receiving ibuprofen plus alprazolam. The study was followed by an open-label extension for 52 patients, who all received a combination of ibuprofen and alprazolam for 8 weeks. At the end of 8 weeks, small but statistically significant improvements were seen in tender point index, depression, and patient and physician global assessment. Quijada-Carrera and coworkers[116] evaluated the efficacy of combination treatment of bromazepam and tenoxicam in 164 patients with FMS. Although no statistically significant difference was seen between combination treatment and placebo, bromazepam and tenoxicam in combination were slightly more effective than tenoxicam alone.

Hench and associates[72] compared the efficacy of amitriptyline, temazepam, and placebo in a double-blind, crossover study of 10 patients and noted that improvements in patient and physician global assessment, sleep disturbance, and morning stiffness were significantly better than placebo when patients received temazepam or amitriptyline. Finally, lorazepam was evaluated by a retrospective chart analysis of fibromyalgia patients with intractable symptoms[74] and in a 1-year follow-up study.[75] Beneficial effect of this drug on pain scores was reported.

From the aforementioned reports, one cannot conclude a definite efficacy of benzodiazepines in FMS. These drugs are not generally recommended for the long-term treatment of FMS because of the potential dependence and withdrawal seizures associated with them.[88] Their usage is limited to selected patients who have significant anxiety.

Hypnotics

In double-blind, placebo-controlled studies, zopiclone and zolpidem were found to be helpful in improvement of subjective sleep complaints and daytime energy, but they were not effective in pain relief.[44, 63, 99]

Tranquilizers

Moldofsky and colleagues[98] compared the efficacy of the major tranquilizer chlorpromazine, 100 mg, with L-tryptophan, 5 g, both given at bedtime in a double-blind, controlled trial of 15 patients. Both drugs significantly increased time spent in stage 4 sleep, but only chlorpromazine improved tender point and subjective pain scores. Chlorpromazine is not recommended in FMS because of its potentially serious neurologic side effects.

Anti-inflammatory Agents

Anti-inflammatory agents are used by 91% of patients[152] despite the fact that there is no evidence of tissue inflammation in FMS.[136, 160] In clinical trials, therapeutic doses of naproxen[58] and ibuprofen[161] were not significantly better than placebo. The combinations of naproxen and amitriptyline,[58] ibuprofen and cyclobenzaprine,[52] ibuprofen and alprazolam,[125] and tenoxicam and bromazepam[116] resulted in slightly more improvement in some of the outcome measures than either drug used alone, which suggests that these combinations may confer slight synergistic analgesic benefit. These differences were not statistically significant. In general, most FMS patients do not get considerable benefit from nonsteroidal anti-inflammatory drugs (NSAIDs), but such agents can take the edge off the pain enough to be therapeutically worthwhile.[135] Moreover, NSAIDs may help concomitant arthritis or dysmenorrhea. However, risk factors for gastrointestinal, renal, or hepatic side effects should be carefully considered before prescribing a nonsteroidal anti-inflammatory drug in FMS.

Prednisone was found to be ineffective in a 2-week, double-blind, placebo-controlled, crossover trial involving 20 patients with FMS.[39] This is consistent with the fact that FMS is not an inflammatory condition and that hypocortisolemia in FMS is of central origin.[159]

Analgesics

Although there is no controlled trial available regarding its efficacy, paracetamol (acetaminophen) is used frequently for pain control in FMS. Wolfe and associates[152] reported that paracetamol was used by 59% of 538 patients with FMS in a 7-year study at six rheumatology centers, whereas 75.5% were reported to have used this drug in another study of 286 patients.[155] In the latter study, 27% of the FMS patients reported paracetamol not to be effective at all, 46% slightly effective, 25% moderately effective and 2% very effective. The patients compared the effectiveness of paracetamol and NSAIDs; 66% reported that paracetamol was less effective than NSAIDs, 26% that it was about the same, and 8% that it was more effective.[155]

The prescription of narcotic analgesics for patients with fibromyalgia should be generally avoided.[31] However, tramadol, a centrally acting analgesic, with both μ-opioid receptor binding and noradrenaline (norepinephrine) and serotonin reuptake inhibition that contribute to its antinociceptive effect, may be useful for the treatment of pain in FMS. Russell and colleagues[124, 126] evaluated the efficacy of tramadol, 50 to 400 mg/day, in 100 patients with fibromyalgia. At the end of an open trial period of 21 days, 69 patients who tolerated tramadol and had adequate pain relief were randomized to receive either tramadol or placebo for 42 days. The time before withdrawal due to inadequate pain relief was significantly longer and the withdrawal rate was significantly lower in the tramadol group than in the placebo group. Statistically significant improvements occurred in patient-reported pain scores and pain relief ratings. Bennett and coworkers[13] examined the efficacy and safety of tramadol in a 6-week, double-blind, placebo-controlled trial. They reported similar results to those of Russell and colleagues.[124, 126] Biasi and associates,[22] employing a single 100-mg intravenous dose of tramadol in a double-blind, placebo-controlled, crossover study of 12 patients, found that the tramadol group had greater pain relief than the placebo group, but the number of tender points did not change. Overall, tramadol seems to be a useful drug in FMS. Results of a larger study on this drug are awaited.

Clinical experience shows that a small dose of codeine, e.g., 15 to 30 mg three times a day, is well tolerated, even on a long-term basis, but it should only be used occasionally, such as during a flare-up.[158]

Other Pharmacologic Agents

Carisoprodol is a muscle relaxant and an analgesic agent. Somadril Compound, a combination of carisoprodol (200 mg), paracetamol (acetaminophen) (160 mg), and caffeine (32 mg), per tablet, given 6 tablets daily was shown to be more effective than placebo in an 8-week, double-blind trial of 58 patients.[143]

Chlormezanone is an effective muscle relaxant that probably acts via reduction of the gamma efferent discharge to motor fibers of muscle spindles. It also has some benzodiazepine-like effects on sleep physiology but does not cause reduction in stage 4 sleep. Pattrick and associates[112] found it to be ineffective in the treatment of FMS.

A combination of malic acid and magnesium (200 mg malic acid plus 50 mg magnesium per tablet), both of which are involved in the generation of adenosine triphosphate, was evaluated in the treatment of FMS, on the presumed basis of deficient high-energy phosphate in muscles in FMS.[127] Symptoms were not alleviated during a 4-week, double-blind, placebo-controlled trial at a dose of three tablets twice daily. A subsequent open-label, dose escalation trial showed improvement in fibromyalgia symptoms. Thus, the efficacy of either malic acid or magnesium in FMS is doubtful.

Bennett and coworkers[17] studied the efficacy of human growth hormone in fibromyalgia patients who had low insulin growth factor–1 (IGF-1) levels. Fifty women were included in a double-blind, placebo-controlled trial of 9 months. An initial dose of 0.0125 mg/kg/day was given for the first month, which was adjusted at monthly intervals to maintain an IGF-1 level of about 250 ng/ml. There was an improvement in Fibromyalgia Impact Questionnaire (FIQ) scores and number of tender points after 9 months of therapy. Pain alone was not evaluated as an outcome measure.

On the basis of serotonin deficiency in patients with fibromyalgia, the serotonin precursor 5-hydroxytryptophan was evaluated in the treatment of FMS in a double-blind, placebo-controlled trial for 30 days,[37] and in a 90-day open study.[115] In both trials, authors reported significant improvements in number of tender points, pain, morning stiffness, sleep, anxiety, fatigue, and patient and physician global assessments.

The blockade of the serotonin receptor subtype 5-HT3 with tropisetron[47, 110, 129] and ondansetron,[76] and of subtype 5-HT2 with ritanserin,[109] was studied in the treatment of fibromyalgia. Limited beneficial effects of these 5-HT receptor blockers were reported. Further studies are needed.

Low-dose (50 IU) sublingual human interferon-alpha (hIFN-α) was found to be beneficial in a 6-week double-blind placebo-controlled study of 112 patients with FMS.[128] In this study, patients received placebo or hIFN-α at 15, 50, or 150 IU. The authors reported that there was no change in the tender point index, pain, and pain threshold at the end of the 6-week trial with any dose of hIFN-α, but morning stiffness and physical function improved significantly in patients who received daily 50 IU hIFN-α.

Several studies evaluated the possible role of melatonin, a pineal hormone, in FMS, because it involves synchronizing circadian systems, and has sleep-promoting properties. Contradictory results have been reported for melatonin levels in patients with FMS in controlled studies, i.e., higher than,[85] lower than,[150] and similar to controls[114]. In a 4-week open study, Citera and coworkers[38] evaluated the effect of melatonin treatment on disturbed sleep, fatigue, and pain among 21 patients with FMS in an open study. Improvements in tender point counts, severity of pain, and sleep disturbances, and patient and physician global assessments were reported with 3 mg melatonin at bedtime. The authors suggested that melatonin could be an alternative and safe treatment for patients with FMS. Further controlled studies with large numbers will be needed to evaluate the efficacy of this nutritional supplement.

Stellate ganglion blockade followed by regional sympathetic blockade was examined in a 28-patient, comparative, blinded trial.[9] Stellate ganglion blockade by bupivacaine was found to be more effective than guanethidine blockade in reducing the number of TPs as evaluated 24 hours after the injection; however, no long-term studies of regional sympathetic blockade are available.

Janzen and Scudds[80] examined the efficacy of sphenopalatine blocks with lignocaine (lidocaine) in the treatment of pain in 42 patients with FMS and 19 with myofascial pain. They reported that 4% lignocaine was no better than placebo. Intravenous lignocaine was studied in a 6-day open-label trial of 10 patients with FMS.[10] Pain relief and improvement in mood scores were reported at 7 and at 30 days' follow-up. No conclusion regarding the efficacy of lidocaine can be reached from this open-label study with a small number of patients.

In small groups of patients, salmon calcitonin,[21] an antidiencephalon immune serum (SER282),[83] and gamma-hydroxybutyrate[132] were reported to have no beneficial effect on mild-to-moderate pain, fatigue, and sleep.

Tender Point Injections

Another therapeutic approach in the treatment of FMS is injections in the tender points—a valuable adjunctive therapy. In an open study of 41 patients with FMS, a mixture of 1% lidocaine, ½ ml, and triamcinolone diacetate, ¼ ml, was injected in tender points.[118] Average duration of pain relief per injected site was 13 weeks. Injection of tender points is particularly useful if the patient can localize one to four areas that are most bothersome. After the injections, patients should apply local ice for several hours and rest the injected areas for 24 to 48 hours to minimize postinjection flare. In our practice, we do not inject tender points more often than every 2 months as a rule. Currently we use only lidocaine because there is no evidence that addition of a corticosteroid preparation is more helpful.

Figuerola and associates[50] found a similar increase in met-enkephalin levels after the injection of tender points by lidocaine, saline, or dry needling. They suggested that some of the benefits of tender point injection might be attributed to mechanistic effects of needling rather than the pharmacologic agent.

Baldry[6] used superficial dry needling in the treatment of myofascial trigger points. He suggested that dry needling alone causes stimulation of A delta nerve fibers in the skin and subcutaneous tissues, which in turn activate pain-inhibiting mechanisms in the spinal cord.[6, 7] Abeles and colleagues[1] examined the effect of needle length, gauge, and solution for injection of tender points both in 25 patients in a single masked, randomized, control trial and in 12 patients in a double-blind, controlled study design. They reported that 8 of 25 patients and 4 of 12 patients responded positively to tender points injections regardless of needle size, solution, or dry needling. The follow-up period and duration of pain relief were not documented.

Nonpharmacologic Interventions

Nonpharmacologic treatments, such as exercise and cognitive behavioral therapy (CBT), are important in FMS in addition to drug therapy.[20] In a recent meta-analysis of FMS treatment interventions, Rossy[122] suggested that drug therapy combined with appropriate nonpharmacologic interventions resulted in better management outcomes.

A number of studies, mostly uncontrolled, examined the efficacy of nonpharmacologic approaches to FMS. Some of them were found to be beneficial in relatively few randomized, controlled studies (Table 2–5), but such benefit was not always maintained at follow-up. However, no blinded and controlled studies exist on the efficacy of commonly employed therapies such as physical therapy alone. In this section we will provide an overview of the results of both controlled and uncontrolled trials of nonpharmacologic approaches in management of FMS.

Physical Fitness Training

The rationale of exercise training in management of FMS included improvement of physical conditioning; resistance to microtrauma; enhancement in strength, endurance, and flexibility; higher levels of general activity; increased sense of control; an antidepressant effect; and relaxation.[15, 92, 134] Additionally, it was expected that exercise would have pain-modulating effects. Following aerobic exercise, increases in β-endorphin–like products, prolactin, and growth hormone were reported, which promoted decreased pain sensitivity.[134] McCain[93] proposed that exercise may normalize the hypothalamic-pituitary-adrenal axis (HPA) dysfunction that plays an important role in the development of pain, fatigue, and sleep difficulties in FMS (see Chapter 1, Fibromyalgia Syndrome: Clinical Features, Diagnosis, and Biopathophysiologic Mechanisms).

McCain and coworkers[94] conducted a randomized, blinded, controlled trial of 42 patients with FMS to compare the efficacy of a 20-week supervised cardiovascular fitness (CVF) training with supervised simple flexibility and stretching exercises (FLEX). At the end of the 20-week program, significant improvements in both patient and physician global assessments and tender point thresholds were recorded in the CVF group, but not in the FLEX group. Visual analogue pain score tended to improve in CVF group, but did not reach statistical significance. Patient reported sleep quality and psychological distress by Symptom Checklist-90-Revised (SCL-90-R) were not different between CVF and FLEX groups at the end of the program. After a mean follow-up of 19 months, only 6 of the original 18 patients in the CVF group had continued their regular exercise; however, 5 patients were lost to follow-up.

Low-intensity endurance training was studied in a randomized trial.[96] During a period of 20 weeks, 18 patients with FMS participated in a 60-minute continuous,

Table 2–5.
Selected Studies on Nonpharmacologic Interventions That Were Found To Be Effective by Controlled Trials in FMS

Intervention	Ref.	No. of Pts.	Study Duration	Control Intervention	Significant Treatment Outcomes
Cardiovascular fitness training (CVF)	94	42	20 weeks	Simple flexibility and stretching exercises	Pain threshold, patient and physician global assessment score, peak work capacity improved in CVF group
Aerobic exercise (AE)	149	60	14 weeks	Usual treatment group	Pain, fatigue, work capacity, patient global assessment improved in AE group
Aerobic, flexibility, and strengthening exercises (AFS)	90	60	6 weeks	Relaxation training	Number of tender points, total myalgic score, and aerobic fitness improved in AFS group
Education and physical training (EPT)	30	99	6 weeks	Waiting list controls	Helplessness, self-efficacy, and quality of life scales improved, and pain and TPs decreased in EPT group
Education and exercise (EE)	61	41	6 weeks	Waiting list controls	6-minute walk distance, well-being, fatigue, self-efficacy, and knowledge improved in EE group
Low-intensity laser	32	86	15 sessions	Sham	Patient and physician global assessment improved in laser group
Balneotherapy (BT)	162	40	2 weeks	Relaxation exercises	Pain and pain threshold improved in BT group
Electroacupuncture	43	70	3 weeks	Sham	Pain, pain threshold, morning stiffness, patient and physician global assessment scores improved in electroacupuncture group
Chiropractic management (CM)	24	21	4 weeks	Waiting list controls	Self reported pain, cervical and lumbar range of motion, and straight leg raise improved in CM group
Hypnotherapy	65	40	12 weeks	Physical therapy	Pain, morning fatigue, sleep and global assessment improved in hypnotherapy group
EMG-biofeedback	49	12	24 weeks	Sham	Pain, TPs, morning stiffness improved in EMG-biofeedback group
Biofeedback/relaxation training/exercise (BRTE)	28	119	6 weeks	Education/attention control program	Self-efficacy for function, TP score, physical activity score improved in BRTE group

EMG, electromyography; TP, tender point.

modified, low-impact aerobic dance program. Training intensity was kept at a heart rate of 120 to 150 beats/minute. As a control group, 17 patients were asked not to change their physical activity level. Eleven (61%) patients in the training group and 14 (82%) in the waiting list group completed the study. At the end of the program, the intensity of pain, fatigue, or sleep had not changed in either group but the patients in the training group reported that exercise had increased their feelings of general well-being. Authors concluded that a modified low-impact aerobic dance program was well tolerated without an increase in pain and fatigue symptoms, and that such a program reduced exercise-induced pain in patients with FMS.

Clark[40] argued that increased pain following exercise may be a result of too much eccentric work (contracting and lengthening a muscle) and/or working at too high an intensity. She suggested educating patients regarding the nature of eccentric work and initially prescribing stretching exercises, followed by activities that minimize eccentric workload. In addition, she emphasized the importance of taking into account a patient's initial fitness level when determining a suitable exercise intensity.

Short- and long-term effects of aerobic exercise were investigated in a controlled, blinded study by Wigers and coworkers.[149] They compared the effects of aerobic exercise, stress management, and "usual treatment" in 60 patients. Patients were randomly placed in one of these 3 treatment groups for 14 weeks. At the end of this time, patients in both the aerobic exercise group and the stress management group improved more than the "usual treatment" group, but 4-year follow-up data showed no obvious group differences in symptom severity. The authors noted a considerable compliance problem with long-term aerobic exercise programs.

Similarly, Martin and associates[90] reported short-term benefit of an exercise program, which included aerobic, flexibility, and strength training exercises in a randomized, controlled, blinded trial of 60 patients. For 6 weeks, patients met 3 times per week for 1 hour supervised exercise or relaxation program. The number of tender points, degree of tenderness, and aerobic fitness level were significantly improved in the exercise group at the end of the study. FIQ, Illness Intrusiveness Questionnaire (IIQ), and Self-Efficacy Questionnaire (SEQ) scores tended to improve in the exercise group, but did not reach the statistically significant level.

The effectiveness of physical training and self-management education was evaluated in a controlled trial.[30] Ninety-nine patients were randomly assigned to one of three groups: Group 1—education (E) only; Group 2—education and physical training (EPT); Group 3—wait-list control. The education program consisted of information on FMS, the role of stress, coping strategies, problem-solving techniques, and relaxation. The physical training program included either walking, swimming, or cycling. The wait-list control group did not receive education or physical training program initially but received both after 12 weeks. Patients completed a 6-week program and were reassessed at the 12th week. The quality of life scale and self-efficacy scale were significantly better in E and EPT groups than the control group, but there was no difference between E and EPT groups. At 6 months (first follow-up after the initial 12-week period), quality of life significantly improved in the EPT group. At second follow-up (4–8 months after the first follow-up), outcome was measured by FIQ only. The EPT group improved in physical functioning, pain, stiffness, morning fatigue, and anxiety and depression subscales of FIQ, the E group improved in physical functioning and general well-being, whereas the wait-list control group (who had received the full program after initial 12 weeks) showed improvement in general well-being and fatigue.

In another randomized controlled trial, Gowans and colleagues[61] evaluated the efficacy of exercise combined with education. Forty-one FMS patients with severe disability, according to the physical impairment subscale of the FIQ and 6-minute walk distance, participated in a 6-week exercise and education program or served as waiting list controls. The physical function, sense of well-being, and self-efficacy of patients in the exercise and education group improved significantly. This improvement was maintained up to the follow-up period of 3 months. However, it was not possible to determine whether exercise or education or both contributed to it. Recently, Ramsay and colleagues[117] compared the efficacy of supervised and home program aerobic exercises in 74 fibromyalgia patients. They reported that 12-week aerobic exercise, in a supervised class or home program, did not help to reduce pain or to improve patient well-being.

Physical Therapy

Numerous physical therapy modalities are widely used as an adjunctive therapy in patients with FMS. These include a variety of hands-on skills, i.e., stretching, strengthening, massage, manipulation, mobilization, and physical energy modalities, such as heat, ice, ultrasound, electrical stimulation, mechanical pressure, light energy, and electromagnetic energy.[121] Some of them can be applied in the patients' own home environment such as heat, ice, acupressure, and stretching and strengthening exercises. These modalities may be useful in achieving muscle relaxation, relieving pain and muscle spasm, and in activating endogenous opioids.[121] However, no controlled studies with adequate sample size and well-designed methodology have confirmed their efficacy in patients with FMS. Only a few open trials with transcutaneous electrical nerve stimulation (TENS),[81] hydrotherapy[64, 162] and electrotherapy[64] showed efficacy to some extent in patients with FMS.

The efficacy of therapeutic low-intensity infrared diode laser therapy was evaluated in a double-blind, placebo-controlled trial.[32] Sixty-eight patients with FMS were included in the study. A total of 15 sessions of therapeutic or placebo diode laser were applied to the tender points. Significant improvements in number of tender points as well as patient and physician global assessment scores were reported in the therapeutic laser group.

TENS was applied to 40 patients with FMS in an open study and was found to produce transient benefit in 70% of the patients.[81]

Hydrogalvanic bath therapy (HBT), which combined a full body immersion in a specific bathtub filled with still tap water of 36° to 37° C and electrotherapy, was compared with progressive muscle relaxation in a 5-week randomized controlled trial of 25 patients with FMS.[64] Outcome was measured by self-reported pain questionnaire. HBT was not found to be effective.

The effect of balneotherapy (warm mineralized bath) and that of relaxation exercises was compared by Yurtkuran and Celiktas[162] in a randomized controlled trial of 40 patients with FMS. In the balneotherapy group, pain and algometer scores were improved significantly at the end of 2 weeks' treatment and 6 weeks' follow-up. No significant changes were observed in the relaxation exercises group.

Manual Medicine Techniques

Chiropractors are the most frequently consulted complementary medicine practitioners reported by patients with FMS.[113] However, there are only two studies that report the efficacy of chiropractic management in FMS.[24, 67] Blunt and associates[24] applied chiropractic management consisting of soft tissue massage, stretching, spinal manipulation, and education, which was administered 3 to 5 times a week for 4 weeks to 21 patients. At the end of the program, in the chiropractic group clinical improvements were observed in the cervical and lumbar ranges of motion, straight leg raising, and self-reported pain severity. However, the nonstandardized treatment protocol and inadequate outcome measurements limit the conclusion of this study. In a recent open-label study, Hains and Hains[67] evaluated the efficacy of chiropractic treatment that included ischemic compression to tender points and spinal manipulation in 15 patients with FMS. Patients received a total of 30 treatments, 2 to 3 times weekly. Pain intensity, fatigue, and sleep quality were measured by visual analogue scales at baseline, after 15 and 30 treatments, and 1 month after the end of the trial. Nine patients (60%) who were classified as responders had a minimum of 50% improvement in total pain score. Pain and fatigue also improved in the respondent group. The authors suggested a potential role for chiropractic care in the management of FMS.

Electromyographic (EMG)-Biofeedback

Ferraccioli and coworkers[49] conducted true EMG-biofeedback or false EMG-biofeedback in 20-minute sessions twice weekly for a total of 15 sessions in 12 patients. They suggested that there was a decrease of plasma adrenocorticotropin hormone (ACTH) and β-endorphin levels during EMG-biofeedback training. However, the blindedness of this study is uncertain. Sarnoch and colleagues[131] conducted an open study in 18 patients, who received 9 training sessions using EMG-biofeedback over a period of 4 weeks. In both trials, improvement in pain was reported.

Acupuncture

DeLuze and associates[43] evaluated the efficacy of electro-acupuncture in a double-blind, controlled trial. Seventy patients were randomized to electro-acupuncture or a sham procedure. Pain intensity, pain threshold, number of analgesic tablets used, regional pain score, sleep quality, and patient and physician global assessment were improved in the electro-acupuncture group. Lewis[89] pointed out the uncertainty of the acupuncture points and the sham procedure in this study.

Sprott and coworkers[139] carried out an open study of 29 patients treated with acupuncture over 6 weeks. They reported decreased pain level and number of tender points, and also an increase of serotonin and substance P levels in serum. Based on these results, the authors suggested a physiologic mechanism of acupuncture for pain relief.

Recently, Berman and associates[19] discussed the results and the methodologic problems of three randomized control trials and four cohort studies of acupuncture in the management of FMS. They suggested that acupuncture had a short-term beneficial effect on FMS; however, further high-quality, randomized trials with long-term follow-up have been suggested.

The National Institutes of Health consensus conference statement on acupuncture[103] also suggested that in some situations, including fibromyalgia, "acupuncture may be useful as an adjunct treatment or an acceptable alternative or may be included in a comprehensive management program."

Hypnotherapy

There is increasing interest in the use of hypnotherapy for the management of chronic pain syndromes,[104] but only one study of this therapy was reported in FMS.[65] Forty patients with FMS were randomized to receive either hypnotherapy or physical therapy for 12 weeks. Pain intensity, morning fatigue, sleep, patient global assessment, and psychological scores were reported to improve significantly in the hypnotherapy group. At 24-week follow-up, beneficial effects were maintained.

Cognitive Behavioral Therapy

Considering the evidence that positive health behaviors and health status are strongly correlated with enhanced self-efficacy,[11] the potential role of CBT in management of FMS has been examined in recent years. CBT includes relaxation training, reinforcement of healthy behavior patterns, reducing pain behavior, coping skills training, and the restructuring of maladaptive beliefs about a person's ability to control pain.[26, 107] A number of studies have reported efficacy of inpatient and outpatient programs of CBT.[26, 69, 107, 137, 145, 148]

Bradley[26] first suggested the possible efficacy of CBT and exercise in FMS. Nielson and associates[107] evaluated CBT among 25 patients with FMS in a preliminary, open study of 3 weeks' duration that included relaxation technique, cognitive techniques (including self-efficacy), aerobic exercise and stretching, pacing and enhancement of pain tolerance, and education of at least one family member regarding the nature of the program. They reported significant improvements in perceived pain severity, psychological distress, and the ability to cope with pain liable to interfere with normal activities. In a follow-up report of this study, White and Nielson[148] noted that improvement persisted 30 months after the treatment. Singh and coworkers[137] showed similar results in an 8-week CBT study. Such findings, however, must be interpreted with caution inasmuch as these reports were not based on randomized, controlled trials.

The effectiveness of cognitive educational treatment was evaluated by Vlaeyen and colleagues[145] in a randomized controlled trial. One hundred thirty-one patients with FMS were randomly assigned to three outpatient programs: cognitive/educational program (ECO); group education and group discussion program (EDI); and waiting list control (WLC); the EDI group did not receive specific cognitive treatment. At post-treatment and compared with the WLC, the EDI group significantly improved in pain control and pain coping, whereas the ECO group showed significant improvement in pain coping and knowledge about FMS. However, further analysis showed no significant difference between the ECO and EDI groups in these variables. The authors concluded that there was no added benefit of cognitive treatment as compared with education/group discussion alone.

Nicassio and associates[106] recently carried out a similar trial. Eighty-six patients with FMS were included in a 10-week treatment and 6-month follow-up program. The behavioral intervention focused on the development of diverse pain coping skills, whereas the control group with education only was presented with information on a range of health-related topics without emphasizing skill acquisition. Similar improvements were found in both groups. Multiple regression analyses revealed that changes in helplessness and passive coping were associated with improvement in some of the clinical outcomes, such as pain and depression.

Buckelew and colleagues[28] compared biofeedback/relaxation treatment with exercise training. They randomized 119 patients to one of four groups: (1) biofeedback/relaxation training; (2) exercise training; (3) a combination treatment; and (4) educational/attention program. Improvement in self-efficacy for physical function was best maintained by the combination group at the end of 2 years' follow-up.

Overall, considering all the published trials as well as our clinical experience, CBT seems helpful in FMS and should be utilized in difficult cases. Further studies with adequate sample size, randomization, blindedness, and follow-up will help to evaluate its beneficial effects in FMS.

Interdisciplinary Group Treatment

Masi[91] has advocated a patient-centered, multimodal psychotherapeutic approach aimed at modifying the effects of life stresses in FMS. He described a combination of physical therapy, medication, and psychological treatment that is likely to improve patients' well-being and TP ratings.

The usefulness of multidimensional group treatment in a 6-month program in 104 patients with FMS was assessed by Bennett and associates.[14] Their program included education, behavior modification, fitness training, muscle awareness training, "spray and stretch" procedures, and management of associated problems, such as depression, anxiety, and irritable bowel syndrome. Total FIQ score, FIQ subscales except days missed work, difficulty with job and physical function, number of TPs, total TP score, quality-of-life index, 6-minute walking distance, Beck depression and anxiety scores, fibromyalgia attitude index, and three coping skills questionnaire subscales, i.e. catastrophizing index, ability to decrease pain, and ability to control pain, were improved significantly at the end of the program. Results were encouraging, but the study was uncontrolled and unblinded.

In a randomized controlled study by Keel and coworkers,[82] 32 patients received either integrated group therapy, including cognitive behavioral strategies, relaxation, physical exercises, and education on chronic pain for 15 weeks, lasting 2 hours per week, or group relaxation training in 15 sessions lasting 45 to 60 minutes. Outcome measurements consisted of medication consumption, number of physical therapies needed, sleep disturbance, pain score, patient global assessment, and severity of general symptoms. At the end of 15 weeks, there was no significant difference between the groups. Patients were asked to continue their program at home. At the end of the 3-month follow-up, 4 patients in integrated group therapy had improvements on at least 4 of 6 outcome measures, but no improvements were reported in the relaxation training group. The authors concluded that psychological inteventions in combination with physiotherapy may have some beneficial effect in FMS.

Turk and colleagues[142] evaluated in an open study the effects of a 4-week outpatient integrated group program of education, exercise therapy, functional re-education, and CBT in 67 patients with FMS. At the end of the program, pain severity, anxiety, depression, affective distress, and fatigue were improved. Discriminant analysis showed that several pretreatment variables, e.g., low levels of depression and perceived disability, high levels of sense of control, and perceived solicitous response from significant others, were significant predictors of improvement in pain severity. The authors emphasized the need for subgrouping of patients in order to maximize benefit from a treatment program, underscoring the need for an individualized approach. At 6-month follow-up, apart from fatigue, the improvements persisted.

In a recent open trial, the long-term efficacy of a package of multidisciplinary nonpharmacologic treatment, which consisted of education/CBT, relaxation/meditation and qi gong movement therapy, was evaluated by Creamer and associates.[42] The intervention comprised 8 weekly sessions, each lasting 2.5 hours. The authors reported that pain, pain threshold, fatigue, function, mood, TPs and Health Assessment Questionnaire scores were improved at the end of the trial, and benefit continued 4 months after the intervention. The improvement in FIQ scores was similar to that seen with antidepressant treatment.

Bennett[11] emphasized the potential benefits of interdisciplinary group treatment in FMS. These benefits included providing patients with basic background information and knowledge about FMS, various treatment options, as well as self-efficacy. Thus, the ultimate goal of interdisciplinary group treatment programs is to complement and maximize subsequent physician-patient interactions.[11] Randomized, blinded, and controlled studies with appropriate sample size are necessary in this area.

Prognosis

The prognosis in FMS is one of chronic pain and disability. Hawley and coworkers[70] evaluated pain, functional disability, and psychological status in 75 patients with FMS by monthly questionnaires for 12 months and found that these parameters remained stable from month to month among the patients as a group, but there was considerable individual variation among the patients. Ledingham and associates[87] also reported that FMS symptoms overall remained unchanged in 72 patients after a mean follow-up period of 4 years (range 1.5–6 years). They noted that 97% of patients still had symptoms, whereas 85% of them fulfilled criteria for FMS at follow-up examination.

In a recent, six-center study in the United States, Wolfe and his associates[153] assessed outcome of symptoms and function among 538 patients with FMS in a longitudinal study over a period of 7 years. Overall, all the parameters evaluated, including pain, fatigue, sleep difficulties, psychological status, global severity, and functional disability, remained unchanged over time. In the same study, a follow-up of 85 patients from the Wichita center over a mean period of 11.5 years was also reported and the outcome was found to be similar.

Kennedy and Felson[84] reported better outcomes. In a prospective follow-up cohort study, 29 patients, whose mean symptom duration was 15.8 years, were interviewed 10 years after diagnosis. It was observed that all patients had persistence of some fibromyalgia symptoms; however, 66% of them reported that their symptoms were better than when first diagnosed. Authors concluded that most patients experienced improvement in symptoms after FMS onset.

Granges and colleagues[62] reported that 47% of 44 patients who were diagnosed and treated with minimal intervention in community rheumatology practice had no longer fulfilled criteria for FMS 2 years after diagnosis, and 24% experienced remission. However, these patients are not representative of usual clinic patients and the results of this study are discordant with other studies employing a large number of patients who were followed for a longer period of time. Granges and colleagues[62] stated that in a significant number of patients, good outcome was associated with simple intervention by a physician who was familiar with the diagnosis and management.

Early diagnosis, younger age,[48] education level,[72] and increased time spent in exercise[62] influence prognosis positively. Factors associated with poor prognosis are the initial degree of global severity and pain, depressed mood, and a large number of pain sites.[48, 62, 73]

Although follow-up studies show that symptoms in fibromyalgia patients as a group do not change significantly overall, there are a lot of variations between individual patients. Many patients have their symptoms improved with appropriate treatment over a relatively short period of time, during which they also experience better function.

Summary

Because biopathophysiologic mechanisms of FMS are incompletely understood, management of this condition remains unsatisfactory in most cases. Various factors interact to produce symptoms, and these factors differ from patient to patient. Therefore, individualization of management according to the patient's symptoms and severity of FMS is essential. The goals of management of FMS are shown in Table 2–6.

Management of FMS includes a variety of nonpharmacologic and pharmacologic interventions. Aerobic exercise, EMG-biofeedback, acupuncture, CBT, and integrated group therapy have been shown to be beneficial by randomized controlled trials in FMS. Although physical therapies such as heat, massage, ultrasound, and TENS are widely used, and some patients report benefit, their efficacy is not proven by controlled studies.

Among pharmacologic agents, studies have focused mainly on serotonergic drugs. Several of these drugs have been shown to be effective by double-blind, controlled trials. Amitriptyline at a dose of 10 to 50 mg at bedtime is beneficial and frequently prescribed in FMS. A combination of amitriptyline and fluoxetine has been reported to be more efficacious than either agent alone. The dose of both drugs should be kept low if used in combination. Cyclobenzaprine and trazadone are the other agents that are used frequently. Benzodiazepines are helpful in anxious patients. Hypnotics may be helpful for sleep disturbance, but they do not help pain. Tramadol appears to be a useful drug. Low-dose codeine may be used during a flare-up and in severe cases. Tender point injection is a very valuable adjunctive therapy.

In a recent meta-analysis of the efficacy of fibromyalgia treatment interventions,[122] antidepressant agents have been reported to be effective in improving physical fitness and self-reported symptoms of FMS. Nonpharmacologic interventions have been

---

Table 2–6.
Goals of Management of Fibromyalgia Syndrome

- **To alleviate pain and other symptoms:** *Medication, TP injection, nonpharmacologic interventions*
- **To eliminate or modify possible aggravating factors:** *Patient education, lifestyle modification, individualization of treatment*
- **To achieve physical fitness:** *Gradual increase of physical activity, stretching and strengthening exercises, aerobic exercise*
- **To improve sleep quality:** *Patient education, medication*
- **To improve patient's coping skills:** *Patient education, reassurance, cognitive behavioral therapy (CBT)*
- **To encourage patients to take an active role in the management:** *Patient education*
- **To improve quality of life:** *Both pharmacologic and nonpharmacologic treatments, including CBT*

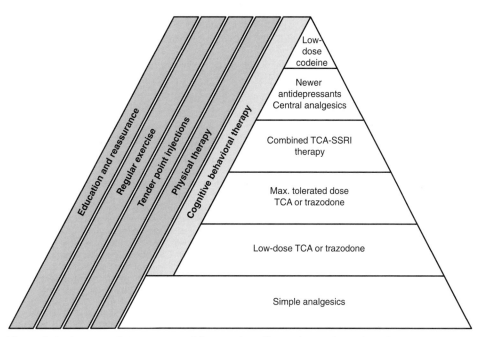

Figure 2–1. A suggested step-up pyramidal approach to fibromyalgia syndrome (FMS) management as a general guideline. Note that patient education and reassurance and regular exercise should be utilized in all stages. Tender point injections and physical therapy can be employed, any time, when necessary. Mildly symptomatic patients usually respond to interventions at lower steps. Items at the higher steps should be considered for severe cases. TCA, tricyclic antidepressants; SSRI, selective serotonin reuptake inhibitors. (Adapted from Yunus MB: Fibromyalgia syndrome: Is there any effective therapy? Consultant 36:1279–1285, 1996.)

found to be beneficial in improving physical status, self-reported symptoms of FMS, psychological status, and daily functioning, with the exception that exercise alone did not significantly improve daily functioning. When compared, a combination of pharmacologic and nonpharmacologic interventions was found to be more efficacious in improving self-reported symptoms of FMS than pharmacologic treatment alone. The authors concluded that optimal management of FMS should include appropriate medical treatment of pain and sleep disturbances in combination with nonpharmacologic interventions, especially aerobic exercises, and CBT.

A pyramidal approach (Fig. 2–1) may be employed, upper steps being reserved for more difficult patients. Acute exacerbation of the symptoms should be treated with reassurance, addressing poor sleep, recent stress, anxiety, or other psychological factors, and with local heat, massage, temporary rest, change of medications or increasing their current dose, and tender point injections. The management plan outlined in this chapter is helpful in most patients.

References

1. Abeles M, Waterman J, Maestrello S: Tender point injections in fibromyalgia [abstract]. Arthritis Rheum 40(9)(Suppl.):S187, 1997.
2. Ahles TA, Khan SA, Yunus MB, et al: Psychiatric status of patients with primary fibromyalgia, patients with rheumatoid arthritis and subjects without pain: A blind comparison of DSM-III diagnoses. Am J Psychiatry 148(12):1721–1726, 1991.
3. Alberts KR, Bradley LA, Alarcon GS: Sertraline hydrochloride (Zoloft) alters pain threshold, sensory discrimination ability, and functional brain activity in patients with fibromyalgia (FM): A randomized controlled trial (RCT) [abstract]. Arthritis Rheum 41(Suppl.):S259, 1998.
4. Anderberg UM, Marteinsdottir I, von Knorring L: Citalopram in patients with fibromyalgia—a randomized, double-blind, placebo-controlled study. Eur J Pain 4(1):27–35, 2000.

5. Arnold LM, Keck PE, Welge JA: Antidepressant treatment of fibromyalgia. A meta-analysis and review. Psychosomatics 41(2):104–113, 2000.
6. Baldry P: Superficial dry needling at myofascial trigger point sites. J Musculoskeletal Pain 3(3):117–126, 1995.
7. Baldry P: Superficial dry needling. In Chaitow L(ed): Fibromyalgia Syndrome: A Practitioner's Guide to Treatment. Edinburgh, Churchill Livingstone, 2000, pp 77–90.
8. Barnes CD, Fung SJ, Gintautus J: Brainstem noradrenergic system depression by cyclobenzaprine. Neuropharmacology 19(2):221–224, 1980.
9. Bengtsson A, Bengtsson M: Regional sympathetic blockade in primary fibromyalgia. Pain 33(2):161–167, 1988.
10. Bennett MI, Tai YM: Intravenous lignocaine in the management of primary fibromyalgia syndrome. Int J Clin Pharmacol Res 15(3):115–119, 1995.
11. Bennett RM: Multidisciplinary group programs to treat fibromyalgia patients. Rheum Dis Clin North Am 22(2):351–367, 1996.
12. Bennett RM: The fibromyalgia syndrome. In Kelley WN (ed): Textbook of Rheumatology. Philadelphia, WB Saunders, 1997, pp 517–518.
13. Bennett RM, TPS-FM Study Group: A blinded, placebo-controlled evaluation of tramadol in the management of fibromyalgia pain [abstract]. J Musculoskeletal Pain 6(Suppl. 2):146, 1998.
14. Bennett RM, Burckhardt CS, Clark SR, et al: Group treatment of fibromyalgia: A 6 month outpatient program. J Rheumatol 23(3):521–528, 1996.
15. Bennett RM, Campbell SM, Burckhardt CS, et al: A multidisciplinary approach to fibromyalgia management. J Musculoskeletal Med 8(11):21–32, 1991.
16. Bennett RM, Clark S, Goldberg L, et al: Aerobic fitness in the fibrositis syndrome: A controlled study of respiratory gas exchange and Xenon 133 clearance from exercising muscle. Arthritis Rheum 32(4):454–460, 1989.
17. Bennett RM, Clark SC, Walczyk J: A randomized, double-blind, placebo-controlled study of growth hormone in the treatment of fibromyalgia. Am J Med 104(3):227–231, 1998.
18. Bennett RM, Gatter RA, Campbell SM, et al: A comparison of cyclobenzaprine and placebo in the management of fibrositis. A double-blind controlled study. Arthritis Rheum 31(12):1535–1542, 1988.
19. Berman BM, Ezzo J, Hadhazy V: Is acupuncture effective in the treatment of fibromyalgia? J Fam Pract 48(3):213–218, 1999.
20. Berman BM, Swyers JP: Complementary medicine treatments for fibromyalgia syndrome. Baillieres Clin Rheum 13(3):487–492, 1999.
21. Bessette L, Carette S, Fossel AH, Lew RA: A placebo-controlled crossover trial of subcutaneous salmon calcitonin in the treatment of patients with fibromyalgia. Scan J Rheumatol 27(2):112–116, 1998.
22. Biasi G, Manca S, Manganelli S, Marcolongo R: Tramadol in the fibromyalgia syndrome: A controlled clinical trial versus placebo. Int J Clin Pharmacol Res 18(1):13–19, 1998.
23. Bibolotti E, Borghi C, Paculli E, et al: The management of fibrositis: A double-blind comparison of maprotiline, chlorimipramine and placebo. Clin Trials J 23:269–240, 1986.
24. Blunt KL, Rajwani MH, Guerriero RC: The effectiveness of chiropractic management of fibromyalgia patients: A pilot study. J Manipulative Physiol Ther 20(6):389–399, 1997.
25. Boghen D, Lamothe L, Elie R, et al: The treatment of the restless legs syndrome with clonazepam: A prospective controlled study. Can J Neurol Sci 13(3):245–247, 1986.
26. Bradley LA: Cognitive-behavioral therapy for primary fibromyalgia. J Rheumatol 19(Suppl.):131–136, 1989.
27. Branco JC, Martini A, Palva T: Treatment of sleep abnormalities and clinical complaints in fibromyalgia with trazodone [abstract]. Arthritis Rheum 39(Suppl.):59, 1996.
28. Buckelew SP, Conway R, Parker J, et al: Biofeedback/relaxation training and exercise interventions for fibromyalgia: A prospective trial. Arthritis Care Res 11(3):196–209, 1998.
29. Burckhardt CS, Bjelle A: Education programs for fibromyalgia patients: Description and evaluation. Baillieres Clin Rheumatol 8(4):935–955, 1994.
30. Burckhardt CS, Mannerkorpi K, Hedenberg L, Bjelle A: A randomized, controlled clinical trial of education and physical training for women with fibromyalgia. J Rheumatol 21(4):714–720, 1994.
31. Buskila D: Drug therapy. Baillieres Best Pract Res Clin Rheumatol 13(3):479–485, 1999.
32. Caballero-Uribe CV, Abuchaibe I, Abuchaibe S, Navarro E: Treatment of tender points in patients with fibromyalgia syndrome (FMS) with therapeutic infrared laser ray [abstract]. Arthritis Rheum 40(9):(Suppl.):S44, 1997.
33. Carette S, Bell MJ, Reynolds WJ, et al: Comparison of amitriptyline, cyclobenzaprine, and placebo in the treatment of fibromyalgia. Arthritis Rheum 37(1):32–40, 1994.
34. Carette S, McCain GA, Bell DA, Fam AG: Evaluation of amitriptyline in primary fibrositis. A double-blind, placebo-controlled study. Arthritis Rheum 29(5):655–659, 1986.
35. Carette S, Oakson G, Guimont C, Steriade M: Sleep electroencephalography and the clinical response to amitriptyline in patients with fibromyalgia. Arthritis Rheum 38(9):1211–1217, 1995.
36. Caruso I, Sarzi Puttini PC, Boccassini L, et al: Double-blind study of dothiepin versus placebo in the treatment of primary fibromyalgia syndrome. J Int Med Res 15(3):154–159, 1987.
37. Caruso I, Sarzi Puttini P, Cazzola M, Azzolini V. Double-blind study of 5-hydroxytryptophan versus placebo in the treatment of primary fibromyalgia syndrome. J Int Med Res 18(3):201–209, 1990.
38. Citera G, Arias MA, Maldonado-Cocco JA, et al: The effect of melatonin in patients with fibromyalgia: A pilot study. Clin Rheumatol 19(1):9–13, 2000.

39. Clark S, Tindall E, Bennett RM: A double-blind crossover trial of prednisone versus placebo in the treatment of fibrositis. J Rheumatol 12(5):980–983, 1985.
40. Clark SR: Prescribing exercise for fibromyalgia patients. Arthritis Care Res 7(4):221–225, 1994.
41. Creamer P: Effective management of fibromyalgia. J Musculoskeletal Med 16:622–637, 1999.
42. Creamer P, Singh BB, Hochberg MC, Berman BC: Sustained improvement produced by nonpharmacologic intervention in fibromyalgia: Results of a pilot study. Arthritis Care Res 13(4):198–204, 2000.
43. DeLuze C, Bosia L, Zirbs A, et al: Electroacupuncture in fibromyalgia: Results of a controlled trial. BMJ 305(6864):1249–1252, 1992.
44. Drewes AM, Andreasen A, Jennum P, Nielsen KD: Zopiclone in the treatment of sleep abnormalities in fibromyalgia. Scan J Rheumatol 20(4):288–293, 1991.
45. Dryson E: Venlafaxine and fibromyalgia. N Z Med J 113(1105):87, 2000.
46. Dwight MM, Arnold LM, O'Brien H, et al: An open clinical trial of venlafaxine treatment of fibromyalgia. Psychosomatics 39(1):14–17, 1998.
47. Faerber L, Stratz T, Michael S, et al: Efficacy and safety of a 5-HT3 receptor antagonist (Tropisetron) in primary fibromyalgia [abstract]. Arthritis Rheum 42(Suppl. 9):S395, 1999.
48. Felson DT, Goldenberg DL: The natural history of fibromyalgia. Arthritis Rheum 29(12):1522–1526, 1986.
49. Ferraccioli G, Ghirelli L, Scita F, et al: EMG-biofeedback training in fibromyalgia syndrome. J Rheumatol 14(4):820–825, 1987.
50. Figuerola ML, Loe W, Sormani M, Barontini M: Met-enkephalin increase in patients with fibromyalgia under local treatment. Funct Neurol 13(4):291–295, 1998.
51. Finestone DH, Ober SK: Fluoxetine and fibromyalgia [letter]. JAMA 264(22):2869–2870, 1990.
52. Fossaluzza V, De Vita S: Combined therapy with cyclobenzaprine and ibuprofen in primary fibromyalgia syndrome. Int J Clin Pharmacol Res 12(2):99–102, 1992.
53. Geller SA: Treatment of fibrositis with fluoxetine hydrochloride (Prozac). Am J Med 87(5):594–595, 1989.
54. Ginsberg F, Joos E, Geczy J, et al: A pilot randomized placebo-controlled study of pirlindole in the treatment of primary fibromyalgia. J Musculoskeletal Pain 6(2):5–17, 1998.
55. Godfrey RG: A guide to the understanding and use of tricyclic antidepressants in the overall management of fibromyalgia and other chronic pain syndromes. Arch Int Med 156(10):1047–1052, 1996.
56. Goldenberg DL: A review of the role of tricyclic medications in the treatment of fibromyalgia syndrome. J Rheumatol 19(Suppl.):137–139, 1989.
57. Goldenberg DL: Fibromyalgia syndrome a decade later. What we have learned? Arch Intern Med 159(8):777–785, 1999.
58. Goldenberg DL, Felson DT, Dinerman H: A randomized, controlled trial of amitriptyline and naproxen in the treatment of patients with fibromyalgia. Arthritis Rheum 29(11):1371–1377, 1986.
59. Goldenberg DL, Kaplan KH, Nadeau MG, et al: A controlled study of stress-reduction, cognitive behavioral treatment program in fibromyalgia. J Musculoskeletal Pain 2(1):53–66, 1994.
60. Goldenberg D, Mayskiy M, Mossey C, et al: A randomized, double-blind crossover trial of fluoxetine and amitriptyline in the treatment of fibromyalgia. Arthritis Rheum 39(11):1852–1859, 1996.
61. Gowans SE, deHueck A, Voss S, Richardson M: A randomized, controlled trial of exercise and education for individuals with fibromyalgia. Arthritis Care Res 12(2):120–128, 1999.
62. Granges G, Zilko P, Littlejohn GO: Fibromyalgia syndrome: Assessment of severity of the condition two years after diagnosis. J Rheumatol 21(3):523–529, 1994.
63. Grönblad M, Nykanen J, Konttinen Y, et al: Effect of zopiclone on sleep quality, morning stiffness, widespread tenderness and pain and general discomfort in primary fibromyalgia patients. A double-blind randomized trial. Clin Rheumatol 12(2):186–191, 1993.
64. Gunther V, Mur E, Kinigadner U, Miller C: Fibromyalgia—the effect of relaxation and hydrogalvanic bath therapy on the subjective pain experience. Clin Rheumatol 13(4):573–578, 1994.
65. Haanen HC, Hoenderdos HT, van Romunde LK, et al: Controlled trial of hypnotherapy in the treatment of refractory fibromyalgia. J Rheumatol 18(1):72–75, 1991.
66. Hagglund KJ, Deuser WE, Buckelew SP, et al: Weather, beliefs about weather and disease severity among patients with fibromyalgia. Arthritis Care Res 7(3):130–135, 1994.
67. Hains G, Hains F: A combined ischemic compression and spinal manipulation in the treatment of fibromyalgia: A preliminary estimate of dose and efficacy. J Manipulative Physiol Ther 23(4):225–230, 2000.
68. Hannonen P, Malminiemi K, Yli-Kerttula U, et al: A randomized, double-blind, placebo-controlled study of moclobemide and amitriptyline in the treatment of fibromyalgia in females without psychiatric disorder. Br J Rheumatol 37(12):1279–1286, 1998.
69. Harding SM: Sleep in fibromyalgia patients: Subjective and objective findings. Am J Med Sci 315(6):367–376, 1998.
70. Hawley DJ, Wolfe F, Cathey MA: Pain, functional disability, and psychological status: A 12-month study of severity in fibromyalgia. J Rheumatol 15(10):1551–1556, 1988.
71. Heymann R, Feldman D, Helfenstein M, et al: Double-blind, randomized, placebo-controlled study of amitriptyline, nortriptyline and placebo in fibromyalgia. Arthritis Rheum 40(9) Suppl:S189, 1997.
72. Hench PK, Cohen R, Mitler MM: Fibromyalgia: Effects of amitriptyline, temazepam and placebo on pain and sleep [abstract]. Arthritis Rheum 32(Suppl.):S47, 1989.
73. Henriksson CM: Long-term effects of fibromyalgia on everyday life: A study of 56 patients. Scan J Rheumatol 23(1):36–41, 1994.

74. Holman AJ: Effect of lorazepam on pain score of refractory fibromyalgia [abstract]. Arthritis Rheum 41(Suppl.):S259, 1998.
75. Holman AJ, Renton WA: Safety and efficacy of lorazepam for refractory fibromyalgia after one year [abstract] Arthritis Rheum 42(9)(Suppl.):S152, 1999.
76. Hrycaj P, Stratz T, Mennet P, Muller V: Pathogenic aspects of responsiveness to ondansetron (5-hydroxytryptamine type 3 receptor antagonist) in patients with primary fibromyalgia syndrome—a preliminary study. J Rheumatol 23(8):1418–1423, 1996.
77. Inanici F, Yunus MB: Management of fibromyalgia syndrome. In Baldry P (ed): Myofascial Pain and Fibromyalgia Syndromes: A Clinical Guide to Diagnosis and Management. London, Churchill Livingstone, 2001, pp 379–398.
78. Jacobsen S, Danneskiold-Samsoe B, Andersen RB: Oral S-adenosylmethionine in primary fibromyalgia. Double-blind clinical evaluation. Scan J Rheumatol 20(4):294–302, 1991.
79. Jaeschke R, Adachi J, Guyatt G, et al: Clinical usefulness of amitriptyline in fibromyalgia: The results of 23 N-of-1 randomized controlled trials. J Rheumatol 18(3):447–451, 1991.
80. Janzen VD, Scudds R: Sphenopalatine blocks in the treatment of pain in fibromyalgia and myofascial pain syndrome. Laryngoscope 107(10):1420–1422, 1997.
81. Kaada B: Treatment of fibromyalgia by low-frequency transcutaneous nerve stimulation. Tidsskrift For Den Norske Laegeforening 109(29):2992–2995, 1989.
82. Keel PJ, Bodoky C, Gerhard U, Muller W: Comparison of integrated group therapy and group relaxation training for fibromyalgia. Clin J Pain 14(3):232–238, 1998.
83. Kempenaers C, Simenon G, Vander Elst M, et al: Effect of an antidiencephalon immune serum on pain and sleep in primary fibromyalgia. Neuropsychobiology 30(2–3):66–72, 1994.
84. Kennedy M, Felson DT: A prospective long-term study of fibromyalgia syndrome. Arthritis Rheum 39(4):682–685, 1996.
85. Korszun A, Sackett-Lundeen L, Papadopoulos E, et al: Melatonin levels in women with fibromyalgia and chronic fatigue syndrome. J Rheumatol 26(12):2675–2680, 1999.
86. Krueger BR: Restless legs syndrome and periodic limb movements of sleep. Mayo Clin Proc 65(7):999–1006, 1990.
87. Ledingham J, Doherty S, Doherty M: Primary fibromyalgia syndrome—an outcome study. Br J Rheumatol 32(2):139–142, 1993.
88. Leventhal LJ: Management of fibromyalgia. Ann Intern Med 7131(11):850–858, 1999.
89. Lewis PJ: Electroacupuncture in fibromyalgia [letter, comment]. BMJ 306(6874):393, 1993.
90. Martin L, Nutting A, MacIntosh BR, et al: An exercise program in the treatment of fibromyalgia. J Rheumatol 23(6):1050–1053, 1996.
91. Masi AT: An intuitive person-centered perspective on fibromyalgia syndrome and its management. Baillieres Clin Rheumatol 8(4):957–993, 1994.
92. McCain GA: Role of physical fitness training in the fibrositis/fibromyalgia syndrome. Am J Med 2981(3A):73–77, 1986.
93. McCain GA: Nonmedicinal treatments in primary fibromyalgia. Rheum Dis Clin North Am 15(1):73–90, 1989.
94. McCain GA, Bell DA, Mai FM, Halliday PD: A controlled study of the effects of a supervised cardiovascular fitness training program on the manifestations of primary fibromyalgia. Arthritis Rheum 31(9):1135–1141, 1988.
95. Mengshoel AM, Forre O, Komnaes HB: Muscle strength and aerobic capacity in primary fibromyalgia. Clin Exp Rheumatol 8(5):475–479, 1990.
96. Mengshoel AM, Komnaes HB, Forre O: The effects of 20 weeks of physical fitness training in female patients with fibromyalgia. Clin Exp Rheumatol 10(4):345–349, 1992.
97. Moldofsky H: Sleep and fibrositis syndrome. Rheum Dis Clin North Am 15(1):90–103, 1989.
98. Moldofsky H, Benz B, Luc F, et al: Comparison of chlorpromazine and L-tryptophan on sleep, musculoskeletal pain, and mood in fibrositis syndrome. Sleep Research 5:76, 1976.
99. Moldofsky H, Lue FA, Mously C, et al: The effect of zolpidem in patients with fibromyalgia: A dose ranging, double-blind, placebo-controlled, modified crossover study. J Rheumatol 23(3):529–533, 1996.
100. Moldofsky H, Scarisbrick P: Induction of neurasthenic musculoskeletal pain syndrome by selective sleep deprivation. Psychosom Med 38(1):35–44, 1976.
101. Montplaisir J, Godbout R, Poirier G, Bedard MA: Restless legs syndrome and periodic limb movements in sleep: Physiopathology and treatment with L-dopa, Clin Neuropharmacology 9(5):456–463, 1986.
102. National Heart, Lung and Blood Institute Working Group on Restless Legs Syndrome: Restless legs syndrome detection and management in primary care. Am Fam Physician 62:108–114, 2000.
103. NIH Consensus Conference: Acupuncture. JAMA 280(17):1518–1524, 1998.
104. NIH Technology Assessment Panel on integration of behavioral and relaxation approaches into the treatment of chronic pain and insomnia. Integration of behavioral and relaxation approaches into the treatment of chronic pain and insomnia. JAMA 276(4):313–318, 1996.
105. Nicassio PM, Schuman C, Kim J, et al: Psychosocial factors associated with complementary treatment use in fibromyalgia. J Rheumatol 24(10):2008–2013, 1997.
106. Nicassio PM, Radojevic V, Weisman MH, et al: A comparison of behavioral and educational interventions for fibromyalgia. J Rheumatol 24(10): 2000–2007, 1997.
107. Nielson WR, Walker C, McCain GA: Cognitive behavioral treatment of fibromyalgia syndrome: Preliminary findings. J Rheumatol 19(1):98–103, 1992.
108. Norregaard J, Volkmann H, Danneskiold-Samsoe B: A randomized controlled trial of citalopram in the treatment of fibromyalgia. Pain 61(3):445–449, 1995.

109. Olin R, Klein R, Berg PA: A randomized double-blind 16-week study of ritanserin in fibromyalgia syndrome: Clinical outcome and analysis of autoantibodies to serotonin, gangliosides and phospholipids. Clin Rheumatol 17(2):89–94, 1998.
110. Papadopoulos IA, Georgiou PE, Katsimbri PP, Drosos AA: Treatment of fibromyalgia with tropisetron, a 5HT3 serotonin antagonist: a pilot study. Clin Rheumatol 19(1):6–8, 2000.
111. Parziale JR: The clinical management of fibromyalgia. Medicine and Health, Rhode Island 82(9):325–328, 1999.
112. Pattrick M, Swannell A, Doherty M: Chlormezanone in primary fibromyalgia syndrome: A double-blind placebo-controlled study. Br J Rheumatol 32(1):55–58, 1993.
113. Pioro-Boisset M, Esdaile JM, Fitzcharles MA: Alternative medicine use in fibromyalgia syndrome. Arthritis Care Res 9(1):13–17, 1996.
114. Press J, Phillip M, Neumann L, et al: Normal melatonin levels in patients with fibromyalgia syndrome. J Rheumatol 25(3):551–555, 1998.
115. Puttini PS, Caruso I: Primary fibromyalgia syndrome and 5-hydroxy-L-tryptophan: A 90-day open study. J Int Med Res 20(2):182–189, 1992.
116. Quijada-Carrera J, Valenzuela-Castano A, Povedano-Gomez J, et al: Comparison of tenoxicam and bromazepam in the treatment of fibromyalgia: A randomized, double-blind, placebo-controlled trial. Pain 65(2–3):221–225, 1996.
117. Ramsay C, Moreland J, Ho M, et al: An observer blinded comparison of supervised and unsupervised aerobic exercise regimen in fibromyalgia. Rheumatology 39(5):501–505, 2000.
118. Reddy SS, Yunus MB, Inanici F, Aldag JC: Tender point injections are beneficial in fibromyalgia syndrome: a descriptive, open study. J Musculoskeletal Pain 8(4):7–18, 2000.
119. Reynolds WJ, Moldofsky H, Saskin P, Lue FA: The effects of cyclobenzaprine on sleep physiology and symptoms in patients with fibromyalgia. J Rheumatol 18(3):452–454, 1991.
120. Richards S, Cleare A: Treating fibromyalgia. Rheumatology 39(4):343–346, 2000.
121. Rosen NB: Physical medicine and rehabilitation approaches to the management of myofascial pain and fibromyalgia syndromes. Baillieres Clin Rheumatol 8(4):881–916, 1994.
122. Rossy LA, Buckelew SP, Dorr N, et al: A meta-analysis of fibromyalgia treatment interventions. Ann Behav Med 21(2):180–191, 1999.
123. Russell IJ: Fibromyalgia syndrome: Approaches to management. Bulletin Rheum Dis 45(3):1–4, 1996.
124. Russell IJ: Efficacy of Ultram (tramadol HCL) treatment of fibromyalgia syndrome: Secondary outcome report. TPS-FM Study Group [abstract]. J Musculoskeletal Pain 6(Suppl. 2):147, 1998.
125. Russell IJ, Fletcher EM, Michalek JE, et al: Treatment of primary fibrositis/fibromyalgia syndrome with ibuprofen and alprazolam. A double-blind, placebo-controlled study. Arthritis Rheum 34(5):552–560, 1991.
126. Russell IJ, Kamin M, Sager D, et al: Efficacy of Ultram (tramadol HCL) treatment of fibromyalgia syndrome: Preliminary analysis of a multi-center, randomized, placebo-controlled study (abstract). Arthritis Rheum 40(Suppl. 9):S117, 1997.
127. Russell IJ, Michalek JE, Flechas JD, Abraham GE: Treatment of fibromyalgia syndrome with Super Malic: A randomized, double-blind, placebo-controlled, crossover pilot study. J Rheumatol 22(5):953–958, 1995.
128. Russell IJ, Michalek JE, Kang YK, Richards AB: Reduction of morning stiffness and improvement in physical function in fibromyalgia syndrome patients treated sublingually with low doses of human interferon-alpha. J Interferon Cytokine Res 19(8):961–968, 1999.
129. Samborski W, Stratz T, Lacki JK, et al: The 5-HT3 blockers in the treatment of the primary fibromyalgia syndrome: A 10-day open study with Tropisetron at a low dose. Materia Medica Polona 28(1):17–19, 1996.
130. Santandrea S, Montrone F, Sarzi-Puttini P, et al: A double-blind crossover study of two cyclobenzaprine regimens in primary fibromyalgia syndrome. J Int Med Res 21(2):74–80, 1993.
131. Sarnoch H, Adler F, Scholz OB: Relevance of muscular sensitivity, muscular activity, and cognitive variables for pain reduction associated with EMG biofeedback in fibromyalgia. Percept Mot Skills 84(3 Pt 1):1043–1050, 1997.
132. Scharf MB, Hauck M, Stover R, et al: Effect of gamma-hydroxybutyrate on pain, fatigue, and the alpha sleep anomaly in patients with fibromyalgia. Preliminary report. J Rheumatol 25(10):1986–1990, 1998.
133. Scudds RA, McCain GA, Rollman GB, Harth M: Improvements in pain responsiveness in patients with fibrositis after successful treatment with amitriptyline. J Rheumatol 19(Suppl.):98–103, 1989.
134. Sim J, Adams N: Physical and other nonpharmacological interventions for fibromyalgia. Baillieres Clin Rheumatol 13(3):507–523, 1999.
135. Simms RW: Controlled trials of therapy in fibromyalgia syndrome. Baillieres Clin Rheumatol 8(4):917–934, 1994.
136. Simms RW: Fibromyalgia is not a muscle disorder. Am J Sci 315(6):346–350, 1998.
137. Singh BB, Berman BM, Hadhazy VA, Creamer P: A pilot study of cognitive behavioral therapy in fibromyalgia. Altern Ther Health Med 4(2):67–70, 1998.
138. Sorensen J, Bengtsson A, Ahlner J, et al: Fibromyalgia—are there different mechanisms in the processing of pain? A double-blind crossover comparison of analgesic drugs. J Rheumatol 24(8):1615–1621, 1997.
139. Sprott H, Franke S, Kluge H, Hein G: Pain treatment of fibromyalgia by acupuncture [letter]. Rheumatology Int 18(1):35–36, 1998.
140. Tavoni A, Jeracitano G, Cirigliano G: Evaluation of S-adenosylmethionine in secondary fibromyalgia: A double-blind study [letter]. Clin Exp Rheumatol 16(1):106–107, 1998.

141. Tavoni A, Vitali C, Bombardieri S, Pasero G: Evaluation of S-adenosylmethionine in primary fibromyalgia. A double-blind crossover study. Am J Med 83(5A):107–110, 1987.
142. Turk DC, Okifuji A, Sinclair JD, Starz TW: Interdisciplinary treatment for fibromyalgia syndrome: Clinical and statistical significance. Arthritis Care Res 11(3):186–195, 1998.
143. Vaeroy H, Abrahamsen A, Forre O, Kass E: Treatment of fibromyalgia (fibrositis syndrome): A parallel double-blind trial with carisoprodol, paracetamol and caffeine (Somadril comp) versus placebo. Clin Rheumatol 8(2):245–250, 1989.
144. Volkmann H, Norregaard J, Jacobsen S, et al: Double-blind, placebo-controlled crossover study of intravenous S-adenosyl-L-methionine in patients with fibromyalgia. Scan J Rheumatol 26(3):206–211, 1997.
145. Vlaeyen JW, Teeken-Gruben NJ, Goossens ME, et al: Cognitive-educational treatment of fibromyalgia: A randomized clinical trial. I. Clinical effects. J Rheumatol 23(7):1237–1245, 1996.
146. Wallace DJ: The fibromyalgia syndrome. Ann Med 29(1):9–21, 1997.
147. Waylonis GW, Ronan PG, Gordon C: A profile of fibromyalgia in occupational environments. Am J Phys Med Rehab 73(2):112–115, 1994.
148. White KP, Nielson WR: Cognitive behavioral treatment of fibromyalgia syndrome: A follow-up assessment. J Rheumatol 22(4):717–721, 1995.
149. Wigers SH, Stiles TC, Vogel PA: Effects of aerobic exercise versus stress management treatment in fibromyalgia. A 4.5 year prospective study. Scan J Rheumatol 25(2):77–86, 1996.
150. Wikner J, Hirsch U, Wetterberg L, Rojdmark S: Fibromyalgia—a syndrome associated with decreased nocturnal melatonin secretion. Clin Endocrinol 49(2):179–183, 1998.
151. Wilke WS: Treatment of 'resistant' fibromyalgia. Rheum Dis Clin North Am 21(1):247–260, 1995.
152. Wolfe F, Anderson J, Harkness D, et al: A prospective, longitudinal, multicenter study of service utilization and costs in fibromyalgia. Arthritis Rheum 40(9):1560–1570, 1997.
153. Wolfe F, Anderson J, Harkness D, et al: Health status and disease severity in fibromyalgia: Results of a six-center longitudinal study. Arthritis Rheum 40(9):1571–1579, 1997.
154. Wolfe F, Cathey MA, Hawley DJ: A double-blind placebo-controlled trial of fluoxetine in fibromyalgia. Scan J Rheumatol 23(5):255–259, 1994.
155. Wolfe F, Zhao S, Lane N: Preference for nonsteroidal antiinflammatory drugs over acetaminophen by rheumatic disease patients. Arthritis Rheum 43(2):378–385, 2000.
156. Wysenbeek AJ, Mor F, Lurie Y, Weinberger A: Imipramine for the treatment of fibrositis: A therapeutic trial. Ann Rheum Dis 44(11):752–753, 1985.
157. Yunus MB: Psychological aspects of fibromyalgia syndrome—a component of the dysfunctional spectrum syndrome. Baillieres Clin Rheumatol 8(4):811–837, 1994.
158. Yunus MB: Fibromyalgia syndrome: Is there any effective therapy? Consultant 36(6):1279–1285, 1996.
159. Yunus MB, Inanici F: Clinical characteristics and biopathophysiological mechanisms of fibromyalgia syndrome. In Baldry P (ed): Myofascial Pain and Fibromyalgia Syndromes: A Clinical Guide to Diagnosis and Management. London, Churchill Livingstone, 2001, pp 351–377.
160. Yunus MB, Kalyan-Raman UP, Masi AT, Aldag JC: Electron microscopic studies of muscle biopsy in primary fibromyalgia syndrome; a controlled and blinded study. J Rheumatol 16(1):97–101, 1989.
161. Yunus MB, Masi AT, Aldag JC: Short term effects of ibuprofen in primary fibromyalgia syndrome: A double-blind, placebo-controlled trial. J Rheumatol 16(4):527–532, 1989.
162. Yurtkuran M, Celiktas M: A randomized, controlled therapy of balneotherapy in the treatment of patients with primary fibromyalgia syndrome. Physikalische Medizin Rehabilitationsmedizin Kurortmedizin 6(2):109–112, 1996.

Chapter 3

Diagnostic Challenges in the Pediatric Patient with Musculoskeletal Pain

Joan T. Gold

Diagnosis of painful conditions of childhood and their management has until recently been given a low priority. Within the past 10 years, attention has been turned to children with postoperative pain, pain related to malignant conditions, and pain related to certain acute features of chronic diseases such as sickle cell disease. Management of painful musculoskeletal conditions such as reflex sympathetic dystrophy of childhood and fibromyalgia has virtually been ignored in the literature and in the curriculum for physiatrists and pediatricians. Even with the advent of the multidisciplinary pediatric pain management clinic, a survey of the 22 existing clinics within the United States revealed that physiatric participation was present in only one of the clinics, clearly compounding the difficulty.[11]

Superimposed upon this problem is the nature of the child; developmental restrictions often do not permit an adequate clinical description of the child's complaints. The younger patient with musculoskeletal discomfort is not easily "labeled" but may be seen as an irritable and "difficult" child with the inability to pay attention to tasks and with sleep disturbances. Diagnosis of such an entity is a formidable task because limb pain accounts for up to 7% of visits to a pediatrician.[128] The diagnosis of a relatively obscure condition without characteristic laboratory data then needs to be teased away from the multiple varied diagnoses for limb pain in childhood.[17] The categories that need to be considered for each child include trauma, collagen vascular and autoimmune disorders such as juvenile rheumatoid arthritis, infections of the musculoskeletal system, neoplastic lesions of the musculoskeletal system, orthopedic conditions of childhood such as slipped capital femoral epiphysis, hematologic disorders such as sickle cell disease, nutritional and endocrinologic conditions, and neurologic conditions such as a peripheral neuropathy or entrapment syndrome.

It is the purpose of this chapter to discuss four diagnostic entities not indicated in the preceding classification. The chapter includes a review of growing pains, reflex sympathetic dystrophy or regional complex pain syndrome, hypermobility syndrome of childhood, and fibromyalgia, with an emphasis on fibromyalgia. More specifically, the chapter seeks to:

- Describe the clinical features of these conditions in the pediatric population
- Discuss how these findings are similar to and different from those of adults with the same condition (when applicable)
- Discuss related conditions and differential diagnoses
- Review the assessments that are of assistance in substantiating the diagnosis, explaining its pathophysiology, and understanding the extent of the child's physical and emotional impairments
- Characterize the unique clinical outcomes in juveniles
- Explore developmentally appropriate treatment options

Growing Pains

Clinical Features

The term growing pains, although descriptive, appears to be somewhat of a misnomer. Although pain does occur in growing children, the intensity of pain does not correlate with the peak periods of growth, or weight or height of the child.[94] Conversely, the pains seem to abate after the age of 13 years in boys just at the start of or prior to their adolescent growth spurt.

Growing pains is not an obscure diagnosis, but the clinical difficulty lies in excluding those conditions that may have common presentations but are more medically serious. When this task is accomplished, the incidence is reported as being from 4.0% up to 12.5% in healthy school boys and 4.7% to 18.4% in healthy school girls. [87, 94]

Several studies over the past 70 years have helped to characterize this condition. Initially, these diffuse, intermittent limb pains were believed, incorrectly, to represent a variation of rheumatic fever[111] or were thought to be attributable to poor posture in association with scoliosis, pes planovalgus, genu valgum/varum, leg length discrepancy, excessive tibial torsion, or femoral anteversion.[56] However, later studies[87, 94] suggested the following criteria:

- Limb pain present for at least 3 months in duration but not present on a constant or daily basis, with pain-free intervals of days to months
- Deep, nonarticular pain with a symmetrical localization, primarily confined to the calves and anterior thighs, with rare involvement of the upper extremities
- Primarily diurnal (64%) or nocturnal (27%) occurrence of the pain
- Pain sufficient to awaken the child from sleep or to cause cessation of usual daily activities
- Absence of functional residuals except for possibly a minimal amount of soreness the day following the episode of pain

Growing pains are most common in children between the ages of 3 and 5 years, but may be present even in infancy.[21] Other studies cite that the most common age of occurrence is 8 to 12 years of age.[87]

Possibly reflecting pathogenesis (see later discussion), pain tends to be exacerbated when the child is tired or has performed vigorous exercise. Other conditions that may increase the occurrence of pain include emotional stressors. Growing pains are associated with a general increase of pain-related symptoms in this population, with headaches and abdominal pain being more frequent in the children so involved, and chronic pain symptoms being more common in the families of these patients.[70, 94]

Differential Diagnosis

Complaints that differ from those described earlier should trigger a list of potential differential diagnoses. Such atypical complaints include asymmetry of the pain, increasing pain especially if present on a daily basis, systemic signs and symptoms such as weight loss or fever or both, decrease in joint range, joint swelling or limp or both. The most serious differential diagnosis category includes neoplastic conditions such as osteogenic sarcoma or other malignant bone tumors, and those involving generalized bone pain, i.e, acute leukemia, neuroblastoma, lymphoma and central nervous system tumors, especially those affecting the spine.[26] Features that suggest a malignancy include nonarticular bone pain, back pain, bone tenderness, severe constitutional symptoms, night sweats, ecchymoses, bruising, abnormal neurologic signs, and a palpable mass. Inflammatory joint diseases such as juvenile rheumatoid arthritis are also within the differential diagnosis. A localized musculoskeletal infection or inflammation such as transient synovitis of the hip should also be considered.[98] A stress fracture may present with recurrent pain, but the pain is generally localized and is asymmetrical. Lastly, certain orthopedic conditions of childhood such as aseptic necrosis of the femoral head(s) (Legg-Perthes disease) in a younger child, slipped femoral capital epiphyses in an older child, as well as Osgood-Schlatter disease and chondromalacia patellae may present with hip and/or knee pains, respectively. The overuse syndromes reported in juvenile athletes may also simulate growing pains but can be differentiated on the basis of history and temporal occurrence with sports activities.[92] Rarely, the presentation of the restless legs syndrome, although atypical in childhood, may be confused with the presentation of growing pains.[131]

Assessment

The most important assessment is not any laboratory examination but the performance of a careful history and physical examination.[98] The elements of such an examination should include the recording of vital signs (especially temperature), observation of the gait and range of motion, manual muscle testing, palpation for masses, measurement for a possible leg length discrepancy, assessment for limb swelling or other signs of inflammation, and overall evaluation of the psychological status of the child and parent-child interaction.

With a typical case of growing pains and a physician familiar with the condition, clinical acumen may be all that is required to make the diagnosis. Diagnostic tests are often undertaken when the presentations are less typical and/or as a matter of reassurance to the physician and parent alike.[76] Family physicians are more likely to order such tests (reportedly in up to 82% of such patients) than are pediatric subspecialists such as pediatric orthopedists and rheumatologists, who, according to one study, order diagnostic testing in only 59% of their patients.[76]

Complete blood counts and sedimentation rates are helpful but not absolute in excluding an infectious condition and/or a hematologic disorder. Serologic testing may be of help only in the presence of a generalized process. Bone scans and x-rays of the limbs may help to distinguish conditions in which there are structural changes in the bones and joints. Only rarely are tomography, arthroscopy, or magnetic resonance imaging (MRI) studies indicated.[98] Abnormalities on more generalized examinations such as an abnormal abdominal ultrasound and an elevated lactic dehydrogenase level are suggestive of a much more serious condition such as a malignancy.[26]

Pathophysiology

The cause of the discomfort in growing pains has not definitively been established. Both the presence of muscle spasm and structural injury to the muscle have been implicated.[1, 39] When local muscle ischemia is produced through repetitive actions, involuntary muscle spasm may occur. This process further exacerbates the reduction in blood flow to the area, with accumulation of metabolites that may further increase the discomfort, although electromyographic studies of such muscles are inconclusive in this regard. Conversely, repetitive muscle use may result in damage to the myofibrils, invoking an inflammatory response that is most intense at 24 to 48 hours following exercise.

Treatment

Inasmuch as this is a self-limiting and benign condition, the most important treatment is reassurance of the parent and child that a serious condition does not exist.

Analgesics may provide some transient relief. Heat may also provide some relief, but is relatively contraindicated in a young and sleepy child who may not appreciate development of a secondary skin lesion, i.e., a burn. Massage may be helpful inasmuch as it might stimulate local muscle circulation. The combination of reassurance, massage, and analgesia is utilized by approximately 37% of physicians, reassurance with massage by 30%, and reassurance with analgesia by 16%.[76]

Muscle stretching by parents may be a proactive way of decreasing the incidence of growing pains by increasing the local circulation to the muscles involved.[36] In a study by Baxter,[5] parents were instructed in a twice-daily, 10-minute regimen of stretching to the quadriceps, hamstrings, and gastrosoleus complex. In the treatment group, there was a decrease from an average of 10 episodes of pain per month to almost 0 by 3 months and 0 by 9 months after the initiation of treatment. In the control group, there was an average of 10 episodes of pain per month initially, and 2 episodes of pain per month persisted 18 months later. The mechanism of relief in the study was attributed to stretching resulting in increased blood flow to the muscles. However, the extra parental attention to the symptomatic child may have also played a role in the resolution of the complaints, given the association of this condition with emotional stressors.

Prognosis

Because this is a self-limited condition, the complaints eventually resolve with cessation of growth if not before. However, the anxiety associated with recurrent episodes and the loss of sleep on a chronic basis may have longer standing implications to the overall development of the child so affected.

Reflex Sympathetic Dystrophy

Clinical Features

Of the four conditions discussed in this chapter, the patient with reflex sympathetic dystrophy (RSD), now more commonly known as regional sympathetic pain syndrome, has the most severe limb pain and most guarded prognosis for recovery. This condition has also been termed as shoulder-hand syndrome, causalgia, reflex neurovascular dystrophy, Sudeck's atrophy, or most recently chronic regional pain syndrome type I. It may represent up to 11% of the cases of limb pain of unknown etiology that present in a pediatric orthopedic setting.[41] It is not a well-known entity in the pediatric literature, and prior to 1978, only 8 cases had been reported.[54] In this context, it is understandable that the average time from presentation to diagnosis has been reported as 9.2 months, with between one and three subspecialists being seen prior to diagnosis.[86, 118]

Unlike in the adult population, there is less likely to have been a precipitating traumatic event; indeed, such an event is found in only about one half of these cases in contrast to adults, in whom trauma almost uniformly has occurred.[67, 86] Out of 49 children with this diagnosis, 31 could recall such an event with the distribution as follows: 7 vehicular accidents, 15 sprains, 5 sports-related injuries, and 4 fractures and postoperative cases.[118] Other, more unusual precipitating insults include infection, thrombosis, foreign body, burn, animal bite, and frostbite.[43]

Unlike in the adult population, there appears to be a predominance of lower extremity involvement. In adults, the areas around the shoulders and hands are preferentially involved.[37] Involvement in pediatric cases occurs with the following distribution: foot and ankle (52%), knee (14%), arm (21%), shoulder (5%), and hand (8%).[37]

The pediatric patient presents with pain in a limb, classified as severe in 61% of the cases,[118] which is often out of proportion to the inciting event or to the physical findings.

Findings on physical examination reflect neurovascular dysfunction and include changes in skin color of the affected extremity with dependent rubor and mottling of the skin (60%), dependent edema (70%), hyperesthesias or hypoesthesia, alterations in skin temperature (either increased or decreased dependent upon the phase of the disease, 58%), reduction in peripheral pulses (16%), altered perspiration (14%), and changes in pattern of hair growth. Of these findings, dysesthesia with light touch is the most common, occurring in 87% of children.[37] Additionally, patients demonstrate weakness due to disuse rather than denervation and decreased range of motion with pain (7%). Trophic changes are present in only 2% of the cases, which is considerably less than in the adult population and which may correlate with the better prognosis in these patients than in adults.[12] A combination of disproportionate limb pain and three or more of the neurovascular signs are seen in at least 75% of the pediatric population.[118]

Another sign of autonomic dysfunction has been described by Dietz[37] and is known as tache cerebrale. On the affected limb, stroking of the skin with a blunt object evokes an erythematous line that persists for 15 to 30 minutes following onset of the stimulus.

In adults, three stages of the disorder have been described. The first is the acute stage, which begins at onset and lasts weeks to months. It is characterized by aching and burning, with the pain restricted to vascular, nerve root, or nerve distribution. The second or dystrophic stage begins about 3 months after onset with extension out of the original dermatome with swelling, hyperesthesia, and muscle wasting and osteopenia present. The chronic or atrophic stage may commence about 6 months after onset, with further exacerbation of the findings in the second stage, wasting of the limb, and further limitation in joint range.[79] Such clinical stages are less reliably described in the pediatric population.

This disorder has a female predominance with a 2:1 ratio in one study[118] and up to 6:1 ratio in others.[37] In adults, the condition occurs equally among men and women. The mean age of presentation is 11 years, with a range of from 3 to 17 years.[37]

Differential Diagnosis

As with the other conditions discussed in this chapter, the etiologies for limb pain in children are multiple. Unlike the other conditions, this is generally a unilateral and therefore asymmetrical condition that generates a differential diagnosis that would be in accordance with such symptoms. Of 38 cases presenting with limb pain and undetermined etiology to a pediatric orthopedic clinic, RSD was a common diagnosis. Other conditions elucidated following imaging and other medical work-up included osteoid osteoma, osteomyelitis, interarticular hemangiomata, slipped epiphyses, and rheumatoid variants. Less uncommon diagnoses included soft tissue hemangiomata, dystonia, and Addison's disease.[41]

Although trauma can present as the precipitating event, post-traumatic lesions may also present with foot and ankle pain and refusal to bear weight, but generally do not have the sudomotor symptoms that are attributable to RSD. Such conditions that may need to be considered include tarsal coalition, sprains, metatarsal, physeal and stress fractures, osteochondritis, and plantar fasciitis.[93] When involvement is localized about the knee, the presentation may be similar to the discomfort noted with chondromalacia patellae.

Space-occupying lesions in the spine may present with radicular findings, weakness, and dysesthesias. Nerve entrapment syndromes may simulate the clinical findings of RSD or may present as a concurrent diagnosis.[96] Patients may ultimately be found to have a tarsal tunnel syndrome or deep peroneal nerve entrapment as a cause of their pain.

Other potential diagnoses that have been cited for consideration in the literature include the following: juvenile rheumatoid arthritis, polymyositis, rheumatic fever, systemic lupus erythematosus, gout, thrombophlebitis, and compartment syndrome.[12]

Assessment

Clearly a good baseline examination of the musculoskeletal and neurovascular system is essential in delineating baseline deficits and response to treatment. This examination includes a determination of range of motion of the affected limb, peripheral pulses, sensory examination, motor power, and the like.

As for the other disorders in this chapter, assessment and diagnosis is largely clinical. There is no standardized test that can definitively diagnose the condition.

Routine blood tests as would be performed for children with limb pain such as complete blood count, sedimentation rate, antinuclear antibodies, and rheumatoid factor are uniformly unremarkable in this condition.

Plain films are obtained to rule out covert injury such as a stress fracture that could present in a similar manner. Such x-rays may also reveal osteopenia over time, probably related to decreased weight bearing in the extremity, but at the onset of the child's complaints osteopenia may not be present. In one study, osteopenia was noted in 15 of 38 radiographs. This frequency is less than the more consistent pattern of osteopenia seen in adults with this disorder and may reflect the increased metabolic activity of bone in growing children.[37] Bone scan results may also be variable[50] and again may help to differentiate the complaints from a stress fracture. Of 24 bone scans performed in the same study, 7 were normal, 11 revealed increased uptake, and 6 revealed decreased uptake.[118] Thus, a child with a normal bone scan is not excluded from this diagnosis.

Thermography may be a way of obtaining diagnostic information without invasive techniques or radiation exposure, certainly an important consideration in the growing child. It can rapidly demonstrate temperature differentials (either warmer or cooler) between the affected and unaffected limb. It takes only a few minutes to perform and may be used in a sequential manner to track responsiveness to physical therapy, medications, and other treatment modalities. [75, 97]

For patients who have significant weakness in a lower extremity and sensory deficits, it may be necessary to perform imaging studies of the spine to evaluate for a spinal mass or a herniated disc. If there is a question of an entrapment syndrome or other possible mechanisms for denervation, electrodiagnostic testing, including somatosensory evoked potentials, can be performed in order to evaluate for such conditions.

If the extremity is cool and peripheral pulses are diminished, especially with discoloration of the limb and edema, there may be suspicion of a vascular compromise of the involved extremity. In such cases, arterial and venous Doppler studies can be performed to better assess the circulation of the limb. It has recently been noted that unilaterally increased blood flow to soft tissue on power Doppler sonography may be confirmatory of a clinical diagnosis of RSD[90]; however, this is not a test that is readily available in most clinical settings.

In Murray's recent study[86] of 46 patients, 43 patients required diagnostic testing prior to diagnosis. Of these, 91% had x-ray studies, 65% had blood test(s), 37% had isotopic bone scans, 9% had ultrasound, 7% had computed tomography (CT) scans, and 13% had MRI studies. There was an average of 2.2 diagnostic studies per patient.

More obscure testing may better assess the autonomic function but is clinically not practical to perform. Resting sweat output, resting skin temperature, and quantitative sudomotor axon reflex test have been cited as diagnostic adjuncts. As a group, they may be predictive of the course of the disease and response to sympathetic block, should this be required.[30]

This condition is highly weighted with psychological issues, and a careful history should be taken in this regard.[112] Often there are periods of stress or change occurring in the life of the child such as parental separation, change in school, or other issues in regard to body image. Parental enmeshment with the child is quite common. Although most children perform well in school, they are often overestimated by their parents to be excellent rather than average students. A few of the cases reported also noted an underlying history of sexual abuse in the children. Concurrent diagnoses of conversion disorder and anorexia nervosa have also been reported.[115] Of 23 children with this diagnosis who underwent psychological assessment, 83% had what was considered as emotional dysfunction.[118] Families are often resistant to the notion that a concurrent emotional problems may be a precipitating or exacerbating factor. They may take offense and feel that although the patient has clear physical findings, he or she is perceived by the medical staff as malingering or having a conversion reaction. Psychological support may be accepted by the patient and parents only if it is presented as a tool for dealing with the severe and abrupt curtailment of the child's usually active physical lifestyle rather than as a separate issue.

Pathophysiology

It is still uncertain if this clinical entity is a result of sympathetic nervous system dysfunction due to increased sympathetic tone as a response to the presence of musculoskeletal pain. Simply, as explained by Schwartzman,[109] an abnormal firing of peripheral nerves, likely related to antecedent soft tissue trauma, occurs due to increased sensitivity of these nerves. There may develop abnormal synapses between sensory afferents and sympathetic efferents, establishing a sort of vicious circle for the perpetuation of pain.[40] This process results in an alteration of the usual response of the spinal cord neuronal pool to the influences of the cortical and brainstem ramifications with dysfunction occurring within the central nervous system as well. The reader is referred to additional sources for other possible explanations, which include the brainstem acting as a "central biasing mechanism" with an inhibitory influence on transmission at synaptic levels[80] and the presence of local sympathetic nervous system overactivity.[64]

Treatment

Treatment is challenging at best, and a large menu of choices is available. The best treatment involves early recognition. If the chronic state of the disease is present and more than 6 to 8 weeks have elapsed since onset, cure may be elusive. Lack of movement and immobilization due to the discomfort would be the choice of most acutely involved patients but this is counterproductive,[12] although up to 50% of patents may initially be treated in this manner.[86] Splinting is utilized only to prevent progressive deformity such as an equinovarus attitude of the foot, or to provide support when there is weakness in a specific muscle group such as the ankle dorsiflexors.

Standard analgesic and anti-inflammatory agents are of little help except as an adjunct to primary therapeutic intervention.

In adults, corticosteroids have been noted to make an improvement in up to 90% of the cases.[65] However, such treatment is rarely if ever utilized in the pediatric population, and the risk-benefit ratio of this treatment has not been determined.[61]

Anticonvulsant drugs with central mediation of pain perception may be utilized for pain control. Initially, phenytoin was used. The mechanism of effect was thought to be related to its ability to regulate and/or stabilize hyperexcitability in both peripheral and central neurons and to facilitate inhibitory mechanisms.[29] Subsequently, carbamazepine was utilized because of a similar mode of action. However, both medications required serial blood tests to determine lack of suppression of the bone marrow, liver function, and therapeutic blood level, which was certainly arduous in the younger population. More recently, gabapentin, also an anticonvulsant, has been utilized for this purpose with a similar clinical efficacy.[79] However, because the incidence of side effects is lower, monitoring of laboratory parameters is less of an issue. Nevertheless, the child still needs to be monitored for side effects, which include sleepiness, dizziness, ataxia, and fatigue.

Both nifedipine, a calcium channel blocker, and phenoxybenzamine, an alpha-channel blocker, have been utilized in adults with RSD.[85] However, their use has not been extended to children, likely out of concern for evoking hypotension, in a group that already has low blood pressures.

The use of EMLA cream, a topical anesthetic agent, has been reported in the literature for treatment for RSD.[99] It may permit some increased desensitization and allow for transient periods of weight-bearing that otherwise might not be possible. However, the need for reapplication and other technical considerations does not permit it to be employed as a long-term treatment strategy.

Local injections to the affected limb are rarely if ever utilized and steroids are rarely prescribed, as is common in adults with shoulder-hand syndrome. Regional sympathetic blockades are used very infrequently in cases otherwise resistant to treatment in the stellate ganglia to control upper extremity pain and in the lumbar region to control lower extremity pain.[95] The initial procedure may be performed as much for diagnostic purposes as it is for pain relief. When performed, the procedure is occasionally done over a series of days on three occasions on an inpatient basis with intensive inpatient physical therapy interspersed between procedures to enhance their efficacy. Complications include Horner's syndrome, hoarseness, and potential pneumothorax with stellate ganglion blocks, and backache with lumbar sympathetic blocks, and hypotension and allergic reaction to the blocking agents such as xylocaine used at either site. Infection and bleeding at the site of injections are also possibilities.[120] In one case in the literature, thoracoscopic electrocauterization of the thoracic sympathetic ganglion at the level of T3 resulted in resolution of symptoms in an 11-year-old girl with RSD.[58]

Spinal cord stimulation has been utilized in the adult population.[59] This technique has not been extended to the pediatric population, and does not appear to be necessary for children, who generally have a better prognosis.

Physical and occupational therapy are the mainstay of treatment. With prompt recognition, immediate referral rather than plaster immobilization from the emergency department should occur.[6] Intervention techniques may include desensitizing massage, progressive weight-bearing beginning with tilt table to initiate the process, gross motor activities, hydrotherapy to augment range of motion, weight-bearing in a gravity-eliminated setting, passive and gentle active assistive range of motion to the affected joints, and use of an adapted bicycle to encourage reciprocal lower extremity movements.

However, in order to be effective, therapy may need to be performed on intensive inpatient basis under the supervision of a multidisciplinary team,[118] with physical therapy being performed two to three times daily. The average length of stay for such a regimen is 21 days, with a range from 7 days to 7 weeks.[12] If emotional stressors are contributory, this strategy also permits the child to be taken out of the home environment, to a place where the medical issues can be more readily resolved.

Traditional therapy may be augmented by the use of transcutaneous nerve stimulation.[99b] When combined with a traditional physical therapy program, 7 out of 10 pediatric patients had full remission of their symptoms within a 2-month period.[61] The mechanism for pain relief is believed to be based on the gate control theory of pain as elaborated by Melzack and Wall.[80] More specifically, by stimulation of large type A afferent fibers, there will be increased inhibition of the cells of the substantia gelatinosa, and a blockage of pain transmission will occur. Massage may be helpful by invoking a similar mechanism.[37]

The use of acupuncture in the pediatric population is beginning to be explored. Tolerance for treatment with needle insertion, heat/moxa, magnets, and cupping was better even in the younger patient. Although the study presented was not controlled and there may be elements of a placebo effect, a good initial response to treatment in the five juvenile patients with RSD was reported.[60] This should not be considered as the mainstay of treatment. Other adjuncts to primary care with physical therapy include biofeedback, guided imagery, and relaxation.

Prognosis

In general the prognosis with noninvasive and nonpharmacologic treatment is good, with success being noted in 78% of cases.[37]

The average time to recovery as reported by Stanton[118] was 9 months with a range of 1 to 36 months noted. The results reported by Murray[86] are significantly reduced, with recovery occurring in an average of 7 weeks (with a range of 1 to 140 weeks) From 5% to 33% of the patients developed subsequent recurrences in the previously affected or a different limb.[86] Approximately 33% had persistent limitations in functional activities at the conclusion of the study. Younger patients and those with an initially colder limb temperature may be at greater risk for recurrences.[127] This is still a better prognosis than that offered for adults.[37]

Young female patients may have a higher risk of severe complications of RSD, especially when there is involvement of a lower extremity.[124] Their cold limbs appear to be more resistant to therapeutic interventions, and a chronic problem may be perpetuated. Additional problems may include secondary infection, ulcers, chronic edema, focal dystonia, and myoclonus, each of which require additional treatment. Baclofen (Lioresal) may need to be employed for the spasms and dystonia that occur.[108]

Hypermobility Syndrome

Clinical Features

Joint hypermobility, in the absence of specific diagnoses such as Marfan, Ehlers-Danlos, or Larsen's syndromes,[71] may still be responsible for diffuse joint pain that results in limitation of activities of the child and adolescent, may be associated with other medical and developmental issues, and may predispose the adult patient to osteoarthritis and increasing functional limitations. This condition was first described by Sutro[121] in young adults presenting with pain in their hypermobile ankles with associated effusions. The hypermobility syndrome was defined by Kirk[62] and was characterized by excessive movement of the joints with musculoskeletal pain attributable to such movement, in the absence of systemic rheumatologic disease or other identifiable syndromes.

The incidence of generalized joint hypermobility in children and adolescence varies with different racial and sexual norms having been established. In a group of white children in England, ages 6 to 11 years, the incidence was 10.5%.[28] This is close to the figures reported by Gedalia[46] as 12% when multiple joints are evaluated according to the criteria noted in the following discussion. Children of Asian ancestry have a higher rate, which may approach 25% in the preschool population. African American children have a rate of ligamentous laxity that is less than 5% and may be related to the slightly earlier onset of achieving gross motor skills. When the incidence of hypermobility in a single joint is assessed, the incidence may be in excess of 47% in the hands of musicians.[68]

The patient population with hypermobility is not always symptomatic, and many may remain without any pain or other manifestations of this disorder. However, a certain subset of the population will develop the syndrome, estimated to be in the range of 40% to 50% of the total.[2, 47] In a group of juvenile patients presenting with joint pain without a recognizable etiology, up to 66% may have joint hypermobility. This presentation has been termed juvenile episodic arthralgia/arthritis.[46] This means that the children so involved may present with joint pain with or without swelling, limitation of range, or pain/tenderness to palpation.

Differential Diagnosis

The list of conditions that cause ligamentous laxity often associated with hypotonia is legion and will not be discussed in detail in this context. Excluded from the diagnoses are those conditions in which a clear syndrome is associated with ligamentous laxity such as in those children with trisomy 21 or Marfan's syndrome. Also excluded are those children who are lax and hypotonic due to underlying and clinically significant weaknesses in their limbs, especially those who cannot lift their limbs against gravity. Such children need to be evaluated in terms of a primary central nervous system disorder such as an anterior horn cell disease (spinal muscular atrophy) or a congenital or other myopathy.

Assessment

Assessment of joint hypermobility can be performed in a variety of ways, including utilization of a machine to measure resistance to passive stretch. However, the criteria developed by Carter[27] and Beighton[7] are most often employed. Those patients who demonstrate three of the five following criteria are accepted as having joint hypermobility. These include the following:

- Ability to hyperextend the fingers so that they lie parallel to the extensor surface of the forearm
- Ability to oppose the thumb to the surface of the forearm
- Ability to hyperextend the elbows to greater than 10 degrees
- Ability to hyperextend the knees greater than 10 degrees
- Ability to forward flex the trunk with the knees unbent, so that the palms rest on the floor

History may be helpful in assessing the population at risk, inasmuch as there is an increased risk of developmental dysplasia of the hip in such patients.

The symptomatic child will need to be assessed for pain and/or swelling of the joints, most commonly occurring at the knee in up to 46% of the cases.[44] Only one or two joints may be involved. The frequency of other joint involvement is as follows: the small joints of the hands (40%); hips, elbows, and feet (each with an incidence of 20%–26%); and the shoulder, mid-back, and temporomandibular joints (each with an incidence of 7%). Pain may occur spontaneously, following exercise, or in association with a growth spurt. As pain is evoked, it is more likely to occur in the late afternoon and evening, different from the morning stiffness characteristic of juvenile rheumatoid arthritis.

Most of the patients who present do so from early childhood. However, a certain group of children and adolescents may develop a more isolated form of ligamentous laxity over time due to repetitive injuries such as those sustained by young dancers.

Given the presentation of multiple joint involvement and joint swelling, laboratory and imaging studies need to be performed to exclude the possibility of a more serious rheumatic disorder, infection, or skeletal neoplasm, as is discussed in the section on growing pains. In one rheumatology clinic where these children were evaluated, the typical diagnostic tests performed included complete blood count, sedimentation rate, rheumatoid factor, antinuclear antibodies, quantitative immunoglobulins, and complement studies, and an ophthalmologic examination, the latter to rule out an association of pauciarticular juvenile rheumatoid arthritis with uveitis.[44]

These patients should have a full neurologic examination as a part of their initial assessment. Patients with Down syndrome are noted to be at risk for subluxation of the cervical spine due to ligamentous laxity, which can predispose them to a myelopathy over time. Potentially, this population is at risk although there is no frank evidence of such in the literature. Certainly any patient with hyperreflexia or any considering contact sports or other activities in which there may be forceful flexion and extension of the neck should be considered for flexion/extension views of the cervical spine. Those patients with lower back pain should have similar imaging studies there to assess for disk protrusion or instabilities, especially if there are ambulatory difficulties or signs of pyramidal tract dysfunction. Lastly, the instability of the joints may predispose certain juveniles to the development of nerve entrapment syndrome. Those patients who have localized pain and sensory deficits should be considered for such an associated diagnosis, such as carpal and tarsal tunnel syndromes.

The patients who are confirmed as having joint hypermobility syndrome should also be assessed for the nonarticular manifestations of the disorder. If a collagen abnormality does exist, it is likely to be present in other parts of the body and would explain the increased risk of mitral valve prolapse in such patients. Mitral valve prolapse may be associated with the development of pain attacks, and these may also be increased in frequency in this population.[78] Other potential complications include increased stretchiness of the skin with increased concern about postsurgical wound healing, and increased laxity of skin about the eyes.[83]

Children with such a condition also need to be assessed in terms of their overall development. There may a delay of early gross motor development in a certain subset of 15% to 17% of this population, including the onset of ambulation. Concurrent delays in fine motor skills may also be documented.[33] Such delays may prompt referral for early intervention services to increase overall strength and coordination. If fine motor delays persist into school age, performance issues become more problematic.

Certain presenting complaints are architectural and relate to pain in the small joints of the hands when writing for longer periods of time, necessitating built-up handles on writing instruments and untimed tests. However, in clinical practice, some perceptual motor deficits may coexist. The reason for their existence is speculative and may relate to a decrease in input from unstretched muscle spindles, which result in proprioceptive and motor planning issues. Such deficits may be amenable to treatment with sensory integration techniques as developed by Jean Ayres.

Pathophysiology

The joint laxity and hyperextensibility that exists is for the most part considered as the upper limit of normal for the general population, with various racial and sex norms recognized as noted earlier.[44] With maturation, and probably with myelination of the nervous system, there tends to be a gradual increase in tone to the normal range, with some improvement possible extending into adulthood. The tendency for tone to improve may also be explained by the tendency of type I collagen to stiffen with age.[31]

Other investigators think that this clinical presentation actually represents abnormalities in the collagen structure that are not yet identified. This information is abstracted by the studies of other connective tissue diseases such as in Ehlers-Danlos syndrome, in which an abnormality exists in the structure of type I or type III collagen.[52, 123] Errors in genes such as collagens IX (COL 9A1, 9A2, and 9A3), XI (COL 11A1 and 11A2), and V (COL 5A1 and 5A2) have been implicated in this process.

Regardless of the quality of the collagen, there is probably excessive motion at the joint, with stretching of the capsule and the ligaments and the soft tissue around it. This results in localized injuries, the pain sensors in these structures are stimulated, and the discomfort occurs.

Treatment

The first step in treatment is identification of the ligamentous laxity, with counseling of parents and children in regard to joint protection techniques so that joint pain does not occur, or, if present, does not exacerbate. For the child younger than 5 years of age, there is a good chance that the problems will resolve with age and little may be required other than watchful waiting. "W" sitting, which places excessive stress on the capsular structures about the hip, should be avoided, and the younger child should be frequently repositioned. Party tricks involving repetitive stressing of the joints, and dislocations of joints and contortions to exhibit other aspects of hypermobility, should be strongly discouraged.

When discomfort does occur, treatment with a mild analgesic such as acetaminophen should be considered in the proper dosage for age and weight. According to Gedalia,[44] nonsteroidal anti-inflammatory agents should not be employed as the first line of treatment because there is no inflammation associated with this disorder.

Patients and parents should be instructed in joint protection techniques. Warm-up exercises that avoid stretching should be avoided because these only compound the problem. However, strengthening exercises for the muscles around the joints may help to compensate for lack of stability due to loose ligaments. Because the knee is the most common site at which signs and symptoms occur, strengthening of the quadriceps with setting and progressive resistive exercises is especially effective. Nonimpact activities such as swimming should also be endorsed.[74] High-impact sports such as football may need to be discouraged, even if taping of the joints or other strategies are suggested by coaches, although definitive recommendations await further clarification.[34] Orthotics for lower extremity alignment and derotational braces for more aggressive activities may need to be considered in some.

However, injuries may need to be treated. Children with ligamentous laxity are more likely to sustain an extension supracondylar fracture of the humerus in a fall on an outstretched arm rather than the usual distal forearm fracture. These include recurrent subluxations and dislocation of joints, ligamentous and muscle tears including epicondylitis and plantar fasciitis, and low back pain due to lumbar disk prolapse, defects of the pars interarticularis, and spondylolisthesis.[52]

Prognosis

The hypermobility syndrome itself is not a dangerous or life-threatening condition. It is also a bit of a double-edged sword, inasmuch as the hypermobility of some children and adolescents is what permits them to perform well as musicians, dancers, and acrobats.[69] However, patients so affected may be at increased risk of ligamentous injuries, especially during sports activities. In a study of football players with hypermobility of the joints, the risk of ligamentous knee injury was eightfold greater than in the non-lax population.[91] Hypermobile ballet dancers also exhibit an increased risk for injury.[63] The actual prognosis is not determined during childhood but rather is dependent upon the increased risk of osteoarthritis that occurs in predisposed adults.[13, 110]

Fibromyalgia

Clinical Features

Fibromyalgia in children in some sectors has been considered as a diagnosis of dubious value, although objective parameters do exist for diagnosis. The criteria for general diagnosis of fibromyalgia as developed by the American College of Rheumatology define the condition as being one with chronic widespread musculoskeletal pain and fatigue without associated inflammation of at least 3 months' duration. Pain must be bilateral, exist above and below the waist, and involve the axial skeleton. More specifically, there should be tenderness to palpation with a pressure of 4 kilograms in at least 11 of 18 sites located symmetrically throughout the body. These sites are described as follows[135]:

- At the occiput, at the insert of trapezius, sternocleiodomastoid, splenius capitus, and/or semispinalis capotis muscles
- At the lower cervical region, at the level of C5 through C7
- At the upper border of the trapezius
- At or near the medial border of the supraspinatus
- Lateral to the costochondral junction of the second rib
- Two centimeters lateral to the lateral epicondyle
- At the anterior edge of the gluteus maximus
- Posterior to the greater trochanter
- At the medial fat pad proximal to the joint line of the knee

The initial descriptions in the literature discussed an adult population, but involvement of juveniles with similar findings was first described in 1985,[139] with multiple reports following. Descriptions vary greatly in terms of incidence figures that may largely be due to the ethnicity and sociopsychological composition of the groups studied. In an assessment of 338 Israeli children, 21 or 6.2% had the diagnosis of fibromyalgia when the aforementioned criteria were employed.[24] However, a study of Mexican children reported an incidence of only 1.2% in children.[32]

Although fibromyalgia is considered an unusual diagnosis, between 7.65% and 45% of the total number of pediatric patients seen in a private rheumatology referral practice carried the diagnosis.[101, 113]

Most pediatric patients with this disorder are female. In the study by Siegel,[113] 41 of 45 of the patients were female. Of this group, 42 were white, although the ethnic/racial distribution of the surrounding community was not noted. The average age of presentation in this group was 13.3 years.

Of the presenting symptoms, over 90% of pediatric patients present with diffuse musculoskeletal pain and sleep disturbances.[113] The musculoskeletal pain is characterized by polymyalgias, and polyarthralgias without swelling or warmth of the affected joints. Other presenting features include headaches in 71%, generalized fatigue in

62%, and morning stiffness in 53%. Other presentations may include difficulty concentrating in school, paresthesias, recurrent abdominal pain sometimes in conjunction with a prior history of irritable bowel syndrome, and/or dizziness.[107] Of a total of a possible 15 symptoms reported by Siegel,[113] most patients had an average of 8 upon presentation.

As described in adults, multiple tender points are present upon examination. These are fewer in number and require more application of pressure than the criteria expressed for adults, possibly because the diagnosis is made earlier in the disease process or because there is an intrinsic difference in the disorder in the younger population. In contrast to adults, where 11 tender points must be present to establish the diagnosis, children and adolescents present with an average of 9.7.[113]

Because this is not an inflammatory disease, the findings of fever, rash, synovitis, or nodules are not seen. There is certainly no evidence of pleuritis or pericarditis, which may exist in some of the more severe systemic cases of juvenile rheumatoid arthritis. In some patients, confusion may exist because juvenile rheumatoid arthritis and fibromyalgia have been reported to exist concurrently.[107] This situation should be considered in patients who do not respond as anticipated to standard pharmacologic treatment for their inflammatory arthritis. Because this is not a neurologic disorder, there are no reflex changes or fixed changes in sensation, although paresthesias have been reported. Weakness and decrease in range of motion may exist as a secondary finding due to inactivity, disuse, and guarding, but there are no focal or unilateral findings. Specific criteria for the amount of reduction and/or strength have not been quantified in the pediatric literature.

Sleep disturbances may include restlessness (especially of the legs), bruxism, somnambulism, and sleep talking.

As in the adult population, there is a significant comorbidity of fibromyalgia in children with depression and irritability, but the depression is not the primary diagnosis.[81] On the basis of clinical findings and projective testing, the incidence of depression in these patients has been reported to be as high as 45.5% of the total population, in contrast with the general pediatric population, in which an incidence figure of 9.7% has been reported.[38] Such changes are not only reported by the patients but are confirmed with consistency by the observations of parents and teachers. In addition to an increased number of anxiety and depressive symptoms, Vandvik reported that children with fibromyalgia had higher than usual desire to achieve academically, high parental expectations, and a higher than usual frequency of parents with chronic diseases.[125] Buskila[22] reported that there is a familial incidence of fibromyalgia in 28% of offspring of patients who are so affected. The contributions of psychological and genetic factors to this incidence are unclear. The average IQ in such a group has been reported as normal.

Despite the presence of clear diagnostic criteria, this is not a diagnosis that is readily made in the pediatric or physiatric community. Up to 67% of patients in one study were seen by three or more physicians prior to diagnosis, and up to 60% may be given an erroneous diagnosis of juvenile rheumatoid arthritis.[101]

Related Conditions and Differential Diagnoses

Hypermobility syndrome is a common associated finding, although a specific ligamentous laxity syndrome need not be identified. Such children have migratory joint pains without swelling, likely due to ligamentous instability with stretching of the joint capsules. Such children will demonstrate their hyperextensibility by demonstrating three or more out of five of the following criteria[28]:

• Hyperextension of the fingers so that they lie parallel with the extensor forearm
• Apposition of the thumbs to lie parallel with the forearms
• Greater than 10 degrees of hyperextension at the elbows
• Greater than 10 degrees of hyperextension of the knees (i.e., genu recurvatum)
• Ability of the child to rest palms on the floor when performing forward flexion

Forty percent of the patients studied by Siegel[113] carried this concurrent diagnosis, and 33% carried the diagnosis of patellofemoral pain syndrome. In an earlier study of 338 children, 43 or 13% were found to have joint hypermobility and 21 or 6% had fibromyalgia. Of the patients with fibromyalgia, 17 or 81% had joint hypermobility and 17 or 40% of the patients with joint hypermobility had fibromyalgia.[48] Findings of fibromyalgia have also been reported with some of the more specific syndromes associated with ligamentous laxity such as the Ehlers-Danlos syndrome.[82]

The chronic fatigue syndrome and fibromyalgia overlap to some extent in both the pediatric and the adult population in terms of presenting symptoms in up to 29.6% of the chronic fatigue syndrome patients.[8] Patients with chronic fatigue syndrome also have complaints of recurrent pharyngitis (in 54%), recurrent adenopathy (in 33%), and recurrent fever (in 28%).[20, 137] In this group, an association has been made with infection with the Epstein-Barr virus. It is therefore of interest that there also may be an association of fibromyalgia with infectious mononucleosis. It is unclear if the fatigue that exists in these patients is due to primary muscular dysfunction or is mediated centrally.

Lyme disease is an infection produced by a tick vector transporting a spirochetal infection. Especially but not exclusively in the northeastern United States, a child who presents with diffuse joint pain will be assessed for this diagnosis. Patients with active disease also have a variety of neurologic, dermatologic, cardiac, and systemic signs and symptoms. Of a study of 488 patients referred to Lyme disease clinics, 23% had active disease, and 20% had evidence of previous infection and another acute process, of which fibromyalgia was the most common. This was especially true in the subgroup of patients who did not respond to antibiotic therapy as would be anticipated.[119] These findings are also supported by a previous study by Sigal,[114] in which 20% of the suspect population was diagnosed with fibromyalgia. Some authors consider those patients with evidence of prior disease as having fibromyalgia as a complication of their previous acute intercurrent infection, although full documentation is not available.

Other acute infectious processes, especially viral illnesses, have been associated with the development of fibromyalgia in children and in adults. One such example is the association of acute mononucleosis, which can occur with an Epstein-Barr virus infection, with findings of fibromyositis in patients acutely in 19% of the total at presentation but only in 3% and 1% at 2 and 6 months following diagnosis.[99a] Other viral infections having an association with this disorder include human immunodeficiency virus,[117] hepatitis C,[25] parvovirus,[88] and coxsackievirus.[73] Such diagnoses should be considered if clinical symptoms dictate. Symptoms of arthralgias and diffuse joint pains have been reported in children following administration of the rubella vaccine. The U.S. Court of Federal Claims has supported this association when signs and symptoms have their onset between 1 and 6 weeks following vaccine administration.[133]

In additional to the aforementioned juvenile rheumatoid arthritis, other conditions that are considered include growing pains, hysteria, and psychological problems.[101] There is a higher than anticipated incidence of emotional stressors, such as final examinations, familial separation, and childhood sexual abuse,[130] the latter occurring in up to 37% of the overall population.[15] The incidence of eating disorders in the population is also increased to 10% vs. 3% in the general population. Accordingly, psychological, nutritional, social services, and possibly gynecological support services are required in certain pediatric patients with this diagnosis.

The family should be assessed for presence of the disorder in other members. In Roizenblatt's study of 34 children, 71% of the mothers were affected, although previously undiagnosed.[100] In a study by Yunus, 74% of siblings, 53% of children, and 39% of parents had a history of the disorder, suggesting a possible inheritance by human leukocyte antigen (HLA) typing.[100]

Assessment

No standard laboratory tests are positive in this disorder, but negative results do assist in excluding other potential differential diagnoses.

The anemia, elevated white count, elevated sedimentation rate, and thrombocytosis that are seen with juvenile rheumatoid arthritis should not be seen unless there is the rare state where both diseases coexist. Similarly, liver function tests should be normal. Because there is no generalized systemic inflammatory disease, there should be no evidence of uveitis or iritis upon slit-lamp examination. Serologic testing for rheumatoid factor and antinuclear antibody testing should also be unrevealing.[107] Lyme disease titers reflective of an infection with *Borrelia burgdorferi* should be negative but may be positive in the crossover group with prior evidence of disease but no active infections.[119]

Dolorimetry is not an assessment that is commonly conducted in the pediatric population; however, patients with this condition do exhibit abnormal results as indicated earlier. Implementation of an easily scaled pain survey for children may help quantify their discomfort and subsequently document responses to treatment.[126] The use of the visual analogue scale for pain grading is developmentally suitable for the younger population and can be reproduced by staff members.[51] The amount of pain has not been correlated with issues of time management of both parent and child or with changes in the functional status of such children. However, from the physiatric viewpoint, documentation of pain is certainly relevant. There is no description in the literature of specific changes in functional status, but the use of the Functional Independence Measure (FIM) or the Wee-FIM for children younger than 7 years of age should provide insight into this topic and should perhaps be studied prospectively.[53]

Sleep studies are not clinically indicated for this disorder but have been described in the literature and help to document the nature of the disorder.[84] Electroencephalographic monitoring during sleep revealed an absence of stage 4 sleep as characterized by the presence of an alpha rhythm in non–rapid eye movement (non-REM) sleep. Similar findings and complaints including muscle hypersensitivity could be induced in sleep-deprived controls. A more recent study[122] also described prolonged sleep latency, shortened total sleep time, decreased sleep efficiency, and increased wakefulness during sleep. Thirty-eight[38] percent also demonstrated an increase in periodic limb movements. No evidence of sleep apnea was documented. The relationship to the underlying physiology of fibromyalgia has not been characterized, but there may be an association with treatment with antidepressant medications, with which some children are treated.

As noted previously, children may exhibit dizziness as a part of this disorder. Although this is clinically disconcerting, extensive testing of 12 affected children failed to reveal any abnormalities of vestibular function.[104] Electronystagmography and sinusoidal harmonic acceleration rotary child testing were within normal limits for all patients so studied. The mechanism for the subjective complaints could not be elucidated, but it was speculated that the patients' muscular dysfunction, especially of the muscles in the cervical area, might result in alterations of proprioception that cause a feeling of imbalance. No findings of orthostasis due to a sedentary lifestyle were documented.

Although the clinical significance is not known, the presence of antipolymer antibodies has been described. These are also seen in the blood of patients with a variety of rheumatologic conditions including osteoarthritis, myopathy, lupus, and systemic sclerosis.[135]

Pathophysiology

Studies of the pathophysiology are limited and have not been specifically studied in the juvenile population as a separate group. Most of the inferences are drawn from the adult literature, which is discussed elsewhere in this text. The incipient event that triggers the onset of fibromyalgia is still unidentified. The common thread from multiple research studies is deemed to be a dysfunction of the neuroendocrine axis.

Cortical motor dysfunction has been described as being abnormal on single and double magnetic stimulation in patients with this disorder.[105] This finding implies that there may be a disturbance in perception of pain centrally as the genesis of the subjective complaints. These findings are not specific to this disorder and have also been reported in patients with rheumatoid arthritis and other chronic painful conditions.

The previously mentioned sleep disturbances may provide a clue as to the pathophysiology of the syndrome. Growth hormone is secreted during stage 4 of sleep. Patients with fibromyalgia have disruption of stage 4 or delta sleep, such that it is possible that less growth hormone is produced by the patients, which correlates with the development of their musculoskeletal pain.[10] Low insulin growth factors have been reported and are thought to be due to a similar mechanism.

A decreased level of serotonin has been documented in patients with fibromyalgia. It is a neurotransmitter that is believed to modulate pain in inhibition.[102] Aberrations in serotonin metabolism have been implicated in the coexistence of fibromyalgia and depression.[102] Adults with fibromyalgia have had positive results in a dexamethasone suppression test, but this finding has not been demonstrated in the pediatric population specifically.

Substance P is a neurotransmitter that is associated with enhanced pain sensation. Studies have noted a threefold increase in this chemical in the cerebrospinal fluid of patients with this disorder.[103]

A reduction in the overall production of cortisol has been noted, which is the antithesis of the findings seen in depressed patients. This finding may explain the patients' poor reactions to stress and the exacerbation of their symptoms at such times.[35] This finding may also be related to the postural hypotension that is experienced in a subset of these patients.[16]

Outcome

In general, the outcome of this disorder is reported as more favorable than in the adult population.[45] This finding may be due to an intrinsic difference in the condition in the younger population or to more prompt recognition and initiation of treatment when the disorder is still less severe. Buskila[23] studied patients over a period of 2.5 years, during which it was reported that 11 of 15 of the patients studied or 73% were no longer considered to have the disease on the basis of the aforementioned diagnostic criteria. In this group, the tenderness threshold of painful sites increased from 4.1 to 6.8 kilograms, and the number of tender points decreased from an average of 11.4 to 3.4. This finding contrasts with the reports in the adult literature, in which from 60% to 85% of adults report continuation of symptoms at a 3- to 4-year period.[42, 72]

In the group of patients studied by Siegel,[113] patients studied over a 2-year period noted an improvement of 4.8 points on a scale from 1 to 10, where 10 represented their most severe pain experienced.

Although this finding is generally accepted as the rule, there is a more negative study as reported by Malleson,[77] who noted a similar finding as in the adult population, with 61% of patients lacking in improvement over a period of up to 4 years. However, the population reported on was heterogeneous and included children with RSD and other uncharacterized disorders.

Treatment Options

The most important treatment in this disorder is to provide reassurance to the patient and his or her family that this is not a more serious or life-threatening disorder, regardless of the degree of discomfort and dysfunction with which the child may present. With this firmly in mind, and with a positive outlook, compliance with treatment program should not be problematic. Effective coping strategies can then be employed.[106]

Because the disease course is relatively self-limited in children in contrast to the adult population, treatment is generally not as intense and long lasting, and appears to have more positive results.

Most treatment regimens provide a combined approach of exercise in moderation, use of antidepressants, and use of nonsteroidal anti-inflammatory agents.

The exercise program chosen should be nonstressful and include rest periods to prevent exacerbation of fatigue. In general, components of slow stretching exercises and strengthening exercises should be utilized. Strengthening exercises need to be performed at least three times weekly (preferably more) in order for them to have a cumulative beneficial effect. Stretching exercises and very vigorous sports should not be performed in the subgroup of the population with associated ligamentous laxity.[66] These children already have too much mobility at the joints and this does not need to be increased; joint instability and pain may occur with such activities, which may further increase their already significant risk of early degenerative joint disease. For similar reasons, high-impact activities should be avoided. Other activities that can be performed include walking, use of a treadmill at a slow speed with close adult supervision in the younger age group, use of a stationary bicycle, and exercises in a pool of the appropriate depth. Again, the latter should be undertaken with close adult supervision given the age of the patients. Initially, given the inconsistencies of childhood, the program should be performed under the direct supervision of a physical therapist. Some younger patients may perform better with their parents in the room and others may perform better when they are excluded. Parents should be taught to supervise a home exercise program. For the younger and uninspired patient, an exercise calendar, possibly with a sticker or other reward system, should be devised.

Heat is not employed as a modality for several reasons. First, in the younger child there are inaccurate reports of pain and temperature that might result in thermal injury. This may be compounded by the child's complaints of paresthesias that alter sensory perception. Lastly, heat is sedating and may exacerbate the fatigue that is already problematic. There is little discussion in the literature of the use of other modalities. In an isolated report of one patient with fibromyalgia localized to one lower extremity, the use of two perifacetal injections of local anesthetics and steroids and application of transcutaneous nerve stimulation was noted to provide significant relief, but this is not the usual treatment methodology employed.[4]

Massage may be of benefit in providing pain relief. In a study of the combined population of patients, such treatment relieved pain in 37% of the population and decreased the amount of reported depression and need for analgesia.[19] Such treatment is likely transient, and prolonged benefit for a period extending over 3 months has not been documented. More aggressive ischemic compression and spinal manipulation[55] should be avoided in this group due to inconsistencies in children's reports of pain, and more importantly due to risk of vascular compromise of the immature pediatric spinal cord. This is a risk factor in patients who have relatively strong vertebrae resistant to fracture, but with pliant ligaments that can be the site of movement.

Prolonged periods of rest should be avoided, and the child should be mobilized as early as tolerated following an intercurrent illness in order to avoid the secondary deleterious effects of such lack of activity. Bed rest has been associated with about a 2% decline in muscle power per day, with an overall loss of 40% to 60% of strength after a 4- to 6-week period,[14] with significant atrophy and ultrastructural changes occurring.

Given the components of headache, musculoskeletal pain, and emotional distress, the use of relaxation exercises can also be of assistance in this patient group. Utilization of developmentally appropriate techniques of progressive muscle relaxation, mental imagery, hypnosis, and centering may provide additional relief.[57, 129]

Good sleep hygiene is important, and sleep time should be regulated, and should be without lights or other disturbances. Vigorous exercise, caffeine, and other stimulants should not be utilized within several hours of retiring.[107]

The injection of trigger points and the use of acupuncture, which are discussed in the adult literature, are not commented on in pediatric-related publications and are not utilized on any consistent basis.

Due to fatigue and discomfort, school performance may be suboptimal and, as previously noted, may be suggestive of an attention deficit disorder. Once psychological testing is performed and this diagnosis is ruled out, other adaptations may still need to be made in terms of school placement and other accommodations. Direct medical services are not guaranteed, but related services as they are needed to maximize the learning and mobility of the child are guaranteed under U.S. Public Law 94-142. Such services may include bus transportation, provision of an extra set of books, exemption from or modification of physical education classes, provision of extra time on tests, rest periods, administration of medications by the school nurse, and provision of physical and occupational therapy and supportive counseling. With parental and student permission, an explanation of the disorder by the patient or health care professional should do much to enhance peer acceptance.

Salicylates are not indicated and children do not respond to them when they are administered for this condition.[101] Nonsteroidals have usually been administrated with limited relief even prior to the diagnosis of the disorder. Although they can be employed for intermittent relief, adjuncts to this treatment are usually required by the time that the diagnosis is finally made.

Cyclobenzaprine (Flexeril) is a medication that is utilized for the relief of muscle spasms. Its method of action is thought to be the reduction of tonic somatic motor activities of the gamma and alpha systems, but exactly how it relates to fibromyalgia specifically is unclear. In one study, up to three fourths of pediatric patients had significant reduction in their signs and symptoms in response to an average dose of 12.75 mg (with a range of 5–25 mg).[101] Inasmuch as the structure of the drug is similar to the tricyclic antidepressants, similar side effects are observed, and it should be utilized with caution in children who are actively being treated with psychopharmacologic agents for depression. The reader is referred to the general literature for a fuller discussion of risks and benefits of this medication. In the study of Siegel,[113] this medication was utilized in 30 of 33 patients identified with beneficial results.

Other medications that could be considered include the use of antidepressants. It should be explained to the patient and his or her family that these are being given for a specific medical disorder and not in the guise of a veiled treatment for a psychiatric condition. Nortriptyline was prescribed in 12 of the 33 patients studied by Siegel[113] with a range of from 10 to 40 mg per evening. Amitriptyline was also used in 8 of the 33 patients, in a dosage range of 5 to 40 mg nightly. Dry mouth, dizziness, and tachycardia are potential side effects about which patient and parents need to be cautioned. Concomitant use of fluoxetine at a dosage of 10 mg in the morning may be synergistic to the use of amitriptyline.[49]

Future pharmacologic treatment may utilize current concepts in regard to pathophysiology, with abnormalities of the neuroendocrine axis. Accordingly, growth hormone supplementation and similar strategies may be of benefit.[9]

Other nontraditional treatments have been utilized as per mention on the Internet and other nonrefereed sources. Dietary modification, use of phototherapy, guaifenesin, dietary supplementation with magnesium and malic acid, and a variety of other substances have been mentioned but have not been endorsed because objective support for their efficacy is lacking.[107]

It should be remembered that children with chronic illnesses grow into adults who have been ill during their formative years or may continue to have pain and disability. Therefore, the transition from high school to college or to vocational training should not be overlooked. The teen should be prepared to develop more instrumental skills of daily living and endurance that allow them to live away from home as well as learn scheduling and energy conservation. Most importantly, the transition should permit teen and young adult patients to become their own well-informed advocate, rather than continuing to have their parents manage their care and unilaterally make medical and lifestyle decisions.

Access to information and provision of support services are certainly an important aspect of care. Unlike in the adult population, there is a general lack of familiarity with the disorder. This problem is reflected in the amount of information that is available to the general public in the quest for diagnosis and treatment. In one survey of the Internet, more than 1200 websites devoted to fibromyalgia and related disorders were found, few of which would qualify as peer-reviewed information, lending speculation to the medical validity of certain treatments. Of these sites, only two were specifically devoted to a discussion of this disorder in children. One geared to parents and older children was not technically challenging and was easily comprehensible, but was more of a personal review of the topic.[133] The second site had a comprehensive list of medical references available through the National Library of Medicine, with specific references and abstracts available, but was highly technical.[89] Neither of these sites was interactive or mentioned the presence of support groups in any local areas for parents and children. Therefore, there is much to be desired and developed in this area to bring this disorder and treatment into the public arena.

References

1. Anrep GV, Blalock A, Samaan A: Effects of muscular contractions upon the blood flow of skeletal muscle. Proc R Soc London 114:233–244, 1934.
2. Arroyo IL, Brewer EJ, Giannini EH: Arthritis/arthralgia and hypermobility of the joints in schoolchildren. J Rheumatol 15:978–980, 1988.
3. Larsson LG, Baum J, Mudholkar GS: Hypermobility: Features and differential incidence between sexes. Arthritis Rheum 30:1426–1430, 1987.
4. Bassan H, Niv D, Jourgenson U, Wientroub S, et al: Localized fibromyalgia in a child. Paediatr Anesth 5:263–265, 1995.
5. Baxter MP, Dulberg C: "Growing pains" in childhood—a proposal for treatment. J Pediatr Orthop 8:402–406, l988.
6. Beattie TF: Reflex sympathetic dystrophy in children; active early physiotherapy is the key to prevention. BMJ 311:1503–1504, 1995.
7. Beighton P, Solomon L, Soskolne CL: Articular mobility in an African population. Ann Rheum Dis 32:413–418, 1973.
8. Bell DS, Bell KM, Cheney PR: Primary juvenile fibromyalgia syndrome and chronic fatigue syndrome in adolescents. Clin Infect Dis 18(Supp. 1):S21–23, 1994.
9. Bennett RM, Clark SC, Walczyk J: A randomized double-blind placebo-controlled study of growth hormone in the treatment of fibromyalgia. Am J Med 104:227–231, 1998.
10. Bennett RM, Clark SR, Campbell SM, Burckhardt CS: Low levels of somatomedin C in patients with the fibromyalgia syndrome: A possible link between sleep and muscle pain. Arthritis Rheum 35:1113–1116, 1992.
11. Berde C, Sethna NF, Masek B, et al: Pediatric pain clinics: Recommendations for their development. Pediatrician 16:94–102, 1989.
12. Bernstein BH, Singsen BH, Kent JT, et al: Reflex neurovascular dystrophy in childhood. J Pediatr 93:211–215, 1978.
13. Bird HA, Tribe CR, Bacon PA: Joint hypermobility leading to osteoarthrosis and chondrocalcinosis. Ann Rheum Dis 37:203–211, 1978.
14. Bloomfield SA: Changes in musculoskeletal structure and function with prolonged bed rest. Med Sci Sports Exerc 29:197–206, 1995.
15. Boisset-Pioro MH, Esdaile JM, Fitzcharles MA: Sexual and physical abuse in women with fibromyalgia syndrome. Arthritis Rheum 38:235–241, 1995.
16. Bou-Holaigah I, Calkins H, Flynn JA, et al: Provocation of hypotension and pain during upright tilt table testing in adults with fibromyalgia. Clin Exp Rheumatol 15:239–246, 1997.
17. Bowyer S, Hollister JR: Limb pain in children. Pediatr Clin North Am 31:1053–1081, 1984.
18. Bowyer S, Roettcher P: Pediatric rheumatology clinic population in the United States: Results of a 3-year survey. J Rheumatol 23:1968–1974, 1996.
19. Brattberg G: Connective tissue massage in the treatment of fibromyalgia. Eur J Pain 3:235–244, 1999.
20. Breau LM, McGrath PJ: Review of juvenile primary fibromyalgia and chronic fatigue syndrome. J Dev Behav Pediatr 20:278–288, 1999.
21. Brenning R: Growing pains. Acta Societatis Medicorum Upsaliensis 65:185, 1960.
22. Buskila D, Neumann L, Hazanov I, Carmi R: Familial aggregative in the fibromyalgia syndrome. Semin Arthritis Rheum 26:605–611, 1996.
23. Buskila D, Neumann L, Hershman E, et al: Fibromyalgia syndrome—an outcome study. J Rheumatol 22:525–528, 1995.
24. Buskila D, Press J, Gedalia A, et al: Assessment of nonarticular tenderness and prevalence of fibromyalgia in children. J Rheumatol 20:368–370, 1993.
25. Buskila D, Shnaider A, Neumann L, et al: Fibromyalgia in hepatitis C infection. Arch Intern Med 157:2497–2500, 1997.
26. Cabral D, Tucker LB: Malignancies in children who initially present with rheumatic complaints. J Pediatr 134:53–57, 1999.
27. Carter C, Sweetnam R: Familial joint laxity and recurrent dislocation of the patella. J Bone Joint Surg 40B:664–667, 1958.

28. Carter C, Wilkinson J: Persistent joint laxity and congenital dislocation of the hip. J Bone Joint Surg 46B:40–45, 1964.
29. Chaturvedi SK: Phenytoin in reflex sympathetic dystrophy. Pain 36: 379–380, 1989.
30. Chelimsky TC, Low PA, Naaessens J, et al: Value of autonomic testing in reflex sympathetic dystrophy. Mayo Clin Proc 70:1029–1040, 1995.
31. Child AH: Joint hypermobility syndrome: Inherited disorder of collagen synthesis. J Rheumatol 12:239–242, 1986.
32. Clark P, Burgos-Vargas C, Medina-Palma P, Lavielle F: Prevalence of fibromyalgia in children: A clinical study of Mexican children. J Rheumatol 25:2009–2014, 1998.
33. Davidovitch M, Tirosh E, Tal Y: The relationship between joint hypermobility and neurodevelopmental attributes in elementary school children. J Child Neurol 9:417–419, 1994.
34. Decoster LC, Vailas JC, Lindsay RH, et al: Prevalence and features of joint hypermobility among adolescent athletes. Arch Pediatr Adolesc Med 151: 989–992, 1997.
35. Demitrack MA, Crofford LJ: Evidence for and pathophysiologic implications of hypothalamic-pituitary-adrenal axis dysregulation in fibromyalgia and chronic fatigue syndrome. Ann N Y Acad Sci 840:684–697, 1998.
36. DeVries HA: Quantitative electromyographic investigation of the spasm theory of muscle pain. Am J Phys Med Rehabil 45:119–134, 1966.
37. Dietz FR, Mathews KD, Montgomery WJ: Reflex sympathetic dystrophy in children. Clin Orthop 1990: 285:225–231.
38. Dolgan JI: Depression in children. Pediatr Ann 19:45–50, 1990.
39. Dorpat TL, Holmes TH: Mechanism of skeletal muscle pain and fatigue. Arch Neurol Psychol 74:628–640, 1955.
40. Drucker WR, Hubay CA, Holden WD: Pathogenesis of posttraumatic sympathetic dystrophy. Am J Surg 97:454–465, 1959.
41. Ehrlich MG, Zaleske DJ: Pediatric orthpaedic pain of unknown etiology. J Pediatr Orthop 6:460, l986.
42. Felson DT, Goldenberg DL: The natural history of fibromyalgia. Arthritis Rheum 29:1522–1526, 1986.
43. Fermaaglich DR: Reflex sympathetic dystrophy in children. Pediatr 60:881–883, 1977.
44. Gedalia A, Brewer EJ: Joint hypermobility in pediatric practice—a review. J Rheum 20:371–374, 1993.
45. Gedalia A, Garcia CO, Molina JF, et al: Fibromyalgia syndrome; experience in a pediatric rheumatology clinic. Clin Exp Rheumatol 18:415–419, 2000.
46. Gedalia A, Person DA, Brewer EJ, Giannini E: Hypermobility of the joint in juvenile episodic arthritis/arthralgia. J Pediatr 107:873–876, 1985.
47. Gedalia A, Press J: Articular symptoms in hypermobile schoolchildren: A prospective study. J Pediatr 119:944–946, 1991.
48. Gedalia A, Press J, Klein M, Buskila D: Joint hypermobility and fibromyalgia in schoolchildren. Ann Rheum Dis 54:494–496, 1993.
49. Goldenberg DL, Mayskly M, Mossey CJ: A randomized double-blind crossover trial of fluoxetine and amitriptyline in the treatment of fibromyaglia. Arthritis Rheum 39:1852–1859, 1996.
50. Goldsmith DP, Vivino FB, Eichenfield AH, et al: Nuclear imaging and clinical features of childhood reflex neurovascular dystrophy: Comparison with adults. Arthritis Rheumat 32:480–485, 1989.
51. Gragg RA, Rapoff MA, Danovsky MB, et al: Assessing chronic musculoskeletal pain associated with rheumatic disease: further validation of the pediatric pain questionnaire. J Pediatr Psychol 21:237–250, 1996.
52. Graham R: Joint hypermobility and genetic collagen disorders: Are they related? Arch Dis Child 80:188–191, 1999.
53. Granger CV, Hamilton BB, Kayton R: Guide for the use of the Functional Independence measure for children (WeeFIM) of the uniform data set for medical rehabilitation. Buffalo, NY, Research Foundation–State University of New York, 1987.
54. Guntheroth WG, Chakakjian S, Brena SC, et al: Posttraumatic sympathetic dystrophy dissociation of pain and vasomotor changes. Am J Dis Child 121:511–514, 1971.
55. Hains G, Hains F: A combined ischemic compression and spinal manipulation in the treatment of fibromyalgia: A preliminary estimate of dose and efficacy. J Manipulative Physiol Ther 23:225–230, 2000.
56. Hawksley JC: The incidence and significance of "growing pains" in children and adolescents. J R Inst Pub Health 1:798–805, 1938.
57. Hobbie C: Relaxation techniques for children and young people. J Pediatr Health Care 3:83–87, 1989.
58. Honjyo K, Hamasaki Y, Kita M, et al: An 11-year-old girl with reflex sympathetic dystrophy successfully treated by thoracoscopic sympathectomy. Acta Paediatr 86:903–905, 1997.
59. Kemler MA, Barendse GA, van Kleef M, Egbrink MG: Pain relief in complex regional pain syndrome due to spinal cord stimulation does not depend on vasodilation. Anesthesiology 92:1653–1660, 2000.
60. Kemper K. Sarah R, Silver-Highfield E, et al: On pins and needles? Pediatric pain patients' experience with acupuncture. Pediatrics 105:941–947, 2000.
61. Kesler RW, Saulsbury FT, Miller LT, Rowlingson JC: Reflex sympathetic dystrophy in children: Treatment with transcutaneous electric nerve stimulation. Pediatrics 82:728–732, 1988.
62. Kirk JA, Ansell BM: Articular hypermobility simulating chronic rheumatic disease. Ann Rheum Dis 26:419–425, 1967.
63. Klemp P, Stevens JE, Isaacs S: A hypermobility study in ballet dancers. J Rheumatol 11:692–695, 1984.
64. Kozin F, Genant H, Berkerman C: The reflex sympathetic dystrophy syndrome: Roentgenographic and scintigraphic evidence of bilaterality of a periarticular involvement. Am J Med 60:332–338, 1976.

65. Kozin F, Ryan LM, Carerra GF: The reflex sympathetic dystrophy syndrome (RSDS). Am J Med 70:23–30, 1981.
66. Kujala UM, Taimela S, Viljanen T: Leisure physical activity and various pain symptoms among adolescents. Br J Sports Med 33:325–328, 1999.
67. Lankford LL, Thompson JE: Reflex sympathetic dystrophy, upper and lower extremity: Diagnosis and treatment. Instr Course Lect 26:163, 1977.
68. Larsson LG, Baum J, Mudholkar GS: Hypermobility: Features and differential incidence between sexes. Arthritis Rheum 30:1426-1430, 1987.
69. Larsson LG, Baum J, Mudholkar GS, Kollia GD: Benefits and disadvantages of joint hypermobility among musicians. N Engl J Med 329:1079–1082, 1993.
70. Lavigne JV, Schulein MJ, Hahn YS: Psychological aspects of painful medical conditions in children II. Personality factors, family characteristics and treatment. Pain 27:147–169, 1986.
71. Laville JM, Lakermance MD, Limouzy F: Larsen's syndrome: Review of the literature and analysis of thirty-eight cases. J Pediatr Orthop 14:63–73, 1994.
72. Ledingham J, Doherty S, Doherty M: Primary fibromyalgia syndrome—an outcome study. Br J Rheumatol 32:139–142, 1993.
73. Leventhal LJ, Naides SJ, Freundlich B: Fibromyalgia and parvovirus infection. Arthritis Rheum 34:1319–1324, 1991.
74. Lewkonia RM: Hypermobility of joints. Arch Dis Child 62:1–2, 1987.
75. Lightman HI, Pochaczevsky R, Aprin H, Ilowite NT: Thermography in childhood reflex sympathetic dystrophy. J Pediatr 111:551–555, 1987.
76. Macarthur C, Wright JG, Srivastava R, et al: Variability in physicians' reported ordering and perceived reassurance value of diagnostic tests in children with "growing pains." Arch Pediatr Adolesc Med 150:1072–1076, 1996.
77. Malleson PN, Al-Matar M, Petty RE: Idiopathic musculoskeletal pain syndromes in children. J Rheumatol 19:1786–1789, 1992.
78. Martin-Santos R, Bulbena A, Porta M, et al: Association between joint hypermobility syndrome and pain disorder. Am J Psychiatr 155:1578–1583, 1998.
79. Mellick GA, Mellick LB: Reflex sympathetic dystrophy treated with gabapentin. Arch Phys Med Rehabil 78:98–105, 1997.
80. Melzack R, Wall PD: Pain mechanisms: A new theory. Science 150:971–979, 1965.
81. Mikkelsson M, Sourander A, Piha J, Salminen J: Psychiatric symptoms in preadolescents with musculo-skeletal pain and fibromyalgia. Pediatrics 100:220–227, 1997.
82. Miller VJ, Zeltser R, Yoeli Z, Bodner L: Ehlers-Danlos syndrome, fibromyalgia and temporomandibular disorder: Report on an unusual combination. Cranio 15:267–269, 1997.
83. Mishra MB, Ryan P, Atkinson P, et al: Extra-articular features of benign joint hypermobility syndrome. Br J Rheumat 35:861–865, 1996.
84. Moldofsky H, Scarisbrick P, England R: Musculoskeletal symptoms and non-REM sleep disturbance in patients with "fibrositis" and healthy subjects. Psychosom Med 37:341–351, 1975.
85. Muizelaar JP, Kleyer M, Hertogs IA, DeLange DC: Complex regional pain syndrome (reflex sympathetic dystrophy and causalgia): Management with the calcium channel blocker nifedipine and/or the alpha-sympathetic blocker phenoxybenzamine in 59 patients. Clin Neurol Neurosurg 99:26–30, 1997.
86. Murray CS, Cohen A, Perkins T, et al: Morbidity in reflex sympathetic dystrophy. Arch Dis Child 82:231–233, 2000.
87. Naish JM, Apley J: "Growing pains." A clinical study of non-arthritic limb pain in children. Arch Dis Child 26:134, 1951.
88. Nash P, Chard M, Hazleman B: Chronic Coxsackie B infection mimicking primary fibromyalgia. J Rheumatol 16:1506–1508, 1989.
89. National Library of Medicine: Fibromyalgia syndrome (FMS) and chronic pain in children and adolescents. 2000. http://www.cfids.org/youth/articles/medical/pain.htm.
90. Nazarian LN, Schweitzer ME, Mandel S, et al: Increased soft tissue blood flow in patients with reflex sympathetic dystrophy of the lower extremity revealed by power Doppler sonography. Am J Radiol 171:1245–1250, 1998.
91. Nicholas AJ: Injuries to knee ligaments: Relationship to looseness and tightness in football players. JAMA 212:701–716, 1970.
92. O'Neill DB, Micheli LJ: Overuse injuries in the young athlete. Clin Sports Med 7:591–610, 1988.
93. Omey ML, Micheli LJ: Foot and ankle problems in the young athlete. Med Sci Sports Exerc 31:S470–486, 1999.
94. Oster J, Nielson A: Growing pains: A clinical investigation of a school population. Acta Pediatr Scand 61:329–334, 1972.
95. Owitz S, Koppolu S: Sympathetic blockage as a diagnostic and therapeutic technique. Mt Sinai J Med 49:282–288, 1982.
96. Paarano E, Pavone V, Greco F, et al: Reflex sympathetic dystrophy associated with deep peroneal nerve entrapment. Brain Develop 20:80–82, 1998.
97. Perelman RB, Adler D, Humphreys M: Reflex sympathetic dystrophy: Electronic thermography as an aid in diagnosis. Orthop Rev 16:561–566, 1987.
98. Peterson H: Growing pains. Pediatr Clin North Am 33:1365–1372, 1986.
99. Rashiq S, Knight B, Ellsworth J: Treatment of reflex sympathetic dystrophy with EMLA cream. Reg Anesth 19:434–435, 1994.

99a. Rea T, Russo J, Katon W, et al: A prospective study of tender points and fibromyalgia during and after an acute viral infection. Arch Intern Med 159:865–870, 1999.

99b. Richlin DM, Carron H, Rowlingson JC, et al: Reflex sympathetic dystrophy: Successful treatment by transcutaneous nerve stimulation. J Pediatr 93:84–86, 1978.

100. Roizenblatt S, Feldman DF, Goldenberg J, Tufik S: Juvenile fibromyalgia-infant-mother association [abstract]. J Musculoskel Rheum 39(Suppl. 1):118, 1995.

101. Romano TJ: Fibromyalgia in children; diagnosis and treatment. W V Med J 87:112–114, 1991.

102. Russell IJ, Michalek JE, Viprais GA, et al: Platelet 3 sup H-imipramine uptake receptor density and serum serotonin levels in patients with fibromyalgia/fibrositis syndrome. J Rheumatol 19:104–109, 1992.

103. Russell IJ, Orr MD, Littman B, Vipraio GA, et al: Elevated cerebrospinal fluid levels of substance P in patients with the fibromyalgia syndrome. Arthritis Rheum 37:1593–1601, 1994.

104. Rusy LM, Harvey SA, Beste DJ: Pediatric fibromyalgia and dizziness: Evaluation of vestibular function. J Dev Behav Pediatr 20:211–215, 1999.

105. Salerno A, Thomas E, Olive P, et al: Motor cortical dysfunction disclosed by single and double magnetic stimulation in patients with fibromyalgia. Clin Neurophysiol 111:994–1001, 2000.

106. Schanberg LE, Keefe FJ, Lefebvre JC, et al: Pain coping strategies in children with juvenile primary fibromyalgia syndrome: Correlation with pain, physical function, and psychological distress. Arthritis Care & Research 9:89–96, 1996.

107. Schikler KN: Is it juvenile rheumatoid arthritis or fibromyalgia? Med Clin North Am 84:967–982, 2000.

108. Schwartzman RJ, Kerrigan J: The movement disorder of reflex sympathetic dystrophy. Neurol 40:57–61, 1990.

109. Schwartzman RJ, McLellan TL: Reflex sympathetic dystrophy: A review. Arch Neurol 44:555, 1987.

110. Scott D, Bird HA, Wright V: Joint laxity leading to osteoarthrosis. Rheumatol Rehabil 18:167–169, 1979.

111. Shapiro MJ: Differential diagnosis of non-rheumatic "growing pains" and subacute rheumatic fever. J Pediatr 14:315, l939.

112. Sherry DD, Weisman R: Psychologic aspects of childhood reflex neurovascular dystrophy. Pediatrics 81:572–578, 1988.

113. Siegel DM, Janeway D, Baum J: Fibromyalgia syndrome in children and adolescents: Clinical features at presentation and status at follow-up. Pediatr 101:377–382, 1998.

114. Sigal LH: Summary of the first 100 patients seen at a Lyme disease referral center. Am J Med 88:577–581, 1990.

115. Silber TJ: Anorexia nervosa and reflex sympathetic dystrophy syndrome. Psychosomatics 30:108–111, 1989.

116. Silber TJ, Majd M: Reflex sympathetic dystrophy syndrome in children and adolescents. Arch Dis Child 142:1325–1330, 1988.

117. Simms RW, Zerbini CA, Ferrante N, et al: Fibromyalgia syndrome in patients with the human immunodeficiency virus. Am J Med 92:368–374, 1992.

118. Stanton RP, Malcolm JR, Wesdock K, Singsen BH: Reflex sympathetic dystrophy in children: An orthopedic perspective. Orthop 16:773–780, 1993.

119. Steere AC, Taylor E, McHigh GL, Logigian EL: The overdiagnosis of Lyme disease. JAMA 269:1812–1816, 1993.

120. Strafford MA, Wilder RT, Berde CB: The risk of infection from epidural analgesia in children: A review of 1620 cases. Anesth Analg 80:234–238, 1995.

121. Sutro CJ: Hypermobility of bones due to overlengthened capsular and ligamentous tissues. Surgery 21:67–76, 1947.

122. Tayag-Kier CE, Keenan GF, Scalzi LV, et al: Sleep and periodic limb movement in sleep in juvenile fibromyalgia. Pediatr 106:70, 2000.

123. Tromp G, Kuivaniemi H, Shikata H: A single base mutation that substitutes serine for glycine 790 of alpha I chain of Type II procollagen exposes arginine and causes Ehler-Danlos syndrome. IV. J Biol Chem 264:1349–1352, 1989.

124. van der Laan L, Veldman PH, Goris RJ: Severe complications of reflex sympathetic dystrophy: Infection, ulcers, chronic edema, dystonia, and myoclonus. Arch Phys Med Rehabil 79:424–429, 1998.

125. Vandvik IH, Forseth KO: A bio-psychological evaluation of ten adolescents with fibromyalgia. Acta Paediatr 83:766–771, 1994.

126. Varni JW, Thompson KL, Hanson V: The Varni/Thompson pediatric pain questionnaire. I. Chronic musculoskeletal pain in juvenile rheumatoid arthritis. Pain 28:27–38, 1987.

127. Veldman PH, Gloris RJ: Multiple reflex sympathetic dystrophy. Which patients are at risk for developing a recurrence of reflex sympathetic dystrophy in the same or another limb. Pain 71:207–208, 1997.

128. Viral and Health Statistics: Patient's reasons for visiting physicians: National Ambulatory Medical Care Survey, U.S., 1977–1978 (DHHS Publication #82-1717). Hyattsville, Md, National Center for Health Statistics, 1981.

129. Walco GA, Ilowite NT: Cognitive-behavioral intervention for juvenile primary fibromyalgia. J Rheumatol 19:1617–1619, 1992.

130. Walker E, Keegan D, Gardner G, et al: Psychosocial factors in fibromyalgia compared with rheumatoid arthritis: II. Sexual, physical and emotional abuse and neglect. Psychosom Med 59:572–577, 1997.

131. Walters AS, Picchietti DL, Ehrenberg BL, Wagner ML: Restless legs syndrome in childhood and adolescence. Pediatr Neurol 11:241–245, 1994.

132. Weibel RE, Benor DE: Chronic arthropathy and musculoskeletal symptoms associated with rubella

vaccines. A review of 124 claims submitted to the National Vaccine Injury Compensation Program. Arthritis Rheum 39:1529–1534, 1996.
133. Williamson M: Fibromyalgia in children. 1996. Available at http://www.mwilliamson.com/children.htm.
134. Wilson RR, Gluck OJ, Tesser JRP: Antipolymer antibody reactivity in a subset of patients with fibromyalgia correlates with severity. J Rheumatol 26:402–407, 1999.
135. Wolfe F, Smythe HA, Yunus MB, et al: The American College of Rheumatology 1990 criteria for the classification of fibromyalgia. Report of the Multicenter Criteria Committee. Arthritis Rheum 33:160–172, 1990.
136. Wright JB, Beverley DW: Chronic fatigue syndrome. Arch Dis Child 79:368–374, 1998.
137. Yunus MB, Masi AT: Juvenile primary fibromyalgia syndrome: A clinical study of thirty-three patients and matched normal controls. Arthritis Rheum 28:138–145, 1985.
138. Yunus MB, Rawlings KK, Khan MA, Green JR: Genetic studies of multicase families with fibromyalgia syndrome (FMS) with HLA typing [abstract]. Arthritis Rheum 36(Suppl.):247, 1995.

Chapter 4

Metabolic and Endocrine Causes of Muscle Syndromes

Louis F. Amorosa, MD

Overview

Disordered metabolism may cause a spectrum of muscle syndromes varying from simple muscle spasms to myalgias, to syndromes as severe as myositis, rhabdomyolysis, and myopathy. The impact of hormonal abnormalities and metabolic disturbances on fascial membranes has yet to be clinically defined. However, disorders affecting protein turnover, membrane composition, and ionic fluxes in muscle would likely affect fascial surfaces. This chapter considers the common metabolic and endocrine disorders resulting in muscle pain and dysfunction.

Statin-associated myalgia-myositis syndrome has become one of the most commonly encountered causes of muscle pain. This new class of drugs for the treatment of hypercholesterolemia has markedly altered the progression of atherosclerosis. Their inhibition of cholesterol synthesis probably alters muscle membrane cholesterol content. This raises the question: Does disordered cholesterol metabolism account for the myalgia-myofascial syndrome associated with high creatine phosphate (CK) and hypercholesterolemia observed in hypothyroidism?

In addition to affecting cholesterol metabolism, thyroid disease affects muscle protein turnover rates and calcium metabolism, causing myopathic weakness. Marked disturbances in calcium and potassium balance associated with parathyroid and adrenal diseases respectively adversely affect muscle performance, resulting in neurospastic signs, myopathy, and paralysis. Diabetes mellitus, the most common hormone disorder, causes a multiplicity of complications resulting from glycosylations of protein and lipid abnormalities. This may result in thickening of subcutaneous tissues, stiffness, and motion pain such as the diabetic stiff shoulder syndrome. Diabetic complications may cause neuromuscular symptoms such as amyotrophy resulting in atrophy.

Use of estrogen replacement in menopause has been observed in some women to relieve nonspecific myofascial symptoms, but such effects do not have an understood physiologic basis. Clearly, much more needs to be learned about how hormones affect muscle and fascia or the perception of myofascial pain by the central nervous system.

Statin-Associated Myalgia-Myositis Syndrome

The cholesterol content of cellular membranes is crucial in maintaining membrane fluidity and structural integrity. Disorder affecting the regulation of cholesterol entry into cells results in hypercholesterolemia, a major risk factor for atherosclerosis—the leading cause of death in North America. Brown and Goldstein, building on basic and clinical observations of Khachadurian, discovered the low-density lipoprotein (LDL) cholesterol-receptor pathway regulating cholesterol synthesis and uptake.[2, 5] Endo's group in Japan and Alberts' at Merck using the Brown and Goldstein model quickly discovered that a class of natural products called statins reduced the synthesis of cholesterol.[1, 4] The statins inhibit the rate-limiting enzyme in cholesterol synthesis, HMGCoA reductase, which is coordinately linked with the LDL-receptor pathway regulating cholesterol entry into cells. Inhibition of the enzyme increases intracellular flux of LDL cholesterol, resulting in significant drops in serum cholesterol levels.

The treatment of hypercholesterolemic patients with statins has revolutionized the management of cardiovascular disease. Because of relatively high compliance compared with other agents, the thresholds for treating hypercholesterolemia with statins have been lowered for patients with risk factors such as diabetes mellitus, hypertension, low levels of high-density lipoprotein, or early death of a parent from atherosclerosis. Thus, statins are widely used. More potent statins have been introduced, making it possible to target profound reductions in LDL cholesterol.

Within the first year following the release of lovastatin, the prototype of the statin class, case reports indicated that rhabdomyolysis could complicate statin therapy. The initial cases were the results of unforeseen drug interactions in the liver. Drugs such as cyclosporin, erythromycin, and ketoconazole increased the serum levels of lovastatin, resulting in myotoxic symptoms.

In subsequent studies, combinations of hypercholesterolemic agents such as statins with high doses of nicotinic acid were linked to clinical myositis and very commonly to elevations of CK, MM fraction with myalgia.[13] CK changes were so widely found in patients on statins that many experts believed that CK levels should not be routinely monitored and should be studied only in symptomatic patients. Considering the benefit of statins in the prevention of atherosclerosis and death, CK thresholds for discontinuing statins in asymptomatic patients are usually four- to fivefold above baseline. However, some patients experience distracting muscular symptomatology with mild CK elevations and even when levels are within normal range.

Symptoms of statin-associated muscle pain are chiefly myalgias about the shoulders or proximal lower extremities. They are likely to occur following exercise or a significant change in the normal physical routine such as raking leaves on a fall weekend.

Some patients have chronic low severity myalgia that is difficult to distinguish from arthralgia of the shoulder area. CK levels may or may not be abnormal. Such symptoms when linked to statins make continued therapy intolerable, and the drug cannot be used. Alternative agents such as fibric acid derivatives, nicotinic acid, and bile acids may have comparable efficacy as statins.

The mechanism of statin-associated muscle syndromes is not well understood. However, some clinical information and animal data suggest a hypothesis linking cholesterol metabolism to muscle membrane integrity. Statin-associated muscle syndromes had been linked to high-dosage therapy, drug interactions that inhibit hepatic clearance of statins, anticholesterolemic drug combinations that dramatically reduce serum cholesterol levels, and inborn errors that delay the clearance of statins from the blood stream. These clinical observations suggest that a build-up of statins and a remarkable reduction in serum cholesterol put muscles at risk.

Many years ago Dietschy's group showed that cholesterol within muscle is primarily regulated by synthesis with little uptake of cholesterol from the serum via the LDL cholesterol-receptor pathway.[12] Thus significant inhibition of cholesterol synthesis by statins active in muscle would make muscles very dependent on serum LDL cholesterol levels to maintain cellular cholesterol content. If serum cholesterol levels are reduced by therapy, muscles do not have an adequate compensatory mechanism to maintain their membrane cholesterol during increased activity associated with exercise. The result is breakdown of muscle membranes and release of CK with myopathic pain.

This syndrome needs to be recognized before myalgias or myositis results in rhabdomyolysis with release of myoglobulin and renal failure. Treatment is discontinuation of the statins, hydration, rest for muscles to recover, analgesics if necessary, and later consideration of alternative drugs to lower cholesterol that are less active in muscles, such as bile acid resins or nicotinic acid.

Thyroid Disorders

Hypothyroidism

Myalgia is a well recognized symptom of hypothyroidism often encountered in patients who demonstrate typical hypothyroid features.[7] Discomfort in shoulder movement may be so distressing as to mimic arthralgias. Patients complain of fatigue, but characteristic facial puffiness associated with pallor from decreased intravascular volume readily suggests the diagnosis of hypothyroidism, which is easily confirmed by finding an elevation of the thyroid-stimulating hormone (TSH) and reduced levels of serum thyroxine (T_4). In such symptomatic patients with typical somatic features, total serum cholesterol, and CK values, MM fractions are usually elevated and readily normalized with thyroxine replacement therapy.

The association of hypothyroid myalgias with elevated cholesterol and CK has not been fully understood. However, the observation of Chait and colleagues that thyroid hormone stimulates LDL cholesterol entry into cells via the LDL-receptor pathway suggests a common mechanism linking hypothyroxinemia to the statin effect.[3] Both would result in decreased cellular cholesterol: hypothyroxinemia by reducing cholesterol uptake while slowing compensatory synthetic pathways; statin by inhibiting cholesterol synthesis. The resulting depletion of cellular cholesterol would compromise membrane integrity, resulting in CK loss into the plasma and muscle symptomatology.

Such symptoms and signs were once typical of hypothyroid patients. In contemporary practice, thyroid function tests are often included in comprehensive profiles used to screen asymptomatic patients or those with vague, nonspecific symptomatology. The diagnosis of hypothyroidism is now made at a much earlier point, when only the TSH is elevated and T_4 is within normal limits. None of the classical clinical features of hypothyroidism such as dry or myxedematous skin, hypothermia, slow pulse, delayed relaxation of the reflexes, hypercholesterolemia, or elevated CK are observed in these subclinical hypothyroid patients. Thus, the clinical significance of finding an isolated TSH elevation is not always clear and often requires endocrinologic consultation to determine if treatment is necessary versus simple follow-up.

The other clinical scenario encountered is an intriguing and controversial challenge. These are patients with myalgias, fibromyalgia, fatigue, and other diffuse symptomatology remotely consistent with hypothyroidism, but whose thyroid function tests are entirely normal. In a previous edition of this book, and in other work, Sonkin suggested that the finding of hypometabolism (reduced basal metabolic rate) and hypercholesterolemia was consistent with partial thyroid hormone resistance syndrome.[10, 11] This syndrome as described did not alter pituitary TSH output as did the classical T_4 resistance syndrome of Refetoff.[8] Thus the syndrome would cause a functional hypothyroidism without altering thyroid function tests. Hypercholesterolemia may be a sign indicative of inadequate T_4 function in the periphery. When there is nothing else to offer the patient, Sonkin suggested that a therapeutic trial with a physiologic dose of thyroxine could produce an efficacious outcome.

Without a proper longitudinal trial, this remains a controversial suggestion. However, the present author has also observed a subset of patients whose nonspecific symptoms have benefited from this approach. It remains unclear whether thyroid hormone action is specific or a euphoric action on the central nervous system similar to the triiodothyronine (T_3) effect that augments the use of antidepressant drugs. Such a therapeutic trial, if attempted, must be carefully monitored by serial thyroid function tests, electrocardiogram (ECG), and bone absorptiometry evaluation to preclude overmedicating the patient. The present author has also noted that the trial often fails to produce improvement in the patient. In these circumstances, T_4 or T_3 therapy should be promptly discontinued.

Hyperthyroidism

The most dramatic myofascial syndrome of this common endocrine disorder is proximal myopathy, usually without pain. This myopathy is secondary to negative nitrogen balance associated with increased muscle turnover rates. Moreover, calcium and potassium turnover in muscle is accelerated, altering action potentials and adversely affecting muscle power. As muscle degradation exceeds muscle build-up and amino acids are lost, even highly conditioned athletic patients begin to experience muscle weakness. They can no longer jog. Older patients note weakness climbing stairs, standing up from a sitting position, or rising from a kneeling position.

More often, hyperthyroidism is dramatic with tachycardia, palpitations, and signs of hypermetabolism. Exophthalmos and diffuse goiter immediately suggest a diagnosis of Graves' disease, the most common etiology of hyperthyroidism. Toxic multinodular goiter or solitary adenomas cause similar symptomatology.

However, not all patients demonstrate this readily recognizable syndrome. The elderly may not demonstrate goiter or experience cardiac and hypermetabolic symptomatology. Instead, they may have a slow, low-grade, chronic form of hyperthyroidism that insidiously wears down the bony and skeletal infrastructure until myopathic weakness occurs. Thus myopathic syndrome of hyperthyroidism is usually a late sign of a more indolent course of hyperthyroidism.

A rare syndrome of intermittent periodic paralysis has been observed in severe hyperthyroidism causing generalized paralysis. The etiologic factor is profound hypokalemia, and potassium levels less than 2.5 mEq/L. The syndrome has been extraordinarily rare in white patients and has been described in Asians, Pacific Islanders, and African Americans. Symptomatology can occur acutely and is reversible by potassium administration. Correction of the hyperthyroid state precludes further episodes of paralysis.

Calcium Disorders

Calcium flux is an essential mechanism of muscle function. Thus, disorders of calcium metabolism may have profound effects on muscles, varying from focal to generalized paroxysmal spasms that can compromise respiration to incapacitating myopathy. Improved life expectancy has placed more emphasis on calcium metabolism and healthy muscle function to prevent the risk and morbidity of osteoporosis associated with advanced age. A quick muscle response of extending the arms and hands to absorb the impact of a fall can prevent a crippling hip fracture. However, the focus on calcium metabolism over the last 15 years has been to preclude bone loss associated with menopause in women, which leads to osteoporosis. More recently men older than 65 years of age have been included in the risk group. Thus, supplemental calcium to maintain dietary calcium intake of 1500 mg/day has been recommended by most nutritional societies for postmenopausal women and men with clinically apparent risk. Pharmacologic treatments including hydrochlorothiazide and bisphosphonates designed to maintain bone vitality may impact on calcium metabolism and exacerbate subtle disorders in calcium regulation. Anecdotal observations by the author suggest that treatment for osteoporosis could result in pain and weakness in proximal muscles in patients with subclinical and subtle hyperparathyroidism.

Hypercalcemia

The causes of hypercalcemia are listed in Table 4–1. Marked hypercalcemia has a profound depressant effect on neuromuscular function, resulting in generalized weakness. Hypercalciuria associated with elevated serum calcium can produce osmotic diuresis leading to hypokalemia, which may also compromise muscle power and may provoke muscle spasms and localized pain.

Table 4–1.
Common Causes of Hypercalcemia

Hyperparathyroidism	Multiple myeloma
Humoral hypercalcemia of malignancy	Hyperthyroidism
Generalized metastatic cancer	Familial hypocalcemic hypercalcemia
Ingestions: drugs and nutritional supplements	Addison's disease
Sarcoidosis	

The inclusion of serum calcium in automated blood screening tests in the 1960s has resulted in a hundredfold increase in the prevalence of hyperparathyroidism, currently at 100/100,000. The large number of these patients remain asymptomatic with mild elevations of calcium from 10.5 to 11.0 mg/dL. Symptomatic patients usually develop renal stone disease, which is an indication for neck surgery. Rarely a patient develops the multisystem dysfunction recognized by Fuller Albright in 1925—marked hypercalcemia greater than 12.0 mg/dL associated with severe hyperparathyroidism.

Thus, hyperparathyroidism may manifest a spectrum of clinical disorders. Patients progressing to symptomatic disease often experience proximal myopathy and myalgia. This finding is readily observed with calcium elevations close to 12 mg/dL. Histologically, changes in muscle have been observed. It has been unclear whether muscle symptoms and changes are related to hypercalcemia or to high parathyroid hormone (PTH) levels. Clinical observations by the author in hyperparathyroid patients being treated for osteoporosis suggest that the widely used bisphosphonate therapy further elevates PTH levels without affecting serum calcium. Some patients so treated develop symptomatic proximal muscle pain and myopathy that dramatically improves following parathyroidectomy. The inference from these anecdotes is that bisphosphonate therapy for osteoporosis when given to patients with generally asymptomatic hyperparathyroidism seems to amplify the disorder, resulting in the classically symptomatic myopathic syndrome described with severe hyperparathyroidism a generation ago.[7]

Other disorders associated with hypercalcemia often have suppressed PTH levels resulting in hyperphosphatemia. If renal disease is present and phosphate excretion is impaired, an increasing calcium phosphate product can result in calcium phosphate complex depositions into soft tissues and muscle, the result of which is foci of pain and stiffness. Treatment of calcium phosphate deposition is calcium diuresis with saline or dialysis and prevention of the syndrome by binding dietary phosphate in the intestine with calcium carbonate or acetate nutritional supplementation.

Hypocalcemia

Profound hypocalcemia causes dysfunction in neuromuscular control resulting in paroxysms distally and around the mouth, carpal and tarsal pedal spasm, generalized muscle rigidity, and ultimately in seizures. The causes of hypocalcemia are listed in Table 4–2. Thyroid surgery for carcinoma resulting in hypoparathyroidism is the most frequently encountered cause of marked hypocalcemia. Thus, thyroid cancer patients are closely monitored postoperatively for calcium changes. However, hypocalcemia may occur many years following total thyroidectomy for carcinoma or other benign entities as vascular changes and fibrosis associated with aging compromise parathyroid glands that were subclinically impaired at the time of surgery.

Insidious progression of hypocalcemia can produce diffuse and nonspecific symptomatology, not only causing neuromuscular symptoms but progressing to an encephalopathic picture if not detected by testing and early diagnosis.

Abnormalities in Potassium Balance

Hyperkalemia

Marked elevation of serum potassium is usually associated with acute and chronic renal disease and causes profound weakness requiring a comprehensive evaluation. Hyperkalemia has a major depressant effect on muscle function and strength. The

Table 4–2.
Causes of Hypocalcemia

Chronic renal disease	Disorders in vitamin D metabolism
Status post thyroidectomy	Primary hypoparathyroidism
Malabsorption syndromes	Pseudohypoparathyroidism

Table 4–3.
Causes of Hypokalemia

Diuretic therapy
Nutritional deficiencies (alcoholism)
Chronic gastrointestinal losses—diarrhea, mucus-secreting tumors
Steroid mediated
   Cushing's syndrome
   Primary hyperaldosteronism
   Congenital adrenal hyperplasia
Nephropathies with renal tubular dysfunction

myopathy is generalized and usually acute as potassium increases over 6.0 mEq/L. Patients with chronic disease such as diabetic nephropathy with hyporeninemic hypoaldosteronism may tolerate potassium levels as high as 6.5 mEq/L asymptomatically. However, these disorders are progressive and generalized weakness eventually occurs. Hyperkalemia will interfere with skeletal muscle action potential. Cardiac depolarization and contractility are impaired, further compromising peripheral muscle function. This acute and generalized muscle weakness is a medical emergency.

Hypokalemia

Significant reductions in serum potassium affect muscle action potential. The earliest effects are muscle cramping or twitches, but as hypokalemia becomes profound, a generalized hyporeflexic weakness occurs that can mimic a neuropathic paralysis. Although endocrine disorders such as hyperaldosteronism and Cushing's syndrome can cause hypokalemia, the effects are rarely profound unless other etiologic factors such as diuretic use or nutritional depletion are in play. Moreover, endocrine disorders causing hypokalemia are associated with hypertension. Cushing's syndrome also causes muscle wasting and fatigue secondary to the diversion of muscle amino acids to gluconeogenesis. Natural causes of Cushing's syndrome are rare, but the efficacy of steroids to treat chronic inflammatory diseases often results in an iatrogenic steroid–induced proximal myopathy.

The disorders causing hypokalemia are listed in Table 4–3.

Diabetes Mellitus

Chronic hyperglycemia caused by diabetes mellitus adversely affects nearly every system in the human body. The peripheral nervous system commonly demonstrates the earliest symptomatology of the disorder. Typically, diabetic neuropathy causes nocturnal paresthesias such as burning, numbness, or tingling in the feet. The symptoms may include cramps in the legs, which patients describe as calf "charley-horses" occurring in the night. These are the result of nerve dysfunction resulting in muscle spasm.

These relatively common and straightforward symptoms may become increasingly difficult to manage if neuropathy affects thoracoabdominal nerve distribution. In this uncommon syndrome, diffuse and intermittent abdominal wall pain occurs. Pain radiates into the proximal lower extremities. Nerve dysfunction can result in bilateral atrophy of the quadriceps with profound myopathy.

The terms to describe these severe neuromuscular syndromes include *diabetic radiculopathy* and *diabetic amyotrophy*. Marked weight loss and depression may occur. Electromyography (EMG) studies are necessary to define the neuropathology. Remarkably, these syndromes are often self-limiting. With stabilization of the disease and proper physical therapy, myopathic and atrophied muscles can significantly recover.

The mechanisms accounting for these syndromes are poorly understood; however, glycosylations of nerve proteins would seem likely. Collagen is known to undergo compositional changes with chronic hyperglycemia. Hands may demonstrate fibrosis of the palms and stiffness of the fingers. After many years, the diabetic heart is known to demonstrate diastolic dysfunction: the inability to relax or stretch during diastole. Thus, the diabetic state readily affects proteins and organs as diverse as connective tissue or the myocardium, suggesting that skeletal muscles or fascial membranes are unlikely to be spared the effects of protein glycosylations. The classic example of this is the diabetic stiff shoulder syndrome, which may occur following injury or without a precipitating event. Patients note pain on movement and slowly progressive loss of full range of motion. Treatment is physical therapy, but many patients cannot initiate therapy until the shoulder motion is passively restored under general anesthesia in the operating room.

Menopause

The loss of cyclic estrogen production in women causes physiologic effects including vasomotor symptomatology, changes in the vagina, reduction in calcium absorption, and loss of protection from atherogenesis. It is not surprising that some women experience adjustment reactions characterized by mood swings or depressive symptomatology that can be dramatically improved with hormone replacement therapy. Sonkin noted that joint and muscle pains and other myofascial symptoms often clear promptly with estrogen replacement. Such observations suggest that estrogen's effects on muscle metabolism are not physiologically defined. However, hormones are known to affect nearly all levels of the central nervous system, where pain thresholds and a state of well-being are perceived.[9] Thus, much more needs to be understood about physiologic and pharmacologic action of hormones in myofascial syndromes.

Metabolic Evaluation for Myofascial, Myopathic Syndromes

Metabolic and hormonal disorders are readily treatable. Thus, they should always be considered in evaluating myofascial, myopathic, or diffuse muscular symptomatology. The conditions discussed earlier are those most commonly associated with muscular involvement. Accordingly, inquiry about the use of cholesterol-lowering drugs is essential. Thyroid function tests initially include TSH and assessment of free T_4. If a suspicion of hyperthyroidism is not confirmed by elevation of T_4, then studies for T_3 are necessary. Hypothyroidism is readily diagnosed by finding an elevated TSH. The hypometabolic syndrome with normal TSH alluded to by Sonkin requires some evidence for impaired T_4 action, which would be suggested by finding a high serum cholesterol and an unexplained increase in CK. If Sonkin's partial T_4 resistance syndrome is considered, determining the basal metabolic rate (BMR) in a pulmonary physiology laboratory could be helpful. An unexplained low value is the basis for a cautious therapeutic trial of T_4.

Potassium, calcium, phosphate, and magnesium are crucial elements in muscle function and action. Deviations from normal values open a broad differential diagnosis, including nutritional factors, renal, parathyroid, and adrenal disease, which require specific studies such as PTH levels and cortisol studies.

Because of the extraordinary prevalence of diabetes and its diverse neuropathic manifestations affecting muscles, disordered glucose metabolism should be looked for routinely. Usually a fasting serum glucose of less than 110 mg/dL excludes the diagnosis of diabetes. However, a random 2-hour postprandial glucose test significantly greater than 140 should arouse suspicion of impairment. A hemoglobin A1C value of greater than 6.0% would increase suspicion for diabetes or at least glucose intolerance.

High hemoglobin A1C values are usually diagnostic, but this method of diagnosis is not standardized. Confirmation of the diagnosis of diabetes mellitus when the fasting glucose values are normal requires the finding of a 2-hour glucose value of 200 mg/dL or greater following ingestion of 75 g of glucose solution.

Finally, menopause or male hypogonadism can be simply diagnosed by finding elevation of the follicle-stimulating hormone (FSH) level.

References

1. Alberts AW: Discovery, biochemistry and biology of lovastatin. Am J Cardiol 62(15):10J–15J, 1988.
2. Brown MS, Goldstein JL: A receptor-mediated pathway for cholesterol homeostasis. Science 232(4746):34–47, 1986.
3. Chait A, Bierman EL, Albers JJ: Regulatory role of triiodothyronine in the degradation of low density lipoprotein by cultured human skin fibroblasts. J Clin Endocrinol Metab 48(5):887–889, 1979.
4. Endo A: 3-Hydroxy-3-methylglutaryl-CoA reductase inhibitors. Methods Enzymol 72:684–689, 1981.
5. Khachadurian AK, Kawahara FS: Cholesterol synthesis by cultured fibroblasts: Decreased feedback inhibition in familial hypercholesterolemia. J Lab Clin Med 83(1):7–15, 1974.
6. Khaleeli AA: Griffith DG, Edwards RH: The clinical presentation of hypothyroid myopathy and its relationship to abnormalities in structure and function of skeletal muscle. Clin Endocrinol (Oxf) 19(3):365–376, 1983.
7. Patten BM, Bilezikian JP, Mallette LE, et al: Neuromuscular disease in primary hyperparathyroidism. Ann Intern Med 80(2):182–193, 1974.
8. Refetoff S: Syndromes of thyroid hormone resistance. Am J Physiol 243(2):E88–98, 1982.
9. Sandman KB, Backstrom CJ: Psychophysiological factors in myofascial pain. J Manipulative Physiol Ther 7(4):237–242, 1984.
10. Sonkin LS: Myofascial pain due to metabolic disorders: Diagnosis and treatment. In Rachlin ES (ed): Myofascial Pain and Fibromyalgia. St. Louis, Mosby-Yearbook, 1994, p 45.
11. Sonkin LS: Paired BMR and serum cholesterol measurements in therapeutic trials with thyroid hormones in patients with normal levels of TSH and/or T4 and symptoms suggesting thyroid deficiency [Abstract 678]. Endocrine Society 60th Annual Meeting, 1978.
12. Spady DK, Dietschy JM: Sterol synthesis in vivo in 18 tissues of the squirrel monkey, guinea pig, rabbit, hamster, and rat. J Lipid Res 24(3):303–315, 1983.
13. Ucar M, Mjorndal T, Dahiqvist R: HMG-CoA reductase inhibitors and myotoxicity. Drug Saf 22(6):441–457, 2000.

Chapter 5

Psychological Considerations in Myofascial Pain, Fibromyalgia, and Related Musculoskeletal Pain

Roy C. Grzesiak, PhD

Author's Note: In preparing an updated and revised version of this work, I attempted to address several questions. First, have we learned much about the complex etiology of fibromyalgia, myofascial pain, and related muscle pain syndromes? Second, have there been any significant advances in diagnosis or treatment? Third, was it a mistake to group fibromyalgia, myofascial pain, and other musculoskeletal pain problems together? Throughout this revision, I will attempt to answer those questions. Overall, little has changed in the way of content. Major additions include a review of cognitive deficits frequently found in these syndromes, my own work on vulnerability to pain syndromes, and a revised focus on the importance of psychotherapy in the multidisciplinary management of chronic pain syndromes.

Clarification of the possible roles of psychological factors in myofascial pain and other musculoskeletal pain problems is a complex undertaking. First, there is a psychology of pain that is complex and multifactorial in nature, suggesting that the role of psychological factors in the etiology of myofascial pain ranges from none to considerable, if not exclusive. The clinician must be attuned to signs that point to possible complicating psychological factors in the patient's presenting behavior. Second, a biopsychosocial perspective on fibromyalgia and myofascial pain indicates that proper treatment and management approaches vary considerably from patient to patient and that progress, or the lack of it, in physical rehabilitation may be the only indication of whether the prescribed treatment program is correct. The focus of this chapter is on a clinical approach to the psychological evaluation and management of individuals with musculoskeletal pain syndromes. After a brief introduction to concepts such as chronic pain and its psychological features, focus will be on *what to look for* in the clinical screening of patients with myofascial and related musculoskeletal pain as well as *what to do* in terms of patient management when psychological or psychosocial factors appear to be complicating the picture. Additionally, an overview of common psychological assessment and treatment approaches is provided. However, to reiterate, the focus is on clinical management.

Chronic Pain and the Pain-Prone Patient

Physicians and other health care professionals who work exclusively with pain patients often develop a skewed and distorted view of chronic pain. Not only do they often end up sounding like psychiatrists,[24] but they frequently fall victim to some form of stereotyping with respect to a favored etiology for chronic pain. The relationship between pain and depression affords an excellent example. The general position on the relationship between pain and depression is that the depression seen in chronic pain patients is a consequence of living with the pain; until recently, there has been only equivocal experimental, empirical, or clinical support for such a notion. Although depression can be either cause of, concomitant with, or consequence of pain,[26, 34, 52] perhaps the earlier bias reflects an implicit apology for the need to include psychological care in the management of people who are "in pain."

One of the facts that is often lost in chronic pain work is that many individuals with persistent pain do not become "chronic pain patients." In other words, they continue to cope, work, love, and embrace life, even with pain. In fact, even within any given sample of chronic pain patients, Turk and Rudy[108, 109] have identified factors that suggest that patients seen in specialty pain clinics/programs are not representative of chronic pain patients as a whole. Studies examining the role of biopsychosocial factors in the development of chronic pain suggest that it is the psychological component of the matrix that leads to chronicity, not the biologic component.[91, 107] In fact, a prospective investigation indicated that anxiety was the psychosocial antecedent that predicted chronicity in herpes zoster (postherpetic neuralgia).[29]

Before considering chronic pain in more detail, it is informative to review the various components of pain. A frequently used schema has been proposed by Loeser (Fig. 5–1).[66, 67] In this scheme, *nociception* refers to the potentially tissue-damaging mechanical, thermal, or chemical energy impinging on specialized nerve endings that can initiate the transmission of a signal into the nervous system. *Pain* is the perception of that signal in the central nervous system. Although pain perception can occur as a consequence of nociception, pain can also be perceived when no tissue-damaging energy has impinged, or continues to impinge, on the nervous system. Pain syndromes reflecting this latter concept would be the various central pain syndromes. *Suffering* is where psychological factors enter the picture. Suffering refers to the negative emotional reactions that can complicate the clinical presentation. *Pain behavior* refers to those observable behaviors that suggest to the observer that the individual is experiencing pain. The concept of pain behavior was proposed first by Fordyce and associates.[40, 41] Considering these multifaceted components of overall pain experience, it is no wonder that patients often present us with complicated and confusing clinical pictures.

What is *chronic* pain? Why is it important to recognize when a continuing pain problem represents a chronic as opposed to an acute condition? Although definitions of chronic pain vary, consensus among pain professionals holds that pain that continues for more than 3 months is the "most convenient point of division between acute and chronic pain."[101] Briefly, chronic pain is pain that continues over time, unresponsive to appropriate medical, surgical, or pharmacologic treatment, lacks biologic utility, is frequently associated with depression, and should not be managed with narcotic analgesics (Table 5–1).[103] In fact, Chapman and Bonica[17] have warned us that the two major dangers in failing to recognize a pain as chronic are unnecessary surgery and risk of addiction.

Even though there is a well-defined distinction between acute and chronic pain, there are potential problems in diagnosis and, hence, in treatment planning as well. Elsewhere I have suggested that the clinician may find it useful to differentiate between acute pain, chronic pain, and chronic pain syndrome.[50] All patients with

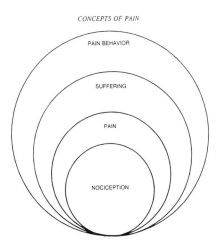

Figure 5–1. Concepts of pain. (From Loeser JD: Concepts of pain. In Stanton-Hicks M, Boas RA [eds]: Chronic Low Back Pain. New York, Raven Press, 1982, pp 145–148, with permission.)

Table 5–1.

Distinctions Between Acute and Chronic Pain

Acute	Chronic
Symptomatic	A disease in itself
Biologically useful	Less diagnostic utility
Induces anxiety	Induces depression
Narcotics indicated; undertreatment is a concern	Narcotics contraindicated
Little potential for addiction	Potential addiction
Pathologic origin recognized	Pathologic origin unclear, often complex interaction
Cure likely	Cure may be impossible

From Tait RC: Psychological factors in chronic benign pain. Current Concepts in Pain 1:10–15, 1983, with permission.

chronic or persistent pain do not suffer from chronic pain syndrome. The individual with chronic pain syndrome demonstrates serious impairment in virtually all biopsychosocial domains. These individuals bring to the clinical situation a heretofore hidden or unconscious "matrix of vulnerability" based on early childhood trauma. The consequence of such trauma is not psychogenic pain in the traditional sense but rather a psychogenic elaboration of sensation and a vulnerability to suffering that feeds on itself to the patient's detriment. We now know that the consequences of early developmental trauma are both enduring and far-reaching, affecting psychological factors such as attachment capacity, resiliency, somatization/somatic awareness, anxiety/panic, and depression, as well as actual changes in neurobiologic functions that affect pain memory, self-regulatory functions, and inability to modulate arousal.[69, 110–112]

An understanding of trauma sequelae, both psychological and neurobiologic, informs and enriches our understanding of chronic pain syndromes. It is conceptually possible to integrate these processes within a neuropsychological model of pain such as Melzack's revised gate-control theory.[73–76] Such an integration then affords psychological and biologic processes equal weight in determining the clinical course of a pain problem.[50]

While there is no singular pain-prone personality, there are certainly pain-prone personali*ties.* The concept of pain-prone personality originated in the work of Engel,[31, 32] who noticed that his patients who lacked definitive physical findings to account for their pain shared a number of common denominators in terms of their early psychosocial/developmental experiences. These early experiences included physically or verbally abusive parents; harsh or punitive parents who then overcompensated with rare displays of affection; cold or distant parents who were only warm and solicitous of the child when the latter was ill; a parent who suffered from chronic illness or pain; and various other parent-child interactions involving guilt, aggression, or pain. Engel proposed that these early developmental events predisposed the individual to pain-proneness. Further, he stated that these pain-prone individuals superimposed an individual psychic signature on their somatically or psychogenically based pain sensation. This individual psychic signature usually complicates symptom presentation. In fact, Engel offered that the more complex the symptom picture, the greater the likelihood that psychological factors came into play. It is important to note that pain-proneness does not reflect a singular personality type but rather is found in a variety of personality and characterological organizations.

Empirical support for the concept of pain-proneness can be found in three studies. Adler and associates[1] compared psychogenic pain patients with three other pain and illness-related control groups and found that the former group recalled significantly more early psychosocial/developmental trauma. In a study investigating the correlation of traumatic psychosocial-developmental events with the outcome of spinal surgery, it was found that these traumatic events had the capacity to severely compromise postsurgical outcomes.[99] Finally, extensive investigations of back pain by Blumer and Heilbronn[9] have demonstrated a similar configuration of early experiences that they believe predispose to depression and subsequently to pain. They have termed this the *dysthymic pain disorder.* These early traumas are frequently not remembered by pain patients and reflect unconscious processes that have been either repressed, dissociated, or otherwise foreclosed from consciousness. It is only when illness, trauma, or pain trigger these early psychodynamic factors that the patient's clinical presentation, course of treatment, and ultimate rehabilitation are affected.[49, 50]

The above thesis should not be taken as suggesting that *all* chronic pain patients have dysfunctional early psychosocial-developmental histories, because that certainly is not the case. But some do. Pain experience reflects the multifactorial interaction of biopsychosocial processes. For example, chronic pain may reflect simple learning, failure to cope, dysfunctional coping capacities, irrational beliefs about pain and suffering, chronic postural problems, musculoskeletal hyperreactivity, as well as more hidden psychological difficulties such as pain-prone tendencies.

Psychological Factors in Myofascial Pain, Fibromyalgia, and Related Musculoskeletal Pains

Turning specifically to myofascial pain syndrome, fibromyalgia, and related musculoskeletal pains, a brief review of the literature is in order. Although a comprehensive review is beyond the scope of this chapter, a number of comprehensive surveys are available.[5, 10, 11, 42, 62, 68, 87] As a whole, although these reviews are thorough and comprehensive, their conclusions are disappointing. For example, they point out that concepts such as primary fibromyalgia, secondary fibromyalgia, fibrositis, myofascial pain syndrome, and psychogenic rheumatism all have considerable overlap and many of the early studies failed to provide clear-cut operational definitions for the syndromes being investigated. Consequently, there is much confusion as to exactly which syndrome is being studied in many of the reports.

There are clear symptom presentation differences between fibromyalgia and myofascial pain syndrome. Although biologic etiologies remain unclear, the consensus of reviews suggests that in fibromyalgia there is some ill-defined physical predisposition that ultimately leads to multisystem dysfunction. Whether this dysfunction is based on peripheral or central factors is unclear, although the evidence suggests a problem in central modulation. For myofascial and other musculoskeletal pain problems, some form of muscle trauma is more clearly implicated.

Similarly, attempts to define psychological and psychiatric variables have been less than clear on methodology, sample characteristics, and illness parameters. Consequently, a more pragmatic approach to presenting this information is to deconstruct it into its component features and present them as summary modules. Accordingly, the following concepts will be summarized: the fibromyalgic personality; depression, in its premorbid, current, and lifetime occurrences; somatization; stress, anxiety, and muscle tension; nonrestorative sleep disturbance; cognitive dysfunction; and phenomenology.

The Fibromyalgic Personality

Historically, persistent pain problems that have ill-defined etiologies have been subjected to personality stereotyping. For example, common terms in the older psychosomatic literature include *migraine personality, rheumatic personality, TMJ (temporomandibular joint) personality,* and so on. So too has there been characterized a *fibromyalgic personality.* Smythe has been an adamant proponent of this concept: "These patients set high standards and are as demanding of themselves as they are of others. They are caring, honest, tidy, committed, moral, industrious—virtuous to a fault (pp 484–485)."[101] Although empirical support for this personality configuration has not been forthcoming, such discrepancy between the empirical and the clinical literature is not unusual. Research efforts to validate personality types as they relate to pain-related and other psychosomatic problems have been plagued by problems of depth of assessment. It may well be that this highly moral, hard-working, perfectionistic type of individual can be found in any subset of pain patients and that the final symptomatic outcome will reflect the interaction of personality type with physical predisposition or diathesis and disease or injury.

Clinicians have found this "workaholic" personality style in many chronic pain sufferers. Sarno[92–97] has stressed chronic character style, avoidance of conflict, and unawareness of anxiety as contributory to neck and back muscular pain. He has noted that many of his patients are conscientious, compulsive, responsible, and hard-working; they are self-motivated and critical of themselves and others. In a paper, Coen and Sarno[23] have explained that one of the primary tension generators in this type of personality is not the psychic conflict proper but rather avoidance of awareness of the conflict so that conscious effort is turned toward external activities, productivity, success, and the like rather than toward one's inner emotional life.

In his most recent effort, Sarno[97] applies his theory of unconscious rage and internal psychodynamic conflict to virtually all persistent pain problems and other debilitating physical conditions such as chronic fatigue, other autoimmune disorders, and cardiac irregularities, to name just a few. In many respects, I agree with his focus on the psychological side of the biopsychosocial matrix. However, his apparent disregard for the biologic side of what is clearly a diathesis-stress model of symptom formation is notable. This disregard may simply reflect the prominence that he places on "mind" within the mind-body equation.

This kind of personality style is also well documented in the research of Blumer and Heilbronn,[8, 9] who have labeled it *ergomanic*. Not unlike Engel's pain-prone personalities,[32] ergomanic individuals work hard to maintain their image as "solid citizens." They have a history of excessive work performance, often hold more than one job, are uncomfortable with time off or vacations, do little to relax, and are pathologically self-reliant. They have maintained this pace from early in life, often having been forced to do so by a dysfunctional family constellation, and when they finally suffer a painful trauma, they have extreme difficulty in allowing themselves to be ill but finally succumb to their dependency needs to such an extent that treatment efforts are foiled. A study by Van Houdenhove[113] surveying a large sample of chronic pain patients for premorbid hyperactivity found a significant number (70%) fit criteria described earlier by Blumer and Heilbronn. A preliminary study by Ciccone and Grzesiak reviewed work history and early psychosocial trauma in a sample of chronic neck and back pain patients. They found significance for the ergomanic traits as well.[21]

It may well be that the so-called fibromyalgic personality is not causal of fibromyalgia or fibrositis but that it is a significant contributor to the overall disablement when an individual does have soft tissue pathology. As such, it is not unique to fibromyalgia or myofascial pain dysfunction but reflects the interaction of a pain-prone premorbid personality with other biologic variables or diatheses for this condition. As Blumer and Heilbronn have suggested, it is clinically most useful to look at the pain problem and the mood as synchronous expressions of the individual's overall state of being.[9]

Depression: Cause, Consequence, or Concomitant

In psychological and psychiatric studies of fibromyalgia and myofascial pain syndrome, depression has been the most extensively studied, although a tally of results leaves us with more questions than answers. Again, definitional problems plague the literature. Myofascial pain syndrome, fibrositis, and fibromyalgia mix together in some of the studies. Furthermore, definitions of depression vary in terms of criteria as do the psychometric and clinical investigative methods used to arrive at results. All that can be done at this point in time in terms of understanding the role of depression in these syndromes is to present the trends that seem apparent in the literature.

It has become commonplace to expect chronic pain patients to be depressed. Many of the studies of depression in fibromyalgia, for example, have used the MMPI (Minnesota Multiphasic Personality Inventory) as the primary psychometric index (the MMPI in psychodiagnostic evaluation will be presented later), and because it was designed for use with psychiatric rather than medical patients, its value is somewhat compromised. Nevertheless, MMPI results constitute a major part of the literature on the psychological aspects of fibromyalgia.

Payne, Leavit, and Garron compared patients with fibromyalgia, mixed arthritis, and rheumatoid arthritis on the MMPI and found that the MMPI profiles of the fibromyalgia group showed greater elevations and more variability. However, only the Hy scale (Hypochondriasis) and the Hs scale (Hysteria) were of clinically significant elevation; the D scale (Depression) was not differentially elevated in the fibromyalgia group.[88] Similarly, Ahles and associates compared patients with fibromyalgia with patients having rheumatoid arthritis as well as with normal controls and found the fibromyalgia group to have higher elevations on Hy, D, and Hs but not to a pathologic degree.[2] Another MMPI study conducted by Wolfe and colleagues found Hy and Hs highest in the fibromyalgia group.[116] So it seems clear that at least part of the so-called neurotic triad of Hypochondriasis, Depression, and Hysteria is more significantly elevated in fibromyalgia patients. However, all three of these MMPI scales load heavily on somatic factors, and individuals with active, painful medical conditions are likely to score higher than either patient controls with painless medical conditions or normal controls. Based on the research presented thus far, it appears that psychological concerns such as somatic preoccupation, symptom endorsement and denial of psychological difficulties figure more prominently in the clinical picture than does depression.

Targeting the relationship between depression and fibromyalgia for study, and using more standardized and structured clinical interview criteria, Hudson and coworkers found that current as well as past episodes of depression were more common in the fibromyalgia group compared with rheumatoid arthritics and controls. Additionally, 64% of the fibromyalgia group recalled experiencing symptoms of depression prior to the onset of their muscle pain.[58] In another study, Kirmayer and coworkers found that fibromyalgia patients had a somewhat greater incidence of lifetime depressive episodes than did patients with rheumatoid arthritis, although the difference did not reach significance. The psychiatric histories of first-degree relatives for both fibromyalgia and rheumatoid arthritis patients were also reviewed; it was found that family histories of those with fibromyalgia had more depression, although not significantly so.[64] Goldenberg proposed that the aforementioned results suggest some form of psychobiologic link between depression and fibromyalgia.[42] Another study used the Zung Depression Scale to compare patients with primary fibromyalgia, rheumatoid arthritis, and healthy controls, attempting to determine if fibromyalgia is a variant of depression. No differences were found for the two clinical groups, although both groups had a subset of patients that appeared to have significant depression.[2]

A recent report addressed the question of depression being antecedent, consequent, or comorbid. In defining *comorbid*, the investigators were referring to depressive episodes, before and after chronic pain, that were seemingly unrelated to the pain itself, such as individuals who appeared predisposed to depression. Although one can find studies that support each position, the studies reviewed were more supportive of both the consequence and "scar" or comorbid relationship between chronic pain and depression.[34]

Although the empirical evidence is meager, it does imply a trend in that many of the studies suggest somewhat greater incidence of premorbid, family, and lifetime incidence of depression in individuals who develop fibromyalgia. The evidence is not sufficient to posit a causal psychosomatic relationship at this time.

Somatization

Closely aligned to the concept of depression is the process of somatization. According to Kellner, somatization disorder is one of the somatoform disorders in the current psychiatric nomenclature.[62] Patients with somatization disorder have multiple somatic complaints (at least 13) beginning before the age of 30. Somatization refers to a subconscious process in which emotional distress is translated into bodily complaints. Although Kellner prefers to restrict the use of either term to those patients who display no evidence of organic illness, the actual DSM-IV (Diagnostic and Statistical

Manual of the American Psychiatric Association, fourth edition) is not so stringent, and patients can be labeled with one of the somatization processes or disorders in the presence of organic pathology if the complaints and resulting social and/or occupational impairments are grossly in excess of what would be expected given the physical findings.

Hudson and associates investigated the presence of somatization disorder in a sample of fibromyalgia patients and found it present in only 6% of cases.[58] Similarly, Kirmayer and coworkers studied the presence and coexistence of depression and somatization in fibromyalgia patients. They found only 5% of their sample met the criteria for somatization disorder. Although only a small percentage of fibromyalgia patients actually meet the criteria for somatization disorder, the authors argue that the fibromyalgia population does have many of the characteristics of somatization disorder, including frequent and varied somatic complaints in multiple organ systems, excessive health care utilization, and many surgeries in systems other than the musculoskeletal. Kirmayer and coworkers argue that it is important to look at somatization not as a disorder but as a process—one of the processes involved in illness behavior—and, from that perspective, gain a richer understanding of how the patient can impose idiosyncratic meaning on his or her symptoms.[64]

Stress, Anxiety, and Muscle Tension

Stress has been implicated as a major factor in the development of many painful conditions, and it has been examined in relationship to fibromyalgia and myofascial pain syndrome. In a major review of orofacial pain syndromes, including myofascial pain dysfunction, Grzesiak found that the literature supported stress as one of the major psychological factors leading to symptom formation or intensification.[48]

Stress leads to muscle tension, and there is ample evidence that prolonged muscle tension leads to pain. Is this a significant factor in fibromyalgia and other myofascial pain syndromes? One of the earliest studies investigating the role of life situations, emotions, and backache was reported by Holmes and Wolff.[57] They studied back pain patients without obvious physical findings to account for their pain and found that both life situations and strong emotions would facilitate back pain. They used both amobarbital (Amytal) interviews and surface electromyographic (EMG) recordings to monitor levels of muscle tension across a variety of muscle groups. Because their subjects were not specifically defined as suffering from myofascial pain syndrome or fibromyalgia, the results may not be directly applicable. However, their findings are important and worth noting because of the implications for virtually all soft tissue pain problems. Most noteworthy is the fact that they found that the majority of their patients engaged in hyperfunctioning of all the skeletal musculature. The subjects tended to be locked in a vigilant "on guard" pattern of sustained muscle contraction. These findings fit nicely with Sarno's observations described earlier in which personality style and psychic conflict generate tension that leads to back pain.

In a study comparing patients with fibromyalgia with both a rheumatoid arthritis group and a normal control group, Ahles and associates found that the fibromyalgia group reported a greater number of stressful life events.[3] Importantly, using the MMPI as a major psychometric index, they found that the fibromyalgia group could be subcategorized and that 31% of the sample showed significant psychological disturbance. In the presence of major stressors, this subgroup was more reactive in terms of symptom pattern. The authors point out that further studies looking at both major stressful life events and minor daily hassles may add another dimension to our understanding of the interaction of stress and muscle pain. Unfortunately, major literature on stress and fibromyalgia does not exist. There is a significant literature on the relationship between stress, muscle tension, and myofascial pain dysfunction of the muscles of mastication and upper quarter.

Nonrestorative Sleep and Symptom Formation

The importance of sleep pattern dysfunction in fibrositis or fibromyalgia was first observed by Moldofsky and associates.[83, 84] Patients with fibromyalgia frequently have a nonrestorative sleep pattern so that they do not awaken feeling refreshed even after what seemed to be a good night's sleep. Additionally, they awaken with generalized musculoskeletal pain and stiffness, fatigue, and localized tender points. Sleep electroencephalograph (EEG) studies have shown that patients with fibromyalgia have an alpha intrusion into their delta or stage 4 sleep.[72] This alpha intrusion is correlated with an increase in muscle tenderness. Furthermore, a study of normal volunteers in whom delta sleep was experimentally disrupted showed the development of fibrositic trigger points.[84] Comparisons of fibromyalgia patients, chronic insomniacs, dysthymics, and normal controls for EEG sleep patterns reveals that the *alpha EEG non–rapid eye movement (NREM) sleep anomaly* is characteristic of fibromyalgia. Whereas normal individuals, insomniacs, and dysthymics average approximately 25% duration in NREM sleep of the alpha EEG sleep, those with fibromyalgia average 60% duration of NREM sleep occupied by the alpha EEG sleep anomaly.[54, 98] According to Moldofsky, alpha EEG sleep may be a sensitive indicator for fibrositis but it is not specific to the disorder. The sleep anomaly has been found in healthy people who are asymptomatic.[81]

Studies that pharmacologically manipulated sleep EEG frequencies using chlorpromazine or L-tryptophan have demonstrated that the alpha and delta frequencies are related to pain, energy, and mood.[82] In a review paper, Moldofsky noted that psychological, environmental, and biologic influences can disrupt sleep and, consequently, a wide range of factors can affect the fibrositis syndrome. Most notable are areas where minor trauma can lead to major changes in musculoskeletal complaints. Stressful life events, for example, motor vehicle accidents, even minor ones, can lead to sleep disturbance, musculoskeletal, and mood symptoms. In addition to trauma, viral illness, immune compromise, and painful articular disease may affect sleep and lead to alpha intrusion and subsequent neuromuscular pain.[81] If one attempts to tie the aforementioned areas together, one gets a sense of the futility clinicians often experience when they try to differentiate biologic variables from psychological ones. Conditions such as fibromyalgia, myofascial pain syndrome, and related musculoskeletal pains do truly reflect the multifactorial interaction of complex biopsychosocial processes.

Cognitive Dysfunction

The experienced clinician evaluating patients with persistent pain—specifically fibromyalgia—expects to find impairments in higher-order cognitive functions irrespective of a history of head injury. Specifically, one finds marked impairments in the areas of attention, concentration, focus, and immediate memory. Surprisingly, one finds very little in the psychological or neuropsychological literature to document or explain this clinical finding. Chronic pain patients in general and fibromyalgia patients in particular show impairments in the attentional axis of cognitive functioning. What is unclear is why? Is it a function of living with pain? Is it a consequence of medication? Do the cognitive impairments remit if the pain is responsive to treatment? Deficits in information processing have been associated with pain, anxiety, depression, and head injury. Goldstein[44] offered a case presentation in which the patient's cognitive impairments were so severe that he was diagnosed as demented on the basis of neuropsychological testing. His cognitive capacities improved as his pain responded to treatment. As a clinician, I have made the same observation innumerable times. In many respects, the patient with fibromyalgia has cognitive impairments that are highly suggestive of mild closed injury. Parenthetically, in patients with acceleration/deceleration (whiplash) injuries, the same cognitive deficits are typically found on neuropsychological examination even if the patient did not lose consciousness in the precipitating event. Goldstein explained that fibromyalgia is best considered as a "neural network disorder" and the cognitive deficits reflect a "biochemical neural network dysfunction" (p. 2).

Phenomenology

In a major review paper, Boissevain and McCain, in addition to reviewing the psychological/psychiatric literature, focused on the phenomenology of fibromyalgia.[11]

Phenomenology refers to experience, and many investigators believe that patients with fibromyalgia experience their symptoms as more painful, global, and debilitating than the pains suffered in other chronic conditions. Pain and physical discomfort are the main symptoms of fibromyalgia. A large number of studies comparing patients with fibromyalgia with those having other chronic pain conditions have documented higher pain and disability ratings for the fibromyalgia group,[117] lower threshold for pain over both tender and nontender points,[15, 101] and more spontaneous and pervasive clinical pain.[37, 43, 116, 117] Boissevain and McCain conclude that the pain of fibromyalgia is more severe and debilitating than the pain of other chronic pain syndromes but that it remains to be clarified what the relative contributions are from psychopathology and pathophysiology.[11]

Identifying the Patient with Potential for Chronic Pain

The majority of primary pain practitioners do not have the luxury of a multidisciplinary team of specialists to evaluate the patient with myofascial pain, fibromyalgia, or other musculoskeletal pain complaints. Therefore, it is important for the clinician to be aware of early signs, symptoms, and behaviors that augur poorly for successful rehabilitation. All individuals with persistent pain problems do not become chronic pain patients in terms of having virtually all areas of psychosocial existence affected by their pain. As noted earlier, it appears that psychosocial factors are the forces that drive any given persistent pain sufferer toward chronic pain syndrome. What are some of the early signs suggesting potential chronicity?

In an earlier paper, I attempted to identify some of the clinical signs that should alert the practitioner to the potential chronicity of his or her patient.[47] The patient who fails to respond to what should be appropriate treatment may be on the road to chronic pain syndrome. Typically, when the patient fails to respond to our ministrations, we question our diagnosis and treatment plan. That is good health care. However, it is also important to consider what the complicating factors may be that prevent improvement. Both excessive anxiety and clinical depression can confound treatment effects. Anxiety is a person's response to real or imagined threat to either self or physical integrity. As such, anxiety is shaped by premorbid personality. Some patients are by nature or character more hysterical or hypochondriacal. Their symptoms will be presented with flair, exaggeration, and drama. However, that does not make their symptoms less real. However, this anxious presentation is likely to confound the clinical picture and result in a clinical picture that is bigger than the sum of its parts. Depression, for example, may inhibit the effectiveness of any given treatment. When the patient appears depressed, it is appropriate for the primary practitioner to inquire about aspects of psychosocial functioning, for example, recent stresses, job changes, mood, marriage, personal losses, and so on. Earlier in this chapter the psychosocial/developmental risk factors for chronicity were reviewed and, particularly when a psychologist or psychiatrist is not a member of the treatment team, the clinician may have to inquire into areas of family history, upbringing, presence of physical, sexual, or emotional abuse, and so on. Was the patient exposed to significant others early in life who had chronic painful illness? Was the patient seriously ill as a child? If so, that patient as a child had the opportunity to learn or take in a repertoire of sick role and illness behaviors that may have laid dormant for many years until recent illness or injury triggered their release from memory and reenactment in the present painful illness. The patient who is drug-seeking may be a potentially chronic patient. When the patient presents with clear physical signs and symptoms but appears more concerned with what prescriptions the physician will write, there may be a hidden drug abuse problem. Patients who are eager to have releases from work or assignment to light duty may or may not be playing out the chronic syndrome. As studies have shown, the role of compensation factors such as litigation for work-related injuries and workers' compensation income often has little or no effect on motivation to return to work, and the evaluation of such potential disincentives must be individualized.[28, 71]

The aforementioned aspects of the patient's clinical presentation are meant to alert the primary practitioner to the possibility of a persistent pain problem on its way to chronic pain syndrome. None of these factors, in and of themselves, is pathognomic of incipient chronicity but should serve as warning signs to the practitioner that a more comprehensive team approach may be necessary.

Psychological Screening and Evaluation

Many pain patients show an initial reluctance to undergo psychological screening or evaluation. This resistance is usually a function of beliefs such as the following: "they think the pain is all in my head," "the psychologist is trying to prove that my problems are mental," and the misinformed notion that a psychologist or psychiatrist can somehow divine just what portion of the patient's problem is mental as opposed to medical. The psychologist on meeting any pain patient for the first time must dispel these myths. On initial meeting I try to deal with this resistance by explaining that there is no scientific way I can determine what, if any, portion of the pain problem is psychological. Instead, I explain that we have learned over the years that when individuals live with pain for extended periods of time and treatments do not alleviate pain, it is not unusual for patients to find themselves upset over this state of affairs. I usually go on to explain that some patients become depressed, others irritable, some rely on medications, others fight with their spouses, and so on. I reassure them that these responses all reflect normal responses to an apparently insoluble situation and that, in the interest of helping them as best we can, we need to have a picture of the entire person. Usually, this introduction is sufficient to enable patients to talk about their pain and its impact on their life. Quite often, I am not able to get through this introduction before patients begin talking about the pain's emotional impact on their life. Patients vary in their degree of psychological sophistication, and it is important to tailor the introduction to the verbal and nonverbal responses coming from the patient.

Clinical psychologists screen and evaluate pain patients using three broad categories of data: (1) interview and observation; (2) psychological/psychometric tests; and (3) psychophysiologic data.[44] Psychologists vary in their preference for one type of data over another; the majority of psychologists use the interview as well as clinical observation, whereas a smaller percentage will include psychological tests as well. A much smaller group will collect psychophysiologic information as part of their assessment.

Clinical Interview and Observation

Psychologists vary in interview style. Some prefer broad, open-ended inquiry, whereas others prefer highly structured and standardized interview formats. As Waldinger has stated, we want our patients to tell us what is wrong.[114] The clinical interview provides the psychologist with basic information on mental status, thought processes, emotions, perceptual functioning, intelligence, and motivation. The psychologist may also glean some information on the presence or absence of more formal psychiatric or psychological dysfunction. However, all of the aforementioned is routine, and the focus will now turn to areas of investigation that are germane to assessment of the patient with pain. Elsewhere, Ciccone and I have provided a set of evaluative questions the physician can use to screen for psychological dysfunction in pain patients. These questions break down into three domains: inappropriate illness behavior; emotional disorder; and premorbid risk factors.[22]

Inappropriate Illness Behavior

1. Is there persistent pain extending beyond the bounds of normal healing time?
2. Is there an identified physical cause for the patient's pain?

3. Does the patient's report of pain appear proportionate to the suspected or identified pathology?

4. Is the distribution of pain, sensory loss, and/or motor weakness consistent with a dermatomal or myotomal distribution?

5. Is the complaint of pain and/or tenderness specific and limited to a single skeletal or neuromuscular structure? (This question may be inappropriate for myofascial and fibrositis patients because the syndrome is diffusely spread across the musculature.)

6. What behaviors does the patient perform to communicate pain and suffering to family members and health care providers?

7. What specific behaviors are performed by the patient's spouse, friends, and/or family in response to the patient's pain behavior?

8. What is the patient's current income and from what sources is it derived?

9. Is the patient using, abusing, or dependent on an addictive drug (narcotic analgesics or tranquilizers)?

10. Does the patient use alcohol as a means of controlling pain?

11. Who performs routine household chores such as grocery shopping, cooking, cleaning, and laundry?

12. How much of the patient's waking day is spent resting or reclining because of pain?

Emotional Disorder

13. Does the patient report or exhibit signs of excessive worry, nervousness, or anxiety?

14. If the pain is of traumatic origin, does the patient dwell on or ruminate about the traumatic incident; experience flashbacks, sleep disturbance, or nightmares; and avoid situations that are reminiscent of the original trauma?

15. Does the patient report discrete periods of heightened anxiety or panic accompanied by such symptoms as shortness of breath, palpitations, feeling faint, or trembling and associated with an intense fear of dying, losing control, or going insane?

16. Does the patient report more frequent loss of temper and/or feelings of hostility following the onset of pain?

17. When pain prevents the patient from engaging in a favorite activity or performing a routine chore, is there a tendency to feel angry and/or aggravated as opposed to frustrated?

18. Is the patient aware of any correlation between the onset of anger and an increase in pain symptoms?

19. Does the patient exhibit symptoms of depression such as prolonged periods of depressed mood, loss of interest or pleasure in most or all activities, disturbance of sleep and/or appetite, psychomotor agitation or retardation, frequent fatigue or loss of energy, diminished concentration, recurrent thoughts of death or suicidal ideation, and feelings of hopelessness and/or worthlessness?

20. If the patient admits to suicidal ideation, has he formulated a plan and does he express serious suicidal intent?

21. When the patient fails to meet social or work-related obligations, does he tend to blame himself or feel guilty?

22. Does the patient frequently perform burdensome or otherwise unpleasant chores with the intent of helping others and/or winning social approval?

Premorbid Risk Factors

23. Does the patient have a premorbid history of hard-driving, work-oriented behavior?

24. Does the patient have a history of depression or other psychiatric disturbance?

25. Does the patient have a history of substance abuse or dependency?

26. Does the patient have a history of chronic pain or other stress-related medical illness?

27. Was the patient exposed to chronic illness during childhood?
28. Did the patient sustain the loss of a loved one early in life?
29. Was the patient a victim of physical or sexual abuse?

By asking the patient questions of this sort, the physician or other health practitioner will develop some understanding for what the patient may be bringing to the clinical situation to make the overall presentation more problematic than it might be. The rationale underlying the above questions can be found in Ciccone and Grzesiak.[22]

Personality traits and states must be assessed to understand the individual with pain. Each patient brings to the pain situation his or her unique premorbid personality. Personality style has implications of emotional expression, cognitive style, behavioral response, and psychophysiologic reactivity. Many of these factors can maintain or exacerbate pain experience. As has been pointed out earlier, many patients with fibromyalgia, myofascial pain syndrome, or ill-defined musculoskeletal pain will present with personality styles that are primarily obsessional and depressive in nature. They are perfectionistic, hypernormal, precociously responsible, aggressive, ambitious, and critical of self and others. They often present with an ergomanic orientation to work and life. The importance of determining developmental events suggestive of pain-proneness is extremely important and will be dealt with later. Suffice it to say that the focus of the interview should be on determining the idiosyncratic or unique meaning that the patient superimposes on the pain sensation.

Premorbid and reactive psychopathology must be evaluated. Both psychological dysfunction and psychiatric illness can play a role in causing or complicating a musculoskeletal pain problem. Earlier it was noted that depression is by far the most common emotional symptom or syndrome presenting along with persistent pain. Such depression may reflect premorbid functioning, be comorbid with the pain, or be a function of attempting to live with a persisting pain problem. In patients with chronic pain, it may be impossible to separate out pain from depression, and, as Blumer and Heilbronn have stated, pain and depression may become synchronous expressions of mood.[9]

For purposes of this presentation, stress responses will be considered as part of reactive psychopathology. Major and minor life events can be stressful, depending on their appraisal by the individual. Major life events, including upheavals such as death of a parent, spouse, or child, serious illness, divorce, marriage, loss of job, and so on, are often associated with the development of medical problems, including pain. Similarly, we have learned that the psychophysiologic and autonomic correlates of stress can build on the basis of repetitive daily hassles leading to stress-related illnesses, including pain. Finally, because so many musculoskeletal pain problems begin with either major or minor trauma, the clinician must be alert to signs of post-traumatic stress disorder (PTSD). PTSD can complicate the patient's clinical presentation and serve as a perpetuator of pain complaints.

A very small number of patients have pain as part of a more serious psychiatric illness. In addition to depression, pain can be a symptom in the anxiety disorders, bipolar illness, hysterical conversions, hypochondriasis, and schizophrenia.[35, 77]

The impact of pain on physical and personal functioning needs to be evaluated as well. In the presence of persistent pain, some individuals continue to live their lives as best they can whereas others will fall victim to a variety of dysfunctions such as unemployment, physical inactivity, medication reliance, and so forth. In other words, they develop a "disability lifestyle." What appears crucial to how dysfunctional any given individual becomes is coping capacity, or the lack of it. As I have said elsewhere, nowhere is the interaction of pain and function more apparent than in the area of inactivity. Pain may spread from one focal area to more generalized and pervasive sites on the basis of disuse and inactivity. This often leads to inappropriate postural adaptations that ultimately lead to more muscular pain and stiffness. Decreased physical functioning because of pain does not lead to less pain in the long run but to more pain.[48]

Psychological Testing

Psychological or psychometric testing adds a more formal and structured dimension to the clinical evaluation. Few psychological tests were developed specifically for the assessment of the individual in clinical pain. Because some psychologists specialize in measurement techniques, they have contributed to the design of procedures for evaluation of pain.

The *Visual Analog Scale* is one of the most popular methods for estimating clinical pain. The Pain Visual Analog Scale (PVAS) is a 10-cm line anchored at one end as "no pain" and on the other end with "unbearable pain."[78] Patients are told to indicate the intensity of their pain by marking on the line between the two extremes. The examiner, if he or she wishes to quantify the results, can convert the mark into a numerical scale, using 0 to 100 mm as the range. Over the years there have been many variations on the PVAS such as using numbers or words rather than the simple line. However, Huskisson has argued that by leaving the line simple with only the two anchor phrases at the extremes, the evaluator is left with a sensitive scale possessing a virtually infinite number of data points.[59] The PVAS can serve as a useful measure of pain as well as a repeated measure to document therapeutic change.

The *McGill Pain Questionnaire* (MPQ) was developed in the mid-1970s by Melzack.[72] Based in part on the components of the gate control theory of pain, the MPQ uses classes of words (verbal descriptors) that have been factorially derived to represent the sensory, affective, and cognitive components of pain experience. The verbal descriptor section of the MPQ provides the evaluator with three kinds of information on the patient's pain: (1) present pain intensity; (2) number of words chosen; and (3) pain rating index. When the MPQ is completed in its entirety, it can also serve as a comprehensive, quasi-structured pain interview.

The *Psychosocial Pain Inventory* is one example of a number of relatively new structured evaluations designed specifically for pain patients.[56] This particular inventory was designed to assess the psychosocial aspects of the pain and, as such, it provides information on pain, psychosocial factors, pain-related treatments, secondary gain, interpersonal factors, and premorbid occupational satisfaction. Because its focus is predominantly psychosocial, it can be used to complement other psychometric procedures that assess personality, such as the MMPI.

The *West Haven-Yale Multidimensional Pain Inventory* was designed to supplement behavioral and psychophysiologic observations.[63] Initially labeled the WHYMPI, it is now better known as the MPI. The MPI provides three broad categories of information on the pain patient: (1) pain dimensions, including pain's interference with various areas of function, role of significant others, pain severity, and mood; (2) specific responses of significant others; and (3) functional activities. The MPI is frequently used in both clinical practice and in research investigations.

The *Minnesota Multiphasic Personality Inventory* (MMPI) is one of the most thoroughly researched and frequently used personality questionnaires with both psychiatric and medical patients. Developed in the 1940s, the MMPI has been a matter of controversy in pain management for years. Critics maintain that its primary focus on personality and psychopathology makes it an inappropriate instrument for the evaluation of chronic pain patients. Rather than discard it from the evaluation process, I think a more practical approach is to understand that interpretation of the MMPI is a sophisticated process that must be accomplished by a skilled clinical psychologist who understands that using the MMPI with medical and pain patients requires some adjustment in interpretation. It is important to know that certain scales, for example, Hypochondriasis, Depression, and Hysteria, are somewhat elevated by virtue of the number of somatic items in them. Interpretation of the MMPI should combine information on the personality and psychopathology dimensions as well as integration of the behaviors and defenses inherent in both high and low elevations on each of the clinical scales. In so doing, the clinician will bring to the diagnostic and treatment planning process useful information on some of the more idiosyncratic aspects of the pain patient's functioning.

Early interest in the MMPI with pain patients began with the publication of a study comparing back pain patients with and without definitive physical findings to account for their pain.[55] Hanvik found that the group of back pain patients with no organic findings produced a composite MMPI profile with elevations on Hy (Hypochondriasis) and Hysteria (Hs), with a D (Depression) score within normal limits. These three scores are called the neurotic triad and the previously noted elevations form a V configuration that has been called the "conversion V" or "psychosomatic V." So for some time it was commonplace to believe that the MMPI could differentiate between "real" pain and so-called psychogenic pain. However, extensive research that will not be detailed here has failed to consistently replicate a capacity to use the MMPI for diagnosis of psychogenic pain.

In 1978 Bradley and associates published the first of several major studies on the MMPI with chronic back pain patients in which multivariate analysis was used to identify consistently recurring clusters of MMPI profile types.[12] Studies such as Hanvik's mentioned earlier used measures of central tendency and, as such, compared the mean scores of one group with those of the other. An unfortunate consequence of such an undertaking is a washing out of individual differences within each group. The Bradley and associates studies found recurring profile types, one of which was the so-called conversion V. To my mind, this remains the prototypical approach to research using psychometric tests with pain patients, and it has two important implications for the clinician. First, these studies demonstrate that individuals with pain bring to the clinical situation their own unique premorbid personalities; some of these personality types are more frequently recurring, suggesting that some personality configurations may be more pain-prone than others. Second, the fact that several personality types have been identified in patients with chronic back pain suggests that this population is not psychologically homogeneous and, further, that psychological evaluation findings should be used to tailor a treatment program unique to the needs of each particular patient.

Other psychological tests have been used with pain patients as well but they will not be detailed here. Suffice it to say that the conclusions based on interview, observation, and psychometric evaluation must be accomplished by a psychologist trained in the clinical assessment of patients with pain. Routine application of psychological tests with pain patients may lead to gross misinterpretations of the results if the extenuating and distorting effects of living with pain are not taken into consideration.

Psychophysiologic Monitoring

As noted earlier, a small number of psychologists also gather information on psychophysiologic functioning as well. In the evaluation of patients with musculoskeletal pain syndromes, the primary method of data collection is surface electrode monitoring of muscle activity. The reader may recall the study mentioned earlier by Holmes and Wolff that used surface EMG recording as one of the measures. In many respects that study is a forerunner of the biofeedback explosion in the late 1960s and early 1970s when EMG biofeedback was applied to problems such as muscle tension headache. Psychophysiologic assessment has come a long way since those early days. Middaugh and Kee have provided a thorough guide for the psychophysiologic assessment of neck, shoulder, and low back pain.[80] They make the important point that static assessment of EMG is often misleading, and proper evaluation of muscle function must involve muscles in function. Accordingly, the Middaugh and Kee program uses a muscle-by-muscle EMG evaluation (Fig. 5–2).

Assessment of neck and shoulder girdle musculoskeletal pain involves a three-component assessment. During the Quiet Sitting Test, patients sit in an armless straight-back chair with their hands on their lap for 2 minutes; this position should allow the muscles being evaluated to become completely relaxed and EMG recordings will be at or very near the inherent noise level of the recording equipment. One is searching for elevated sitting baselines in the muscles being monitored. Second, patients do the Shrug/Return Test in which they are asked to shrug both shoulders up, hold this position for 3 seconds, and then let the shoulders back down. The

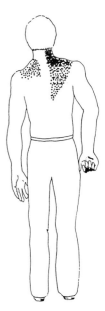

Figure 5–2. Common areas of reported pain in patients with chronic cervical and shoulder girdle pain. (From Middaugh SJ, Kee WG: Advances in electromyographic monitoring and biofeedback in the treatment of chronic cervical and low back pain. In Eisenberg MG, Grzesiak RC [eds]: Advances in Clinical Rehabilitation, vol 1. New York, Springer, 1987, pp 137–172, with permission.)

muscles are then monitored for 1 minute to assess recovery to baseline. This procedure is repeated three times. This component of the evaluation is the muscle's capacity to recover in a timely fashion. According to Middaugh and Kee, ". . . the significant finding is a failure on the part of the individual patient to recover his own sitting baseline level within 30 seconds on two of three trials" (p. 150). Such findings are indicative of muscle hyperactivity and irritability. The third area of assessment involves the Abduct/Return Test, in which sitting patients are asked to raise (abduct) the arms straight out to the side to the horizontal position, hold that position 3 seconds, and then lower the arms to lap to resume baseline. Muscle activity is again observed for 1 minute, and this procedure is repeated three times. Failure to recover to baseline after this test is another indication of irritability in the muscles being monitored.

The example in Figure 5–3 from Ciccone and Grzesiak illustrates three different parameters of muscle abnormality.[20] Comparing right and left shoulder shrugs and recovery to baseline suggests marked differences; the right shoulder is more active

Figure 5–3. Dynamic electromyographic (EMG) assessment of upper trapezius muscle activity before, during, and after shoulder shrug provocation. (From Ciccone DS, Grzesiak RC: Chronic musculoskeletal pain: A cognitive approach to psychophysiologic assessment and intervention. In Eisenberg MG, Grzesiak RC [eds]: Advances in Clinical Rehabilitation, vol 3. New York, Springer, 1990, pp 197–215, with permission.)

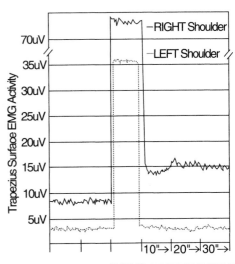

(hypertonic), is reactive when the muscles are at work (hyperactive), and fails to return to baseline in a timely manner (persistence).

Dynamic psychophysiologic assessment of the low back is similar to that of the shoulder girdle. Two or four muscle sites are evaluated on each patient; right and left lumbar paraspinous muscles and right and left lower thoracic paraspinous muscles, with electrode placements being parallel to the spine and approximately 1 inch from midline (L4 and T8–T12, respectively). Each patient undergoes a standing baseline in which he or she is asked to stand still, as straight as possible, with weight equally distributed between the two legs. The test is positive for muscle hyperactivity if one or both sides shows sustained muscle activity. Trunk rotation is used to establish the absence or presence of inappropriate reciprocal activity between left and right as the trunk rotates in either direction. Trunk flexion is used to assess poor relaxation (muscle irritability), asymmetry, continued contraction, and failure to recover baseline. Middaugh and Kee point out that although shoulder muscle irritability is common (65%), only 26% of low back pain patients show similar irritability. Overall, they point out that these simple tests often identify problems of inappropriate and inefficient use of low back muscles for posture and movement. Both overuse and underuse of appropriate musculature is common.[80]

Other psychophysiologic parameters are occasionally used in assessment of the patient with musculoskeletal pain; perhaps the most frequent other parameter is temperature, on the premise that the persistent pain is tied into autonomic dysregulation. However, that assessment tactic is not frequently used and will not be elaborated on here.

Taken as a complete package, the results of clinical interview and observations, psychological test findings, psychophysiologic assessment, the psychologist can make a substantial contribution to understanding the cognitive, behavioral, affective, and psychophysiologic dimensions of any given pain patient's problem. We will now turn to how to use this information in the psychological treatment of patients with musculoskeletal pain.

Approaches to Psychological Treatment

One of the major failings in behavioral medicine so far has been its inability to use psychological findings to do differential treatment planning. Turk has argued for customizing treatment plans, and he states many pain programs fall victim to what he calls the "patient uniformity myth" and the "treatment uniformity myth."[105] It should be clear by now that all persistent musculoskeletal pain patients, whether they have myofascial pain syndrome or fibrositis, do not present with a similar psychology and physiology. People are different, yet few reports in the pain treatment literature address those differences in any significant way.

All patients with persistent pain do not require psychological treatment although, in an ideal program, all should have a psychological evaluation. We must customize treatment. An early example of defining treatment on the basis of affirmative and negative physical and psychological findings was offered by Brena and Koch when they subdivided their patients on the basis of behavioral and tissue pathology findings into four groups: (1) pain amplifiers (high pain behavior—low tissue pathology), (2) pain verbalizers (low pain behavior—low tissue pathology), (3) chronic sufferers (high pain behavior—high tissue pathology), and (4) pain reducers (low pain behavior—high tissue pathology).[13] Clearly, each of these groups requires a treatment plan that weighs differently on medical and psychological interventions.

Psychological treatment approaches are diverse. Exactly how to divide them into reasonably discrete packages is no mean feat. For our purposes, the following section is divided into three components; psychotherapy (including the small but meaningful empirical information on psychoactive medication), self-regulatory approaches (relaxation, biofeedback, and hypnosis), and multidisciplinary pain management.

Psychotherapy

In this section, behavioral management, cognitive therapy, and integrative psychody-namic psychotherapy will be presented as well as some information on the use of psychoactive medication. Psychoactive medication does not fall within the purview of the psychologist. Yet, frequently the medical team will seek out information on possible psychopharmacologic interventions from the psychologist. Ideally, a psychiatrist with psychopharmacologic expertise and an interest in pain management should be a member or a consultant to the treating physician or team, but such specialists are few and far between.

Behavioral management of the patient with musculoskeletal pain is an important component of any psychological treatment. Years ago, Fordyce stated that pain behavior became chronic because it was rewarded while efforts the individual might make to engage in well or healthy behavior went unnoticed or were actually discouraged.[39] Therefore, the rewards or contingencies for displaying pain behavior were greater than those for healthy behavior. It is not my intention to present a behavioral management program here. However, key patient behaviors that are most appropri-ately managed with behavioral methods are activity levels, exercise performance, and medication intake. Chronic musculoskeletal pain patients often have had months, if not years, of inactivity and muscle disuse. Exercise is incompatible with pain behavior. The psychologist can assist the physician and the physical therapist in designing an exercise program in which the patient is unlikely to experience failure; a major impediment to rehabilitative progress is attempting to advance the patient in his or her activities too quickly. With both reconditioning and individualized therapeutic exercises, it is important to determine the patient's baseline level of performance. After identifying that level of performance, a systematic schedule of slowly increasing activity goals can be established, enabling the patient to improve his or her perfor-mance without experiencing failure. When medication use is a problem, it is important to determine just how much pain medication is needed to cover the patient's discom-fort so that he or she does not have breakthrough pain during participation in the rehabilitation program. As activity and exercise levels increase, pain medications are slowly decreased.

One area in which I take issue with an orthodox behavioral approach is in the attribution of responsibility. It is generally believed that instrumental learning can take place without thinking being involved. Therefore, the manipulation of behavior change can be viewed as a thoughtless process in which environmental contingencies are the sole shapers of behavior. Such an attitude takes away from the patient responsibility for his or her behavior. I believe it is better for patient motivation to educate the patient that, even though these environmental contingencies have an impact on behavior, it is the patient's own responsibility to determine the course of the rehabilita-tion program; responsibility for change can then become an internalized process.

Cognitive or cognitive-behavior therapy is by far the most commonly used of the psychotherapies in the management of patients with chronic pain. Turk and associates have been the foremost proponents of the cognitive-behavioral position.[106] Cognitive-behavioral theory is not so much a theory as it is a pragmatic integration of a variety of psychological techniques borrowed from such diverse areas of psychology as behaviorism, social learning, rational-emotive therapy and cognitive psychology. A focal concept in the cognitive-behavioral position is the idea that what people think about their illness and pain is actually more important than the illness or pain itself. Turk and associates have stated: "affect and behavior are largely determined by the way in which the individual construes the world." Patients often maintain an inner dialogue with themselves, have automatic thoughts, self-statements, and private conceptualiza-tions that add to their symptomatic distress. Although affect, behavior, and cognition are given equal weight in the cognitive-behavioral position, a focus on behavior change is still believed to be the most efficient way to alter emotion and thought as well. A major focus of cognitive-behavior therapy is coping; people often believe they have little or no control over what is happening to them. Cognitive-behavior therapy is active, educative, and interactive. The components of cognitive-behavioral therapy as applied to pain are as follows. First, there is developed a shared conceptualization of the patient's problems so that a psychologically based treatment is feasible. The scientific validity of this conceptualization is less important than its plausibility to the patient. Until both patient and therapist have a consensual understanding of how the treatment will work and what it aims to accomplish, treatment efforts are likely to work at cross-purposes. After reaching this shared conceptualization, therapy proceeds to the acquisition of necessary cognitive coping skills and behavioral strategies for managing pain-related dysfunction. Skill deficiencies are identified, new or improved cognitive skills are defined, rehearsed in the clinical setting, and applied to mutually agreed upon goals, and plans for implementing generalization and maintenance are developed. Although this sounds relatively simple, it is not in the actual clinical situation.

A somewhat similar cognitive approach to treatment of the chronic pain patient has been put forth by Eimers.[30] He uses the acronym PADDS to define his approach to pain management. PADDS refers to five components of his cognitive therapy approach. The first letter, P, stands for pacing. The importance of setting appropriate therapeutic goals and moving toward them in an orderly and nonexhaustive manner has been mentioned earlier. Too often patients fail in their physical rehabilitation because they attempt to do too much, too fast. Pacing is an important component of any physical restoration program. The A stands for anxiety management; many of the techniques for anxiety management will be spelled out later in the section on self-regulatory techniques. At this point it is sufficient to state that anxiety can negatively affect both pain experience and treatment participation. The D stands for distraction. The patient in pain can easily become focused and enmeshed in the overall pain experience, adding anxiety and augmenting the pain sensation. Distraction techniques change the gate on pain sensation, for example, selective inattention, attention diversion, reinterpretation of sensation, and so forth can be used to modify the interactive effects of anxiety and pain sensation. The next D stands for the disputation of negative thoughts. This procedure, similar if not identical to what will be discussed in the next section on rational-emotive cognitive therapy, involves identifying underlying automatic thoughts and irrational beliefs and then challenging their validity. The final letter S stands for stopping negative thoughts and images through a cognitive technique called thought stopping.

A cognitive therapy based on Ellis's rational-emotive psychotherapy has been presented by Ciccone and Grzesiak.[18–20] This approach does not set behavior, affect, and cognition on an equal footing but rather proposes that central to all affective, behavioral, and psychophysiologic dysfunctions are cognitions that are based on irrational beliefs and distorted interpretations of the meaning of pain. Using Ellis's ABC model of how irrational beliefs impact on behavior and emotion, these authors spell out how to do cognitive analysis and treatment. Among the more common cognitive errors that lead to coping failure and inability to adapt to pain are "awfulizing," demandingness, low frustration tolerance, conditional self-worth, and attributing responsibility to external sources. By changing how one thinks about pain, one can modify adaptation to it as well as dampen the negative impact of pain on virtually all functional activities (Fig. 5–4). In addition to its utilization as a cognitive psychotherapy, Ciccone and Grzesiak have also demonstrated how cognitive therapy and dynamic EMG assessment and treatment can be integrated.[20]

Integrative psychodynamic psychotherapy for patients with chronic pain has been proposed by Dworkin and Grzesiak.[27] Their integrative approach combines self-regulatory approaches and behavioral prescription with psychotherapy. The psychotherapeutic interventions vary on a continuum from supportive to insight-interpretive depending on patient needs. According to the authors, if psychological involvement in chronic pain is conceptualized as varying from minimal to maximal, as potentially involving cognitive, behavioral, affective, psychophysiologic, and intrapsychic (unconscious) components, and as playing a role as cause, consequence, or concomitant, then the value of being able to bring an integrative psychotherapy to bear on the chronic pain patient's pain and suffering becomes clear. The authors stress the usefulness of

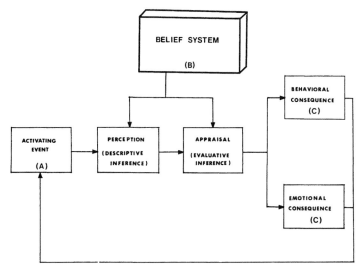

Figure 5–4. A cognitive model of human behavior and emotion. (From Ciccone DS, Grzesiak RC: Chronic musculoskeletal pain: A cognitive approach to psychophysiologic assessment and intervention. In Eisenberg MG, Grzesiak RC [eds]: Advances in Clinical Rehabilitation, vol 3. New York, Springer, 1990, pp 197–215, with permission.)

this form of psychotherapy for working with pain patients who have psychopathology and personality disorder; they also stress the value of using adjunctive psychoactive medications when indicated.

There are only two major studies evaluating the usefulness of psychotherapy with musculoskeletal pain problems. Both demonstrate significant success. Draspa studied patients with muscular pain, many of them apparently having fibrositis or "psychogenic rheumatism," who underwent extensive psychological evaluation and then psychological treatment combining active and passive relaxation, education (reassurance that the pain was muscular and not medically dangerous), and insight-oriented psychotherapy. The insight-oriented focus was on demonstrating how their stress and inner psychological world were contributing to musculoskeletal strain and consequently pain. Two groups with muscle pain were used; one group received psychological treatment plus physical therapy, while the other received physical therapy only. Almost twice as many patients in the treatment group became pain-free compared with the pain controls.[25]

The other study was completed by Pomp, who did not use a control group but who selected myofascial pain patients who failed to respond to conventional treatment. Symptom remission occurred during brief psychotherapy in 15 out of 23 patients, with an additional 2 patients becoming pain-free after psychotherapy was completed. According to the author, the aspects of psychotherapeutic process that led to symptom remission included relief from strong negative emotion, recognition of an invalid and unrealistic self-concept, development of a greater sense of self-competence or efficacy, and changes in the stress-creating aspects of the individual's environment.[90] Both of the aforementioned studies suggest that in selected musculoskeletal pain patients, one must deal with the interaction of personality, defense, coping style, and environment to attain pain relief.

Two clinical reports using psychotherapy with chronic pain patients have made similar points. Not unlike cognitive therapy, Shutty and Sheras[100] have used clinical examples to demonstrate the value of brief strategic psychotherapy to reframe problems faced by chronic pain patients in such a way as to provide them with new coping options. From a more psychoanalytic perspective, Whale[115] reported on the successful use of brief psychoanalytic psychotherapy with chronic pain patients. Each of her cases revealed underlying blocked anger and an inability to mourn important losses. However, even when evaluation findings suggest psychologic dysfunction or psychiatric disturbance, psychotherapy may not prove to be an appropriate treatment. Tunks and

Merskey have stressed the importance of differentiating between the need for support-ive or insight-oriented individual psychotherapy, group psychotherapy, and family therapy.[104]

Psychopharmacologic intervention has achieved a prominent place in the pain management armamentarium. The tricyclic antidepressants, in particular, are now used routinely in the management of chronic pain. Turning specifically to the use of psychoactive medications in fibromyalgia and fibrositis, there is only a meager literature supporting efficacy. In a controlled comparison of chlorpromazine and L-tryptophan for pain and mood symptoms in a sample of fibrositis patients, Moldofsky and Lue[82] found chlorpromazine to be more effective. In a double-blind study comparing amitriptyline and placebo, the group receiving the former showed improvements in morning stiffness, pain, sleep, and global functioning.[16] Goldenberg and associates conducted a double-blind study of amitriptyline, naproxen, a combination of amitripty-line and naproxen, and placebo on fibromyalgic symptoms. They found the amitripty-line groups showed significant improvement on all measures. The combination of amitriptyline and naproxen was not better than amitriptyline alone.[43] In the final study to be reviewed here, Bennett and associates studied cyclobenzaprine (cyclobenzaprine is structurally related to the tricyclic antidepressants) with placebo in a study compar-ing therapeutic response between a group with fibromyalgia and a control. The fibromyalgia group showed significant improvement in pain intensity as well as a nonsignificant improvement in fatigue, tender point pain, and muscle tightness.[6]

In terms of psychopharmacologic intervention in fibromyalgia and myofascial pain syndrome, results are not promising, with the exception of using amitriptyline in low doses. The mechanisms by which this tricyclic antidepressant are effective remain unclear but appear to involve improvement in sleep pattern and serotonin uptake.

Self-regulatory Approaches: Relaxation, Biofeedback, and Hypnosis

Relaxation and biofeedback are commonly used with chronic pain patients. It is most appropriate to consider relaxation and biofeedback together because they both allow the patient to experience a modicum of control over pain sensations. Hypnosis, on the other hand, is often viewed by patients as a surrendering of control, and hypnotic techniques often meet greater resistance than the other self-regulatory approaches.

Relaxation training is perhaps the most benign of the behavioral interventions. The rationale for relaxation training with musculoskeletal pain patients involves the notion that it is impossible to be relaxed and augmenting one's pain at the same time. Relaxation training is so widespread in behavioral medicine that it has been called the "aspirin of behavioral medicine."

It is unfortunate that relaxation training is often viewed as a simple, rather straight-forward technique. One should not look to the pain literature to understand the varieties of relaxation but to the stress management literature. In contemporary practice, relaxation training is usually one component of a much more comprehensive treatment package.

The origins of contemporary relaxation training lie in the work of Jacobson[60] but few practitioners actually use a Jacobsonian protocol because it is time-consuming and not fitted to the rather short-term treatment focus seen in most pain management settings. Nevertheless, relaxation approaches have proven useful in the overall manage-ment of diverse chronic pain problems, including musculoskeletal pain. Using a Jacobsonian protocol, McGuigan has pointed out that one must relax all the complexly interacting systems of the body. By directly relaxing the skeletal musculature, one also "relaxes" the central nervous system as well as the various components of the auto-nomic nervous system.[70] A key to relaxation training is not attempting to relax but in "turning off the power" to various muscle groups. In the Jacobson method, one works with only one muscle group at a time and, consequently, the process is quite extended over time.

More popular with psychologists working in pain management are the abbreviated forms of relaxation training. One of the more popular versions is that of Bernstein and Borkovec,[7] who have divided the muscles into 16 major groups. The patient is taught to relax each of these groups using a tense/relax strategy. When the patient is proficient with relaxation at this level, a briefer version is introduced that combines some of the interrelated groups. When the patient is proficient with the combined muscle groups, instructions focus on relaxation by recall, therefore eliminating the need to go through the tense/relax paradigm. The final step is to induce a relaxed state by counting.

Another version of relaxation, a simple relaxation method, was introduced by French and Tupin, who added a meditation-like imagery component.[36] This approach involves deep breathing, abbreviated tense/relax training for major muscles, and relaxing imagery. Grzesiak applied this approach to chronic pain secondary to spinal injury and, in a clinical case follow-up study, found it successful in the majority of cases.[45] One of the major values of relaxation training is that it enables the patient to develop a better sense of body functioning or somatic awareness. However, as the patient becomes more attuned to internal cues, the clinician must be aware of the possibility of untoward side effects. Jacobsen and Edinger have reported on two patients who developed anxiety symptoms apparently related to underlying psychodynamic conflicts that were released by the relaxation paradigm.[60] Relaxation approaches have been quite effective in the management of headache and back pain.[51]

Biofeedback is a form of psychophysiologic treatment that has developed a nearly overwhelming literature over the last two decades. The section on psychophysiologic assessment provided a brief introduction into how surface electrode EMG monitoring could be used to assess muscle functions. Before considering specific applications of biofeedback to problems of myofascial pain and fibromyalgia, some introductory comments are in order. In a brief review article, Grzesiak pointed out that the use of biofeedback in pain management can be conceptualized as involving two targets. The first involves using biofeedback as a generalized relaxation or quieting procedure; the second involves using biofeedback to target specific areas of dysfunction believed related to the pathophysiology of the pain problem itself.[46] There is a relatively extensive literature on using biofeedback for tension headache, low back pain, and myofascial pain but only one study on the biofeedback treatment of fibromyalgia. The extensive research on biofeedback applications to headache will not be included in this presentation.

Biofeedback involves monitoring a physiologic system of which we are not ordinarily aware, converting it electronically into signals (usually visual or auditory), and feeding back that information to the subject so that he or she can become aware of it and develop internal strategies for its modification. The use of static EMG biofeedback in the management of back pain has not had a particularly good record. Using as a rationale for the application of biofeedback the idea of muscle spasm/tension/pain, Nouwen and Solinger reported a controlled study of lumbar paraspinal EMG feedback. After a 20-session feedback period, they found that the treatment group had lowered EMG levels as well as lowered pain reports. However, on 3 month follow-up they found that although the treatment group continued to report improved pain, the resting paraspinal muscles had returned to baseline levels of activity.[86] This suggests that factors, possibly nonspecific therapeutic ones, were responsible for the pain improvement, not lowered levels of paraspinal muscle tension. A somewhat more sophisticated study was conducted by Large and Lamb, who used a counterbalanced design to treat chronic musculoskeletal pain patients (neck, low back, and fibrositis) with actual EMG biofeedback, an EMG control, and a waiting list control. For patients with focal pain complaints, site-specific EMG was used and for those with more generalized complaints, frontalis EMG was used. Interestingly, only those patients who began treatment with actual EMG feedback were able to achieve linear levels of improvement. The EMG control (a bogus feedback) actually had the lowest pain levels.[65] Both of these studies suggested the need for more research on the relationship between pain and muscle tension.

Because of equivocal findings such as the above, Nouwen and Bush conducted a major review of the relationship between EMG levels and pain.[85] They broke the data down on the basis of seven hypotheses:

- The hypothesis that resting levels of paraspinal EMG will be higher in low back pain patients has minimal support.
- The hypothesis that paraspinal EMG levels will be higher in low back pain patients during various movements and postures does have some support.
- The hypothesis that low back pain patients have more reactive paraspinal musculature under stress has not been supported.
- The hypothesis that lowered paraspinal EMG levels is associated with lower pain levels has not received consistent support.
- The hypothesis that low back pain patients will have higher levels of paraspinal EMG while other muscle groups remain normal has not been supported.
- The hypothesis that low back pain patients will have greater general muscular and autonomic reactivity has not been supported.
- Finally, the hypothesis that low back pain patients will respond better to biofeedback-enhanced relaxation training than to simple relaxation training has not been supported.

So one of the only areas where paraspinal muscle tension may play a role in back pain involves the differential patterning of paraspinal EMG. Return, if you will, to the data presented earlier on psychophysiological assessment using dynamic EMG assessment. Middaugh and Kee, for example, provide a comprehensive EMG treatment program for cervical and low back pain based on their dynamic assessment.

Biofeedback treatment of myofascial pain and muscle tension has an equivocal track record. There appear to be more successful studies involving myofascial syndromes of the upper quarter. For example, Peck and Kraft compared the outcomes of EMG treatment for a small group of tension headache, back, shoulder, and jaw pain; although treatment outcomes were satisfactory for the tension headache group, the results were far less promising for the other pain problems.[89] Another study compared relaxation training with biofeedback in the treatment of myofascial pain dysfunction syndrome. Relaxation treatment appeared effective in reducing pain. Adding biofeedback to the relaxation program did not enhance effectiveness.[14] Overall, it does appear that either relaxation training or EMG biofeedback is a promising treatment for myofascial pain of the upper quarter.

There is only one biofeedback study on fibromyalgia. Ferraccioli and associates used EMG biofeedback to treat the pain associated with fibromyalgia. They found that 56% of their treatment group achieved long-lasting clinical benefit. Looking at those who failed to benefit from treatment, they found the subgroup that failed to benefit was clinically depressed. This study calls attention for the need to deal with both mind and muscle.[38] Many appropriate and potentially effective treatments will fail if psychopathology is not taken into consideration.

Hypnosis is probably one of the oldest nonmedicinal treatments known, and, despite such an extended history, controversy continues over just what hypnosis is and how it works. One of the more common definitions of hypnosis is that it is a state of focused attention or heightened concentration.[118] Some refer to the hypnotic state as a dissociation phenomenon whereas others equate it more to a relaxation response. Neither position is likely correct. Because the capacity to be hypnotized varies widely, it is most probable that a small percentage of the population can be put in a deeply dissociated state of mind in which they are amenable to suggestion whereas, at the other extreme, there are a small number of people who simply cannot surrender any personal control whatsoever. In the middle range are those individuals to whom hypnosis is the equivalent of a relaxation response. Hypnotic applications to clinical pain are extensively documented but, for the most part, involve clinical case reports and anecdotal tales.

Four common hypnotic suggestions for modifying clinical pain have been reviewed by Wolskee.[118]

- The first involves direct suggestion of analgesia. In the hypnotic trance, suggestions are given of pain relief as well as imaginative transfer of sensation from pain to some other sensation such as numbness.
- The second group of suggestions involves filtering of pain. These suggestions often combine imagery with sensation to provide the patient with a sense of the pain being filtered through or out of the body.
- The third group of suggestions involves dissociation of the pain from the body. Again, with this approach, use of imagery is helpful and the patient is encouraged to stand aside or away from his or her pain.
- The fourth set of suggestions involves displacement of the pain sensation to another part of the body.

These suggestions can be very effective in pain management. Evans has counseled care in assessment of the patient who is a candidate for hypnotic pain relief. He is particularly concerned about the pain masking depression. If such is the case, too rapid or complete a removal of pain can lead to increased overt depression and suicidality.[33]

Hypnotic techniques can be combined with other forms of psychological intervention as well. Techniques such as hypnotherapy and hypnoanalysis are often used to determine the deeper meanings and idiosyncratic aspects of how the patient's psychology interacts with pain sensation.

Patients can be taught self-hypnosis. Again, this is similar to training the relaxation response and it enables the patient to have yet another positive coping skill for dealing with the more intense of pain sensations. Both relaxation and self-hypnosis need to be learned and practiced at times when the pain is less intense. Intense pain is disruptive of concentration and the patient may be unable to engage in the induction.

All of the self-regulatory techniques require intensive training. One of the failures often seen in pain management is too limited a trial of any one of the methods discussed earlier. One cannot teach relaxation, biofeedback, or self-hypnosis in one or two sessions. Yet, in my experience, many patients report that is exactly what happened to them.

Multidisciplinary pain management is often the only reasonable approach to managing the intractable pain patient. Specialty centers frequently use the services of physicians, psychologists, and physical therapists, in addition to an array of consultants that are called on an as-needed basis. As persistent pain continues, it may take on more psychological features. The nonpsychiatric physician rarely has the time, training, or inclination to listen to the patient in the same way that the psychiatrist or psychologist does. A team approach to evaluation, treatment planning, and implementation of that plan provides the patient with the most comprehensive care available. In the absence of a multidisciplinary setting, the physician managing these complicated cases of fibromyalgia, myofascial syndrome, and other related musculoskeletal pain should attempt to have access to both skilled physical therapy services and a psychologist or psychiatrist with an interest in pain problems.

Summary

The role of psychological factors in fibromyalgia, myofascial pain syndrome, and related musculoskeletal pain is extremely variable. Although there is some evidence that depression is more prevalent in the personal and family histories of patients with fibromyalgia, the empirical and experimental support is neither consistent nor strong. Patients should also be assessed with attention to anxiety, stress, somatization, cognitive impairment, and nonrestorative sleep disorder. It is important to remember that all patients with persistent pain do not develop chronic pain syndromes in which virtually all areas of psychosocial activity are compromised. Those patients who do develop chronic pain syndromes are more likely to have a history that includes developmental and psychosocial risk factors. Careful screening of the patient may provide clues as to which patients may require more comprehensive management, including psychological services. Both biofeedback and psychotherapy have shown promise in the comprehensive management of the patient with musculoskeletal pain.

References

1. Adler RH, Zlot S, Hurny C, et al: Engel's "Psychogenic pain and the pain-prone patient: A retrospective, controlled clinical study." Psychosomatics 51:87–101, 1989.
2. Ahles TA, Yunus MB, Masi AT: Is chronic pain a variant of depressive disease? The case of primary fibromyalgia syndrome. Pain 29:105–111, 1987.
3. Ahles TA, Yunus MB, Riley SD, et al: Psychological factors associated with primary fibromyalgia syndrome. Arthritis Rheum 27:1101–1106, 1984.
4. Anderson DA, Hines RH: Attachment and pain. In Grzesiak RC, Ciccone DS (eds): Psychological Vulnerability to Chronic Pain. New York, Springer, 1994, pp 137–152.
5. Arnoff GM: Myofascial pain syndrome and fibromyalgia: A critical assessment and alternate view. Clin J Pain 14:74–85, 1998.
6. Bennett RM, Gatter RA, Campbell SM, et al: A comparison of cyclobenzaprine and placebo in the management of fibrositis. Arthritis Rheum 31:1535–1542, 1988.
7. Bernstein DA, Borkovec TD: Progressive relaxation training. Champaign, Ill, Research Press, 1973.
8. Blumer D, Heilbronn M: Chronic pain as a variant of depressive disease: The pain-prone disorder. J Nerv Ment Dis 170:381–405, 1982.
9. Blumer D, Heilbronn M: Dysthymic pain disorder: The treatment of chronic pain as a variant of depression. In Tollison CD (ed): Handbook of Chronic Pain Management. Baltimore, Williams & Wilkins, 1989, pp 197–209.
10. Boissevain MD, McCain GA: Toward an integrated understanding of fibromyalgia syndrome. I. Medical and pathophysiological aspects. Pain 45:227–238, 1991.
11. Boissevain MD, McCain GA: Toward an integrated understanding of fibromyalgia syndrome. II. Psychological and phenomenological aspects. Pain 45:239–248, 1991.
12. Bradley LA, Prokop CK, Margolis R, et al: Multivariate analysis of the MMPI profiles of low back pain patients. J Behav Med 1:253–272, 1978.
13. Brena SF, Koch DL: "Pain estimate" model for quantification and classification of chronic pain states. Anesthesiol Rev 2:8–13, 1975.
14. Brooke RI, Stenn PG: Myofascial pain dysfunction syndrome: How effective is biofeedback-assisted relaxation training? In Bonica JJ, Lindblom U, Iggo A (eds): Advances in Pain Research and Therapy, vol 5. New York, Raven, 1983, pp 809–812.
15. Campbell SM, Clark S, Tindall EA, et al: Clinical characteristics of fibrositis: A "blinded" controlled study of symptoms and tender points. Arthritis Rheum 26:817–824, 1983.
16. Carette S, McCain GA, Bell DA, et al: Evaluation of amitriptyline in primary fibrositis: A double-blind, placebo-controlled study. Arthritis Rheum 29:655–650, 1986.
17. Chapman CR, Bonica JJ: Chronic pain. Kalamazoo, Mich, Upjohn, 1985.
18. Ciccone DS, Grzesiak RC: Cognitive dimensions of chronic pain. Soc Sci Med 19:1339–1345, 1984.
19. Ciccone DS, Grzesiak RC: Cognitive therapy: An overview of theory and practice. In Lynch NT, Vasudevan S (eds): Persistent Pain: Psychosocial Assessment and Intervention. Boston, Kluwer, 1988, pp 133–161.
20. Ciccone DS, Grzesiak RC: Chronic musculoskeletal pain: A cognitive approach to psychophysiologic assessment and intervention. In Eisenberg MG, Grzesiak RC (eds): Advances in Clinical Rehabilitation, vol 3. New York, Springer, 1990, pp 197–115.
21. Ciccone DS, Grzesiak RC: Psychological vulnerability to chronic pain: A preliminary study. Paper presented at the Annual Meeting of the American Pain Society, October 1990, St. Louis.
22. Ciccone DS, Grzesiak RC: Psychological dysfunction in chronic cervical pain: An introduction to clinical assessment. In Tollison CD, Satterthwaite JR (eds): Painful Cervical Trauma: Diagnosis and Rehabilitative Treatment of Neuromusculoskeletal Injuries. Baltimore, Williams & Wilkins, 1992, pp 79–92.
23. Coen SJ, Sarno JE: Psychosomatic avoidance of conflict in back pain. J Am Acad Psychoanal 17:359–376, 1989.
24. Crue BL Jr: Evaluation of chronic pain syndromes (Tape T 155). New York, BioMonitoring Applications, 1978.
25. Draspa LJ: Psychological factors in muscular pain. Br J Med Psychol 32:106–116, 1959.
26. Dworkin RH, Gitlin MJ: Clinical aspects of depression in chronic pain patients. Clin J Pain 7:79–94, 1991.
27. Dworkin RH, Grzesiak RC: Chronic pain: On the integration of psyche and soma. In Stricker G, Gold GR (eds): Comprehensive Handbook of Psychotherapy Integration. New York, Plenum, 1993, pp 365–384.
28. Dworkin RH, Handlin DS, Richlin DM, et al: Unraveling the effects of compensation, litigation, and employment on treatment response in chronic pain. Pain 23:49–59, 1985.
29. Dworkin RH, Hartstein G, Rosner HL, et al: A high-risk method of studying psychosocial antecedents of chronic pain: The prospective investigation of herpes zoster. J Abnorm Psychol 101:200–205, 1992.

30. Eimers BN: Psychotherapy for chronic pain: A cognitive approach. In Freeman A, Simon KM, Beutler LE, et al (eds): Comprehensive Handbook of Cognitive Therapy. New York, Plenum, 1989, pp 440–465.
31. Engel GL: Primary atypical facial neuralgia: A hysterical conversion symptom. Psychosom Med 13:375–396, 1951.
32. Engel GL: "Psychogenic" pain and the pain-prone patient. Am J Med 26:899–918, 1959.
33. Evans FJ: Hypnosis and chronic pain management. In Burrows G, Elton D, Stanley G (eds): Handbook of Chronic Pain Management. Amsterdam, Elsevier, 1987.
34. Fishbain DA, Cutler R, Rosomoff HL, Rosomoff RS: Chronic pain associated depression: Antecedent or consequence of chronic pain? A review. Clin J Pain 13:116–137, 1997.
35. France RD, Krishnan KRR: Pain in psychiatric disorders. In France RD, Krishnan KRR (eds): Chronic Pain. Washington, DC, American Psychiatric Press, 1988, pp 117–141.
36. French AP, Tupin JP: Therapeutic application of a simple relaxation method. Am J Psychother 28:282–287, 1974.
37. Felson DT, Goldenberg DL: The natural history of fibromyalgia. Arthritis Rheum 29:1522–1526, 1986.
38. Ferraccioli G, Ghirelli L, Scita F, et al: EMG-biofeedback training in fibromyalgia syndrome. J Rheumatol 144:820–825, 1987.
39. Fordyce WE: Behavioral methods for chronic pain and illness. St. Louis, Mosby, 1976.
40. Fordyce WE, Fowler RS, deLateur BJ: Application of behavior modification technique to problems of chronic pain. Behav Res Ther 6:105–107, 1968.
41. Fordyce WE, Fowler RS, Lehmann J, et al: Some applications of learning to problems of chronic pain. J Chron Dis 21:179–190, 1968.
42. Goldenberg DL: Psychiatric and psychologic aspects of fibromyalgia syndrome. Rheum Dis Clin 15:105–114, 1989.
43. Goldenberg DL, Felson DT, Dinnerman HA: A randomized controlled trial of amitriptyline and naproxen in the treatment of patients with fibromyalgia. Arthritis Rheum 29:1371–1377, 1986.
44. Goldstein JA: Betrayal By the Brain: The Neurologic Basis of Chronic Fatigue Syndrome, Fibromyalgia Syndrome, and Related Neural Network Disorders. New York, Haworth, 1996.
45. Grzesiak RC: Relaxation techniques in treatment of chronic pain. Arch Phys Med Rehab 58:270–272, 1977.
46. Grzesiak RC: Biofeedback in the treatment of chronic pain. Current Concepts in Pain 2:3–8, 1984.
47. Grzesiak RC: Strategies for multidisciplinary pain management. Compendium of Continuing Education in Dentistry 10:444–448, 1989.
48. Grzesiak RC: Psychological aspects of chronic orofacial pain: Theory, assessment and management. Pain Digest 1:100–119, 1991.
49. Grzesiak RC: Unconscious processes and chronic pain: On the foundations of pain-proneness. Paper presented at the Annual Meeting of the American Psychological Association, August 1992, Washington, DC.
50. Grzesiak RC: The matrix of vulnerability. In Grzesiak RC and Ciccone DS (eds): Psychological Vulnerability to Chronic Pain. New York, Springer, 1994, pp 1–27.
51. Grzesiak RC, Ciccone DS: Relaxation, biofeedback and hypnosis in the management of pain. In Lynch NT, Vasudevan S (eds): Persistent Pain: Psychosocial Assessment and Intervention. Boston, Kluwer, 1988, pp 163–188.
52. Grzesiak RC, Perrine KR: Psychological aspects of chronic pain. In Wu W (ed): Pain Management: Assessment and Treatment of Chronic and Acute Syndromes. New York, Human Sciences, 1986, pp 44–69.
53. Grzesiak RC, Ury G, Dworkin RH: Psychodynamic psychotherapy with chronic pain patients. In Gatchel RJ, Turk DC (eds): Psychological Approaches to Pain Management: A Practitioner's Handbook. New York, Guilford, 1996, pp 148–178.
54. Gupta M, Moldofsky H: Dysthymic disorder and rheumatic pain modulation disorder (fibrositis syndrome): A comparison of symptoms and sleep physiology. Can J Psychiatry 31:608–616, 1986.
55. Hanvik LJ: MMPI profiles in patients with low back pain. J Consult Psychol 15:350–353, 1951.
56. Heaton RK, Lehman RAW, Getto CJ: Psychosocial Pain Inventory. Odessa, Fla, Psychological Assessment Resources, 1980.
57. Holmes TH, Wolff HG: Life situations, emotions, and backache. Psychosom Med 14:18–33, 1952.
58. Hudson JI, Hudson MS, Pliner LF, et al: Fibromyalgia and major affective disorder: A controlled phenomenology and family history study. Am J Psychiatry 142:441–446, 1985.
59. Huskisson EC: Measurement of pain. Lancet 2:1127–1131, 1974.
60. Jacobsen R, Edinger JD: Side effects of relaxation treatment. Am J Psychiatry 139:952–953, 1982.
61. Jacobson E: Modern Treatment of Tense Patients. Springfield, Ill: Charles C Thomas, 1964.
62. Kellner R: Psychosomatic syndromes and somatic symptoms. Washington, DC, American Psychiatric Press, 1991.
63. Kerns RD, Turk DC, Rudy TE: The West Haven-Yale Multi-dimensional Pain Inventory (WHYMPI). Pain 23:345–356, 1985.
64. Kirmayer LJ, Robbins JM, Kapusta MA: Somatization and depression in fibromyalgia syndrome. Am J Psychiatry 145:950–954, 1988.
65. Large RG, Lamb AM: Electromyographic (EMG) feedback in chronic musculoskeletal pain: A controlled trial. Pain 17:167–177, 1983.
66. Loeser JD: Concepts of pain. In Stanton-Hicks M, Boas RA (eds): Chronic Low Back Pain. New York, Raven, 1982, pp 145–148.

67. Loeser JD, Black RG: A taxonomy of pain. Pain 1:81–90, 1975.
68. McCain FA, Scudds RA: The concept of primary fibromyalgia (fibrositis): Clinical value, relation and significance to other musculoskeletal pain syndromes. Pain 33:273–287, 1988.
69. McFarlane AC: Resiliency, vulnerability, and the course of posttraumatic reactions. In Van Der Kolk BA, McFarlane AC, Weisaeth L (eds): Traumatic Stress: The Effects of Overwhelming Experience on Mind, Body and Society. New York, Guilford, 1996, pp 155–181.
70. McGuigan FJ: Progressive relaxation: Origins, principles, and clinical applications. In Woolfolk RL, Lehrer PM (eds): Principles and Practice of Stress Management. New York, Guilford, 1984, pp 12–42.
71. Mendelson G: Compensation, pain complaints, and psychological disturbance. Pain 20:169–177, 1984.
72. Melzack R: The McGill Pain Questionnaire: Major properties and scoring methods. Pain 1:277–299, 1975.
73. Melzack R: Phantom limbs. Regional Anesthesia 14:208–211, 1989.
74. Melzack R: Central pain syndromes and theories of pain. In Casey KL (ed): Pain and Central Nervous System Disease: The Central Pain Syndromes. New York, Raven, 1991, pp 195–210.
75. Melzack R: Phantom limbs. Scientific American, April 1992:120–126.
76. Melzack R, Wall RD: Pain mechanisms: A new theory. Science, 150:971–979, 1965.
77. Merskey H: Psychiatric patients with persistent pain. J Psychosom Res 9:299–309, 1965.
78. Merskey H: The perception and measurement of pain. J Psychosom Res 17:251–255, 1973.
79. Merskey H (ed): Classification of chronic pain: Descriptions of chronic pain syndromes and definitions of pain terms. Pain (Suppl. 3), 1986.
80. Middaugh SJ, Kee WG: Advances in electromyographic monitoring and biofeedback in the treatment of chronic cervical and low back pain. In Eisenberg MG, Grzesiak RC (eds): Advances in Clinical Rehabilitation, vol 1. New York, Springer, 1987, pp 137–172.
81. Moldofsky H: Sleep and fibrositis syndrome. Rheum Dis Clin 15:91–103, 1989.
82. Moldofsky H, Lue FA: The relationship of alpha delta EEG frequencies to pain and mood in "fibrositis" patients with chlorpromazine and L-tryptophan. Electroencephalogr Clin Neurophysiol 50:71–80, 1980.
83. Moldofsky H, Scarisbrick P: Induction of neurasthenic musculoskeletal pain syndrome by selective sleep stage deprivation. Psychosom Med 38:35–44, 1976.
84. Moldofsky H, Scarisbrick P, England R, et al: Musculoskeletal symptoms and non-REM sleep disturbance in patients with "fibrositis" syndrome and healthy subjects. Psychosom Med 37:341–351, 1975.
85. Nouwen A, Bush C: The relationship between paraspinal EMG and chronic low back pain. Pain 20:109–123, 1984.
86. Nouwen A, Solinger JW: The effectiveness of EMG biofeedback training in low back pain. Biofeedback Self Regul 4:8–12, 1979.
87. Okifuji A, Turk DC: Fibromyalgia: Search for mechanisms and effective treatments. In Gatchel RJ, DC Turk (eds): Psychosocial Factors in Pain: Critical Perspectives. New York, Guilford, 1999, pp 227–246.
88. Payne TC, Leavit F, Garron DC, et al: Fibrositis and psychologic disturbances. Arthritis Rheum 25:213–217, 1982.
89. Peck CL, Kraft GH: Electromyographic biofeedback for pain related to muscle tension: A study of tension headache, back and jaw pain. Arch Surg 112:889–895, 1977.
90. Pomp AM: Psychotherapy for the myofascial pain-dysfunction syndrome: A study of factors coinciding with symptom remission. J Am Dent Assoc 89:629–632, 1974.
91. Rudy TE, Turk DC, Zaki HS, et al: An empirical taxometric alternative to traditional classification of temporomandibular disorders. Pain 36:311–320, 1989.
92. Sarno JE: Psychogenic backache: The missing dimension. J Fam Pract 1:8–12, 1974.
93. Sarno JE: Chronic back pain and psychic conflict. Scand J Rehab Med 8:143–153, 1976.
94. Sarno JE: Psychosomatic backache. J Fam Pract 5:353–357, 1977.
95. Sarno JE: Etiology of neck and back pain: An autonomic myoneuralgia. J Nerv Ment Dis 169:55–59, 1981.
96. Sarno JE: Mind over back pain. New York, Berkeley Books, 1984.
97. Sarno JE: The mind-body prescription: Healing the body, healing the pain. New York, Warner Books, 1998.
98. Saskin P, Moldofsky H, Lue FA: Sleep and posttraumatic pain modulation disorder (fibrositis syndrome). Psychosom Med 48:319–323, 1986.
99. Schofferman J, Anderson D, Hines R, et al: Childhood psychological trauma correlates with unsuccessful lumbar spine surgery. Spine 17:138–144, 1992.
100. Shutty MS, Sheras P: Brief strategic psychotherapy with chronic pain patients: Reframing and problem resolution. Psychother 28:636–642, 1991.
101. Simms RW, Goldenberg DL, Felson DT, et al: Tenderness in 75 anatomic sites: Distinguishing fibromyalgia patients from controls. Arthritis Rheum 31:182–187, 1988.
102. Smythe HA: Non-articular rheumatism and psychogenic musculo-skeletal syndromes. In: McCarty DJ (ed): Arthritis and Allied Conditions, 11th ed. Philadelphia, Lea & Febiger, 1988, pp 1241–1254.
103. Tait RC: Psychological factors in chronic benign pain. Current Concepts in Pain 1:10–15, 1983.
104. Tunks ER, Merskey H: Psychotherapy in the management of chronic pain. In Bonica JJ (ed): The Management of Pain, vol II, 2nd ed. Philadelphia, Lea & Febiger, 1990, pp 1751–1756.
105. Turk DC: Customizing treatment for chronic pain patients: Who, what, and why? Clin J Pain 6:255–270, 1990.

106. Turk, DC, Meichenbaum D, Genest M: Pain and behavioral medicine: A cognitive-behavioral perspective. New York, Guilford, 1983.
107. Turk DC, Rudy TE: Toward an empirically derived taxonomy of chronic pain patients: Integration of psychological assessment data. J Consult Clin Psychol 56:233–238, 1988.
108. Turk DC, Rudy TE: Neglected factors in chronic pain treatment outcome studies—referral patterns, failure to enter treatment, and attrition. Pain 43:7–25, 1990.
109. Turk DC, Rudy TE: Neglected topics in the treatment of chronic pain patients—relapse, noncompliance, and adherence enhancement. Pain 44:5–28, 1991.
110. van der Kolk BA: The complexity of adaptation to trauma: Self-regulation, stimulus discrimination, and characterological development. In van der Kolk BA, McFarlane AC, Weisaeth L (eds): Traumatic Stress: The Effects of Overwhelming Experience on Mind, Body and Society. New York, Guilford, 1996, pp 182–213.
111. van der Kolk BA: The body keeps the scare: Approaches to the psychobiology of posttraumatic stress disorder. In van der Kolk BA, McFarlane AC, Weisaeth L (eds): Traumatic Stress: The Effects of Overwhelming Experience on Mind, Body and Society. New York, Guilford, 1996, pp 214–241.
112. van der Kolk BA, van der Hart O: The intrusive past: The flexibility of memory and the engraving of trauma. American Imago 48:425–454, 1991.
113. Van Houdenhov B: Prevalence and psychodynamic interpretation of premorbid hyperactivity in patients with chronic pain. Psychother Psychosom 45:195–200, 1986.
114. Waldinger RJ: Psychiatry for medical students. Washington, DC, American Psychiatric Press, 1984.
115. Whale J: The use of brief focal psychotherapy in the treatment of chronic pain. Psychoanalytic Psychother 6:61–72, 1992.
116. Wolfe F, Cathey MA, Kleinheksel SM, et al: Psychological status in primary fibrositis and fibrositis associated with rheumatoid arthritis. J Rheumatol 11:500–506, 1984.
117. Wolfe F, Smythe HA, Yunus MB, et al: The American College of Rheumatology 1990 criteria for the classification of fibromyalgia. Arthritis Rheum 33:160–172, 1990.
118. Wolskee PJ: Psychological therapy for chronic pain. In Wu W (ed): Pain Management: Assessment and Treatment of Chronic and Acute Syndromes. New York, Human Sciences, 1987, pp 201–215.

Chapter 6

Disability Evaluation and Management of Myofascial Pain

Matthew Monsein, MD

Unfortunately, not all patients with myofascial pain syndromes respond successfully to treatment. There exist a small but significant number of patients who despite undergoing extensive treatment continue to complain of severe and often disabling pain. Often characterized as having a chronic pain syndrome, these patients can be recognized by their clinical unresponsiveness to standard medical care, the presence of numerous psychosocial contributing factors, and the frustration confounding their physicians, themselves, and the medical-legal systems with which they are frequently involved. In spite of treatment, they continue to complain of pain, often greater than one would expect based on the clinical findings alone.

Associated with their complaints of pain are often a number of dysfunctional behaviors. These may include excessive alcohol use; overdependence on narcotics and over-the-counter medications; histrionic behaviors, i.e., grimacing, groaning, bizarre posturing, or touch-me-not reactions in response to even the lightest palpation; and depression, anxiety, and other psychological distress. These patients have often developed extremely sedentary lifestyles secondary to their experience of pain and are physically deconditioned. Most important, from the patient's perspective and that of society's, they have become socially isolated, given up a number of recreational activities, and claimed disability from work secondary to their experience of pain.

The reasons for this type of behavior remain unclear.[44] Simons suggests that these patients have developed a post-traumatic hyperirritability of their nervous system and of their trigger points. Each patient has suffered trauma, usually from an automobile accident or fall severe enough to damage the sensory pathways of the central nervous system. The damage apparently acts as an endogenous perpetuating factor susceptible to augmentation by severe pain, additional trauma, vibration, loud noises, prolonged physical activity, and emotional stress. From the date of the trauma, coping with pain typically becomes the focus of life for these patients who previously paid little attention to pain. They are unable to increase their activity substantially without increasing their pain level.[40]

Others suggest that it is the psychosocial factors that are the dominant feature in the evolution of this pattern of behavior. Addressing these factors is at the heart of successful rehabilitation of these patients.[3, 26, 35, 39] Assessing the clinical status of this group of patients, providing appropriate guidance toward rehabilitation, and interfacing with the various disability systems remain an extremely challenging task for the physician.

Physicians often feel inadequate in addressing issues that society has demanded of them with the establishment of the various disability systems. Disability assessment is not a standard part of medical school or residency training. Physicians often resent the requirements of filling out lengthy forms and the involvement of attorneys. Finally, they may have concerns about their own ability based on their training and knowledge to delineate issues for society such as disability, percentage of bodily impairment, functional limitations, and the patient's ability or inability to work.[9] These determinations are extremely vexing, particularly when they are based to a large degree on the patient's subjective experience.

In 1955, congressional hearings were held to establish whether physicians were able to determine disability by standard medical examinations. Physicians from almost every state and medical society were interviewed. A substantial majority of physicians believed that they were unable to determine disability purely on a medical basis. Moreover, most thought that intervening in the disability process would be in conflict with their therapeutic relationship with the patient.

> *Disability certification for purpose of cash benefits required the physician to mediate between the patient and the government's interest. In such gate-keeping rules, physicians would be "caught in a squeeze" and forced to "serve two masters." Patients could and would simply shop around for a doctor willing to provide evidence of their impairments, and friends and family, as well as patients, would put unbearable pressure on physicians, reducing their ability to make good clinical judgments. Introducing such extensions into the doctor patient relationship would undermine its therapeutic effectiveness.*[29]

Nevertheless, in spite of these objections, most disability systems do place considerable, if not total, dependence upon the treating physician's evaluation.

In the area of pain—particularly myofascial pain—this issue is even more problematic. By definition, pain is simply a personal and subjective experience known only to the patient. As clinicians, we can only observe the outer manifestations of this experience or the patient's pain behaviors. We are dependent on the patient's subjective complaints in assessing the severity of the problem.

In myofascial pain disorders, there are no agreed-on objective standards for assessing the anatomic severity of the condition. Specifically, although data exist to support the reliability and validity of pressure algometry, questions remain as to their sensitivity because they are still reliant on the patient's subjective response.[34] Furthermore, neither pressure algometry nor the more controversial thermography[10] has been accepted as a reliable standard by medical organizations such as the American Medical Association (AMA) or the American Academy of Orthopaedic Surgeons, or by the various disability systems such as Social Security disability or workers' compensation.

Although Simons[40] believes that a palpable hardening of taut bands of muscle fibers passing through the tender spot in a shortened muscle and a local twitch response of the taut band are objective indications of myofascial pain, assessment of these findings depends on the sensitivity and clinical acumen of the examiner. Thus, at the present time, assessing a patient's level of pain and dysfunction, as well as determining how to help this select group of patients with myofascial pain syndromes who claim disability, remains a challenge.

The purpose of this chapter is threefold: first, to discuss various disability systems in the context of myofascial pain; second, to describe in more detail the psychosocial characteristics of patients who present with disability secondary to myofascial pain syndromes; and finally, to present a model for rehabilitation to assist these patients in returning to a more normal and functional lifestyle.

Disability Systems

Most patients with myofascial pain are covered under one of four systems: Social Security Disability Insurance (SSDI), workers' compensation (WC),[31] personal injury (PI), or long-term disability (LTD). Each system has its own characteristics established either through legislation, in the case of SSDI and WC, or in PI and LTD cases through a combination of legislation and individual policy formulation. In order to understand the implication of myofascial pain each specific system, it is important to review the concept of impairment and its relationship to pain and disability.

Definitions

Impairment

Impairment is defined as any loss or abnormality of psychological, physiologic, or anatomic structure or function that can be defined in terms of objective medical

Table 6–1.
Comparison of Impairment (Disability)

System	Symptoms	ROM	Diagnosis	Other Physiologic	Functional Evaluator
Social Security	X	X		X	
California (WC)	X	X	X	X	X
Minnesota (WC)	X		X		
American Medical Association		X	X		
American Academy of Orthopedic Surgeons	X	X	X		

ROM, range of motion; WC, workers' compensation.
Modified from Mayer TG, Mooney V, Gatchel RJ, et al: Contemporary Conservative Care for Painful Spinal Disorders: Impairment Evaluation Issues and the Disability System. Philadelphia, Lea & Febiger, 1991, p 533, with permission.

evidence such as radiographs or laboratory tests, standardized psychological tests, and objective clinical findings such as range of motion, muscle atrophy, sensory changes, and so forth.[8] It should be noted that trigger points are generally not included in the various systems that define medical impairment. Furthermore, the patient's subjective complaints, although vitally important in defining disability and functional capacity, may or may not be considered in the establishment of a medical impairment, depending on the system (Table 6–1). At times, physicians are asked only to assess whether the patient has a physical or psychological condition and at other times are asked to actually give a percentage of impairment. The rationale for this concept dates back to models used in determining casualty and property damage in which an insurance adjuster, for example, was capable of estimating the percentage of fire damage to a building. The premise is that a physician has the same capability in terms of defining a percentage of damage to the body of an individual. Although one may argue the reasonableness of this idea, as long as the current legal system remains, physicians will continue to be held responsible for defining impairment as a percentage of the whole person or of an individual extremity.[4]

In an attempt to gain some uniformity, several systems of impairment or disability determination have emerged. The factors utilized in determining impairment vary based on each individual system. For example, the AMA *Guides to the Evaluation of Permanent Impairment*,[9] which was first published in 1958 and is now in its fourth edition, is based primarily on anatomic features but does include diagnosis as well. This is also true of the American Academy of Orthopaedic Surgeons system, which was a modification of the AMA model.[22] The latter does, however, incorporate a scale for pain in patients with documented organic disorders. In Minnesota, WC impairment is defined in the state regulations and is based primarily on range of motion and radiographic findings, although clinical symptoms are also included.[49]

With specific regard to the issue of myofascial pain, let us take an example of someone with a cervical strain or whiplash injury. Using the AMA guidelines, two specific areas would be utilized in determining the percentage of impairment. First, as defined in Figure 6–1A, assuming that the patient does not have any degenerative radiographic changes, he or she would receive a 4% permanent partial impairment of the whole person for the diagnosis of a cervical strain. This is based on the observation that not only does the patient have pain but there is clinical evidence of recurrent muscle spasm or rigidity. Assuming that there is loss of motion, there would be an additional percentage of impairment based on the findings as indicated in Figure 6–1B to D. Adding these together and using what the AMA calls a Combined Values Chart, one would be able to determine the actual percentage of physical impairment. It is of interest that myofascial pain is not included in the index.

However, in the fourth edition, unlike its predecessors, there is a chapter that specifically addresses pain and estimating impairment. Although the authors acknowledge that pain in and of itself can be considered an impairment, they suggest that a

Disorder	% Impairment of the whole person		
	Cervical	Thoracic	Lumbar
I. Fracture:			
A. Compression of one vertebral body			
0%–25%	4	2	5
26%–50%	6	3	7
>50%	10	5	12
B. Fracture of posterior element (pedicle, lamina, articular process, transverse process). *Note:* An impairment due to compression of a vertebra and one due to fracture of a posterior element are *combined* using the Combined Values Chart. Fractures or compressions of several vertebrae are *combined* using the Combined Values Chart.	4	2	5
C. Reduced dislocation of one vertebra. If two or more vertebrae are dislocated and reduced, *combine* the estimates using the Combined Values Chart. An unreduced dislocation causes impairment until it is reduced: The physician should then evaluate the impairment on the basis of the subject's condition with the dislocation reduced. If no reduction is possible, the physician should evaluate the impairment on the basis of the range of motion and the neurologic findings according to criteria in this chapter and the nervous system chapter.	5	3	6
II. Intervertebral disc or other soft-tissue lesion			
A. Unoperated on, with no residual signs or symptoms.	0	0	0
B. Unoperated on, stable, with medically documented injury, pain, and rigidity associated with *none to minimal* degenerative changes on structural tests, such as those involving roentgenography or magnetic resonance imaging.	4	2	5
C. Unoperated on, stable, with medically documented injury, pain, and rigidity associated with *moderate to severe* degenerative changes on structural tests; includes unoperated on herniated nucleus pulposus with or without radiculopathy.	6	3	7
D. Surgically treated disk lesion without residual signs or symptoms: includes disk injection.	7	4	7 8
E. Surgically treated disk lesion with residual, medically documented pain and rigidity.	9	5	10
F. Multiple levels, with or without operations and with or without residual signs or symptoms.	Add 1% per level		
G. Multiple operations *with* or without residual symptoms: 1. Second operation	Add 2%		
2. Third or subsequent operation	Add 1% per operation		
III. Spondylolysis and spondylolisthesis, not operated on			
A. Spondylolysis or grade I (1%–25% slippage); or grade II (26%–50% slippage) spondylolisthesis, accompanied by medically documented injury that is stable, and medically documented pain and rigidity with or without muscle spasm.	6	3	7
B. Grade III (51%–75% slippage) or grade IV (76%–100% slippage) spondylolisthesis, accompanied by medically documented injury that is stable and medically documented pain and rigidity with or without muscle spasm.	8	4	9

Figure 6–1. A–D, Determining the percentage of impairment due to specific disorders of the spine. (From Doege TC [ed]: Guides to the Evaluation of Permanent Impairment, 4th ed. Chicago, American Medical Association, 1993, with permission.)

A *Continued*

	% Impairment of the whole person		
Disorder	Cervical	Thoracic	Lumbar
IV. Spinal stenosis, segmental instability, spondylolisthesis, fracture, or dislocation, operated on			
A. Single-level decompression *without* spinal fusion and *without* residual signs or symptoms.	7	4	8
B. Single-level decompression *with* residual signs or symptoms.	9	5	10
C. Single-level spinal fusion with or without decompression *without* residual signs or symptoms.	8 10	4 5	9 12
D. Single-level spinal fusion with or without decompression *with* residual signs or symptoms.	10	5	12
E. Multiple levels, operated on, with residual, medically documented pain and rigidity with or without muscle spasm.	Add 1% per level		
1. Second operation	Add 2%		
2. Third or subsequent operation	Add 1% per operation		

*Instructions:
1. Identify the most significant impairment of the primarily involved region.
2. The diagnosis-based impairment estimates and percents shown above should be combined with range of motion impairment estimates and with whole-person impairment estimates involving sensation, weakness, and conditions of the musculoskeletal, nervous, or other organ systems.
3. List the diagnosis-based, range of motion, and other whole-person impairment estimates on the Spine Impairment Summary Form.
The words "with medically documented injury, pain, and rigidity" imply not only that an injury or illness has occurred, but also that the condition is stable, as shown by the evaluator's history, examination, and other data, and that a permanent impairment exists, which is at least partly due to the condition being evaluated and not only due to preexisting disease.

B

Abnormal Motion Average range of flexion and extension is 110°. The proportion of all cervical motions is 40%.			
a.	**Flexion** from neutral Position (0°) to:	Degrees of cervical motion		% Impairment of the whole person
		Lost	Retained	
	0° 15° 30° 50°	50 30 15 0	0 15 30 50	5 4 2 0
b.	**Extension** from neutral Position (0°) to:			
	0° 20° 40° 60°	60 40 20 0	0 20 40 60+	6 4 2 0
c.	**Ankylosis** Region ankylosed at:			
	0° (neutral position) 15° 30° 50° (full flexion)			12 20 30 40
	Region ankylosed at:			
	0° (neutral position) 20° 40° 60° (full extension)			12 20 30 40

Figure 6–1 *Continued*

Illustration continued on following page

C

Abnormal Motion
The average range of lateral flexion is 90°.
The proportion of all cervical motions is 25%.

a.	**Right lateral flexion** From neutral position (0°) to:	Degrees of cervical motion		% Impairment of the whole person
		Lost	Retained	
	0°	45	0	4
	15°	30	15	2
	30°	15	30	1
	45°	0	45	0
b.	**Left lateral flexion** From neutral position (0°) to:			
	0°	45	0	4
	15°	30	15	2
	30°	15	30	1
	45°	0	45+	0
c.	**Ankylosis** Region ankylosed at:			
	0° (neutral position)			8
	15°			20
	30°			30
	45° (full right or left lateral flexion)			40

D

Abnormal Motion
Average range of rotation is 160°; the proportion of all cervical motion is 35%.

a.	**Right rotation** from neutral position (0°) to:	Degrees of cervical motion		% Impairment of the whole person
		Lost	Retained	
	0°	80	0	6
	20°	60	20	4
	40°	40	40	2
	60°	20	60	1
	80°	0	80+	0
b.	**Left rotation** from neutral position (0°) to:			
	0°	80	0	6
	20°	60	20	4
	40°	40	40	2
	60°	20	60	1
	80°	0	80+	0
c.	**Ankylosis** Region ankylosed at:			
	0° (neutral position)			12
	20°			20
	40°			30
	60°			40
	80° (full right or left rotation)			50

Figure 6–1 *Continued*

numerical rating should be given only if "the pain can itself be evaluated according to the criteria applicable to a particular organ system." The presence of trigger points is not considered an objective criterion of organ system pathology.

Thus the presence of pain in and of itself is not considered to be ratable in this example. Pain associated with the soft tissue injury is not ratable but is recognized as a factor that will contribute to decreased range of motion. In fact, pain, fear of injury, and neuromuscular inhibition are considered to be factors that may diminish range of motion due to either diminished effort or guarding, and in order for range of motion to be considered accurate, reproducibility is required. Specifically "the examiner must take at least three consecutive mobility measurements which fall within ± 10 percent or 5 percent (whichever is greater to be considered consistent)."[8]

In Minnesota, under the workers' compensation system, a person with a cervical strain would receive only a 3.5% permanent partial impairment, assuming that there were no abnormalities on radiographs and that there was documented muscle spasm or rigidity associated with loss of motion (Fig. 6–2). Although one can certainly argue about the fairness of these various systems, they do point out the inconsistencies and ambiguities associated with the evaluation of impairment with myofascial pain.[49]

In persons involved with personal injury cases, defining impairment may or may not be required depending on the legislative statutes and the wishes of the attorneys. Often, in persons with soft tissue injuries in which pain is a major component of disability, physicians are asked only to give their medical opinion regarding whether the injury is permanent.

In long-term disability, although an impairment needs to be established, a much more crucial issue is the determination of the patients' functional capacities. This includes the ability to return either to their previous profession or, if this is not possible, to return to any type of gainful employment.

Under Social Security disability, one must demonstrate an inability to return to gainful employment on a sustained basis. To qualify for Social Security disability, claimants must prove, based on their impairment as well as other factors such as age, education, and psychological functioning, that they are incapable of performing any job on a full-time basis.

Thus, in conclusion, impairment is a definable loss of structure or function. It is not synonymous with disability. There are certainly some individuals with significant impairments who in spite of their illnesses are able to function relatively normally in terms of performing activities of daily living and working full time whereas others with a minimal medical impairment will find themselves extremely disabled owing to a combination of psychological, social, and behavior factors, in addition to their impairment and experience of pain.

Disability

Disability is defined as the limiting loss or absence of a person's capacity to meet personal, social, or occupational demands, or to meet statutory or regulatory

---

> **Subp. 3. Cervical pain syndrome.**
> A. Symptoms of pain or stiffness in the region of the cervical spine not substantiated by persistent objective clinical findings, regardless of radiographic findings, zero percent.
> B. Symptoms of pain or stiffness in the region of the cervical spine, substantiated by persistent objective clinical findings, that is, involuntary muscle tightness in the paracervical muscle or decreased passive range of motion in the cervical spine, but no radiographic abnormality, 3.5 percent.
> C. Symptoms of pain or stiffness in the region of the cervical spine, substantiated by persistent objective clinical findings, that is, involuntary muscle tightness in the paracervical muscle or decreased passive range of motion in the cervical spine, and with any radiographic, myelographic, CT scan, or MRI scan abnormality not specifically addressed elsewhere in this part:
> (1) single vertebral level, seven percent;
> (2) multiple vertebral levels, ten percent.

Figure 6–2. Determining the percentage of impairment in cervical spine injury: the Minnesota system. (From 2000 Minnesota Statutes, Section 5223.0370, Subp. 3.A.B.C.1.2.)

requirements.[35] Disability reflects loss of function and is usually defined operationally in terms of an inability to participate in social or recreational activities, other activities of daily living, and most important, in the individual's inability to perform work, based on functional limitations.[42] Disability is a reflection of the patient's psychological and physical perception of his or her underlying condition or illness. Disability may result from a medical impairment, but the degree of disability does not necessarily conform to the extent of the pathologic findings.

In terms of work, for example, a professional piano player who loses a little finger would have the same impairment as a truck driver with a similar injury. The former, however, would be totally disabled with respect to going back to work as a piano player, whereas the truck driver would not be affected in terms of his ability to return to his pre-injury job. Moreover, in understanding disability, psychological and social factors need to be evaluated and integrated into the disability assessment.

In patients with myofascial pain syndromes, their psychological status, i.e., their level of anxiety and depression; their personality style, i.e., whether they have a dependent or histrionic personality; the meaning of pain to that person, i.e., the fear of re-injury, concerns about having a more serious underlying medical condition; motivational factors, i.e., desire to return to work; relationship with their employer; litigation; other potential secondary gain factors; cultural issues; and family modeling, i.e., other family members with a history of disability—all can have a significant impact on the way patients perceive and express their condition. In terms of determining work-related disability, the patient's age, education, intelligence, the economic status of the community, work experience, and job availability are crucial. The fact that the patient's symptoms of pain and subsequent disability are greater than what might be expected based on the clinical findings alone does not mean that the patient is malingering or consciously exaggerating his or her symptoms.[35] Obviously then, the determination of disability is an extremely complex and multifaceted process.[16]

Whereas impairment is a medical decision, disability is a legal one. Physicians are trained to assess illness. Although the physical examination, history, and laboratory and imaging studies can establish the existence of an abnormal condition (impairment), the psychosocial factors mentioned earlier are crucial in determining an individual's level of disability. In the case of myofascial pain and disability, a patient's functional capacity is by definition a self-limited phenomenon secondary to the patient's perception of pain and his or her interpretation of that perception. This is ultimately what defines the patient's ability to perform activities of daily living, including work. In order for the physician to evaluate the patient's level of disability, obviously the accuracy of the patient's self-report is vital. Confirmation of the patient's reported limitations by family members can be helpful in defining functional limitations.

Another useful source of information regarding the patient's functional abilities is through the use of a standardized self-assessment questionnaire. Although currently there does not exist a specific instrument that has been established as the gold standard in the assessment of disability and pain, there are a number of instruments (i.e., the Symptom Inventory Profile [SIP], Multidimensional Personality Inventory [WHYMPI], West Haven Yale Oswestry and Integrated Multidimensional Patient Assessment Tool for Health [IMPATH], Short Form 36 [SF36])),[27] that are currently in use. These instruments and others have undergone validity and reliability testing. They provide information to the clinician or the disability evaluator, reflecting the patient's level of function compared with a "normal" population. While they provide a system of standardization, one serious criticism of the use of these instruments in determining disability is that they reflect wholly the claimant's subjective, personal, and potentially biased view. Even though some instruments have built-in "lie" scales, similar to the MMPI, to identify exaggerated responses, they still rely wholly on what the claimants state and therefore lack objectivity.

Another method for assessing disability is the functional capacity evaluation.[17, 18] This is performed by either a physical therapist or an occupational therapist and consists of a minimum of a 2- to 3-hour assessment up to a weeklong assessment of the patient's physical and functional capabilities. Patients are asked to perform a number of activities on a repetitive basis. Repetitive testing is performed to maintain consistency and test for reliability. A skilled therapist is able to distinguish limitations due to physiologic capacities, i.e., muscle fatigue as opposed to pain-limited functions. While testing may be capable of measuring consistency of effort, the observation that inconsistencies are present does not distinguish between a poor outcome secondary to the patient consciously making a poor effort, versus a poor outcome due to unconscious factors. The former obviously implies malingering, whereas the latter may reflect the fear of increased pain, anxiety, or other psychological factors.

A well-performed functional capacity evaluation can certainly provide important data as to a person's functional capacities and identify work restrictions. On completion of a functional capacity evaluation, information is provided as to the patient's capacities regarding sitting, walking, standing, ability to perform repetitive motions, as well as lifting and carrying capacities. Moreover, a well-performed functional capacity evaluation can also provide important data as to which patients, owing to physiologic limitations or pain behaviors, may be candidates for more intensive work-hardening programs, intensive pain rehabilitation, or other types of functional restoration programs.[19, 20] Information gathered by the physical therapist (Fig. 6–3) allows the physician to generate restrictions required for a return-to-work plan (Fig. 6–4).

Social Security Administration

Since the Social Security Administration adjudicates the single largest disability system in this country, it is relevant to discuss how it goes about assessing patients with myofascial pain and fibromyalgia.

Over 1.5 million people apply each year for Social Security disability. Of these, approximately 10% are considered to have a chronic pain syndrome. This implies that they have pain as their primary complaint.

In order to qualify for Social Security disability, a claimant has to prove that he or she is unable "to engage in any substantial gainful activity by reason of a medically determinable, physical, or mental impairment which can be expected to result in death or can be expected to last for a continuous period of not less than 12 months."[29] Furthermore, a physical or mental impairment is further defined as that which "would result from anatomic, physiologic, or psychological abnormalities that can be shown by medically acceptable clinical and laboratory techniques,"[23] and by regulation must be established by medical evidence consisting of symptoms, signs, and laboratory findings.

The Social Security regulations go on to define *symptoms* as the patient's own perception of his or her physical or mental impairment, and *signs* as being anatomic, physiologic, or psychological abnormalities that can be observed with medically acceptable clinical techniques. *Laboratory findings* are manifestations of anatomic, physiologic, or psychological phenomena demonstrable by replacing or extending the perceptiveness of the observer's senses. They include chemical, electrophysiologic, roentgenologic, and psychological tests.[29, 41]

In order to qualify for Social Security disability benefits, the claimant must go through a standardized procedure. First, he or she files a claim with one of the more than 1300 federal, district, and branch offices of the Social Security Administration. The claim is then referred to a state agency—the Disability Determination Service (DDS). Each claim is reviewed by a two-member team composed of a physician and disability examiner who make the initial decision regarding qualification for disability, the physician evaluating for medical impairment and the disability evaluator being responsible for legal and administrative requirements. The team is required to assess the claimant based on a method established by regulation and known as the five-step sequential evaluation process (Fig. 6–5A).

Step one asks whether the patient is engaging "in sustainable gainful activities." This has been defined as earnings greater than $300 per month. Those persons not involved in substantial gainful activity progress to the second step. This asks whether the patient has a severe impairment. Impairment is defined as being severe when it is

Item	Percent of 8-hour Day					Restrictions	Recommendations
	0	1–5	6–33	34–66	67–100		
WEIGHT CAPACITY IN LBS.							
Floor to waist lift							
Waist to overhead lift							
Horizontal lift							
Push							
Pull							
Right carry							
Left carry							
Front carry							
Right hand grip							
Left hand grip							
FLEXIBILITY/POSITIONAL							
Elevated work							
Forward bending/sitting							
Forward bending/standing							
Rotation sitting							
Rotation standing							
Crawl							
Kneel							
Crouch-deep static							
Repetitive squat							
STATIC WORK							
Sitting tolerance							
Standing tolerance							
AMBULATION							
Walking							
Stair climbing							
Step ladder climbing							
Balance							
COORDINATION							
R. upper extremity							
L. upper extremity							

Client

Date

Evaluator   Date

Copyright 1989, Isernhagen Work Systems, Duluth, MN

Figure 6–3. A functional capacity evaluation in subacute spinal disorders. (From Mayer TG, Mooney V, Gatchel RJ, et al: Contemporary Conservative Care for Painful Spinal Disorders: Impairment Evaluation Issues and the Disability System. Philadelphia, Lea & Febiger, 1991, p 533, with permission.)

PATIENT: _____

I estimate this person is able to:

	Never	Occasionally (1-33%)	Frequently (34-66%)	Continuously (67-100%)

1. LIFT:
   a. up to 10 lb.   _____   _____   _____   _____
   b. 11-25 lb.   _____   _____   _____   _____
   c. 26-35 lb.   _____   _____   _____   _____
   d. 36-50 lb.   _____   _____   _____   _____
   e. 51-75 lb.   _____   _____   _____   _____
   f. 76-100 lb.   _____   _____   _____   _____

2. CARRY:
   a. up to 10 lb.   _____   _____   _____   _____
   b. 11-25 lb.   _____   _____   _____   _____
   c. 26-34 lb.   _____   _____   _____   _____
   d. 36-50 lb.   _____   _____   _____   _____
   e. 51-75 lb.   _____   _____   _____   _____
   f. 76-100 lb.   _____   _____   _____   _____

3. CAN THE PERSON PERFORM
   THE FOLLOWING TASKS:
   Push/Pull—Seated   _____   _____   _____   _____
   Push/Pull—Standing   _____   _____   _____   _____
   Bend   _____   _____   _____   _____
   Squat   _____   _____   _____   _____
   Crawl   _____   _____   _____   _____
   Climb   _____   _____   _____   _____
   Reach above shoulder level _____   _____   _____   _____

4. CIRCLE THE NUMBER OF HOURS FOR EACH ACTIVITY:
   Note: Does not have to total 8 hours.

										Continuously	With Rest
Sit	1	2	3	4	5	6	7	8	(hrs)	_____	_____
Stand	1	2	3	4	5	6	7	8	(hrs)	_____	_____
Walk	1	2	3	4	5	6	7	8	(hrs)	_____	_____
Sit/Stand	1	2	3	4	5	6	7	8	(hrs)	_____	_____

5. CAN PERSON USE HANDS FOR REPETITIVE ACTION SUCH AS:

	Simple Grasping	Firm Grasp	Fine Manipulating
Right	Yes _____ No _____	Yes _____ No _____	Yes _____ No _____
Left	Yes _____ No _____	Yes _____ No _____	Yes _____ No _____

6. CAN PERSON USE FEET FOR REPETITIVE MOVEMENTS, AS IN OPERATING FOOT CONTROLS?

Right	Left	Both
Yes _____ No_____	Yes _____ No _____	Yes _____ No _____

7. ANY RESTRICTIONS OF ACTIVITIES INVOLVED?

8. CAN PERSON NOW RETURN TO FORMER JOB?

   Yes _____ No _____

   CAN PERSON RETURN TO OTHER WORK ACCORDING TO RESTRICTIONS DEFINED ABOVE?

   Yes _____ No _____

   IF NOT, GIVE ESTIMATED DATE FOR RETURN TO WORK _____

   Work part time?   _____ hrs/day   Work full-time?   Yes _____ No _____
   Disability rating   _____% (if applicable)

9. COMMENTS: _____
   _____
   _____
   _____
   _____
   _____
   _____

_____   _____
          Physician   Date

Figure 6–4. Workers' compensation functional capacity form. (From Mayer TG, Mooney V, Gatchel RJ, et al: Contemporary Conservative Care for Painful Spinal Disorders: Impairment Evaluation Issues and the Disability System. Philadelphia, Lea & Febiger, 1991, pp 330–331, with permission.)

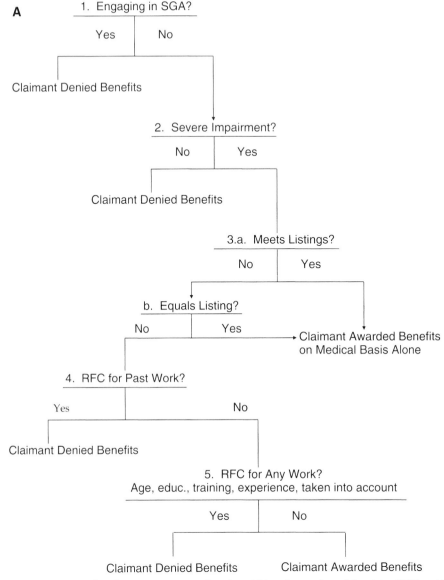

Figure 6–5. Sequential evaluation process. A, Algorithm. SGA, substantial gainful activity; RFC, residual functional capacity.

"judged to have a significant effect on the individual's capacity to perform work activities." By this definition, myofascial pain falls somewhere in between the lines. Specifically, there currently are no medically acceptable laboratory techniques by which the diagnosis can be made, and clinically both myofascial pain and fibromyalgia are considered, at least in the context of pain and disability, to be controversial diagnoses.

In 1984, Congress mandated the Secretary of the Department of Health and Human Services to appoint a commission for the evaluation of pain with the primary task of studying current pain policy and to recommend appropriate changes.[35] In addition, the commission was mandated to work in consultation with the National Academy of Sciences, and through the Institute of Medicine a more detailed study was commissioned. There was discussion and debate on the issue of myofascial pain. There was no consensus. According to the report, the discussion on this topic was

B

Disorders of the Spine

A. Arthritis manifested by ankylosis or fixation of the cervical or dorsolumbar spine at 30° or more of flexion measured from the neutral position, with X-ray evidence of:
 1. Calcification of the anterior and lateral ligaments; OR
 2. Bilateral ankylosis of the sacroiliac joints with abnormal apophyseal articulations; OR

B. Osteoporosis, generalized (established by X-ray) manifested by pain and limitation of back motion and paravertebral muscle spasm, with X-ray evidence of either:
 1. Compression fracture of a vertebral body with loss of at least 50 percent of the estimated height of the vertebral body prior to the compression fracture, with no intervening direct traumatic episode; OR
 2. Multiple fractures of vertebrae with no intervening direct traumatic episode: OR

C. Other vertebrogenic disorders (e.g., herniated nucleus pulposus, spinal stenosis) with the following persisting for at least 3 months despite prescribed therapy and expected to last 12 months. With both 1 and 2:
 1. Pain, muscle spasm, and significant limitation of motion in the spine; AND
 2. Appropriate radicular distribution of significant motor loss with muscle weakness and sensory and reflex loss.

Active rheumatoid arthritis and other inflammatory arthritis. With both A and B.

A. Persistent joint pain, swelling, and tenderness involving multiple joints with signs of joint inflammation (heat, swelling, tenderness) despite therapy for at least 3 months, and activity expected to last over 12 months; AND

B. Corroboration of diagnosis at some point in time by either:
 1. Positive serologic test for rheumatoid factor; OR
 2. Antinuclear antibodies; OR
 3. Elevated sedimentation rate.

Figure 6–5 *Continued. B,* Listings for musculoskeletal impairments. (From Osterweis M, Kleinman A, Mechanic D [eds]: Pain and Disability: Clinical, Behavioral, and Public Perspectives. Washington, DC, National Academy, 1987.)

"very heated," although all the clinicians acknowledged the existence of muscular involvement in musculoskeletal pain; some expressed strong doubts about the existence of myofascial trigger points. Similarly, others expressed strong doubts that the orthopedic view of the pathogenesis of back pain (disc rupture, nerve compression, etc.) is correct. Although advocates of the view that trigger points and referred pain are primary elements in the pathogenesis of many common pain symptoms, they acknowledged the absence of controlled clinical trials. However, they pointed to a rapidly growing literature reporting that the diagnosis is useful and common and asserted that efficacious treatment approaches have been developed. The committee did not reach agreement on this. Because of the debate, and in light of the increasing prominence of myofascial pain syndrome in clinical reports, the committee believed that the topic and the controversy should be "brought to the attention of clinicians and researchers."[35] Ultimately, the Institute's publication on pain and disability included a discussion of myofascial pain syndromes by Simons,[40] but the issue of myofascial pain as an entity or as a cause of an impairment, in the context of Social Security disability, remains controversial.

Over the last few years, there have been several court decisions mandating that the Social Security Administration take into account the patient's complaints of pain. In order to conform to these decrees, the Social Security Administration now recognizes the presence of tender points in the case of fibromyalgia, and active trigger points in myofascial pain as an objective indicator of an impairment. If indeed a patient is found to have these findings, by his or her treating physician and if necessary by an independent consultant, then the patient is recognized as having a bona fide impairment and qualifies to go on to step number two. If these findings are not substantiated by the physical examination, then the patient does not qualify as having an impairment, and therefore his or her claim will be denied.

The third step of the sequential evaluation process deals with whether the individual's impairment meets or equals the listings. In the case of musculoskeletal impairments, this generally includes findings associated with significant arthritis, ankylosis of joints, disc herniation, spinal stenosis, and osteoporosis. If the patient's impairment meets the listings, he or she would qualify for disability. By definition, persons with myofascial pain or fibromyalgia would not meet the listings (Fig. 6–5B). However, if an individual does not qualify based on this category, this does not mean that he or she does not qualify for Social Security disability. Rather, the claimant then moves to the next step (step four) in the sequential evaluation process, which has to do with residual functional capacity, i.e., does the patient's residual functional capacity allow him or her the ability to perform past relevant work? Essentially, a functional residual capacity is determined by the program physician on the basis of the limitations caused by the patient's impairment and symptoms. This determination is made by review of the medical records as well as information from the patient, family members, and other sources that will allow the adjudicators to establish the severity of the patient's functional limitations. If it is determined that the patient is unable to return to past relevant work, the final question (step five) is whether the patient is able to perform "any work that exists in the national economy." At this point, in addition to the functional impairment, age, education, training, and past work experience are also taken into account.

It is in the area of the fourth and fifth steps that pain becomes a factor. Case law has determined that the adjudicator may not disregard the claimant's subjective complaints solely because objective medical evidence does not fully support them. Adjudicators must give full consideration to all of the evidence presented relating to subjective complaints. This includes the patient's prior work record and observations by third parties and treating and examining physicians relating to such matters as the claimant's daily activities; the duration, frequency, and intensity of pain; precipitating and aggravating factors; doses, effectiveness, and side effects of medication; and functional restrictions. These recommendations have largely been incorporated in the Social Security Administration's current assessment of pain and disability.[29, 41]

Thus, the determination of disability due to pain remains a challenge. Because pain is subjective, there always exists the possibility of conscious fabrication or exaggeration of symptoms by the claimant. More common, and of a deeper complexity, is the role of the various psychosocial variables and how they influence the claimant's perception of pain and ultimate disability. More specifically, does the granting of Social Security benefits for these individuals truly provide a safety net for the disabled, or does it merely represent a mechanism that fosters dependency on a governmental system and only serves further to disable individuals potentially capable of rehabilitation by legally authenticating their position? The answer remains unknown. Until further research is done, one can only surmise that a large part of the so-called chronic pain syndrome population does in fact fall into the category of myofascial pain patients.

Myofascial Pain vs. the Chronic Pain Syndrome

Patients with myofascial pain who despite appropriate medical treatment fail to respond and who continue to demonstrate significant pain behaviors, whose clinical presentation appears to be exaggerated, and whose time for healing is prolonged fall into the category of chronic pain syndrome. In order to understand these patients and the clinical evolution of their syndrome, an extensive history with the focus on psychosocial contributing factors is essential. Identifying and addressing the psychosocial factors often serves as the key to successful rehabilitation.[7, 12, 13, 30, 45] Although an exhaustive discussion of the many psychosocial issues interfering with the treatment and rehabilitation of patients with chronic myofascial pain is beyond the scope of this chapter, there are several crucial risk factors that can be identified as part of the history and that certainly can predispose a person to the development of a chronic pain syndrome (Fig. 6–6). Furthermore, if these issues are not taken into account as

---

Chronic pain risk factors

Instructions: Place a checkmark next to each risk factor that is present.

---

1 Medical history
- ☐ Pain that persists despite appropriate treatment
- ☐ Physical deconditioning or prolonged inactivity
- ☐ Unrealistic expectations from treatment
- ☐ History of conflicting medical opinion
- ☐ Anger or dissatisfaction with medical care
- ☐ Life-long history of health problems

---

2 Pain behavior
- ☐ Dramatic description or display of pain
- ☐ Dependency on paraphernalia (canes, collars, etc.)
- ☐ "Doctor shopping"

---

3 Chemical dependency
- ☐ Overuse or preoccupation with medications
- ☐ Use of alcohol for pain
- ☐ History of alcohol or drug abuse and/or CD treatment

---

4 Emotional reactions
- ☐ Depression, social withdrawal
- ☐ Anxiety, worry, fear
- ☐ Anger, resentment, blaming, "power struggles"
- ☐ Overreaction to stress
- ☐ Complacency, too comfortable with disability

---

5 Vocational
- ☐ Job dissatisfaction or anger at employer
- ☐ Injured near retirement age
- ☐ Loss or threatened loss of job
- ☐ Unstable work history
- ☐ Limited education

---

6 Secondary benefits
- ☐ Avoidance of stressful situations
- ☐ Increased attention from family, including overprotection
- ☐ Financial compensation for disability
- ☐ Prospect of gain through litigation

---

7 Stress factors
(Prior to or developing after the onset of pain)
- ☐ Role changes (retirement, "empty nest")
- ☐ Financial problems
- ☐ Marital discord, separation, divorce
- ☐ Illness or death in family
- ☐ Chemical dependency in family

---

8 Personality factors
- ☐ Passive or dependent
- ☐ Hypochondriacal or hysteroid
- ☐ Perfectionist or "workaholic"

---

9 Childhood trauma
(Between birth and 16 years)
- ☐ Death, disability, or serious illness in family
- ☐ Chemical dependency in family
- ☐ Verbal or physical abuse in home

© Pilling Pain Clinic/Fairview Southdale Hospital.

Figure 6–6. Checklist for chronic pain risk factors. CD, combination drug. (From Pilling LF, Clift RB: Instructions for use of the chronic pain risk factors checklist. Modern Medicine 54:83–84, 1986, with permission.)

part of the assessment process, the likelihood of any type of intervention proving successful is decreased significantly. Certainly, if a patient with acute myofascial pain has not responded to treatment in a reasonable time period, then it is likely that a referral to either a psychologist with extensive experience in pain assessment or to an interdisciplinary pain clinic for an evaluation is appropriate.

The appropriate length of time for the use of passive treatment modalities in defining the end of normal tissue healing is difficult. Physicians often err on the safe side, which only leads to further physical deconditioning and dysfunctional pain behaviors on the part of the patient. In Minnesota, a task force of the Department of Labor and Industry charged with defining this issue for workers' compensation cases has suggested that no passive therapy, i.e., passive physical therapy (PT), chiropractic care, massage, and such, should continue for more than 90 days following the date of the acute injury.

Clinically, the majority of patients with myofascial pain syndromes, when the problem becomes chronic, manifest findings associated with depression,[11, 36] i.e., sleep disturbance, irritability, fatigue, and anhedonia. In fact, Blumer and Heilbronn believe that chronic pain may be simply a variant of a depressive disorder.[2] Frequently, in obtaining a history on these patients, one finds a pattern of significant social disruption predating the injury. Often, there is a history of chemical dependency in the family system, a history of physical or sexual abuse, loss of a parent at an early age, or some event that placed the patient in the role of a victim. Patients who are injured and become involved with disability systems often respond to this process either with a sense of hopelessness or anger. With time, they often develop a hostile dependent relationship with their physician and the various disability systems. They express their frustration and anger at their lack of improvement and their dependency on the system, yet they continue to seek relief of their symptoms through further diagnostic tests, medications, or the use of passive PT modalities, e.g., trigger point injections, massage, heat, and so on, which produce at best temporary improvement without any long-lasting benefit, and thus they remain stuck in the disability process. Recognition of the role of family dynamics in the patient's social environment often provides vital information regarding the clinical expression of a painful condition. This is illustrated by the following vignettes:

Case 1: A 47-year-old woman with a 12-month history of back pain diagnosed as a strain was referred to a multidisciplinary pain clinic because of her lack of response to PT. Physical examination revealed trigger point tenderness over the right gluteal muscle. Radiographs, including a computed tomography (CT) scan, were negative. *Her history revealed a long-standing pattern of physical abuse by her husband.* After she was injured, her husband had stopped beating her.

Case 2: A 57-year-old laborer, father of five, with an eighth-grade education, suffered a cervical strain. Spinal films demonstrated multilevel degenerative disc disease. During the history, the patient's college-educated wife answered most of the questions directed toward the patient. She described him as being severely disabled and indicated that it was her opinion that he would never return to work. She said that her husband "couldn't even do anything" around the house and that she and her children had taken over essentially all of his former activities such as lawn care, car care, and driving. On physical examination, palpation of the cervical muscles elicited grimacing and groaning on the part of the patient's wife. When asked what was the matter, her response was, "You're hurting him."

Case 3: A 37-year-old factory worker with a 9-month history of back pain was evaluated. The physical examination showed trigger point tenderness over the quadratus and gluteal muscles with some decreased range of motion. His neurologic examination was normal and spinal films showed no degenerative changes. In spite of appropriate, conservative care, the patient remained disabled. During the history, he began a long diatribe regarding his work environment. His company had been sold to a large conglomerate and his boss of 15 years had been replaced "by a punk kid." He had told his new supervisor about a potential hazard associated with an oil spill on the floor, but was ignored. Then one day while carrying a box of parts, he had slipped on that oil spill, injuring his back.

In each of these cases, psychosocial factors clearly influence the meaning of the painful experience to the patient and by inference the clinical expression of that condition. No amount or type of somatically oriented treatment will affect these factors. Even identification of these issues, however, does not guarantee that they can be successfully addressed. Asking patients to confront and modify long-standing behavior patterns or identify repressed emotions can be extremely challenging. Thus, for many of these patients, ongoing counseling and appropriate follow-up are essential to maintain any gains made in an intensive rehabilitation center and to ensure long-term success.

Fear is a major component in the clinical presentation. Patients are often frightened that because they have not improved, they can only get worse. They are afraid that, despite undergoing multiple diagnostic tests, there must be some underlying condition that no one has been able to diagnose. They doubt their ability to return to gainful employment, fear that they may be "spied upon" by investigators working for the insurance carrier, and are petrified about losing their benefits, which serve as the barrier against poverty.

For many people involved with disability systems, their pain and resultant pain behaviors represent their only leverage in dealing with the complex medical-legal system in which they have become disempowered, being now fully dependent on the insurance carrier for their paycheck, on their physician for relief of their symptoms as well as affirmation of their disabled status, and on their attorney for future security. With time, the majority of these patients become extremely deconditioned. In our patient population, we have found that, from an aerobic or cardiovascular standpoint, pain patients are more deconditioned than persons undergoing cardiac rehabilitation following a myocardial infarction. As patients continue with their extremely sedentary lifestyles, limiting themselves in terms of activities of daily living, weight gain is common, muscle mass and strength decrease, and endurance lessens.

These patients require a holistic or biopsychosocial model of intervention. Because of the complexity of their clinical presentation, either a team approach utilizing active PT (i.e., exercise and reconditioning), psychological support, and appropriate medical supervision, or involvement in a more intensive pain management or functional restoration program integrating these components is mandatory.[23]

Pain Management vs. Pain Treatment

Although some would argue this contention, the primary role of a chronic pain rehabilitation program is not pain amelioration but rather functional restoration. Eliminating the patient's dependency on the physician, passive PT modalities, and the use of ineffective medications is the primary goal. Empowering patients to regain functional activities, return to work, release their anger, and address their sense of indignation and victimization are crucial. Shifting the focus from pain relief to normalization of living, as well as helping patients overcome their fears of re-injury, is the hallmark of a successful rehabilitation model.

As part of our assessment, patients are told that they are the ones responsible for getting well. If their pain actually lessens or goes away, we jokingly tell them that there won't be any extra charge and they should consider it a bonus. Deflecting the issue of pain relief and shifting the responsibility for eliminating pain from the clinician to the patient is empowering. The dynamic of searching for the magic bullet, which has not proved effective up to this point, is now diffused.

Pain management is not an isolated treatment intervention. Many pain rehabilitation programs use biofeedback, injections, physical therapy, and so forth without success in eliminating or reducing pain. These modalities are best presented from the perspective that they will help the patient better manage stress, improve his or her level of physical conditioning, and assist in a return to a functional lifestyle, rather than reduce or eliminate the pain.[6] This approach needs to be viewed in opposition to the traditional acute model in which the patient is treated like an infant and the responsibility for success or failure lies with the clinician in terms of making a proper diagnosis and prescribing treatment (Fig. 6–7A and B).

In order for patients to benefit from a pain rehabilitation program, proper screening is required. This should consist of a review of relevant medical records; an extensive history, with emphasis on identifying psychosocial contributing factors described previously; physical examination; review of the appropriate laboratory findings; and development of a treatment plan that is agreed upon by all concerned parties. In addition, absolute contraindications such as primary substance abuse and psychosis need to be ruled out.

Medical Records

Unfortunately, patients with chronic pain are not the best historians. They have often seen numerous physicians and undergone multiple diagnostic studies. In addition, if medication dependency or compensation issues are involved, they may intentionally leave out significant details. Thus, obtaining previous medical records from treating physicians, or at least an adequate summary of medical data, is mandatory.[23, 28]

The History

As discussed earlier, the history should include, with careful documentation, the onset of the patient's problems with special emphasis on causation, the previous treating physicians, previous treatments, and the patient's response. The issue of causation is extremely important, particularly in the determination of workers' compensation and PI cases. In addition to describing the patient's current symptoms, documentation of alterations in lifestyle and social and recreational activities, as well as current activities, is essential. Identification of various psychosocial stressors is mandatory. These include job dissatisfaction, history of abuse and family discord, psychological status, drug and chemical usage including caffeine and nicotine, economic factors such as litigation, and previous pain problems. All of these contributing factors can complicate and influence the clinical manifestations of the patient's condition.[24]

An MMPI or other appropriate psychometric testing, as well as evaluation by a competent psychologist or psychiatrist, should be considered in assessing a patient as a potential candidate for a pain rehabilitation program. Usually, a careful history will reveal important psychosocial factors that provide the key elements in understanding the clinical presentation of the patient.

Physical Examination

In terms of the physical examination, two important determinants need to be kept in mind. First, one wants to make sure that the diagnosis of myofascial pain is correct.[10] In general, by the time patients are referred to a pain rehabilitation program, they have undergone extensive diagnostic tests, including radiographs and electrophysiologic evaluations, to rule out entrapment syndromes. However, the possibility of sympathetic-mediated pain is frequently overlooked. Therefore, it is key to look for signs of skin temperature change, asymmetry, discoloration, swelling, and other signs associated with complex regional pain disorder (Type I, reflex sympathetic dystrophy, or Type II, causalgia) when evaluating a patient.

The other important aspect of the physical examination is identifying nonphysiologic responses that suggest psychological distress and somatization. Findings such as Waddell's signs[47] (Table 6–2), exaggerated grimacing, or bizarre posturing suggest either conscious or unconscious exaggeration of symptoms. Although nonphysiologic findings on physical examination are important to observe, they do not mean that the patient is malingering. Malingering implies conscious premeditated exaggeration, or confabulation on the part of the patient. Most experts in the field of pain consider malingerers

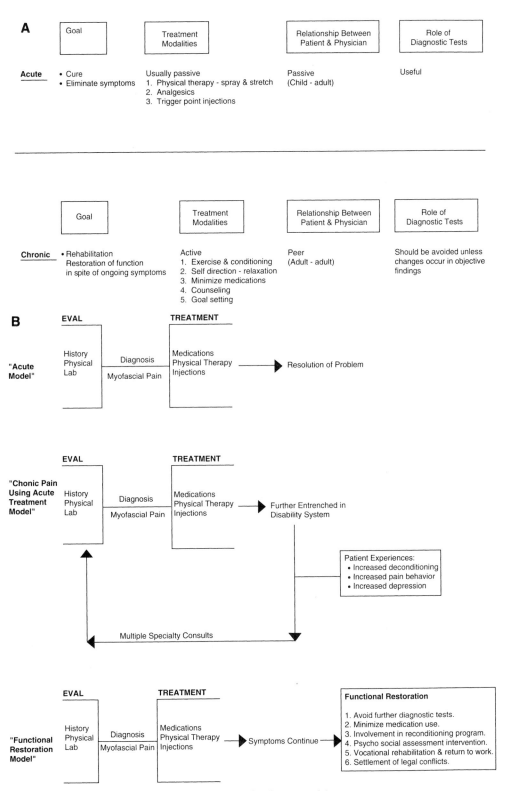

A

Goal	Treatment Modalities	Relationship Between Patient & Physician	Role of Diagnostic Tests

Acute
- Cure
- Eliminate symptoms

Usually passive
1. Physical therapy - spray & stretch
2. Analgesics
3. Trigger point injections

Passive
(Child - adult)

Useful

Goal	Treatment Modalities	Relationship Between Patient & Physician	Role of Diagnostic Tests

Chronic
- Rehabilitation
  Restoration of function
  in spite of ongoing symptoms

Active
1. Exercise & conditioning
2. Self direction - relaxation
3. Minimize medications
4. Counseling
5. Goal setting

Peer
(Adult - adult)

Should be avoided unless
changes occur in objective
findings

B

EVAL   **TREATMENT**

"Acute Model"

History
Physical
Lab

Diagnosis

Myofascial Pain

Medications
Physical Therapy
Injections

Resolution of Problem

EVAL   **TREATMENT**

"Chonic Pain Using Acute Treatment Model"

History
Physical
Lab

Diagnosis

Myofascial Pain

Medications
Physical Therapy
Injections

Further Entrenched in
Disability System

Patient Experiences:
- Increased deconditioning
- Increased pain behavior
- Increased depression

Multiple Specialty Consults

EVAL   **TREATMENT**

"Functional Restoration Model"

History
Physical
Lab

Diagnosis

Myofascial Pain

Medications
Physical Therapy
Injections

Symptoms Continue

Functional Restoration

1. Avoid further diagnostic tests.
2. Minimize medication use.
3. Involvement in reconditioning program.
4. Psycho social assessment intervention.
5. Vocational rehabilitation & return to work.
6. Settlement of legal conflicts.

Figure 6–7. A and B, The acute vs. the chronic model in pain management.

Table 6–2.

Comparison of Symptoms and Signs of Physical Disease and Abnormal Illness Behavior in Chronic Low Back Pain

	Physical Disease and Normal Illness Behavior	Magnified or Inappropriate Illness Behavior
Symptoms		
Pain	Localized	Whole leg pain, tailbone pain
Numbness	Dermatomal	Whole leg numbness
Weakness	Myotomal	Whole leg giving way
Time pattern	Varies with time	Never free of pain
Response to treatment	Variable benefit	Intolerance of treatment, emergency admissions to hospital
Signs		
Tenderness	Localized	Superficial, widespread, nonanatomic
Axial loading	No lumbar pain	Lumbar pain
Simulated rotation	No lumbar pain	Lumbar pain
Straight leg raising	Limited on distraction	Improves with distraction
Sensory	Dermatomal	Regional
Motor	Myotomal	Regional, jerky giving way
General response	Appropriate pain	Overreaction

From Waddell G, Bircher M, Finlayson D, et al: Symptoms and signs: Physical disease or illness behaviour?: Br Med J (Clin Res Ed) Sep 22; 289(6447)740, 1984, with permission.

to represent a small minority of chronic pain patients. A much higher percentage of these patients truly have an exaggerated pain perception and pain behaviors, often due to psychological factors. They may well be histrionic personality types or for various reasons have extremely poor pain thresholds. Psychometric testing reveals elevations on scales measuring histrionic or hysterical behavior or hypochondriasis.[15]

Radiologic Examination

No radiographic findings exist that can establish the diagnosis of myofascial pain syndrome. The fact that a spinal film may show degenerative changes such as facet hypertrophy or a bulging disc does not exclude the diagnosis of myofascial pain. The development of sophisticated imaging methods, particularly magnetic resonance (MR), comes as a mixed blessing for many of these patients. Although providing excellent imaging, particularly of the anatomy of the disc, MR and CT scans often demonstrate abnormalities that are not clinically significant.[48] Although physicians recognize the importance of correlating symptoms with the physical examination and radiologic findings, this is not necessarily true of plaintiff attorneys, unsophisticated patients, or administrative judges who often have the final say as to the relative clinical importance of these findings from the standpoint of disability and impairment ratings.

Moreover, patients who lack the sophistication to understand the significance of x-ray findings commonly become frightened when they find that there are some structural changes on their radiographs. It is not uncommon to find a patient presenting not with a complaint of back or neck pain, but rather with a complaint of a bulging disc or stenosis. Once the patient has been told that there is an abnormality on the x-ray film, it is often difficult to reassure the patient that even with these findings, he or she can return to a functional lifestyle.

Developing a Rehabilitation Plan

Once the patient has been evaluated, a specific rehabilitation plan needs to be established. While specific modalities vary among pain rehabilitation programs, all have certain features in common. The primary goal is returning the patient to a functional lifestyle, including work. It is important that, at the end of treatment, a functional capacity evaluation be obtained and appropriate functional restrictions be imposed. The patient needs to be told this and also that he or she will be supported in returning to work despite the continuing discomfort. The message that is communicated is simply that chronic pain may indeed cause hurt and discomfort, but that it is not necessarily harmful.

Working closely with the employer, as well as with other members involved in the rehabilitation process, such as the rehabilitation counselor, is required. In the Pain Rehabilitation program at Sister Kenny Rehabilitation, there is one full-time vocational counselor whose primary function is to interface with patients, employers, and insurers in helping to establish a return-to-work plan.

Although pain management programs make various claims about how they are helping chronic pain patients deal with their pain, from the insurer's perspective, the only true measure of success is whether that patient returns to work. In this regard, there will always be a subgroup of pain patients who clearly have no intention of going back to work for their current employer, if at all. Either they wish to retire or they have developed an extremely adversarial relationship with their employer. In these cases, as in a marriage in trouble, counseling may save the relationship. At other times the best solution for both parties is a divorce. Likewise, in the vocational realm, at times the relationship between the employer and employee can be saved, differences can be worked out, and the patient can be successfully returned to work. In other instances, however, the degree of anger, resentment, and mutual enmity is so great that any attempt at resolution will be met with failure. At this point, it may be in everyone's best interest to resolve their differences through an administrative settlement. Particularly in the area of workers' compensation in which adversarial relationships exist between employer and employee, each side will attempt to exert whatever leverage is available to gain an advantage. In the case of the employer and the insurer, they are the ones that pay the bills and often direct medical care. The employer can certainly attempt to provide a job position within the restrictions of the individual's condition.

The patient has fewer options in terms of leverage. In fact, the primary one is pain behavior. If a situation exists that the patient does not like, e.g., being placed in a monotonous light-duty position, the patient's only option is to hurt more. Since pain by definition is subjective, it is impossible to either substantiate or disprove this position. Again, this does not imply malingering, but merely represents a mechanism for survival from the patient's perspective. Acknowledging the patient's feelings, yet not necessarily acquiescing to the patient's position, is a difficult act of diplomacy.

In addition to help for the patient in returning to work, modalities that foster a sense of independence and self-sufficiency on the part of the patient are helpful. An exercise program that emphasizes flexibility, strength, and cardiovascular conditioning is crucial to a reconditioning program. Again, the focus of exercise is not on the resolution of pain but rather on restoration of function.[38] Patients need to be reassured that during the early part of any type of physical reactivation program, they can expect to experience increased soreness. This does not mean that their condition is worse. On completion of an intensive 3- or 4-week pain rehabilitation program, continued involvement in a comprehensive conditioning program is vital. It may be another 3 to 6 months, if ever, before the patient actually notes diminution in pain.

Medications

Narcotics, benzodiazepines, and other potentially addictive drugs should be avoided in the long-term management of patients with myofascial pain.[28] Although the use of narcotics is controversial in the management of nonmalignant pain syndromes,[1, 25, 32, 43] in general, patients with myofascial pain do not need chronic narcotics or benzodiazepines for pain management (Table 6–3). The chronic use of these medications can and often does enhance depression and lethargy, and can affect motivation to return to work. In addition, the patient's ability to concentrate may be affected by the long-term use of these medications. Attempts should also be made to reduce the use of

Table 6–3.
Indications for Long-Term Narcotic Use

Factors Indicating Poor Candidates for Long-Term Narcotic Use	Factors Indicating Possibly Appropriate Candidates for Long-Term Narcotic Use
1. No or minimal indications of structural pathologic changes, inflammation, or active disease process to substantiate pain complaints.	1. Clear clinical, anatomic, and laboratory data to substantiate the diagnosis of a painful condition.
2. History of previous alcoholism, substance abuse, or family history of substance abuse or involvement in chemical dependency treatment.	2. No history either of chemical dependency on the part of the patient or on the part of the family.
3. Inappropriate or dramatic pain behaviors or inappropriate use of canes, braces, or other supportive devices.	3. Pain behaviors appear to be appropriate to the clinical condition.
4. History of previous psychological problems, especially depression or hysteria.	4. No premorbid psychological dysfunction.
5. Evidence of dependent personality style, e.g., heavy caffeine or nicotine use or compulsive overeating.	5. The patient is not a heavy smoker, heavy caffeine user, nor does he or she demonstrate other signs of a compulsive lifestyle or dependent behavior pattern.
6. No evidence that using narcotic medications allows the patient to improve function with respect to activities of daily living and vocational pursuits.	6. The patient does function reasonably in spite of pain, but using narcotic medications appears to improve the level of functioning significantly.
7. Unstable work history.	7. Previous stable work history.
8. History of physical, sexual, or emotional abuse.	8. No history of physical, sexual, or emotional abuse.
9. Poor family support system or a history of a dysfunctional family system.	9. Good family support system.
10. Noncompliance with treatment recommendations.	10. All other reasonable attempts at pain control have failed, and the patient has demonstrated compliance.

other medications, including nonsteroidal anti-inflammatory drugs (NSAIDs) and over-the-counter analgesics. Although these medications may be useful in acute flare-ups, they have potential adverse side effects. It is my experience that many patients with myofascial pain can be weaned from addictive medications and NSAIDs. Usually, they do not notice any major increase in their pain.

Antidepressants have been demonstrated to be useful in the treatment of myofascial pain syndromes. In patients with sleep disturbance and without major depressive symptoms, response has been favorable to very low doses of tricyclics. Amitriptyline (Elavil) 5–50 mg, or nortriptyline (Pamelor) 5 to 50 mg, or trazodone (Desyrel) 25–50 mg slowly titrated up to a level that allows the patient to sleep without undue side effects can prove quite effective. A more normal sleep pattern often has a positive effect on the patient's general functional ability as well as pain management. After 2 to 3 months, assuming the patient is back to a more functional lifestyle, is exercising, and utilizing other stress management strategies, an attempt can be made to decrease the antidepressant. Some patients, however, may require small amounts of antidepressant medication on a long-term basis.

Patient Expectations

Before recommending a comprehensive pain rehabilitation program, it is important to negotiate with the patient and clearly define expectations. If the patient is looking for a quick fix or miracle cure, a functional restoration approach is not appropriate. The patient needs to find out for himself or herself whether acupuncture, chiropractic, myofascial therapy, or some other type of passive modality will actually eliminate the symptoms. Attempting to force a reluctant or unwilling patient into a pain rehabilitation program often leads to increased mistrust and anger on the part of the patient, and all attempts to support this person's rehabilitation will be met with resistance.

Typically, patients at the Pain Rehabilitation Program at Sister Kenny Rehabilitation are asked to sign an agreement that outlines what can and cannot be offered. Thus, even before admission, the message is made clear that the patient is the one responsible for success. The job of the staff is not to "fix" the patient but to support him or her in making the necessary behavioral and perceptual changes required to deal with pain in a more functional manner and to return to a normal lifestyle (Fig. 6–8). By setting appropriate boundaries from the start, there is far less of a chance of getting caught up in the patient's dependent and manipulative behaviors.

The Role of Self-Regulation Techniques

Self-regulation techniques, such as self-hypnosis, relaxation training, and biofeedback, can be helpful adjuncts in the treatment of myofascial pain syndromes. Stress, anxiety, and tension all increase levels of muscle tension and can certainly aggravate if

---

ABBOTT NORTHWESTERN HOSPITAL/SISTER KENNY INSTITUTE
CHRONIC PAIN REHABILITATION PROGRAM

PATIENT/STAFF AGREEMENT

The purpose of the Chronic Pain Rehabilitation Program is to create an opportunity for individuals experiencing chronic or long-term pain to improve the quality and enjoyment of their lives, to gain skills to manage their pain, and to return to a more productive lifestyle. The success or failure of the Program depends on the willingness of the individual to apply these pain management concepts to his or her everyday life.

In order to achieve this purpose, I understand and I am willing to follow these guidelines:

1. To participate fully in all scheduled activities. This includes being on time for classes, staying to the end of each day, attending evening sessions (for residents), and arriving by 9:00 PM Sunday night prior to the beginning of each week, with the exception of the first Sunday orientation from 3:00–4:00 arrival.
2. To review all prescribed medications and over-the-counter medications at a scheduled private meeting with a staff nurse. To wean or minimize use of narcotic and other medications according to the recommendations of the medical staff.
3. To abstain from alcohol, marijuana, or other nonprescribed drugs for the three-week period of time *(including weekends)* in order to allow my system to properly respond to pain management techniques. Periodic urine screening may be required.
4. To be open to reducing caffeine and nicotine consumption.
5. To strive to improve physical and emotional health in order to return to work, normal activities, and/or a more productive lifestyle. This includes a monitored exercise and pool therapy program.
6. To be open to learn and practice pain and stress management techniques. These include acupressure, relaxation, imagery, breathing techniques, and/or biofeedback.
7. To participate in the Aftercare Program following completion of the three-week program, including a Final Aftercare session.
8. To understand that family participation is extremely important. I agree that at least one family member or significant friend will participate in the scheduled Family Day activities. Phone contact will be made in specific cases where scheduled time at the Program cannot be arranged.
9. To remain on campus of Abbott Northwestern Hospital (for my own safety and security) except on weekends, unless I have received permission to leave from a staff member.
10. To respect everyone's diverse backgrounds; to not interfere with the progress of fellow patients; and to not compare my individual treatment plan to someone else's plan.

These issues are critical to the success of pain management and rehabilitation.

I, _____ HAVE READ, UNDERSTAND FULLY, AND AGREE TO COMPLY WITH THE STATEMENTS LISTED ABOVE.
(Signature implies a self-responsibility commitment.)

ADDITIONAL AGREEMENTS:

Figure 6–8. The patient-staff agreement. (Courtesy of Abbott Northwestern Hospital/Sister Kenny Rehabilitation, Minneapolis, Minn.)

not precipitate a myofascial pain problem.[5, 37] Patients are taught basic relaxation and particularly breathing techniques, emphasizing that these techniques be used throughout the day, rather than occasionally.

Teaching patients how to breathe in a controlled and rhythmic manner using their diaphragm often provides immediate reduction of stress and anxiety. After all, breathing is both an autonomic and a voluntary function. Persons under stress often demonstrate shallow breathing patterns, breathing from the chest as opposed to the diaphragm. This is not only inefficient, in that there is poorer oxygenation, but is also associated with fear and anxiety. Diaphragmatic breathing, on the other hand, is a more natural and efficient way of breathing. It is almost impossible to breathe diaphragmatically in a slow and rhythmic manner and experience tension and anxiety.[33]

Cognitive Psychotherapy

The subject of psychological intervention with chronic pain patients needs to be approached carefully. As mentioned, patients with chronic pain are often resistant to looking at psychological factors. Recognition of psychological factors implies that the pain is not in their bodies, but "in their heads." They have a difficult time understanding how their feelings and emotions can affect their current situation. They are often extremely defensive about seeing a clinical psychologist or psychiatrist, or taking an MMPI. However, unless the issues associated with anger, family problems, job dissatisfaction, fear, mistrust, and other self-defeating behaviors are addressed, it is difficult to help the patient move forward. I have found that our most effective therapists are not necessarily Ph.D.'s or M.D.'s, but peer counselors who themselves have chronic pain and have successfully completed a pain program. Patients do need to work through their anger and depression. Following an injury, there is a loss. Patients have a right to be angry, but the challenge is how to help them refocus their anger in a positive and constructive way and assume responsibility for their underlying condition rather than blame an external force, i.e., their employer, physician, insurer, and the like, or themselves.

A metaphor applicable to chronic pain is similar to that expressed by Kubler-Ross[21] in dealing with dying patients.[14] Initially, following an injury, there is a loss. Patients often deal with this loss with a sense of denial, a belief that their symptoms will go away, and that they will get better. As time goes on, and the condition does not improve, they are often left with a sense of anger and depression. When patients are helped to move through this position to a point of acceptance, they are able to deal with their injury in a healthier manner.

Conclusion

Myofascial pain is a common,[46] perhaps the most common, cause of chronic musculoskeletal pain and disability. In one study, 85% of 283 patients presenting to a chronic pain clinic were diagnosed as having myofascial pain syndromes.[11] In another study of 296 patients presenting with head and neck pain, 55.4% had a primary diagnosis of myofascial pain.[14]

The cost to society is enormous. Although no specific estimates regarding myofascial pain exist, it has been estimated that the total annual cost of low back care, including vocational retraining, medical care, compensation, and legal fees, approaches 40 to 50 billion dollars. The cost of medical care alone is $16 billion, half of that going to surgical treatment. Combining the prevalence data with the economic costs certainly establishes a tremendously high social and economic cost to society for myofascial pain syndromes. By the time the condition becomes chronic, psychosocial factors and physical deconditioning have played a major role in the manifestation of the condition and subsequent disability. Identification of psychosocial risk factors, supporting the patient in developing healthy coping skills, and focusing on functional restoration rather than symptomatic relief are often the key to successful pain management.

Approaches to management should include limiting passive modalities to the acute stages or aggravations of a condition; avoiding long-term use of narcotics, benzodiazepines, NSAIDs, and over-the-counter drugs; reinforcing physical reactivation through a home exercise and conditioning program; and teaching appropriate stress management. Educating the patient on the interrelationships between stress, fear, depression, and deconditioning in terms of overall function is crucial. For evaluating patients with a chronic pain syndrome, only by assessing the patients from a biopsychosocial perspective, addressing the individual biologic, psychological, and social contributing factors, can one truly empower these persons to cope more effectively with their pain and maximize their potential for rehabilitation.

References

1. Bannwarth B: Risk benefit assessment of opioids in chronic noncancer pain. Drug Saf 21(4):283–296, 1999.
2. Blumer D, Heilbronn M: Chronic pain as a variant of depressive disease: The pain prone disorder. J Nerv Ment Dis 170:381–406, 1982.
3. Boisset-Pioro MH, Espaile JM, Fitzcharles M: Sexual and physical abuse associated with outpatient health care utilization and pain medication usage in women with fibromyalgia syndrome. Arthritis Rheum 38:235–241, 1995.
4. Brigham CR, Babitsky S: Independent medical evaluations and impairment ratings. Occup Med 13(1):209–213, 1998.
5. Cailliet R: Soft Tissue Pain and Disability. Philadelphia, FA Davis, 1977.
6. Chapman SL, Jamison RN, Sanders SH, et al: Perceived treatment helpfulness and cost in chronic pain rehabilitation. Clin J Pain 16(2):169–177, 2000.
7. Demetier SL: Disability evaluation. Occup Med 13(2):315–323, 1998.
8. Doege TC (ed): Guides to the Evaluation of Permanent Impairment, 4th ed. Chicago, American Medical Association, 1993, pp 113, 118, 120, 122.
9. Engel G: "Psychogenic" pain and the pain-prone patient. Am J Med 26:899–915, 1959.
10. Fischer AA: Documentation of myofascial trigger points. Arch Phys Med Rehabil 69:286–291, 1988.
11. Fishbain DA, Goldberg M, Meagher R, et al: Male and female chronic pain patients categorized by DSM-III psychiatric diagnostic criteria. Pain 26:181–197, 1986.
12. Flor H, Turk DC, Scholz OB: Impact of chronic pain on the spouse: Marital, emotional, and physical consequences. J Psychosom Res 31:63–71, 1987.
13. Fordyce WE: Pain and suffering. Am Psychol 43:276–283, 1988.
14. Fricton J, Kroening R, Haley D, et al: Myofascial pain syndrome of the head and neck: A review of clinical characteristics of 164 patients. Oral Surg Oral Med Oral Pathol 60:615–623, 1985.
15. Frymoyer JW: Back pain and sciatica. N Engl J Med 318:291–298, 1988.
16. Frymoyer JW, Rosen JC, Clements J, et al: Psychologic factors in low back pain disability. Clin Orthop 195:178–184, 1985.
17. Harten JA: Functional capacity evaluation. Occup Med 13(1):209–213, 1998.
18. Isernhagen SJ: Functional capacity evaluation and work hardening perspectives. In Mayer TG, Mooney V, Gatchel RJ (eds): Contemporary Conservative Care for Painful Spinal Disorders. Philadelphia, Lea & Febiger, 1991.
19. Isernagen SJ: The comprehensive guide to work injury management. Gaithersburg, Md, Aspen, 1995.
20. Keeley J: Quantification of function. In Mayer TG, Mooney V, Gatchel RJ (eds): Contemporary Conservative Care for Painful Spinal Disorders. Philadelphia, Lea & Febiger, 1991, pp 290–307.
21. Kubler-Ross E: On Death and Dying. New York, Macmillan, 1969.
22. Manual for Orthopaedic Surgeons in Evaluating Permanent Impairment. Chicago, American Academy of Orthopaedic Surgeons, 1966.
23. Mayer TG, Gatchel RJ: Functional Restoration for Spinal Disorders: The Sports Medicine Approach. Philadelphia, Lea & Febiger, 1988.
24. McDermid AJ, Rollman GB, McCain GA: Generalized hypervigilance in fibromyalgia; evidence of perceptual amplification. Pain 66(2–3):133–144, 1996.
25. McQuay H: Opioids in pain management. Lancet 353:2229–2232, 1999.
26. Merskey H: Psychosocial factors and muscular pain. In Fricton J, Awad EA (eds): Advances in Pain Research and Therapy, vol 17: Myofascial Pain and Fibromyalgia. New York, Raven, 1990.
27. Monsein M: Soft tissue pain and disability. In Fricton J, Awad EA (eds): Advances in Pain Research and Therapy, vol 17: Myofascial Pain and Fibromyalgia. New York, Raven, 1990.
28. Nies KM: Treatment of the fibromyalgia syndrome. J Musculoskeletal Med 9:20–26, 1992.
29. Osterweis M, Kleinman A, Mechanic D (eds): Pain and disability: Clinical, behavioral, and public policy perspectives. Washington, DC, National Academy, 1987, pp 6, 25, 35, 38–41, 198, 280.

30. Pape MH, Rosen JC, Wilder DG, et al: The relation between biomechanical and psychological factors in patients with low back pain. Spine 5:173–178, 1980.
31. Plumb JM, Cowell JWF: An overview of worker's compensation. Occup Med 13(2):241–272, 1998.
32. Portenoy RK: Opioid therapy for chronic noncancer pain: The issue revisited. American Pain Society Bulletin 1:4–7, 1991.
33. Rama S, Ballentine R, Hymes A: Science of breath: A practical guide. Honesdale, Pa, The Himalayan International Institute of Yoga Science and Philosophy, 1979.
34. Reeves JL, Jaegen G, Graff-Radford SB: Reliability of the pressure algometer as a measure of myofascial trigger point sensitivity. Pain 24:313–321, 1986.
35. Report of the Commission on the Evaluation of Pain (Social Security Administration Publication No. 64-031). Washington, DC, Government Printing Office, 1987.
36. Romano JM, Turner JA: Chronic pain and depression: Does the evidence support a relationship? Psychol Bull 97:18–34, 1985.
37. Sarno JE: Etiology of neck and back pain: An autonomic myoneuralgia? J Nerv Ment Dis 169:55–59, 1981.
38. Sherman C: Managing fibromyalgia with exercise. The Physician and Sportsmedicine 20:166–172, 1992.
39. Sherman JJ, Turk DC, Okifuji A: Prevalence and impact of post traumatic stress disorder-like symptoms on patients with fibromyalgia. Clin J Pain 16:127–135, 2000.
40. Simons DG: Myofascial pain syndromes due to trigger points. In Osterweis M, Kleinman A, Mechanic D (eds): Pain and Disability: Clinical, Behavioral, and Public Policy Perspectives. Washington, DC, National Academy, 1987, pp 285–292.
41. Social Security Regulations Title II 404.1529, Title VI 416.929. Sections 216(i), 223(d), and 1614(a)(3) of the Social Security Act, as amended; Regulations No. 4, sections 404.1505, 404.1508, 404.1520, 404.1528(a), 404.1529, 404.1569a, and subpart P, appendix 2; and Regulations No. 16, sections 416.905, 416.908, 416.920, 416.924, 416.928(a), 416.929, and 416.969a, 1996.
42. Stone D: The Disabled State. Philadelphia, Temple University, 1984.
43. Turk DC, Brody MC: Chronic opioid therapy for persistent noncancer pain: Panacea or oxymoron? American Pain Society Bulletin 1:4–7, 1991.
44. Turk DC: Customizing treatment for chronic pain patients: Who, what and why? Clin J Pain 6:255–270, 1990.
45. Turk DC, Rudy TE: Assessment of cognitive factors in chronic pain: A worthwhile enterprise? J Consult Clin Psychol 54:760–768, 1986.
46. Verhaak PFM, Kerssens JJ, Pekker J, et al: Prevalence of chronic benign pain disorder among adults: A review of the literature. Pain 77:231–239, 1998.
47. Waddell G: Clinical assessment of lumbar impairment. Clin Orthop 221:110–120, 1987.
48. Wiesel SW, Tsourmas M, Feffer HL, et al: A study of computer-assisted tomography: 1. The incidence of positive CAT scans in an asymptomatic group of patients. Spine 9:549–551, 1984.
49. Worker's Compensation Permanent Partial Disability Schedule. St. Paul, Minn, Minnesota Medical Association, 1984.

Chapter 7

Functional Diagnosis of Musculoskeletal Pain and Evaluation of Treatment Results by Quantitative and Objective Techniques

Andrew A. Fischer, MD, PhD

This chapter is an update of "Pressure Algometry (Dolorimetry) in the Differential Diagnosis of Muscle Pain" from the first edition of this book[9] and following publications such as "Algometry in Quantification of Diagnosis and Treatment Outcome" in *Muscle Pain Syndromes and Fibromyalgia*[13] and others.[10, 12–13, 52] However, it does not replace them because substantial information on reliability and technical details are not repeated.

Recently, so much progress has been achieved in functional diagnosis for musculoskeletal pain that in addition to updating the information on pressure algometry, it seemed useful to add a description of newly introduced tests,[14, 15] such as quantified pinch and roll (P&R), electric skin conductance (ESC), and quantified diagnosis of microedema.

The first part of this chapter describes pain diagnostic instruments and their employment. The second part describes the most efficient, sensitive, and precise system for testing sensory nerve fiber dysfunction, specifically dermatomal involvement. Finally, the clinical diagnosis of *spinal segmental sensitization (SSS)*, a very important condition because it is consistently associated with musculoskeletal pain, will be described. Chapter 13[16] describes the treatment of SSS by a new technique, the paraspinous block (PSB), which along with other injections essentially improved results in management of musculoskeletal pain.

Summary of Previous Study

Clinical findings and treatment results in 120 patients with low back, neck, and extremity pain were reported.[15] The results of this study regarding diagnostic aspects can be summarized as follows:

A battery of tests was described that renders a quantitative and objective diagnosis of radicular dysfunction. The diagnostic sensitivity of the tests exceeds the conventional neurologic examination. In addition, the tests are more efficient, saving considerable time required for the examination.

1. The tests include a system of sensory examination using scratching instead of pinprick as nociceptive stimulus: The P&R technique explores the subcutaneous tissue and renders the highest diagnostic sensitivity for detection of nerve fiber sensitization and referred pain. Electric skin conductance diagnoses objectively and quantitatively nerve fiber dysfunction (sensitization) and its normalization immediately following paraspinous blocks. The diagnostic sensitivity of ESC is higher than the subjective reaction to pinprick.

Table 7–1.
Pain Diagnostic Instruments and Their Employment

Instrument	Measured Quality	Employment
1. Pressure algometers	Pressure pain sensitivity	Diagnosis of tenderness Evaluation of treatment results
2. Tissue compliance meter	Muscle tone, consistency	Dx. of muscle spasm Taut bands
3. Dynamometer	Muscle strength	Weakness

4. Electric skin conductance meter	Electric skin conductance	Sensory fiber irritation
		Sympathetic hyperactivity, objective dx
		  of local tissue damage (dysfunction)
		  and radiculopathy, SSS

2. Using these more sophisticated tests, a pentad of signs were described that are frequently the cause of musculoskeletal pain. *The pentad of discopathy-radiculopathy-paraspinal spasm and supra-interspinous ligament sprain* consists of:
   a. Narrowed disc space and neural foramen on imaging; this is manifested clinically by: Narrowed space between spinous processes and sprained (tender) supraspinous and interspinous ligaments.
   b. There is palpable paraspinal muscle spasm, which causes: Radicular compression and dysfunction (sensitization). Consequently, spinal segmental sensitization develops and can be diagnosed as will be described later.
3. The pentad was identified as the cause of symptoms in 82% of patients.
4. Diagnosis of radicular or spinal segmental dysfunction can be made exclusively by Keegan's dermatomal charts. This conclusion is based on the established fact that only the dermatomes described by Keegan[30] are correct because they consistently correlate with pain and sensory neurologic findings.
5. Findings of neurologic deficit such as numbness, decreased sensation of pinprick, and diminished reflexes failed to demonstrate any correlation with pain. Positive, irritative neurologic findings in the form of hyperactivity, irritation, and sensitization are consistently present in painful areas. They consist of tingling, buzzing, feeling of pins and needles, and hyperalgesia to scratch (pinprick), P&R of subcutaneous tissue, and point tenderness in muscles.
6. Myofascial pain is frequently a manifestation of spinal segmental sensitization.

Pain Diagnostic Instruments for Quantification of Physical Findings

Five pain diagnostic instruments° are described along with their employment for quantification of physical findings as well as documentation of treatment outcome. In addition to quantification of physical finding related to pain, the tissue compliance meter renders objective data, i.e., independent of the patient's reaction regarding muscle tone and spasm. ESC also objectively documents dysfunction of sensory fibers, including their sensitization and improvement by treatment (desensitization) (Table 7–1).

Table 7–2 describes acronyms used in this chapter.

1. **The Pressure Threshold Meter** (10-kg range, 0.1-kg divisions). The pressure threshold meter (Fig. 7–1) consists of a rubber disk attached to the pole of a pressure (force) gauge. The gauge is calibrated in kilograms and pounds. The kilogram scale is used for clinical purposes. Since the surface of the rubber tip is exactly 1 cm², the readings are expressed in kilograms per square centimeter

°Note: Pain diagnostic instruments, algometers, tissue compliance meter, and the like are distributed by Pain Diagnostics & Treatment, Inc., 233 East Shore Road, Suite 108, Great Neck, NY 11021.

Table 7–2.
Acronyms Used in this Chapter

ESC:	Electric skin conductance
FM:	Fibromyalgia syndrome
MSkP:	Musculoskeletal pain
MPS:	Myofascial pain syndrome
MSp:	Muscle spasm
N&I:	Needling and infiltration of taut band. A special trigger point injection technique that breaks up the abnormal tissue.
P&R:	Pinch and roll. A technique for testing the sensitivity of subcutaneous tissue.
PIB:	Preinjection block. An injection technique for blocking sensation from TrP to be injected
PPT:	Pressure pain threshold.
PSB:	Paraspinous block. Interrupts sensation from supra/interspinous ligaments and desensitizes the SSS.
SSS:	Spinal segmental sensitization. A state of hyperactivity, facilitation of spinal segment in reaction to an irritative focus.
SSP/IS:	Supra/infraspinous ligaments.
RPZ:	Referred pain zone. A specific area in which pain caused by trigger point is perceived.
TB:	Taut band associated with trigger points and tender spots
TrP:	Trigger point. A tender spot that spontaneously or on irritation shoots pain into a distant referred pain zone.
TS:	Tender spot. A small tender area under the finger pointing at the most intensive pain.
VAS:	Visual analog scale of pain intensity.

(kg/cm^2). A maximum hold feature maintains the indicator on the highest pressure achieved. Pressing the zeroing knob returns the indicator to the original resting position, which is not necessarily 0. Deviations of resting position do not affect the precision of measurements. The range of the meter is 0 to 10 kg, with 0.1-kg divisions.[9, 12, 13]

2. **The Pressure Tolerance Meter** (20-kg range, 0.2-kg divisions). The tolerance gauge has a similar construction as the pressure threshold meter, with two important differences. The range of the tolerance gauge is extended to 20 kg, as compared to 10 kg with the threshold meter. Consequently, the divisions on

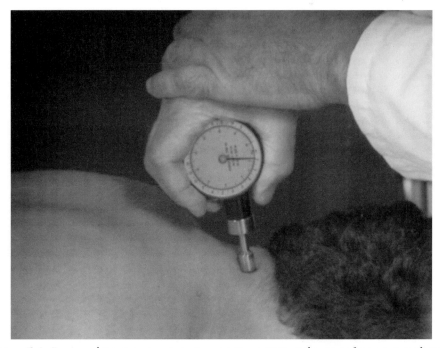

Figure 7–1. Pressure algometer measuring pressure pain sensitivity at the point of maximum tenderness.

the tolerance gauge are also larger (0.2 kg vs. 0.1 kg on the threshold meter). The tolerance meter, by gaining a higher range, lost somewhat in precision of measurement. The threshold meter, although more precise than the tolerance gauge, lacks sufficient range for high normal threshold and tolerance measurements. Therefore, for best results, the use of both gauges—one for threshold (10 kg) and one for high threshold and for tolerance (20 kg)—is recommended.

Pressure tolerance is the highest pressure that the person can endure under the conditions of the examination. Pressure tolerance expresses the subject's sensitivity to pain.[9–13] This type of dolorimeter rendered the best results.[54, 55]

3. **Tissue Compliance Meter for Objective Quantitative Documentation of Alterations in Muscle Tone (Spasm, Taut Bands, and Hypotonia).** The tissue compliance meter (TCM, Fig. 7–2) is a hand-held mechanical instrument that measures the consistency of soft tissues.[6] Muscle tone and its alterations including spasm, tension, spasticity, and taut bands associated with trigger points and tender spots can be documented objectively. Figure 7–3 shows objective and quantitative recording of muscle spasm in left infraspinatus muscle, where lower pressure threshold, 4.5 kg/cm^2 vs. 8.0 kg over the control side, indicated the presence of trigger point. Several authors showed consistency of TCM results, and normal values were established in paraspinal muscles for each segment.[63] Patients with fibromyalgia syndrome (FMS) demonstrated increased muscle tone in paraspinal muscles.[20] This finding adds two important new dimensions to the diagnosis of FMS; namely, the increased muscle tone and its objective and quantitative documentation by TCM.

Increased resistance (decreased softness or compliance) in the form of a taut band is recognized as a diagnostic finding of myofascial trigger points. The presence of a harder consistency in trigger points, which were diagnosed by lower pressure threshold, can be corroborated objectively using tissue compliance measurement.[6, 15]

4. **Dynamometer for measurement of muscle strength. The Universal Handheld Dynamometer** can be employed in clinical practice for strength measurements of any muscle in extremities.[9, 10] The dynamometer consists of a

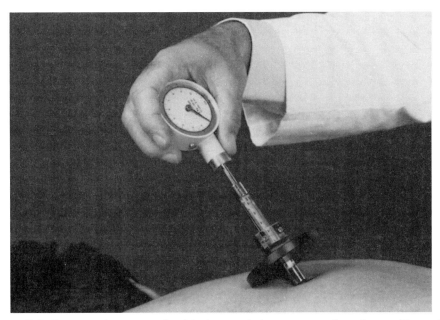

Figure 7–2. Tissue compliance meter for objective quantitative assessment of muscle tone. The method documents muscle spasm as well as taut bands associated with trigger points.

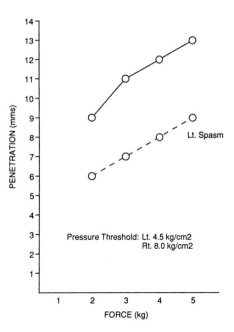

Figure 7–3. Objective and quantitative recording of muscle spasm by tissue compliance meter. X axis shows the applied force. Y axis indicates the compliance, i.e., depth of penetration of the probe in millimeters. On the left side, over the trigger point showing decreased pressure threshold (4.5 kg/cm² as compared to 8.0 kg on control side), there is decreased compliance (harder consistency), indicating muscle spasm.

30-kg range gauge with a large footplate that provides the resistance to the measured body part. Dynamometry is useful for quantification of functional impairment and documentation of recovery in the course of treatment.

5. **Electric Skin Conductance Meter.** ESC can be employed in daily clinical practice of pain management for diagnosis and for instantaneous, as well as long-term, evaluation of treatment results.[15, 33–35, 39, 49] ESC has two very important advantages as compared with the sensory examination by pinprick or scratch. First, ESC is an objective and quantitative method providing unique information about sensory nerve dysfunction without the need to rely on a patient's subjective response. Second, ESC frequently shows positive findings when the subjective response to pinprick or scratch is negative, indicating a higher diagnostic sensitivity of the method. In most cases, however, the territory of subjective response to scratch, in terms of *hyperalgesia, corresponds exactly to the increased ESC*. The method is based on the measurement of an electric current passing between a reference electrode that the patient holds in either palm, and an explorative electrode that is dragged across the examined dermatomes. The use of a pointed explorative electrode allows for the combination of scratching that represents a painful stimulus and solicits the patients' subjective response with the objective quantitative data collection by ESC. In addition, the simultaneous use of both methods saves considerable time.

The sensitivity of the meter for clinical purposes should be at least 50 microamperes. Increased ESC is recorded over hyperalgesic areas where the scratch or pinprick causes pain.[15] The sudden increase in conductance is best detected by a change in the pitch of a sound generated by the alteration of current. The mechanism of higher skin conductance over the sensitized dermatomes or other areas supplied by the sensitized nerve fibers can be explained by increased sympathetic activity inducing sweating, which lowers skin resistance.[15, 33–35, 49] Antidromic impulses traveling from the irritated and sensitized sensory nerve fibers toward the periphery can switch by the axon reflex to sympathetic fibers.[56, 57] Their excitation causes increase of sweating and augmented electric skin conductance. This mechanism can explain the identical territories of ESC abnormalities and that of subjective responses to painful stimuli, particularly if the findings correspond to dermatomes.

Use of Pressure Algometry for Quantification of Diagnosis and Treatment Outcome in Musculoskeletal Disorders

Pressure algometry (PA) (dolorimetry) is a method that measures pressure pain threshold (PPT), i.e., the minimal pressure that causes pain. PA quantifies the examiner's subjective impression of tenderness. The method is being employed for quantitative diagnosis of painful conditions, particularly myofascial pain (MP),[9–13] fibromyalgia (FMS),[40, 50] and tenderness related to inflammation.[14, 36, 40–42] Pressure pain threshold measurement has also proved to be instrumental for documentation of treatment outcomes: PA successfully evaluated the immediate effects of therapy, particularly different injection techniques.[13, 15, 16] Efficacy of preinjection blocks, which anesthetize the sensitive, tender areas to be injected, can be monitored.[15] Most importantly, long-term outcome of treatment modalities, particularly that of needling and infiltration of tender spots (TSs), trigger points (TrPs), and local pathology that are the immediate cause of pain could be documented successfully by PA.[13–15]

Pressure threshold measurement quantifies tenderness, i.e., pressure pain sensitivity of tender spots and trigger points. *Pressure threshold* is the minimum pressure (force) that causes pain. Threshold is measured over hypersensitive spots (tender points, tender spots, or trigger points) in order to diagnose their location and to quantify the degree of pressure sensitivity that expresses their level of *activity*. If the patient is asked to indicate by pointing with one finger where the most intense pain is, in over 90% of cases a tender spot can be palpated exactly underneath the pointing finger.[15] This is called a *tender spot (TS)*, as opposed to a trigger point (TrP), which is also a small, exquisitely tender area, but causes pain in a distant part, called referred pain zone (RPZ). Each TrP has a specific RPZ.[13, 47, 53, 58] The crucial determination as to whether tenderness should be considered abnormal is assisted by PA. Table 7–3 summarizes the clinical and research applications of pressure algometry.

Table 7–4 summarizes normal values of pressure pain threshold.

Abnormal focal tenderness is the most important, decisive, reliable, and reproducible criterion for diagnosis of *myofascial trigger points (MTrPs)* and *tender spots*.[9, 14, 15, 44] Experimental results show that all other criteria for the establishment of the diagnosis of MTrPs are both inconsistent and less reliable than point tenderness.[9, 19, 44, 45] The criterion for abnormal tenderness used to establish the diagnosis of *fibromyalgia (FMS)* is an absolute PPT value of 4 kg over 11 out of a possible 18 established tender points.[50, 65] In contrast, an abnormal PPT for diagnosis of MTrPs has been established in terms relative to normosensitive areas in the same patient. A PPT that is lower by 2 kg/cm² relative to a normosensitive control site, usually on a corresponding contralateral side, is considered abnormal tenderness.[7, 9] It is important to note that physicians

---

Table 7–3.
Clinical Applications of Pressure Algometry

I. Diagnosis
   A. Trigger Points and Tender Spots in muscles, ligaments, and other soft tissues
   B. Fibromyalgia
   C. Activity of Arthritis
   D. Subcutaneous Tissue Sensitization = quantification of pinch
   E. Diffuse Muscle Tenderness—characteristic of endocrine disorders (thyroid or estrogen deficiency). Muscle PPT decreases below shin bone levels.
   F. Medicolegal Documentation of abnormal tenderness quantitatively. Consistent results assure reliability of results.
   G. Pain Tolerance measurements
II. Evaluation of Treatment Results
   A. Immediate Effect of injections, preinjection blocks, physical therapy, spray, stretch, relaxation, manipulation
   B. Long-term Outcome of treatment
   C. Effect of Medications and Balneologic Procedures

Table 7–4.
Normal Values for Pressure Pain Threshold

1. *For diagnosis of tender spots and trigger points.* Criterion of abnormal pressure pain threshold (PPT) is 2 kg/cm² lower than a control point with normal sensitivity usually over the corresponding opposite side.
2. Measurement of *subcutaneous tenderness* (quantification of pinch and roll). Criterion has not been established yet specifically, therefore identical norm is used as in #1, i.e., lower than a control point by 2 kg/cm²
3. *Fibromyalgia (FMS).* Criterion is a PPT of 4 kg absolute value over 11 out of 18 specific tender points diagnostic of FMS. In addition, widespread pain should be present. In children, PPT is lower and equals 3 kg.
4. *Tenderness of muscles vs. bones* (deltoids vs. shin bones). Basic criterion is that PPT over muscles is normally higher than that over the bones. Reversal of this relation indicates abnormal muscle tenderness.

using digital compression as a diagnostic technique were unable to provide exactly 4 kg/cm² of pressure to a region, nor were they able to reproduce the same level of pressure on repeated attempts.[13] This fact alone indicates the need for algometry to quantify tenderness.

Another advantage of the use of PA in pain management is that it facilitates communication among clinicians and researchers and allows quantitative comparison of their findings.

Pressure algometry also assists in the *evaluation of treatment results.* Both the immediate effects of treatment, as well as long-term outcomes, have been successfully monitored quantitatively.[13–15] A good correlation can be found between the improved pressure threshold values and the degree of pain alleviation, with the latter usually assessed by visual analog scales (VAS).[12–15] This indicates that the treated TSs/TrPs were the immediate cause of the patient's complaints. On the other hand, the lack of correlation between PPT changes and alterations in pain intensity may indicate that the measured tender areas were not the main cause of pain. Hence, evaluation of treatment results by PA requires precise localization of the TSs or TrPs that are causing the pain.

Pressure algometry has been successfully used to evaluate different treatments for myofascial and musculoskeletal pain, including systemic medications,[46] transcutaneous electrical nerve stimulation, various injection types, various injected medications,[13–15] and physical modalities,[23, 26–29] healing[8] and manipulation.[62]

Several studies have proved that PA is effective in differentiating MTrPs from nontender control tender points.[24, 48] Several authors[24, 45, 48] independently proved the validity, reliability, and reproducibility of PA measurements.

Sensitization of Nerves—The Cause of Tenderness and Pain

Tenderness, i.e., increased *pressure pain sensitivity,* is quantified by a decrease in the pressure threshold. *Pressure pain threshold,* defined as the minimum pressure that induces pain, is the point at which the patient reports that the feeling of pressure changes into a painful sensation. Tenderness is the leading diagnostic sign of inflammation.[1, 2, 5] Normal tissues do not generate real pain on pressure. *Sensitization* refers to the process that changes the reactivity of the nerve fibers making the mechanical pressure painful.[1, 2, 5, 42, 43, 51] It is known that cell *damage* causes release of substances that induce a chemical cascade and inflammation, resulting in pain and sensitivity to pressure.[1, 2, 5, 42, 43, 51] The main inflammatory mediators causing hyperalgesia and excitation of nociceptors include adenosine, bradykinin, interleukin-1 and -8, leukotriene B4, norepinephrine, 5-hydroxytryptamine, prostaglandin E_2 and I_2, serotonin and substance P and a high concentration of potassium.[42, 43, 51] Prostaglandins of the E type and bradykinin itself[42, 43] potentiate further the action of this group. Increased sympathetic activity can release prostaglandins that further potentiate the effect of other inflammatory substances.[42, 43] It is obvious that the identical process of sensitization, which can be measured by decreased pressure pain threshold, causes spontaneously occurring pain in the injured tissue, as well as its tenderness on pressure. Pressure threshold measurement thus reflects the activity of the chemical inflammatory process and degree of nerve fiber sensitization. Dolorimetry makes it possible to quantify in clinical practice the increase of nerve sensitivity, which is the most frequent cause of musculoskeletal pain.

Fibromyalgia: Diagnosis of Fibromyalgia by Quantification of Tender Point Sensitivity and Objective Documentation of Muscle Tension

The diagnosis of fibromyalgia is based on three main components.[40, 50, 65]

1. *Widespread pain* that includes pain in the upper body and lower body, as well as on the right and left half of the body.
2. In addition, so-called *axial pain* that is over the sternum and spine is required to qualify as widespread pain.
3. Tenderness at a pressure of 4 kg over *11 out of 18 tender points*. The tender points are nine pairs of points that demonstrate specifically more tenderness in patients with FMS. The nine points illustrated can be divided into two groups. First, tender points *over muscles,* which include trapezius (upper border), supraspinatus, and gluteus medius. The rest of the tender points are not located over muscles, and include suboccipital, space between C5 and C7 transverse processes, second costochondral junction, 2 cm distal from the lateral epicondyle, greater trochanter, and medial fat pad of knees proximal to the joint line.[65]

The clinical diagnosis of tenderness relies on the examiner's subjective judgment, guessing how much pressure equals 4 kg. A study of 34 physicians was conducted,[11, 13] and a second study consisting of 16 more physicians rendered identical results. It was shown that a subjective estimate of 4 kg pressure exerted by a digit is not precise. The physicians were asked to press the algometer blindly, without seeing the dial, and attempt to exert a pressure of 4 kg. The results were scattered far above and below the 4 kg level. In addition, on twice-repeated attempts, the examiners rarely reproduced the results. The *conclusion* is that exerting digital pressure at 4 kg pressure used for diagnosis of FMS is not reliable and *quantification of the critical pressure by algometry is necessary.*

In addition, using the tissue compliance meter, Australian researchers demonstrated *increased muscle tension* of the paraspinal muscles at the third thoracic level in patients with FMS.[20] This is the first objective and quantitative clinical finding for diagnosis of FMS. It also demonstrated for the first time presence of muscle tension in this puzzling condition.

Diagnosis of Specific Muscle Tenderness by Pressure Pain Sensitivity of Deltoid Muscle vs. Shinbone

Comparison of the pressure pain threshold over the deltoid muscle and shin bone is an indicator of tenderness specifically affecting only muscles. If both values are decreased below normal levels, then generalized low pain tolerance syndrome is present. If the values of deltoid muscle are lower relative to the shinbone, then *specific muscle tenderness* is considered. This is a typical finding in endocrine disorders, particularly in the case of low thyroid or estrogen production or peripheral resistance to the thyroid hormone.[1, 12, 13, 56] These conditions are frequent causes of specific muscle tenderness. Normal values for pressure threshold over deltoid are somewhat higher than over tibia.[9–12]

The clinical importance of the abnormal specific pressure sensitivity over the muscles is underscored by the fact *that it is the only test that indicates muscle dysfunction due to peripheral resistance to hormones* on which normal muscle metabolism depends.[13, 56] Measurement of muscle pressure pain sensitivity in relation to the tibia is also very useful in *evaluation of treatment results with hormonal replacement.*

Improved Examination Techniques for Diagnosis of Sensory Nerve Fiber Dysfunction

A system of sensory neurologic evaluation for painful stimuli has been introduced. *Scratching the skin* is a technique that is superior to pinprick for testing *sensitivity to painful stimuli.* Scratching the skin is performed with a sharp object, such as an opened paper clip. The subjective response to scratching the skin can be combined with the objective measurement of electrical skin conductance if a sharp, exploring electrode is employed. These tests are far superior to conventional examination techniques using pinprick because they render more precise territorial diagnosis of the involved spinal segmental (radicular), as well as other nerve fiber dysfunction. In addition, testing by scratch has a higher diagnostic sensitivity than the conventional pinprick method and can be performed in a fraction of the time.

The P&R technique tests subcutaneous tissue and therefore is the most sensitive method for diagnosis of nerve fiber sensitization. Our experience supports the experimental data of Vecchiet and colleagues[59-61] that the subcutaneous tissue is the most sensitive reactor to nerve irritation. We found that *P&R is also the most sensitive method for diagnosis of spinal segmental (radicular) or other peripheral nerve fiber dysfunction.* The technique of P&R consists of pinching the skin between the thumb and index finger and making a fold over a nonpainful area.[15] Without releasing the pressure, the skinfold is rolled while the thumb and index finger of the other hand take over the pinching and continue the rolling.[37, 38] Areas with sensitized nerve fibers are very painful. The degree of sensitization can be quantified using a pressure algometer (Fig. 7–4).[13, 15]

Electric skin conductance combined with simultaneous evaluation of reaction to painful stimuli in the form of scratching is a major improvement in sensory evaluation, as has been described earlier.

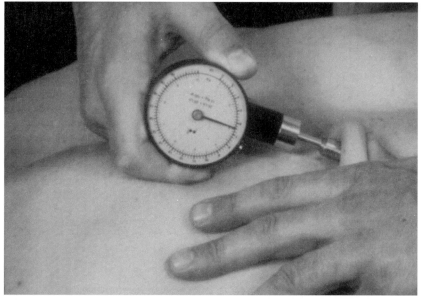

Figure 7–4. Quantification of pinch and roll test using pressure algometer. A skinfold is created and the algometer provides tangential pressure over the base of the skinfold, being opposed by the examiner's thumb, which has a stabilizing effect without pressing against the measuring tape.

Sensory Evaluation Tracks for Efficient and Precise Diagnosis of Spinal Segmental Sensitization and Nerve Fiber Dysfunction

The dermatomes that were described by Keegan and Garrett[30] corresponded exactly to findings in 600 examinations using the most precise methods. These included scratch, P&R, as well as ESC. The only correct dermatomes are presented in Figure 7–5. Dermatomes described by other authors are incorrect.[3, 17, 27]

Figure 7–6 shows *sensory evaluation tracks* developed by the author superimposed over the dermatomal chart. Using the tracks, the diagnosis of hypersensitive and hyposensitive dermatomes can be performed with a *minimal amount of testing, while the results are more precise and more reliable*. The improvement of results is considerable and is achieved in a fraction of the time required for examination by conventional technique. The sensory evaluation tracks can be used for testing by pinprick, scratch, P&R, as well as by ESC. Most advantageous is the simultaneous application of scratch and ESC.

Each track is numbered and carries a name describing its location. Examination of the extremities is performed in the shape of circles. *Basic sensory evaluation tracks* represent the minimal number of tracks needed to establish a diagnosis in the upper or lower body.

For the *lower body,* the minimum basic tracks include the Tr1 (below knee), which explores L3 to L5 and S1, S2 segments; and Tr2 (below groin), which in addition to L3 to S2 also tests the L1 and L2 segments. In addition, the paraspinal tracks starting at the T1 level going down to S5 level should be tested bilaterally. The Tr3 (buttock) that examines L1 to S5 dermatomes is useful to correlate the level of pentad with sensitized peripheral dermatomes.

For the *upper body,* the basic tracks consist of Tr6 (below elbow) and Tr7 (above elbow), both testing the C5 to T1 dermatomes. In addition, the cervical and thoracic paraspinal tracks have to be tested. Tr6 (midclavicular) explores the thoracic ventral rami. Tr9 (behind ear) tests C2 to C3 dermatomes and is used for diagnosis of SSS related to *headache and neck pain.* In addition, paraspinal testing of the upper body is necessary, starting on the head (C2) and descending to low back (T12) level.

Referred Pain Zones

Referred pain zones from trigger points and dermatomes overlap. Referred pain is a manifestation of spinal segmental sensitization. Referred pain zones[15, 53, 58] from myofascial trigger points, as described by Travell and Simons,[58] and their relation to dermatomes are shown in Figures 7–7 through 7–11. RPZs from ligamentous trigger points, as described by Hackett,[22] are shown in Figures 7–12 and 7–13. It is obvious that the referred RPZs from both muscles and ligaments overlap with individual dermatomes. This finding, which is contrary to previous belief, indicates that *referred pain is a manifestation of spinal segmental sensitization.*

Figures 7-7 through 7–13 are very useful to identify the cause of pain: When the patient points to a location of pain, the RPZs indicate which TrP is causing the symptoms. Treatment should be focused on this TrP. However, because musculoskeletal pain is connected with SSS, the Figures 7–7 through 7–13 also show to which sensitized spinal segment the TrP and its RPZ belong. Best results are achieved when the SSS is treated first by paraspinous block.[15, 16]

Diagnosis of Spinal Segmental Sensitization in Clinical Practice

Spinal segmental sensitization (SSS) is a hyperactive, facilitated state of a spinal segment that develops in reaction to an *irritative focus (IF)*, which constantly bombards the sensory ganglion with nociceptive stimuli.[1, 4] The IF usually consists of a

Text continued on page 164

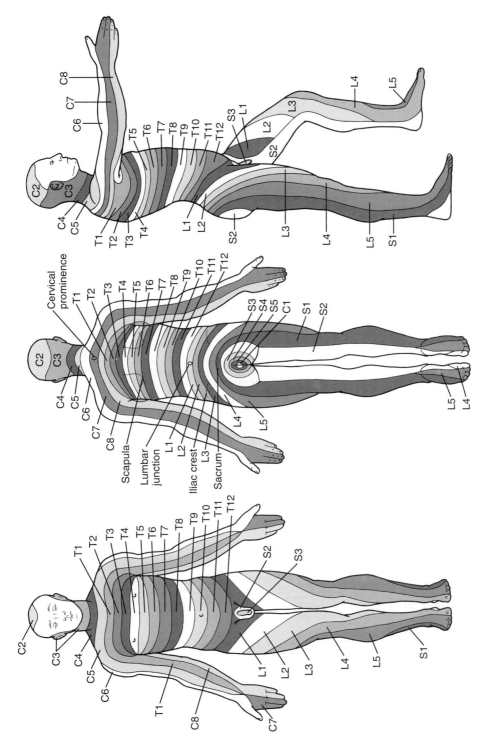

Figure 7–5. Dermatomes according to Keegan and Garrett.[30] This dermatomal chart has proved to be the only correct chart corresponding exactly to hyperalgesic and hypoalgesic areas as measured by the most sensitive quantitative and objective methods for testing sensory nerve fibers: pinch and roll, electric skin conductance, and scratching of skin.

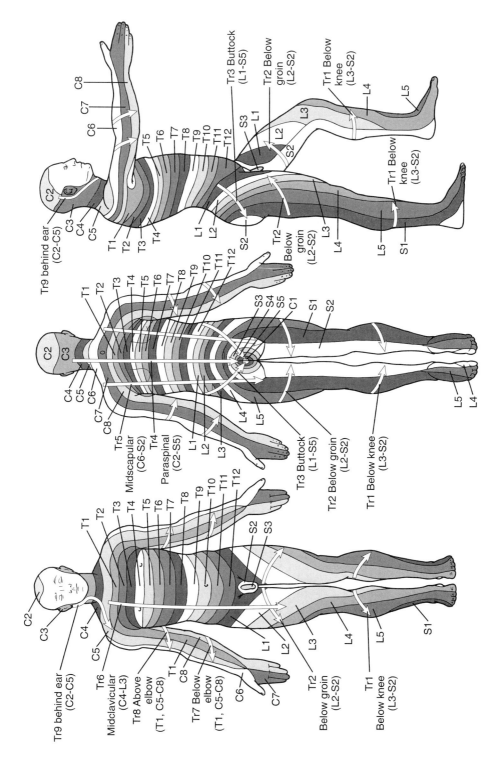

Figure 7–6. Tracks for fast and precise testing of sensory dysfunction, particularly dermatomal involvement. The arrows superimposed across the dermatomal borders indicate the tracks and direction of testing. Each track (Tr) carries a name and number. The dermatomes tested by each track are indicated in parentheses.

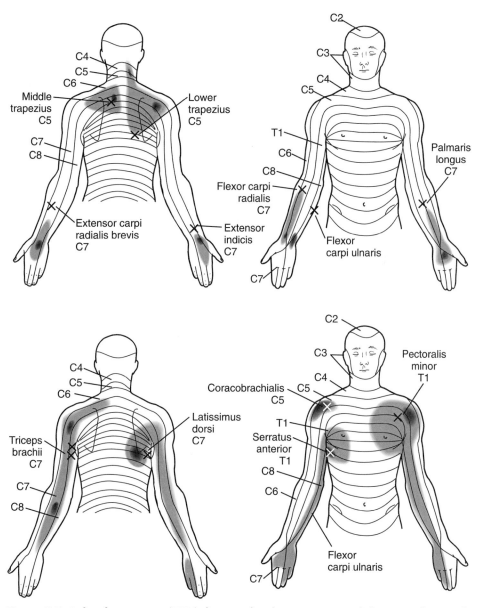

Figure 7–7. Referred pain zones (RPZs) from myofascial trigger points and their coincidence with dermatomes. Panel 1 shows the upper body. Figures 7–7 through 7–15 show that RPZs represent a portion of spinal segmental sensitization because they overlap exactly with segments of the corresponding dermatomes. The RPZ that overlaps a dermatome is usually caused by a muscle, which is innervated by the identical spinal segment as the dermatome itself.

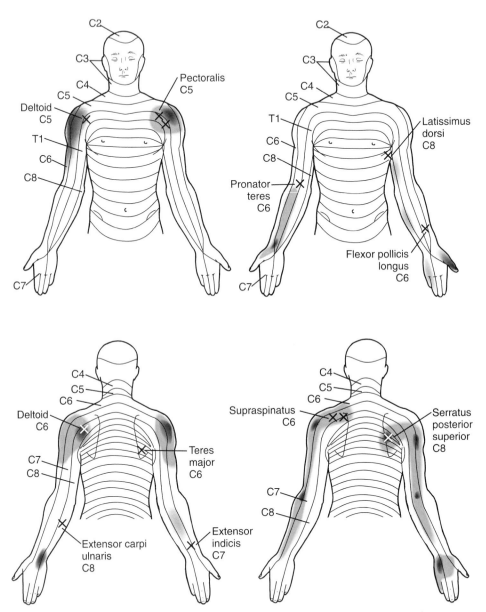

Figure 7–8. Referred pain zones from myofascial trigger points and their coincidence with dermatomes. Panel 2 shows the upper body, continued.

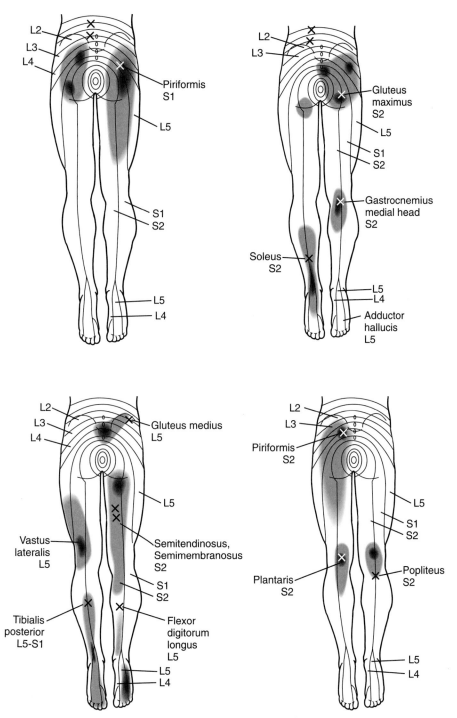

Figure 7–9. Referred pain zones from myofascial trigger points and their coincidence with dermatomes. Panel 3 shows the lower body.

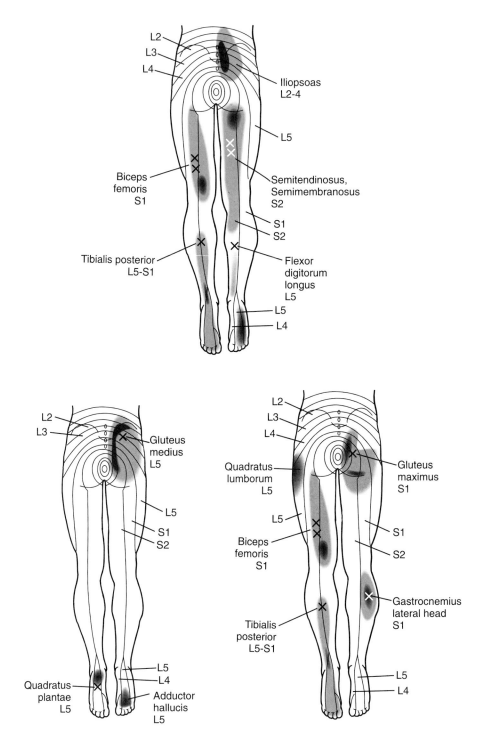

Figure 7–10. Referred pain zones from myofascial trigger points and their coincidence with dermatomes. Panel 4 shows the lower body, continued.

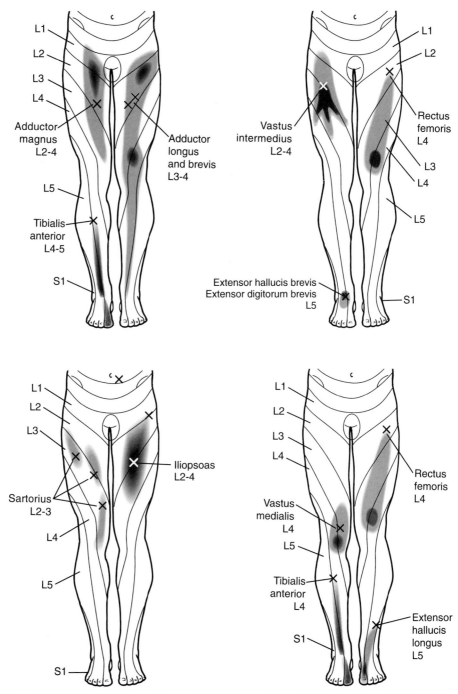

Figure 7–11. Referred pain zones from myofascial trigger points and their coincidence with dermatomes. Panel 5 shows the lower body, continued.

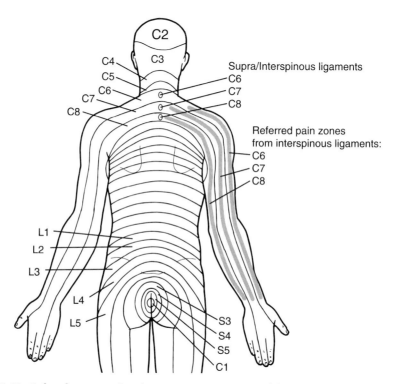

Figure 7–12. Referred pain zones from ligamentous trigger points and their coincidence with dermatomes. Panel 1 shows the upper body. The exact overlapping of dermatomes and RPZs from ligaments as described by Hackett[22] proves that the referred pain is part of spinal segmental sensitization.

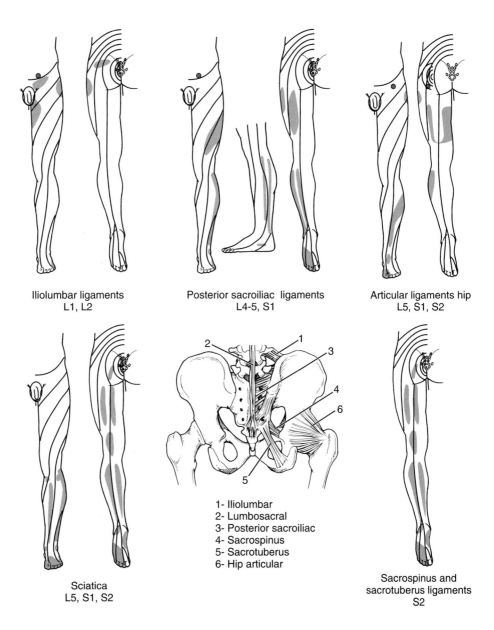

Iliolumbar ligaments
L1, L2

Posterior sacroiliac ligaments
L4-5, S1

Articular ligaments hip
L5, S1, S2

Sciatica
L5, S1, S2

1- Iliolumbar
2- Lumbosacral
3- Posterior sacroiliac
4- Sacrospinus
5- Sacrotuberus
6- Hip articular

Sacrospinus and
sacrotuberus ligaments
S2

Figure 7–13. Referred pain zones from ligamentous trigger points and their coincidence with dermatomes. Panel 2 shows the lower body.

small area of damaged or dysfunctional tissue where peripheral sensitization, irritation of the nerve fibers, generates the continuous nociceptive stimuli causing sensitization of the central nervous system.[66] This *central sensitization* starts with the spinal segment. The most frequently affected segments are C5 and C6, as well as L5 and S1. A frequent irritative focus causing SSS is sprain of the supra/interspinous ligaments[14, 15, 18, 31] that can be treated by paraspinous blocks (PSB).[14, 15]

Peripheral sensitization is the pathophysiologic process that changes the reactivity of sensory nerve fibers to stimuli. The usual mechanism of sensitization consists of local tissue damage producing sensitizing, inflammatory irritating substances, such as prostaglandins and bradykinin, as described earlier.[2, 4, 42, 43, 64]

SSS affects in clinical practice all functional components of the spinal segment; namely, the dermatome (sensory), myotome (motor), and sclerotome (bones along with the attachments of ligaments to bones, tendons, and joint capsules). A sympathetic component of the segment can also be involved.

Figures 7–14 and 7–15 on the left-hand side show the *dermatomes* according to Keegan and Garrett.[30] In the middle selected *myotomes* are presented,[32] and on the right-hand side sites of *typical sclerotomal involvement* in individual SSS are illustrated.[37] The pictures facilitate clinical diagnosis of SSS.

Diagnosis of Sensory Segmental Involvement

The most sensitive method for the diagnosis of sensory fiber or segmental sensory dysfunction is the *P&R technique*, which tests the sensitivity of subcutaneous tissue. P&R can be quantified by an algometer (see Fig. 7–4). Second in diagnostic sensitivity for sensory dysfunction is the increased *ESC*, which also has the advantage of being objective and quantitative. The least sensitive and least reliable of the sensory tests is pinprick or scratching of the skin, which relies on the patient's subjective response. The precision and reliability of *scratching* surpasses that of pinprick and is suitable also to use with the sensory diagnostic tracks described in this chapter, which saves considerable time and improves the precision of sensory examination

Diagnosis of Spinal Segmental Sensitization Affecting the Myotome

Motor, myotomal involvement is very consistently present as part of SSS and most frequently is the *presenting complaint*.

In the myotome the SSS manifests by three typical and consistent findings that include mainly TSs/TrPs with associated taut bands and muscle spasm. The incidence is approximately 9 TSs for each TrP.[15] Both TSs and TrPs are located within a taut band, which is the most important diagnostic finding for several reasons. First, a taut band represents an *objective finding* on palpation. Second, the taut band is present consistently around TSs or TrPs. Even in latent TrPs, i.e., in the period when the patient has no pain or other symptoms caused by the TSs/TrPs, the taut band indicates the presence of pathology.

Taut bands are diagnosed by palpating across the length of the affected muscle fibers. The characteristic findings, which are actually pathognomonic, consist of a group of muscle fibers that demonstrate *harder consistency and tenderness* on compression. Tenderness is a recognized symptom of nerve fiber sensitization (allodynia). The hard consistency of TBs consists of two components that were differentiated by the effect of sensory blocks: A neurogenic contraction that is released by the block is responsible usually for about 80% of the taut band. The remaining 20% of the taut band, which fails to relax after the block, demonstrates on palpation and needle penetration very hard consistency, characteristic of fibrotic tissue. Therefore, we call this structure the *fibrotic core*.

Taut bands are frequently missed because the examined muscle is not relaxed. Contraction of the antagonist induces most effective relaxation of the examined muscle that harbors the taut band, and the pathology becomes prominent instantaneously.

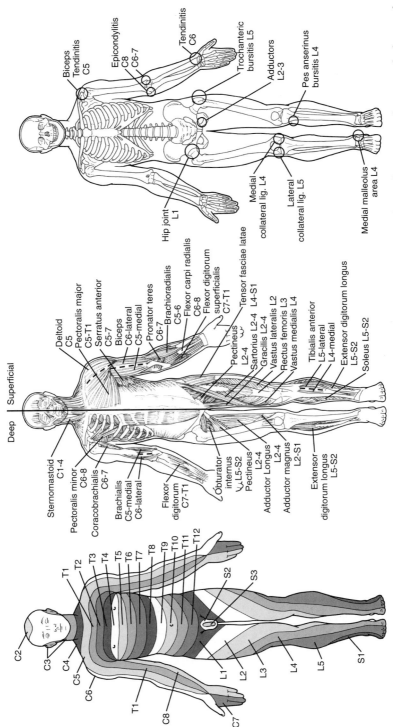

Figure 7–14. Diagnosis of spinal segmental sensitization (SSS) by its components: dermatomes, myotomes and most frequent manifestations of sclerotomal involvement. The innervating spinal segments are indicated on each figure. Front view.

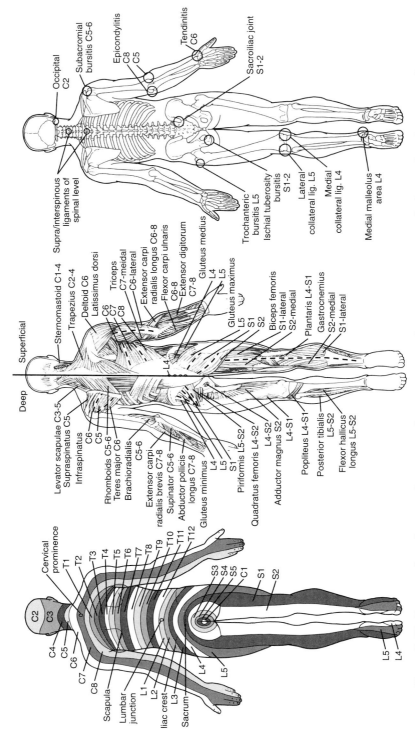

Figure 7–15. Diagnosis of spinal segmental sensitization by its components: dermatomes, myotomes and sclerotomal involvements. Back view.

Within the taut band there is one most sensitive point, which is the *TrPs/TSs*. Another consistent finding, which affects the entire myotome, is *muscle spasm*. Two identical palpatory findings, namely increased muscle tone and tenderness are characteristic of both muscle spasms and taut bands. The extent of findings is what differentiates the two conditions: In the case of muscle spasms the tenderness and increased tone extend over the *entire muscle*, whereas in the taut band findings are limited to a *group of muscle fibers only.* The tissue compliance meter can diagnose muscle spasms and its relief by treatment objectively and quantitatively,[6, 10, 11, 63] as shown on Figure 7–3.

Use of Dermatomes for Determination of Which Part of a Muscle Is Innervated by the Identical Spinal Segment

For treatment of TrPs/TSs and taut bands employing the PSB it is not sufficient to know the segment innervating the myotome because part of each muscle is supplied by one spinal segment only. For example, the S2 segment innervates the medial part of the gastrocnemius muscle, whereas the S1 level supplies the lateral part of the same muscle. Consequently, TrPs and spasm in the lateral part of the gastrocnemius muscle will respond exclusively to paraspinous block of S1, whereas blocking of the S2 level would be ineffective for treatment of the S1-supplied part of the muscle.

Figures 7–16 and 7–17 are back and front views respectively of muscles with superimposed dermatomes. The pictures are useful for identification of which muscle or even part of a muscle is innervated by a spinal segment. Identical spinal segment usually supplies the part of a muscle that is covered by the corresponding dermatome. There are few exceptions to this rule as, for example, supra-infra-spinatus, teres minor, and the like.

Manifestations of Sclerotomal Involvement in Spinal Segmental Sensitization

The most consistent finding related to sensitization of sclerotome is *enthesopathy* (inflammation at the attachment of tendons to bones) supplied by the involved segment.

The enthesopathy is not distributed equally over the entire tendon, but affects mainly and specifically the attachment of taut bands to the bone. Other manifestations of sclerotomal sensitization include *bursitis, tendinitis, pericapsulitis, and epicondylitis*. Each condition is located within the sensitized spinal segment, usually covered by the hyperalgesic dermatome, and the tendinitis belongs to the corresponding myotome. Figures 7–14 and 7–15 on the right-hand side show typical sclerotomal segmental sensitizations and their relation to dermatomes.

Neurogenic inflammation is the best explanation for the mechanism that causes segmental sclerotomal involvement that consists of extravasations (microedema) and tenderness (sensitization). The fact that pain and tenderness affecting these sclerotomal structures is alleviated when paraspinous blocks eradicate SSS confirms that neurogenic inflammation plays a role in the development of sclerotomal sensitization. The sensitized, hyperactive, irritated sensory fibers convey antidromic impulses (traveling in the opposite direction than normal nerve conduction) from the sensitized central nervous system to the periphery. At the end of sensory fibers, sensitizing substances are produced that induce inflammation.[57]

Sympathetic Components of Spinal Segmental Sensitization
Increased Skin Conductance and Trophoedema

Sympathetic dysfunction, as part of SSS, consists of *increased ESC in dermatomal distribution* and the presence of *microedema (trophoedema)* in subcutaneous tissue of the affected segment.

Increased values of ESC are caused by augmentation of sweating by sympathetic hyperactivity. The moisture increases the ESC. If the ESC changes correspond to the

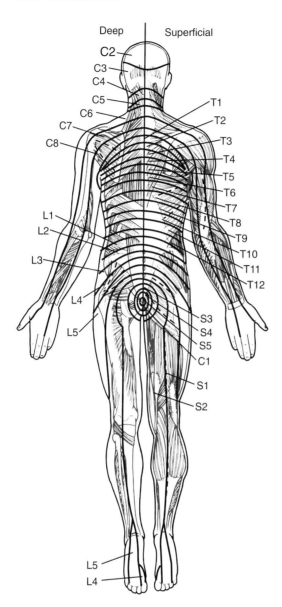

Figure 7–16. Dermatomes superimposed over muscles assist in identifying which specific spinal segment innervates a muscle or part of it. The identical spinal segment usually innervates parts of muscles located underneath a dermatome. For example, underneath the S2 dermatome lie the medial gastrocnemius muscle and medial hamstrings. Therefore, the S2 spinal segment also supplies these muscle parts. In contrast, the lateral parts of the same muscles are covered by S1 dermatome, and consequently are innervated by the S1 segment. There are some exceptions to this rule, the migrating muscles. Back view.

territory of a dermatome, the increased sympathetic activity is the result of antidromic impulses spreading over the sensory fibers from the center toward the periphery, where it activates the sympathetic fibers causing sweating.[33–35, 39, 57] Changes in ESC are a sensitive and objective indicator confirming the subjective response of hyperalgesia.[15]

Trophoedema (microedema) is a consistent sign of local tissue injury, as well as of spinal segmental sensitization. Microedema is a local sign that is always present at the site of any, even minimal, tissue injury. Therefore, it is an *extraordinarily useful sign for objective diagnosis and for locating the underlying pathology.* A lesser degree of microedema is present over the sensitized dermatome and is particularly obvious on P&R maneuver.

Microedema is diagnosed by an indentation caused by pressing into the skin a sharp object, such as the nails of the examiner or the tip of a key. Over the normal tissue the indentation returns to the initial level within seconds, whereas over the microedema, it takes much longer (sometimes a minute or two). Using the pressure algometer and applying 3 kg of pressure for 3 seconds can quantify this test.[15]

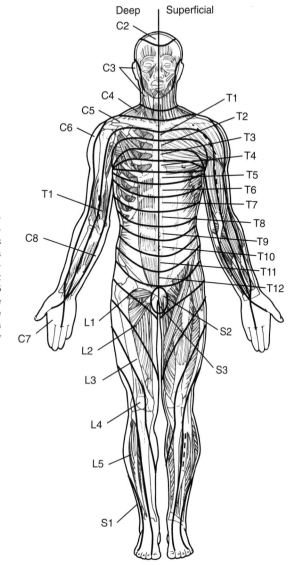

Figure 7–17. Dermatomes superimposed over muscles. Front view. The picture is useful in identifying the muscles and their parts, which are supplied by a spinal segment, as explained in the previous figure. For example, the lateral part of the deltoid muscle is covered by C6 dermatome and is innervated by the identical spinal segment. However, the ventral part of the muscle lies underneath the C5 dermatome; it is innervated by the same spinal segment.

Employing the algometer, the microedema becomes an objective and quantifiable, absolutely consistent finding indicating very precisely the area of damaged tissue where needling and infiltration should take place. This applies particularly in ligament sprain, bursitis, tendinitis, and pericapsulitis. The mechanism of microedema is most probably venous spasm due to sympathetic hyperactivity[15] and possibly neurogenic inflammation.[57]

Evidence That Spinal Segmental Sensitization Is the Pathophysiologic Basis of Referred Pain

At least three arguments serve as evidence for the conclusion that SSS constitutes the pathophysiologic basis of referred pain from any structure:

1. *Overlapping of referred pain zones (RPZs) with dermatomes.* RPZs from myofascial trigger points, as described by Travell and Simons,[58] and their relation to dermatomes are shown in Figures 7–7 through 7–11.

RPZs from ligamentous trigger points, as described by Hackett,[22] are shown in Figures 7–12 and 7–13. It is obvious that the referred RPZs from both muscles and ligaments overlap with individual dermatomes. This finding, which is contrary to previous belief, indicates that *referred pain is a component of the SSS.*

2. *Whenever referred pain was present in patients with musculoskeletal disorders, SSS corresponding to the painful area was also diagnosed.* The hyperalgesia, increased sensitivity to pinprick and scratch, and allodynia, i.e., tenderness on P&R and compression, were always present within the dermatome that corresponded exactly to the pain of musculoskeletal origin. The MSkP that was part of the sensitized spinal segment can be referred pain from TrPs within muscle or ligament or from any other structures. In addition, all kinds of MSkP originating from any tissue were found to be also consistently associated with SSS. The conditions included pain from local inflammation or injuries such as bursitis, tendinitis, enthesopathy (inflammation of the muscle attachment to bones), epicondylitis, overuse syndrome, pericapsulitis, and arthritis. Still, the most frequent condition is muscle pain caused by TSs/TrPs and taut bands. The second most frequent cause of musculoskeletal pain consists of ligament sprains, also manifested by TSs/TrPs.

3. The third evidence that SSS is the pathophysiologic basis of musculoskeletal pain consists of the *reversal of SSS to normal sensory findings by paraspinous block (PSB).* This injection *simultaneously relieves pain of musculoskeletal origin.* Both the referred pain, as well as pain caused by peripheral nerve fiber sensitization located within the sensitized spinal segment, is alleviated by the PSB. Hyperalgesia and tenderness, the hallmarks of sensitization, revert to normal sensitivity immediately following the PSB. At the same time, the pain in the treated segment is also alleviated. These results are so consistent that it is our routine procedure to test normalization of sensory findings within the treated dermatome immediately after the PSB in order to assess its efficacy.

Significance of Spinal Segmental Sensitization for Pain Management

SSS has been established as a consistent component associated with musculoskeletal pain caused by a wide variety of etiologic factors.[1, 2] Therefore, the diagnosis of SSS has been proven to be of crucial importance for understanding a variety of conditions causing musculoskeletal pain. In addition, such diagnosis of SSS is of great value in the management of musculoskeletal pain because new injection techniques, such as paraspinous block, represent an effective treatment for SSS, frequently reversing the hyperalgesic segment to normal sensitivity.[14, 15] Gunn[21] and Maigne[37] partially described concepts corresponding to SSS.

Summary

Pain diagnostic instruments were described for quantitative functional diagnosis of conditions associated with neuromuscular and skeletal pain. The *pressure algometer* quantifies the pressure pain sensitivity (tenderness), which is the manifestation of nerve fiber sensitization. *The tissue compliance meter* measures objectively and quantitatively the muscle tone and its changes, particularly muscle spasm, and its relief by treatment. The universal *hand-held dynamometer* measures muscle strength in a clinical setting. *Electric skin conductance (ESC)* documents objectively and quantitatively sensory and sympathetic nerve dysfunction in clinical practice. ESC is useful for objective and precise delineation of sensitized hyperactive dermatomes. The subjective response in hyperalgesia can be confirmed objectively by ESC values.

Using the pain diagnostic instruments, a battery of tests is described for objective and quantitative diagnosis of nerve and muscle dysfunction. Local *peripheral sensitization* by inflammatory substances can be documented quantitatively by pressure algometry over tender spots. The *pinch and roll (P&R) technique* tests the subcutaneous tissue that is the most sensitive reactor to nerve irritation, and it is the most sensitive method for detection of peripheral sensitization. P&R can be quantified also by a pressure algometer. *ESC* is more sensitive than the subjective response to pinprick. A system of sensory testing is described that is most efficient and saves considerable time while rendering more precise and reliable results. *Spinal segmental sensitization (SSS)* is a hyperactive, facilitated state of the spinal segment. The hyperexcitability usually affects all four components of the spinal segment (sensory, motor, skeletal, and sympathetic). SSS develops as a reaction to an irritative focus of peripheral sensitization, which sends continuous nociceptive impulses to the sensory ganglion. The author and his trainees found that SSS is consistently present in a variety of musculoskeletal pain (MSkP). Therefore SSS is considered a component of and the pathophysiologic basis of MSkP.

Acknowledgments

The assistance of Hy Dubo, MD, in preparation of the manuscript is appreciated.

References

1. Bonica JJ: The Management of Pain. Philadelphia, Lea & Febiger, 1990.
2. Carlsson CA, Nachemson A: Neurophysiology of back pain: Current knowledge. In Nachemson A, Jonsson E (eds): Neck and Back Pain. Philadelphia, Lippincott Williams & Wilkins, 2000, pp 149–163.
3. Chusid JG, McDonald JJ: Correlative Neuroanatomy and Functional Neurology, 13th ed. Los Altos, Lange, 1967.
4. Coderre TJ, Melzack R: Cutaneous hyperalgesia: Contributions of the peripheral and central nervous systems to the increase in pain sensitivity after injury. Brain 404:95–106, 1987.
5. Fields HL: Pain. New York, McGraw-Hill, 1987.
6. Fischer AA: Clinical use of tissue compliance meter for documentation of soft tissue pathology. Clin J Pain 3:23–30, 1987.
7. Fischer AA: Pressure algometry over normal muscles: Standard values, validity and reproducibility of pressure threshold. Pain 30:115–126, 1987.
8. Fischer AA: Pressure threshold: A valuable method in evaluation of stump problems and healing. Arch Phys Med Rehabil 69:732, 1988.
9. Fischer AA: Pressure algometry (dolorimetry) in the differential diagnosis of muscle pain. In Rachlin ES (ed): Myofascial Pain and Fibromyalgia: Trigger Point Management. St. Louis, Mosby, 1994, pp 121–141.
10. Fischer AA: Quantitative and objective documentation of soft tissue abnormality: Pressure algometry and tissue compliance recording. In Nordhoff LS: Motor Vehicle Collision Injuries. Gaithenburg, Md, Aspen, 1996, pp 142–148.
11. Fischer AA: New developments in diagnosis of myofascial pain and fibromyalgia. Phys Med Rehabil Clin North America 8:1–21, 1997.
12. Fischer AA: Algometry in the daily practice of pain management. J Back Musculoskeletal Rehabilitation 8:151–163, 1997.
13. Fischer AA: Algometry in diagnosis of musculoskeletal pain and evaluation of treatment outcome: An update. In Fischer AA (ed): Muscle Pain Syndromes and Fibromyalgia. New York, Haworth Medical, 1998, pp 5–32.
14. Fischer AA: Treatment of myofascial pain. J Musculoskeletal Pain 7:131–142, 1999.
15. Fischer AA, Imamura M: New concepts in the diagnosis and management of musculoskeletal pain. In Leonard TA (ed): Pain Procedures in Clinical Practice, 2nd ed. Philadelphia, Henley & Belfus, 2000, pp 213–229.
16. Fischer AA: New injection techniques for treatment of musculoskeletal pain. In Myofascial Pain and Fibromyalgia: Trigger Point Management, 2nd ed. Philadelphia, WB Saunders (in press).
17. Foerster O: The dermatomes in man. Brain 56:1–39, 1933.
18. Fujiwara A, Tamai K, An HS, et al: The interspinous ligament of the lumbar spine. Spine 25:358–363, 2000.
19. Gerwin RD, Shannon S, Hong CZ, et al: Interrater reliability in myofascial trigger point examination. Pain 69:65–73, 1997.
20. Granges G, Littlejohn GO: A comparative study of clinical signs in fibromyalgia/fibrositis syndrome, in healthy and exercising subjects. J Rheumatol 20:344–351, 1993.

21. Gunn CC: The Gunn Approach to the Treatment of Chronic Pain. New York, Churchill Livingstone, 1996.
22. Hackett GS: Ligament and tendon relaxation treated by prolotherapy, 3rd ed. Springfield, Ill, Charles C Thomas, 1958, pp 27–36, 70.
23. Hong C-Z, Chen Y-C, Pon CH, Yu J: Immediate effects of various physical medicine modalities of pain threshold of an active myofascial trigger point. J Musculosketal Pain 1(2):37–53, 1993.
24. Hong C-Z: Algometry in evaluation of trigger points and referred pain. J Musculosketal Pain 6(1):47–59, 1998.
25. Hong C-Z: Considerations and recommendations regarding myofascial trigger point injection. J Musculoskeletal Pain 2:29–59, 1994.
26. Hseuh T-C, Yu S, Kuan T-S, Hong C-Z: The immediate effectiveness of electrical nerve stimulation and electrical muscle stimulation on myofascial trigger points. Am J Phys Med Rehabil 76:471–476, 1997.
27. Inman VT, Saunders JB deC: Referred pain from skeletal structures. J Nerv Ment Dis 99:660–667, 1944.
28. Jaeger B, Reeves JL: Quantification of changes in myofascial trigger point sensitivity with the pressure algometer following passive stretch. Pain 27:203–210, 1986.
29. Jensen K, et al: Pressure pain threshold in human temporal region. Evaluation of a new pressure algometer. Pain 25:313–323, 1986.
30. Keegan JJ, Garrett FD: The segmental distribution of the cutaneous nerves in the limbs of man. Anat Rec 102–109, 1948.
31. Kellgren JH: On the distribution of pain arising from deep somatic structures with charts of segmental pain areas. Clin Sci 4:35–46, 1939–1942.
32. Kendall FP, et al: Muscles. Testing and Function. Baltimore, Williams & Wilkins, 1993, pp 408–410.
33. Korr IM, Thomas PE, Wright HM: Patterns of electrical skin resistance in man. Acta Neurovegetativa 64:77–96, 1958.
34. Korr IM, Wright HM, Chace JA: Cutaneous patterns of sympathetic activity in clinical abnormalities of the musculoskeletal system. Acta Neurovegetativa 25:589–606, 1964.
35. Korr IM, Wright HM, Thomas PE: Effects of experimental myofascial insults on cutaneous patterns of sympathetic activity in man. Acta Neurovegetativa 23:329–355, 1962.
36. Lansbury J: Methods for evaluating rheumatoid arthritis. In Hollander JL (ed): Arthritis and Allied Conditions. Philadelphia, Lea & Febiger, 1967, pp 269–291.
37. Maigne R: Diagnosis and Treatment of Pain of Vertebral Origin. Baltimore, Williams & Wilkins, 1996.
38. Maigne R: Pain syndromes of the thoracolumbar junction. A frequent source of misdiagnosis. Phys Med Rehab Clin North Am 8:87–100, 1997.
39. Mamichev RV: An objective method for observing neuritis of the sciatic nerve. Klinicheskaya Meditsina 32:47–51, 1954.
40. McCain GA: Fibromyalgia and myofascial pain syndromes. In Wall PD, Melzack R (eds): Textbook of Pain, 3rd ed. Edinburgh, Churchill Livingstone, 1994, pp 475–493.
41. McCarthy DJ Jr, Gatter RA, Phelps P: A dolorimeter for quantification of articular tenderness. Arthritis Rheum 8:551–559, 1965.
42. Mense S: Pathophysiologic basis of muscle pain syndromes. Phys Med Rehab Clin North Am 8:23–53, 1997.
43. Mense S, Simons DG: Muscle Pain. Philadelphia, Lippincott Williams & Wilkins, 2000, pp 92–95.
44. Njoo KH: The occurrence and inter-rater reliability of myofascial trigger points in the quadratus lumborum and gluteus medius: A prospective study in non-specific low back pain patients and controls in general practice. Pain 58:317–323, 1994.
45. Pontinen PJ: Reliability, validity, reproducibility of algometry in diagnosis of active and latent tender spots and trigger points. J Musculosketal Pain 6(1):61–71, 1998.
46. Pratzel HG: Application of pressure algometry in balneology for evaluation of physical therapeutic modalities and drug effects. J Musculoskeletal Pain 6(1):111–137, 1997.
47. Rachlin ES: Trigger points. In Rachlin ES (ed): Myofascial Pain and Fibromyalgia: Trigger Point Management. St. Louis, Mosby, 1994.
48. Reeves JL, Jaeger B, Graff-Radford SB: Reliability of the pressure algometer as a measure of myofascial trigger point sensitivity. Pain 24:313–321, 1986.
49. Richter CP, Woodruff BG: Lumbar sympathetic dermatomes in man determined by the electrical skin resistance method. J Neurophysiol 8:323–338, 1945.
50. Russell IJ: The reliability of algometry in the assessment of patients with fibromyalgia syndrome. J Musculoskeletal Pain 6(1):139–152, 1998.
51. Simone DA: Peripheral mechanisms of pain perception. In Miller RD (ed): Atlas of Anesthesia. Vol VI: Pain Management (Abram SE, vol ed) Philadelphia, Churchill Livingstone, 1998, pp 1.1–1.11.
52. Simons DG, Fischer AA: Myofascial pain. In Fields HL (ed): Core Curriculum for Professional Education in Pain, 2nd ed. Seattle, ASP Press, 1995, pp 79–81.
53. Simons DG, Travell JG, Simons LS: Myofascial Pain and Dysfunction. The Trigger Point Manual Vol. 1. Upper Half of Body, 2nd ed. Baltimore, Williams & Wilkins, 1999.
54. Smythe HA, et al: Control and fibrositic tenderness. Comparison of two dolorimeters. J Rheumatol 19:768–771, 1992.
55. Smythe HA, et al: Relation between fibrositic and control tenderness; effects of dolorimeter scale length and footplate size. J Rheumatol 19:284–289, 1992.
56. Sonkin LS: Myofascial pain due to metabolic disorders: Diagnosis and treatment. In Rachlin ES (ed): Myofascial Pain and Fibromyalgia. St. Louis, Mosby, 1994, pp 45–60.

57. Sorkin L, Yaksh TL: Mechanisms of Pain Processing. In Miller RD (ed): Atlas of Anesthesia. Vol VI: Pain Management (Abram SE, vol ed). Philadelphia, Churchill Livingstone, 1998, 2.1–2.13.
58. Travell JG, Simons DG: Myofascial Pain Dysfunction: The Trigger Point Manual: The Lower Extremities, vol 1. Baltimore, Williams & Wilkins, 1983.
59. Vecchiet L, Dragani L, De Bigontina P, et al: Experimental referred pain and hyperalgesia from muscles in humans. In Vecchiet L, Albe-Fessard D, Lindblom U (eds): New Trends in Referred Pain and Hyperalgesia. Amsterdam, Elsevier, 1993, pp 239–249.
60. Vecchiet L, Giamberardino MA: Referred pain. Clinical significance, pathophysiology, and treatment. Phys Med Rehabil Clin North Am 8:119–136, 1997.
61. Vecchiet L, et al: Differentiation of sensitivity in different tissues and its clinical significance. J Musculosketal Pain 6(1):33–45, 1998.
62. Vernon HT, et al: Pressure pain threshold evaluation of the effect of spinal manipulation in the treatment of chronic neck pain: A pilot study. J Manipulative Physiol Ther 13:13–16, 1990.
63. Waldorf T, Devlin L, Nansel DD: The comparative assessment of paraspinal tissue compliance in asymptomatic female and male subjects in both prone and standing positions. J Manipulative Physiol Ther 14:457–461, 1991.
64. Wall PD, Melzack R (eds): Textbook of Pain, 3rd ed. Edinburgh, Churchill Livingstone, 1994, pp 997–1023.
65. Wolfe F, Smythe HA, Yunus MB, et al: The American College of Rheumatology 1990 criteria for classification of fibromyalgia. Arthritis Rheum 33:160–172, 1990.
66. Woolf CJ: A new strategy for treatment of inflammatory pain. Prevention or elimination of central sensitization. In Drugs 47(Suppl 5):1–9, 1994.

Chapter 8

Diagnosis and Management of Musculoskeletal Orofacial Pain

Harold V. Cohen, DDS ▪ Richard A. Pertes, DDS

Orofacial pain (OFP), especially if the problem is chronic, presents a diagnostic and management challenge to all health practitioners. OFP is classified into one of the three basic pain categories: somatic, neuropathic, or psychogenic. Somatic pain results from noxious stimulation of normal neural structures. Neuropathic pain is caused by a structural abnormality in the nervous system. Psychogenic pain arises from psychic causes; there is no apparent physiologic or organic basis for the pain. Further differential diagnosis becomes a challenge as the clinician must determine from which tissue system the pain is arising: intracranial, extracranial, musculoskeletal, neurovascular, or neurogenous, or whether it is psychological. The finite neural circuitry of the fifth cranial nerve, the trigeminal nerve (CNV), provides sensory innervation to most of the head. This extensive neural mapping adds further complexity to the process of diagnosing and managing OFP.

This chapter focuses on the diagnosis and management of orofacial myofascial pain.

Sensory Innervation of the Head and Face

Approximately two thirds of the face receives sensory innervation from the CNV, the trigeminal nerve. However, the dorsal third of the upper head is innervated by the second cervical nerve (C2) and the lower third of the face beneath the pinna of the ear receives innervation from the second and third (C3) cervical nerves (Fig. 8–1).

CNV provides sensory innervation to the following structures via the ophthalmic (V1), maxillary (V2), and mandibular (V3) divisions[17]:

- Face
- Scalp
- Conjunctiva
- Mucous membranes of the oral cavity (including general sensory and the anterior two-thirds of the tongue), nasal passages, and paranasal sinuses
- Teeth and supporting structures
- Part of the external tympanic membrane
- Meninges of the anterior and middle cranial fossae

Sensory information from the three divisions of CNV passes through the gasserian ganglion, which is located in a depression called Meckel's cave in the middle cranial fossa. Nerve fibers enter the central nervous system (CNS) at the pons in a manner similar to other afferent fibers of the peripheral nervous system (PNS). The CNV analogue of the spinal dorsal horn is a unique elongate structure known as the trigeminal spinal nucleus. This structure extends from the pontine level caudally to cervical segments C2 to C3. Within this relay center occurs pain and temperature integration from the face, dura mater, large blood vessels of the brain, eyeball (cornea), ear, paranasal sinuses, oral cavity, tongue, and cervical spine structures.[13] Also included in this intermix is a barrage of signals from the oral cavity, teeth, facial muscles, and temporomandibular joint (TMJ). The neurophysiologic principle of convergence of afferent neurons on second-order neurons within the trigeminal nucleus is crucial in the processing of incoming information. From the second order neuron in the nucleus,

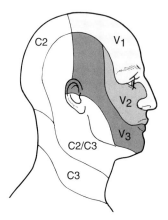

Figure 8–1. Dermatomes for sensory innervation of face.

information ascends to thalamic and cortical levels. Projection to the cortical level often leads to patient misinterpretation of the pain source, and patients may describe pain symptoms as emanating from areas other than the actual pain source (Fig. 8–2).

The Relationship of Cervical Spine Disorders to Facial Pain

As part of an OFP examination, aspects of the cervical spine should be assessed. The cervical spine can produce pain within the cranial and orofacial regions via neural innervation of the cervical plexus or referred pain from the musculature. The neuroanatomic basis for referred cervical muscle pain is convergence within the trigeminal spinal nucleus (multiple first order neurons synapsing on second order neurons).

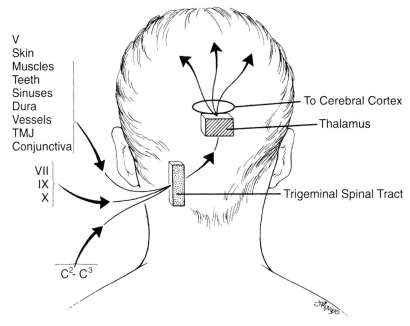

Figure 8–2. Schematic of sensory convergence to the trigeminal spinal nucleus.

Assessment of the Orofacial Pain Patient

Because of the complex neural networking of the facial and oral regions, the clinician must apply a logical differential approach in attempting to reach a diagnostic impression. Table 8–1 presents a differential diagnosis of orofacial pain. The following is a suggested diagnostic sequence to guide the clinician's thinking:

1. Dental or other intraoral pathology
2. Headache disorder
3. Paranasal sinus disorder
4. Temporomandibular disorder (TMD)
5. If dental pathology, headache, and TMD are ruled out, a thorough medical differential diagnosis is indicated.

To further guide the clinician, the following is a suggested list of questions that can be used to aid in further focusing the assessment:

1. Have you noticed an increase in headaches, neckaches, or toothaches?
2. Have you had recent dental work or a recent injury to your head, jaw, or neck?
3. Do you have increased tooth sensitivity to cold or hot?
4. Do you feel that your bite has changed?
5. Do you have pain on chewing or when opening your mouth?
6. Do you have difficulty opening your mouth or have your jaws ever locked?
7. Are there any associated symptoms with your facial pain? (This question may guide the clinician to expand the differential diagnosis into other medical areas).
8. Do you have new headaches or headaches that are different from those in the past?
9. Have there been any other changes in your medical history or medication profile?

The screening examination for OFP or TMD would include:

1. History
2. Physical examination
3. Cranial nerve screen

A comprehensive examination would include the addition of:

4. Imaging studies (dental, panoramic, computed tomographic [CT] scans, magnetic resonance imaging [MRI])
5. Laboratory studies
6. Local anesthetic diagnostic blocks
7. Behavioral assessment
8. Evaluation of a pain log or diary provided by the patient

Odontogenic Pain

Dental and periodontal assessment should be the first evaluation in the differential diagnosis of pain in the orofacial area. Most OFP originates in the teeth and supporting

Table 8–1.
Categories of Orofacial Pain

Extracranial	Neurovascular
Teeth and supporting structures	Migrainous headache, cluster headache
Temporomandibular disorders	Giant cell arteritis
Temporomandibular joints	Neuropathic
Masticatory musculature	Paroxysmal disorders
Eyes, ears, nose, throat, sinuses, tongue, glandular tissue	Continuous disorders
Intracranial disease	Psychogenic
Neoplasm	Endogenous disorders
Arteriovenous malformations	Reactive processes

periodontal and alveolar structures. Difficulties can be encountered in the localization of dental pain that can be further complicated by pain referral patterns within the CNV spinal nucleus. Acute dental pain can mimic neurologic phenomena, whereas chronic dental disease may have characteristics of low-grade muscular pain. As a toothache increases in intensity, the proximal facial muscles may develop pain due to central convergence resulting in pain referral. It should be noted that myofascial trigger points in the masticatory muscles can also refer pain to dental structures.

Paranasal sinus diseases are a common cause of facial pain. Most often this occurs in the maxillary sinuses, but both the sphenoidal and ethmoidal sinuses can be pain sources. When the maxillary sinuses are involved, clinical characteristics are a constant mild, nonpulsatile, or aching pain that can extend from the maxillary canine area to the third molars. As opposed to dental pain, this type of discomfort rarely refers to the mandibular arch. The patient usually has a history of a recent upper respiratory infection that was antecedent to the development of the facial pain. The patient often reports tenderness of the maxillary bicuspid and/or molar teeth or a toothache localized to these teeth.

Intracranial lesions can also cause facial pain. The patient may not present with obvious neurologic signs or deficits; the pain can be referred to the dental arches or face and thus be confused with toothache. Patients with intracranial lesions such as neoplasm or arteriovenous malformation may first appear at the dental office complaining of dental pain. If a differential assessment is negative for the more common pathologies such as dental, muscular, and sinusoidal, neurologic evaluation should be strongly considered. Age and health status are crucial factors that should be included when evaluating the patient.

Neurovascular pain disorders, most commonly migraine and tension-type headaches, can also be expressed as facial pain. Migrainous episodes tend to be short term (hours to days) with remittances between episodes, often accompanied by related neurologic phenomena and nausea. Tension-type headaches, usually described by the patient as the nonprogressive day-after-day headache, are included in this grouping because current research suggests a neurophysiologic relationship between these headaches and migrainous syndromes. Acute headache discomfort can also lead to reflex muscle tightening within the face or neck, which creates more pain. This self-sustaining loop presents diagnostic difficulty for the clinician as both the headache and muscular processes must be analyzed and treated. Another less common headache that can present as facial pain is cluster headache. This pain is usually short lived, tends to recur over time spans, and then remits for a prolonged period. The character of the pain in cluster headache is unilateral, intense, and most often accompanied by marked autonomic symptoms such as nasal drainage and eye tearing.

Neuropathic pain disorders are thought to be related to alterations in neuronal function and conduction properties in both the peripheral and central nervous system. These disorders exhibit temporal pain qualities that can be grouped as either paroxysmal or continuous. Paroxysmal neurogenic pain can be initiated by a primary functional disturbance within the nervous system (e.g., trigeminal neuralgia, glossopharyngeal neuralgia) or can also be associated with neoplasms or demyelinating disease. Neuropathic disorders of the continuous type can include neuroma formation after injury, deafferentation pain, and traumatic neuropathy. Neuropathic pain will often have overlying muscular responses. Here again, the astute clinician must sort out both the primary and secondary processes.

Psychogenic pain refers to the development of pain in the absence of a true pain source. It originates in the mind. These patients have an emotional or personality disorder, and pain complaints do not follow reasonable biologic principles. Somatoform disorders encompass those syndromes in which people experience physical symptoms (pain) in the absence of a physical cause.[7] For additional information, the reader is referred to the *Diagnostic and Statistical Manual of Mental Disorders* (DSM-IV) by the American Psychiatric Association. As an additional consideration, psychological factors may also alter a patient's response to a true pain problem. Thus comprehensive therapy should include management of both the physical and psychological factors.

When one considers the multitude and complexity of OFP disorders, it becomes mandatory that in a complete examination the presence of more than one disorder at a time should be suspected.

Temporomandibular Disorders

Temporomandibular disorders are a group of related conditions that present with symptoms in the masticatory system. TMDs should not be viewed as a single syndrome. Thus a wide variety of treatments are available depending on the level of knowledge and experience of the health care provider. Other considerations related to TMD that have received much attention in the literature include:

1. The predominance of females presenting for treatment
2. The comorbidity of TMD and widespread pain such as fibromyalgia[12]
3. The relationship of depression to the presence of TMD

Patients with TMD and widespread pain tend to be more debilitated by these disorders and exhibit high rates of depression and somatization.[12] However, whereas antecedent depression has been thought to be a factor in the onset of chronic pain conditions, newer research has concluded that chronic myofascial pain may be more of a consequence of living with chronic pain.[3]

TMD is classified as a somatic pain disorder with muscular and/or articular (TMJ) components:

1. Muscular problems due to pain or disorders of the masticatory musculature
2. Temporomandibular joint (TMJ) disturbances including articular disc displacements, degenerative bony changes, inflammatory processes, altered growth and development, and systemic arthropathies

Often there is both an articular and a muscular component.

The etiology of TMD can be multifactorial:

1. Microtrauma—bruxism, major occlusal discrepancies
2. Macrotrauma (e.g., a traumatic blow to the mandible)
3. Emotional tension
4. Systemic arthritides

Traditionally, oral parafunctional habits have been viewed as prime contributors to these disorders. These deleterious habits include tooth clenching, tooth grinding (bruxism), nail or cuticle biting, and gum chewing. These cause repetitive microtrauma to the TMJs; the persistent adverse loading can cause adaptive and degenerative changes in the TMJs and also produce a painful masticatory muscle disorder. Bruxism during sleep can be defined as an intense, high-frequency, rhythmic side-to-side jaw movement, although at times, the patient may clench without the side-to-side movement.[2] At the present time, the true basis of nocturnal bruxism is not well defined. Sleep studies have shown that bruxism tends to occur during the transition from deep to lighter states of sleep (rapid eye movement [REM] sleep) but other studies have found it to occur during stage 2 (non-REM sleep). Transient, nonintense nocturnal clenching activity during stressful life events should be differentiated from true nocturnal bruxism.[2]

Bruxism may or may not be associated with pain. The presence of jaw pain on morning awakening may be related to nocturnal clenching/bruxism. However, many patients have no pain on arising and develop masticatory muscle pain as the day goes on, usually peaking in the mid to late afternoon. These patients often report an awareness of daytime clenching or increased tension in the masticatory muscles.

Some diagnosticians consider the presence of wear facets on the teeth as correlating with these deleterious habits. However, the presence of wear facets in an asymptomatic dental population raises a doubt as to their etiologic significance.

It should be noted that some research studies do not support the link between pain and masticatory muscle hyperactivity.[14] The majority of clenchers do not have pain.

Electromyographic (EMG) studies of the masseter muscle have shown that there is not a significant correlation with pain complaints, and that, in fact, the activity of painful muscles may be weaker than that of nonpainful muscles. Therefore one would expect reduced muscle activity in patients with painful jaws.

Macrotrauma sustained in a mandibular injury can also lead to TMJ arthropathies. Additionally, as listed later in the TMD classification, there can be congenital, developmental, and acquired defects in this articular complex.

Emotional tension is often associated with TMD. The tensional issue may stem from an endogenous psychological problem or it may be a response to a pain process. In either case, elevated facial muscle stress levels ensue and are commonly (but not always) accompanied by clenching or bruxism, or both, and subsequent TMD.

The Relationship of Malocclusion and Other Dental Disorders to the Etiology of Temporomandibular Disorders

Dental malocclusion and missing teeth have long been subjects of controversy as to their role in masticatory muscle and TMJ problems. Malocclusion (as commonly assessed in the pediatric or adolescent dental patient) should not be considered a cause of myofascial dysfunction. Anecdotal reports of this interrelationship of occlusion and TMD have not held up when subjected to scientific scrutiny.

Recent changes in the dental occlusion (as with new bridgework) can trigger dysfunctional pain problems, but these complaints may be due to patient inability to accommodate and should not necessarily be attributed to faulty restorations.

Dental disease can also affect the temporomandibular complex indirectly. The presence of loose or tender teeth may lead to altered chewing patterns. Periodontal or painful tooth pulpal disease can also lead to compromised jaw function along with referred dental pain throughout the face. These patients with painful dental problems may develop defensive chewing patterns that can also be contributory to altered mandibular function leading to signs and symptoms of TMD.

A screening or comprehensive examination for a temporomandibular disorder is similar to those described previously for OFP. However, particular attention should be paid to the masticatory and cervical musculature, the presence of TMJ noises, and the mandibular range of motion in opening, lateral, and protrusive excursions.

Disc Disorders of the Temporomandibular Joint

The masticatory muscles are involved in providing mandibular movement for opening, closing, mastication, and speech. The articulations around which these muscles function are the bilateral temporomandibular joints (TMJs). This arrangement is unique in that the two joints are intimately connected in function through the body of the mandible; muscular effects on one joint are reflected in compensating stresses or movements in the other. In addition, because of the day-long habits of breathing, swallowing, chewing, and talking, the temporomandibular articulation is rarely at rest.

A common finding in patients is the presence of jaw clicking emanating from one or both TMJs. Clicking is usually indicative of anterior displacement of the articulating disc, whereby the mandibular condyle must traverse over the back end of the disc in order to accomplish the opening movement; it will then slip off the back end of this disc as the jaw closes to full occlusion. The clicking noises occur when the condyle jumps over the back end of the disc on opening and when it slips off the back end on jaw closure. The opening noise is more commonly heard than the closing noise and the sounds can be intermittent. This sequence of events is termed *anterior disc displacement with reduction* (Fig. 8–3).

If the clinician desires to precisely define the position of the articular disc, MRI studies provide the most accurate views. Figure 8-4 includes MRI studies showing both a normal disc position (Fig. 8–4A) and a markedly displaced disc (Fig. 8–4B).

In some patients, this is a painless process, as the tissues adapt well to the altered disc-condyle relationship. However, many patients experience pain in the TMJ because

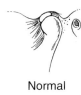

Normal

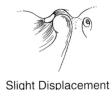

Slight Displacement

Figure 8–3. Variations of temporomandibular joint disc position.

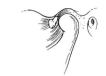

Advanced Displacement

the cushioning effect of the displaced disc is lost and the tissues now supporting the mandibular condyle do not adapt but rather stay persistently inflamed and painful. There is often associated muscular pain.

Patients may also report episodes of persistent interference on opening as more advanced disc displacement starts to interfere with mandibular translation and the condyle cannot slip over the back end of the disc. The patient can usually maneuver the mandible to slip onto the disc, thus allowing for continued jaw translation. In the advanced degenerative stage, the articular disc may displace to a point at which it permanently interferes with mandibular opening. This sudden event is termed *anterior disc displacement without reduction* or *closed lock* (see Fig. 8–3). Conservative approaches by a dentist can aid the patient in regaining an acceptable opening range, but at times an arthroscopic or surgical approach may be indicated.

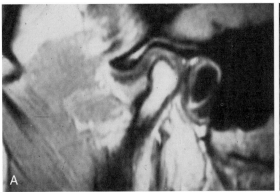
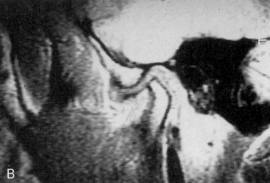

Figure 8–4. A, MRI showing normal condyle and normal disc position. **B,** MRI showing displaced disc and degenerative bony surface of condyle.

Precautions in Interpreting Temporomandibular Joint Noise

1. The presence of joint noise cannot always define the particular dysfunction (e.g., disc displacement or surface discrepancy).

2. TMJ noise that is not associated with pain and does not interfere with function does not require treatment.

3. Untreated TMJ noises or disc displacements most often do not progress to more degenerative conditions.

4. Most TMD patients experience more pain from muscle rather than from the TMJ.

The TMJ is also subject to additional congenital, developmental, and acquired disorders as are other orthopedic joints. These include condylar hyperplasia, hypoplasia, aplasia, condylolysis, neoplasms, and fractures.

If a TMD is not suspected or a TMD evaluation is not indicative of such a disorder, a thorough examination for another pain source must be accomplished or the patient should be referred to the appropriate health care professional. Additionally, assessment for a cervical disorder should also be considered.

It is crucial that the clinician also consider the age and previous medical/dental history of the patient. Facial pain presenting as TMD is often accompanied by headache disorder, which should be assessed from its own diagnostic approach. TMD tends to be a problem that occurs most often in the early to middle years. In an older patient with no previous history of TMD, a total medical differential assessment should be done.

Masticatory Muscle Pain Disorders

Categories of masticatory muscle pain include:

- Myofascial pain
- Fibromyalgia
- Myositis
- Myospasm
- Local myalgia
- Muscle contracture (myostatic, myofibrotic)

Myofascial Pain

Myofascial pain (MFP) is a regional muscle disorder that is one of the most common causes of persistent pain in the head, face, and neck regions. MFP is characterized by the presence of one or more hyperirritable sites within the muscle known as myofascial trigger points (TrPs). A myofascial TrP is defined as a localized deep tenderness in a taut band of skeletal muscle, tendon, or ligament that has the ability to refer pain to another region known as a zone of reference (i.e., area of pain complaint). Although the zone of reference can be distant from the involved muscle and may not be in the same dermatome, the pattern of pain referral is reproducible and consistent and can serve as a guide to locate TrPs.

Clinical Characteristics of Myofascial Pain

MFP can be very localized involving one or two TrPs, or more generalized as the result of muscle injury. It is often comorbid with other conditions such as chronic "whiplash" pain including those with facet joint injury or discogenic pain.

The TrP itself is an exquisitely tender area, 2 to 5 mm in diameter, that is usually located within a taut band of muscle. Taut bands can be found in all skeletal muscles and are not specific for myofascial pain. However, palpation of a TrP within a taut band using sustained deep, single fingertip pressure of 2 kg for 6 to 10 seconds will elicit an alteration in pain intensity (increase or decrease) in the zone of reference.

This response may occur immediately or be delayed by several seconds. Firm palpation of a TrP will also cause a characteristic behavioral response on the part of the patient—the jump sign. This is a spontaneous reaction to palpation that can manifest itself as a verbal response or withdrawal of the patient's head. The jump sign should be distinguished from a local twitch response (LTR), which is a rapid, contractile motor effect elicited by "snapping palpation" of the taut band at the location of the TrP.

In addition to local tenderness and referred pain, the jump sign and twitch response, MFP is characterized by other symptoms including increased muscle fatigue and stiffness, a mildly restricted range of motion, pain when the muscle is stretched, and a subjective feeling of weakness. Sensitization of autonomic nerves may result in various autonomic phenomena such as excessive lacrimation, nasal congestion, sweating, flushing, and cutaneous vasomotor effects (e.g., cutaneous hyperthermia or hypothermia).

Two types of TrPs are present: active and latent. Both types are sensitive when palpated but only an active TrP causes spontaneous referred pains during muscle use. Although a latent TrP is not as tender to palpation as an active TrP, it is still more tender than normal muscle tissue. A latent TrP does not cause referred pain during muscle use but will elicit referred pain symptoms when palpated. Normally, TrPs cycle between an active and latent state. However, various perpetuating factors such as stress may not allow an active TrP to become latent.

Theories of Referred Muscular Pain

Several theories have evolved over the years as to the nature of referred pain. Classic concepts of pain referral still center on convergence in the CNS of afferent stimuli from muscle, skin, joints, and viscera and misinterpretation by the cerebral cortex of the pain source.

Another concept by Mense[9] hypothesizes that referred pain is due to the unmasking of latent connections. These connections are composed of interneurons from one level to another within the trigeminal system (spinal cord) and branches of neurons entering the CNS. Activation of these connections is believed to result from action of the neurochemical substance P and calcitonin gene–related peptide (CTRP) resulting in N-methyl-D-aspartate (NMDA) receptor changes. In particular, long-lasting stimuli resulting from muscle pain are believed to cause depolarization of these normally quiet CNS neurons as well as autonomic and motor central excitatory effects.

Chronic myofascial pain is understandably more difficult to manage. Peripheral pain sites such as the trigger points have traditionally been looked on as primary sources of chronic muscular pain. Here again, neuroscientists have looked with more interest at changes in CNS pain processing, notably the NMDA receptor. This receptor exhibits irreversible functional changes that are now believed to be associated with chronic pain states. Such changes in neuronal function have caused chronic pain to be viewed as a disease entity of its own with its own particular pathophysiology. As expressed by Sternbach, acute pain is a symptom of disease whereas chronic pain is a disease unto itself.[14]

Fibromyalgia

Although fibromyalgia (FM) is a systemic pain syndrome that produces more general pain throughout the body, it can also involve the masticatory muscles and is thus included in this classification.

Whereas MFP is a disorder involving regional muscles, FM is a generalized systemic condition that is characterized by widespread aching or pain throughout the body, notably in the weight-bearing muscles. To be included in the diagnosis of FM, this pain should be located in all four quadrants of the body or along the entire spine, and must have been present for a minimum of 3 months. Both MFP and FM share muscle pain as a symptom and have localized areas of tenderness to palpation as a clinical sign. However, myofascial TrPs can refer pain to distant sites, but the tender points (TePs) of FM do not.

Current inclusionary criteria for FM requires the presence of 11 out of 18 specifically defined TePs in addition to generalized pain. The pain of FM is often accompanied by the presence of unusual fatigue, morning stiffness, and a sleep disturbance. FM is often found in association with other conditions such as chronic fatigue syndrome, TMD, and irritable bowel syndrome. Although patients present with documentable physical symptoms, no specific pathology has been defined and there are no routine clinical markers, imaging studies, or diagnostic tests that are useful for diagnosis. Therefore, the standard for diagnosis depends on the clinical history and the tender point examination.

Comparison of Myofascial Pain with Fibromyalgia

Although MFP and FM have some features in common, there are significant differences. MFP can occur equally in men and women, but FM occurs primarily in women. MFP usually starts with a specific muscle problem such as strain, overuse, or trauma; FM begins insidiously and develops as a generalized pain except when trauma is involved. The pain of MFP is usually unilateral as opposed to the pain of FM, which is bilateral and symmetrical.

Despite these differences, it has been suggested by some authors that MFP may be a regional expression of FM. In their view, the pain of FM could initially present as a few localized TrPs (i.e., MFP) and then spread through dysfunctional muscle units to other areas of the body as the condition became chronic. In other words, FM could be a chronic version of MFP. To quote Gerwin, "It is simplistic and inappropriate to use widespread pain as a feature that distinguishes FMS from FM."[5] Obviously, the final answer to the relationship between MFP and FM is still unknown and awaits the results of future research.

Pathophysiology of Fibromyalgia

In the past, FM patients were considered to be healthy complainers without positive clinical signs. Later they were considered to be depressed patients who translated their emotional distress into bodily complaints through the process of somatization. Both explanations now appear to be inadequate. Although the mechanisms involved in FM are still not well understood, there is increasing evidence that central amplification of nociceptive processing is important. Two neurotransmitters that appear to have a significant role in FM are substance P (SP) and serotonin (5-HT).

In FM patients, low concentrations of tryptophan, the precursor of 5-HT, have been found in serum and cerebrospinal fluid. Also, FM patients have a low serum level of 5-HT due to low levels of platelet 5-HT. Adequate levels of 5-HT are important because it is involved in the regulation of pain perception and deep sleep. Elevated levels of SP were found in the cerebrospinal fluid of FM patients. Although the specific mechanisms of SP involvement in nociceptive processing are still controversial, it appears to facilitate nociception at the level of second-order neurons.

Management of Fibromyalgia

Pharmacotherapy has produced mixed results in the management of FM. Both amitriptyline (10–35 mg) and cyclobenzaprine (2.5–10 mg) have been found to be effective. Other medication groups that can be used include SSRIs, NSAIDs, topical capsaicin, anxiolytics, GABA agonists, and anticonvulsants. However, studies supporting their specific use for fibromyalgia remain to be done.

Nonpharmacologic treatments (e.g., cardiovascular fitness training, EMG biofeedback training) produced significant improvement in objective and subjective measurements of pain in patients with primary FM (i.e., no organic cause). Cognitive behavioral therapy produced mixed results with some major improvement in pain severity and some psychological variables. However, it was possible that some of these changes could also have been the result of an educational program that accompanied the behavioral intervention. It is possible that nonpharmacologic treatment helps FM and MFP patients by giving them a sense of control and mastery over life circumstances.

Myositis

Myositis is an inflammation of muscle resulting from local cause. A common cause of myositis is inflammation from a local anesthetic injection. The injury may be due to the needle itself or to the irritating qualities of the local anesthetic. Other causes of myositis include mild muscle strain or dental infection following a difficult third molar extraction.

Clinically, myositis presents as a more-or-less continuously painful muscle that may be accompanied by swelling, redness, increased temperature, and diffuse tenderness over the entire muscle. Involvement of mandibular elevator muscles will cause a moderate to severe limited opening, referred to as mandibular trismus.

Therapy for myositis includes use of analgesics, anti-inflammatories, and appropriate antibiotics if an infection is present. Muscle injections are contraindicated for myositis because injection procedures can aggravate the problem.

Myospasm

Myospasm (muscle spasm) is a relatively uncommon acute disorder of a muscle or a group of muscles that is characterized by an involuntary sudden contraction resulting in a shortened muscle. It can occur from acute overuse, strain, or overstretching of a muscle that was previously weakened.

The pain of myospasm can vary from a dull ache to intense pain with movement. Occasionally, the pain may be accompanied by a sharp, shooting pain. The acutely shortened muscle may result in a markedly reduced range of motion. If mandibular elevator muscles are affected, a normal jaw opening of 40 to 55 mm could be decreased to as little as 10 to 20 mm. An acute malocclusion may be present if the lateral pterygoid muscle is involved. Because myospasm is a continuous contraction, there is an increase in EMG activity even at rest.

Historically, muscle spasm was thought to arise from a pain-spasm-pain cycle in which muscle pain led to increased muscle hyperactivity resulting in more muscle pain. However, new studies have revealed that a painful muscle exhibits reduced activity rather than hyperactivity as previously thought. These findings invalidate the pain-spasm-pain cycle theory.

Management consists of restricting the jaw within pain-free limits. In the acute stage, ice may be of some benefit. Adjunctive pharmacologic therapy using muscle relaxants and analgesics is often of value. If the symptoms do not subside in a few days, a local anesthetic block often relieves the pain and allows muscle length to be restored. Usually the spasm will subside, but if it is sustained, it may result in myostatic contracture, a painless but reversible shortening of a muscle belly due to structural alteration in the sarcomeres.

Local Myalgia

This category includes other masticatory pain disorders that do not have adequate distinguishing characteristics to enable them to be listed as a separate clinical entity. Local myalgia includes muscle co-contraction and muscle soreness.

Muscle co-contraction (i.e., muscle splinting) is a reflex protective response that is mediated through the CNS. It results in muscle tightening (i.e., guarding) to protect the injured part. Usually there is no pain until the injured part is moved. However, when that part is threatened, the degree of muscle splinting and pain is proportional to the extent of the strain on the affected structure.

In contrast to muscle spasm, in which EMG activity is always present, EMG activity in muscle co-contraction is low when the injured part is at rest.

Muscle co-contraction is characterized by local muscle soreness, restricted range of motion, pain that is increased with movement of the injured part, and a subjective feeling of weakness when the part is threatened. Because the primary problem is not the muscle, management of muscle co-contraction is directed at allowing the injured part to heal as opposed to treating the muscle itself.

Delayed onset muscle soreness (DOMS) is a postexercise muscle pain that may result from unusually heavy chewing. It can be present in facial muscles on awakening because of muscle hyperactivity during sleep and is thought to be due to the release of algogenic substances such as bradykinin and substance P. Although pain-producing neurochemicals are involved, there is no evidence of localized cellular change and no change in electromyography of the involved muscles.

Presenting symptoms include muscle stiffness, palpable tenderness, and pain with active muscle contractions. Symptoms usually subside within a short period of time without any residual effects. DOMS is more likely to occur in patients with episodic bruxism than in individuals who exhibit chronic bruxism. Individuals who constantly contract their muscles usually have well-developed muscles that are pain-free, similar to any individual who exercises regularly. In contrast, individuals who only occasionally contract their muscles may develop DOMS through overexertion of poorly developed muscles. However, some patients with chronic sleep bruxism will develop muscle symptoms for reasons that are still not understood.

Muscle Contracture

Muscle contracture is a painless shortening of a muscle that does not interfere with the muscle's ability to contract further. Involvement of mandibular elevator muscles will result in a persistent restricted opening. There are two types of contracture: myostatic and myofibrotic.

Myostatic contracture is a reversible shortening of a muscle belly that is painless unless the muscle is forcibly stretched. It occurs when a muscle is kept from reaching its full resting length for a prolonged period of time and gradually shortens to accommodate the degree of opening. This condition is usually reversible with passive stretch exercises. *Myofibrotic contracture* is a chronic condition that results from fibrosis of the muscle fibers, tendons, or ligaments. This condition is also painless unless the muscle is forcibly stretched. It can follow an inflammatory muscle condition such as myositis or trauma. Myofibrotic contracture is reversible only with surgical intervention.

The Primary Masticatory Muscles: Anatomy, Physiology, and Myofasical Trigger Point Referral Pattern
Motor and Sensory Innervation to the Masticatory Muscles

Lower motor neuron innervation to the muscles of mastication is unique in that there is bilateral innervation to these muscles via the corticobulbar tract.[6] Thus an upper motor neuron lesion may not present with a visible deficit. Lower motor neuron lesions to the masticatory muscles are not common and thus asymmetrical jaw function should be viewed as a product of local cause. Further control of masticatory muscle function is mediated by muscle spindle and Golgi tendon organ input as in other skeletal muscles. Trigeminal motor function is also influenced by proprioceptive responses in the mesencephalic nucleus of CNV, which receives proprioceptive input from the masticatory muscles. Unique to trigeminal motor function is input from the periodontal ligaments of the teeth, which provides additional proprioceptive input to the mesencephalic nucleus.

As previously discussed, sensory innervation of the masticatory muscles is via trigeminal afferents.

The total facial muscle complex consists of the muscles of mastication and the accessory muscles of facial expression. The primary muscles of mastication are the masseter, temporalis, medial pterygoid, and lateral pterygoid. The digastric and mylohyoid muscles are also involved in mandibular function but are usually not considered primary masticatory muscles. In the assessment of orofacial-myofascial disorders, most attention should be directed toward the primary masticatory muscles and the associated trigeminal innervation.

Orofacial Muscle Pain

"It hurts when I chew!" "I can't open my jaw all the way!" "My jaws hurt when I talk a lot and cause a headache (or exaggerate an existing headache)!" "My jaw makes noise when I chew." These quotes represent the usual complaints given by patients with facial myofascial trigger points. Although pain can be present when the jaws are not used, most commonly it is jaw function that elicits or exaggerates the complaint. Restricted vertical range of mandibular motion accompanied by pain on jaw movement is a consistent finding in patients with facial trigger points. Although intracapsular (TMJ) pain can be present, most often the main source of pain is the masticatory musculature.

The patient with muscle pain (myalgia) from guarding or spasm may also present with limited opening. Differentiating myalgic pain from trigger point discomfort can be difficult; as a general rule, the sore muscle has a generalized aching pattern without the presence of the taut bands or twitch responses commonly found in trigger points. Well-defined pain referral patterns are more common with trigger point provocation.

For the myofascial pain patient, reasonable opening range is attainable after pain reduction through the use of anesthetic injection, vaporized coolant spray, or medications. These diagnostic and therapeutic steps can help in differentiating muscle-induced restraint from intracapsular TMJ restrictions due to disc interferences.

Examination of the masticatory muscles is done by direct palpation of accessible areas and functional manipulation of deeper-lying muscles. Because of the unique bilateral nature of the mandibular attachment to the maxilla, examination should include both the side ipsilateral to the chief pain complaint and also the contralateral musculature. Mandibular movements are the sum total of bilateral muscular and TMJ function. Treatments may have to encompass both sides and should give consideration to all possible involved structures, both muscle and joint.

The masticatory muscle most commonly involved in myofascial problems is the masseter muscle (Fig. 8–5). Its prime function is to elevate the mandible and bring the teeth to maximum contact. It consists of two segments. The *superficial belly* originates on the zygomatic arch and inserts on the external surface of the angle of the mandible and the lower half of the ramus. A second portion, the *deep belly*, also originates on the zygomatic arch and inserts on the superior half of the ramus.[16] Muscle fibers from the deep belly have been found within the capsule of the TMJ, which may account for some of the confusion in differentiating facial myofascial pain from TMJ arthralgia.

Patients who present with limited opening and pain with mandibular function invariably have a component of a masseter problem. In the symptomatic patient, it is rare that palpation is negative for masseter pain.

Masseter myofascial trigger point pain referral patterns are based in which belly the trigger point is located: superficial masseter pain is commonly felt locally under the examiner's hand or it may exhibit trigger point referral patterns to the teeth, maxilla, and mandible. Referred pain patterns from the deep belly of the masseter are commonly felt in the periauricular area or ear, and can be mistaken for TMJ arthralgia or otalgia. Clinical signs will be limited opening, usually accompanied by pain, discomfort on chewing, and a fatigued feeling with brief jaw use, particularly after meals.

Temporalis Muscle

This large fan-shaped muscle originates on the temporal bone and temporal fascia in the temporal fossa and inserts on the coronoid process of the mandible (Fig. 8–6).[16] It functions to elevate and retract the mandible. Temporalis trigger points are commonly associated with masseter myofascial triggers. Pain in this muscle is often

MASSETER MUSCLE-
SUPERFICIAL & DEEP BELLIES

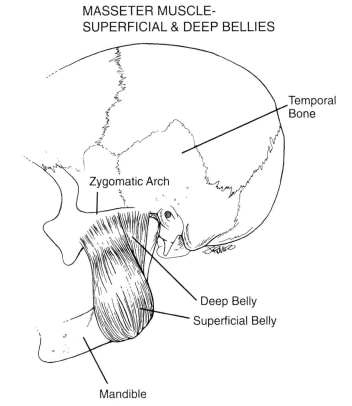

Figure 8–5. Masseter muscle.

interpreted by the patient as "headache." Differentiating myofascial trigger points from a primary headache process is essential because different therapeutic approaches are indicated for each condition. Temporalis pain referral patterns extend to the maxillary teeth and mid temple area.[16]

Temporalis pain is also readily palpable by the examiner and may exhibit trigger point referral patterns to the vertex, maxilla, and upper teeth. The tendinous insertion

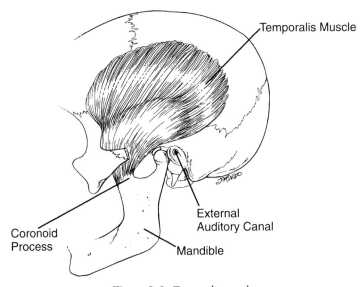

Figure 8–6. Temporalis muscle.

on the coronoid process is often sore to intraoral finger palpation. Because this area has little submucosal tissue, examination should be done judiciously because the mucosa is tightly attached to the underlying bone and can be exquisitely sensitive to excessive finger pressure. Temporalis trigger points can cause pain described as "headache," and soreness in the temples on opening, chewing, or talking.

Medial Pterygoid Muscle

The medial pterygoid muscle originates on the lateral pterygoid plate and attaches at the medial angle of the mandible (Fig. 8–7). It functions to elevate the jaw and assist in lateral and protrusive motions. This muscle, when symptomatic, can contribute to restricted jaw opening, along with the masseter.

Medial pterygoid pain referral patterns include the tongue, throat, TMJ, and nose.[16]

Medial pterygoid assessment is more of a challenge because the muscle is not easy to palpate and many patients will manifest a gag response to the examiner's finger. Here again, the patient may describe a deeper soreness with mandibular use and a sense of having a sore throat. Pain deep to the ear can also be reported. Pain at the inferior border of the mandible can be reported in the area of the medial pterygoid attachment but may be difficult to differentiate from soreness at the masseter insertion. It is *not* common to find the medial pterygoid as a primary sore muscle in a facial trigger point analysis; masseter discomfort is invariably present and usually predominates.

Lateral Pterygoid Muscle

The lateral pterygoid muscle consists of two bellies that affect mandibular movement (Fig. 8–8). The inferior belly functions to depress the mandible on jaw opening (along with the digastric). This portion originates on the lateral pterygoid plate and inserts on the neck of the mandible. The superior belly originates on the sphenoid bone and inserts into the anterosuperior portion of the condylar neck just below the

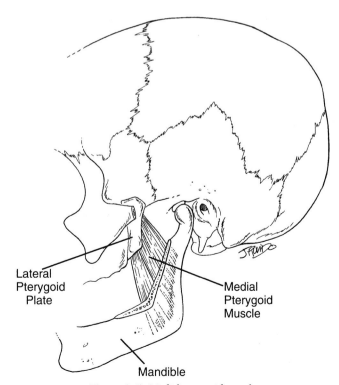

Lateral Pterygoid Plate

Medial Pterygoid Muscle

Mandible

Figure 8–7. Medial pterygoid muscle.

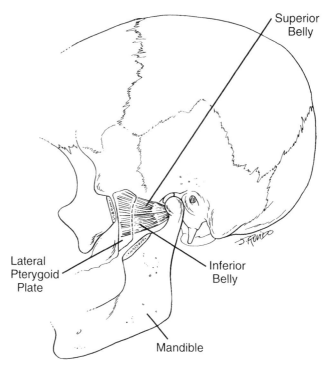

Figure 8–8. Lateral pterygoid muscle.

condyle, with attachment fibers also inserting into the articular disc. The two muscle bellies function reciprocally. The inferior belly protrudes and depresses the mandible when contraction is bilateral. When contraction is unilateral, the inferior belly moves the mandible to the opposite side; this occurs because of the medial position of the inferior belly. The superior belly contracts as the teeth come to maximum intercuspation serving to "brace" the mandible against the articular disc and glenoid fossa.

Intraoral palpation of this muscle is difficult because of its high and medial position. Functional manipulation, as described by Bell,[1] provides the most consistent diagnostic approach to assessing this muscle. The clinician asks the patient to protrude the mandible or go into a lateral excursion and at the same time the clinician uses a hand to resist this movement. As the mandible moves against the hand resistance, the lateral pterygoid is activated and pain may be elicited if the muscle is symptomatic.

Lateral pterygoid pain referral patterns (for both bellies) are to the maxillary sinus and TMJ.[16]

Cervical Musculature

Cervical structures, as part of the upper quarter (head, neck, and shoulder girdles), have the potential of causing pain in an adjacent or functionally related area. Forward head posture can disrupt the high degree of finely coordinated muscle balance necessary to support the head and neck. This is usually accompanied by referral of myofascial trigger point pain to the face, the physiology of which is mediated through the V spinal tract. The clinician needs only to provoke a trapezius trigger point to have the patient report ipsilateral temporal pain. The sternocleidomastoid muscle is a common source of myofascial pain referred to multiple areas of the face. Therefore, differential diagnosis of nonspecific orofacial complaints may often involve diagnostic anesthetic injection of cervical muscles. Trigger points within the cervical musculature can refer pain to the facial areas via defined reference fields. Secondary or satellite trigger points in the face may occur as a product of continuous input from the cervical region, and treatments addressing only the secondary sites may not resolve the patient's complaints.

Therapies for Orofacial Myofascial Trigger Points

Diagnostic and therapeutic approaches to orofacial myofascial trigger points can be frustrating to both the clinician and the patient. The bilateral influence of multiple muscles creates complex pain and functional patterns that can be difficult to assess. In addition, as previously stated, the mandible is rarely at rest inasmuch as normal functional demands of chewing and talking are often complicated by dysfunctional habits (clenching). The latter problem often continues uncontrolled throughout the sleep period. The therapeutic approaches to orofacial myofascial disorders are:

1. Trigger point injections—anesthetic, dry needling
2. Physical therapy
3. Intraoral orthotics
4. Pharmacologic management
5. Behavioral modification

Treatment sequencing of the aforementioned steps will vary depending on the severity of the initial symptom presentation and whether the problem is acute or chronic. Acute episodes can be aborted with use of trigger point injections and appropriate medications. Intramuscular injections are used to eradicate trigger points and restore more comfortable functional patterns. However, patients are often resistant to the injection or medication approach. These patients may be amenable to the use of an intraoral occlusal appliance. Behavioral modification can be added to prevent recurrence.

Injection Techniques

Injection of facial muscle trigger points provides a rapid and convenient approach to management. Physicians tend to be more comfortable with extraoral injections, whereas dentists are understandably more familiar with the intraoral route. Extraoral techniques are preferable because they allow access to all four of the primary masticatory muscles and enable manipulation of the syringe at various angles. With proper injection techniques and understanding of the anatomy, complications, if any, are few and easily managed.

Few patients look forward to the discomfort usually associated with intraoral injections for dental treatment. Although most patients are initially alarmed at the thought of receiving injections to the external face, discomfort tends to be less than that experienced with intraoral injections. Once the initial anesthetic is deposited, the clinician will be surprised at patient tolerance to prolonged manipulation of the syringe following needle entry.

General Considerations in Facial Injections

Risks of untoward side effects due to masticatory muscle injections are relatively low. With application of anatomic considerations for each masticatory muscle being treated, problems can be kept to a minimum. The occurrence of hematoma and prolonged muscle inflammatory response is not unusual and is easily managed. Important considerations for the outpatient are cosmetic disturbances due to the injections and anesthetic effects that may affect the patient's ability to drive home from the office. As in any medical or dental technique, *informed consent* is mandatory.

Armamentarium

Because masticatory muscle mass is small in comparison to other major body muscles, a 25-gauge needle is sufficiently wide to provide for trigger point needling without excessive muscle tissue damage. Smaller-gauge needles will deflect in these muscles and not allow for operator control; also, false-negative aspiration is more likely with the narrower gauge. The masseter and temporalis muscles are amenable to needles of 1 1/2-inch length, whereas muscles medial to the mandible, the medial and lateral pterygoid may require a longer needle to access them from the extraoral route. The shorter-length needle will suffice for intraoral approaches.

Recommended syringe techniques for trigger point ablation usually include injection of anesthetic, saline, or no solution at all (dry needling technique). Because of the sensitive nature of the face and the proximity of crucial structures, local anesthetic is the preferred vehicle because the numbness will allow for needle manipulation without the potential danger of face or eye injury due to patient movement.

Anesthetics of choice are those without vasoconstrictor, most commonly procaine, mepivacaine, lidocaine, or bupivacaine. Mepivacaine and lidocaine are readily available in multidose vials or dental cartridges and will provide sufficient facial anesthesia for trigger point needling and increased range of mandibular motion in the absence of pain. The duration of action for mepivacaine and lidocaine is short. This feature may be valuable as temporary anesthesia of the facial nerve commonly occurs as a side effect of solution dispersion, which may compromise the patient's ability to drive home (see later discussion). Bupivacaine can be used for prolonged anesthesia, but patients should be accompanied by another adult if they are to leave the office after the procedure.

Many clinicians employ injectable corticosteroid when injecting trigger points with local anesthetic.[8] Although the exact mechanisms of corticosteroid action on myofascial TPs are not well defined, it may relate to the inherent inflammation-reducing effect of the steroid. Other proposed theories have focused on stabilization of neuronal membranes, thus inhibiting the conduction of nociceptive impulses. As with any steroid, expecially when placed over bony structures, judicious short-term use is preferable.

Often, patients are at risk for a subacute bacterial endocarditis (SBE) when certain dental or oral surgical procedures are performed and thus they require prophylactic antibiotic therapy for dental visits. Typically, these patients present with a history of mitral valve prolapse with regurgitation confirmed by echocardiogram, hypertrophic cardiomyopathy, or other condition creating a risk for SBE. However, in the dental office, antibiotic prophylaxis is not indicated for every dental procedure, and this decision is left to the discretion of the dental practitioner depending on the particular medical status of the patient and the procedure to be performed. As to myofascial TrP injections into the masticatory muscles, prophylactic antibiotic therapy (to prevent SBE) is not indicated when giving TrP injections to these muscles. This holds true when injecting masticatory muscles in patients who have prosthetic joint replacements. (As in any medical condition, the final determination is made at the discretion of the treating clinician with appropriate medical consultation as needed.)

Another frequent consideration exists with the patient on warfarin therapy. There is always the risk of a hematoma when doing TrP injections, and the clinician may want to consider the patient's prothrombin time and International Normalized Ratio (INR) before proceeding with injection therapy.

Skin preparation before needle penetration can be accomplished with povidone-iodine (Betadine) wipes. Patients will appreciate removal of the orange color with an additional alcohol wipe. Surfaces are then sprayed to an initial frost using a vaporized coolant spray such as Fluori-Methane spray (Gebauer Pharmaceutical Co., Cleveland, Ohio). Because of the proximity of the eye and ear to the refrigerant stream, the operator or assistant should provide hand protection to both these structures (Fig. 8–9).

Needle penetration at the site of the frost is usually painless, and a small amount of anesthetic solution is deposited followed by a pause to allow for initial localized numbness (Fig. 8–10).

Initial aspiration is done and is repeated throughout the injection process. The needle can then be advanced slowly while expressing anesthetic solution to further

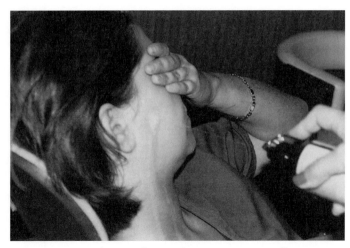

Figure 8–9. Application of vapocoolant spray prior to needle insertion.

widen the anesthetized area. The pause is repeated and this can then be followed by fanning out with the syringe and needling of trigger points. On completion of the injection-needling procedure, pressure is applied to promote hemostasis and a small bandage is placed over the site of needle penetration. This is followed by bilateral stretch and spray of the involved muscles. The patient should be kept in the office under observation for at least 30 minutes, and anti-inflammatory medication should be prescribed for 1 to 3 days. The patient is then referred for physical therapy management starting on the following day. Either ice or warm moist compresses can be applied over the injection site. The patient will express a preference for either cold or hot, which acts to reduce pain input.

Masseter Muscle

The size and superficial location of this muscle allow for efficient trigger point injection procedures. Pain in the superficial belly is usually reported in the midportion

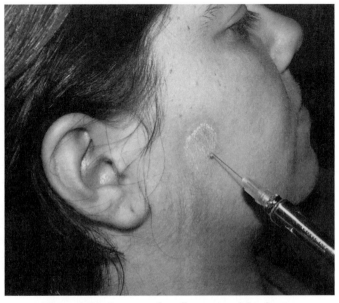

Figure 8–10. Insertion of needle at point of skin frosting.

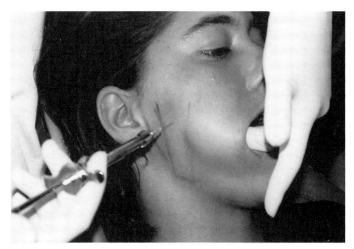

Figure 8–11. Needle insertion into superficial belly of masseter muscle.

with fewer complaints noted toward the zygomatic origin or insertion point on the mandibular border. Because of the relatively large size of this muscle, multiple sore areas will be found and the clinician will have to differentiate trigger point sites from surrounding myalgia. When the deep belly is symptomatic, the patient usually reports marked pain on palpation just inferior to the tragus.

For needle insertion into the superficial belly, the patient is asked to open the mouth as wide as possible and the doctor's free hand index finger is placed intraorally to locate the anterior border of this belly. This should provide a guide for needle insertion that will prevent needle entrance into the oral cavity (Fig. 8–11).

If the patient cannot open, direct insertion of the needle to contact the midlateral surface of the mandibular ramus will provide a sufficient starting landmark. After superficial deposition of anesthetic, the needle is rapidly advanced to contact the bony ramus. The importance of making this contact is to be sufficiently deep within the muscle area, thus avoiding injection into the parotid gland. The needle is then fanned out through the large muscle belly to break up trigger points (Fig. 8–12). The facial artery and the parotid gland are the prime structures to avoid.

For deep belly needle insertion, the prime landmark is the posterior border of the condylar neck just below the ear. The needle is inserted just anterior to this until bony contact with the neck or lateral surface of the ramus is reached (Fig. 8–13).

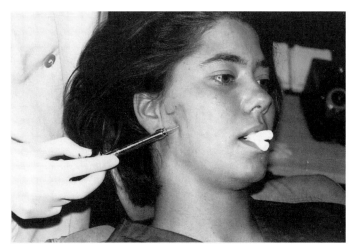

Figure 8–12. Fanning of needle within masseter muscle to disrupt trigger points.

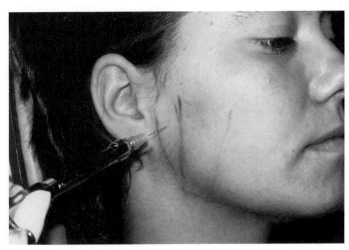

Figure 8–13. Injection of deep belly of masseter muscle.

Having the patient open slightly may allow for better palpation of landmarks. It is essential to contact bony landmarks, thus avoiding untoward injection into the coronoid notch of the mandible or deeper soft tissue structures within the neck.

The most common, usually benign, side effect of masseter injection is that associated with anesthesia of the facial nerve as it passes through the parotid gland. This is more common with deep belly injection and the patient should be advised before starting the procedure that he or she may lose the ability to close or blink the ipsilateral eye for about 40 minutes subsequent to the injection. In order to protect conjunctival and corneal structures, the patient should be given safety glasses or the eye should be taped closed for the duration of anesthesia. The patient should then wait in the office until motor function returns.

Temporalis Muscle

Most trigger point pain in the temporalis muscle will be felt in the anterior portion and is easily provoked by palpation. Tenderness in this muscle can be confused with a potential headache process of central origin. It is not routine practice to shave this area before injection, and surface wiping with disinfectant will not totally clean epithelial surfaces below the hair. However, the potential for complications from a compromised surface preparation is low. The clinician should insert the syringe fully until contacting the bony surface of the temporal bone and then withdraw the needle followed by a subsequent fanning-out motion to broach trigger points. The superficial temporal artery is the main complicating anatomic part to be avoided (Fig. 8–14).

Medial Pterygoid Muscle

Intraoral trigger point injection of the medial pterygoid muscle is feasible but can present difficulties because of restricted opening range, the gag reflex, and limited ability to manipulate the needle. If the intraoral route is desired, the patient is asked to open the mouth as wide as possible and a prop is then inserted between the teeth on the opposite side to stabilize the mandible. The needle is inserted just medial to the pterygomandibular raphe about midway between the upper and lower teeth. The needle should also be held horizontal and parallel to the ramus.[4] After insertion into the muscle, trigger points can be approached by redirecting the needle, although syringe manipulation may be limited by space available in the oral cavity.

There are two extraoral techniques for injection of the medial pterygoid. The inferior portion may be approached under the inferior ramus of the mandible just anterior to the angle of the jaw.[11] Injecting through the coronoid notch of the mandible provides direct access to the muscle belly, especially when the patient presents with

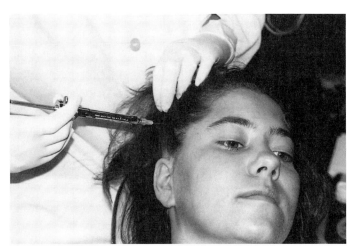

Figure 8–14. Injection of temporalis muscle.

severely restricted opening.[16] The mouth is propped open if possible, and the needle is inserted through the coronoid notch in an inferior and slightly caudad direction until the muscle belly is penetrated. The pterygoid plexus of veins lies just medial to the mandible and lateral to the lateral pterygoid muscle; hemorrhage can be avoided by smoothly and rapidly passing the needle through this plexus (Fig. 8–15).

Lateral Pterygoid Muscle

Intraoral approaches to injection of the lateral pterygoid muscle are not recommended because the high and medial position of this large muscle body prevents direct access with the needle. The extraoral route through the coronoid notch provides good access to both bellies of the lateral pterygoid. The patient's mouth is propped open and the syringe is passed through the coronoid notch in an upward direction until contact with the lateral pterygoid plate is made. The needle is withdrawn slightly, and the inferior and superior bellies may be injected by altering needle direction. Again, rapidly passing the needle through the pterygoid plexus will prevent a bleeding episode. The other possible vascular event may be nicking of the maxillary artery, which runs in close proximity to the muscle bellies. Because of the size and deep

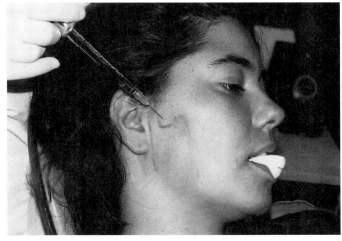

Figure 8–15. Injection of medial pterygoid muscle.

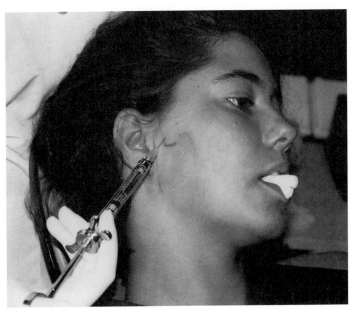

Figure 8–16. Injection of lateral pterygoid muscle.

location of this muscle, false-negative results may occur with this injection technique (Fig. 8–16).

Physical Therapy

Physical therapy care can be prescribed for both short- and long-term management of chronic myofascial trigger points. Stretch and spray techniques using vaporized coolant are effective in eliminating trigger points and can be first-line therapy to obviate the need for needling procedures.[10] Restoration of reasonable jaw function and continued management for recurrent muscular pain problems can be accomplished within the physical therapy setting, perhaps avoiding the necessity of further injections or medication treatments.

Intraoral Orthotics

Adjunctive care for facial trigger point management can include use of a removable intraoral plastic orthosis to help manage parafunctional habits. This appliance covers the occlusal surfaces of the teeth with a thin layer of acrylic. It is placed preferably over the maxillary teeth, but can be placed on the mandibular arch. The result is usually a reduction in clenching habits and some reflex relaxation of the masticatory musculature. These orthoses provide varying degrees of improvement in different patients and, when successful, may obviate the need for supplemental medications. The true physiologic mechanisms of these appliances are not known but effects may be due to alteration of occlusal proprioception, change in muscle length, or placebo.

If the patient has a major TMJ disc displacement disorder that interferes with jaw opening, repositioning of the mandible with an occlusal appliance may allow for more acceptable joint function in a few selected cases (Fig. 8–17). This is accomplished by changing the bite pattern on the orthosis to bring the mandible forward, thus moving the condyle forward onto the displaced articular disc. However, wearing this orthosis for extensive time periods can lead to irreversible tooth movement and a permanent change in mandibular position, necessitating additional dental rehabilitation procedures. This clinical approach should be done with extreme caution. As in any arthropathy that is refractory to nonsurgical management, arthroscopic or open joint surgery remains an option.

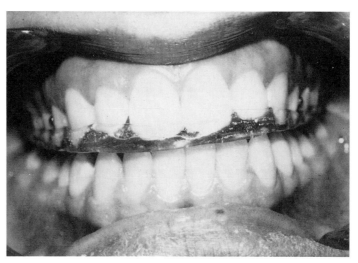

Figure 8–17. Intraoral bite plate: maxillary flat plane design.

Pharmacologic Management

Medications are a valuable adjunct in the management of myofascial trigger point pain. Drug selection is based on the pharmacologic objective, medical history, and the length of time that the patient will be taking the drug. Medications include nonsteroidal anti-inflammatory drugs (NSAIDs), anxiolytics, skeletal muscle relaxants, and antidepressants.

Nonsteroidal Anti-inflammatory Drugs

NSAIDs can have both short-term and long-term application within trigger point management. For brief periods of acute pain, NSAID management can provide sufficient analgesia to allow for better mandibular function. They should be prescribed routinely after trigger point injections to reduce postoperative discomfort. Longer-term use may be indicated for prolonged problems, but this will require closer patient monitoring, notably for the added risk of adverse gastrointestinal side effects. Pregnancy, asthma, and a history of gastrointestinal disorders are major medical considerations in use of these drugs. Cox-2 inhibitor NSAIDs may be employed for the medically at-risk patient, but studies verifying their efficacy in the management of myofascial pain are lacking.

Anxiolytics

Anxiolytic medication may provide more predictable muscle relaxation effects than that attained by use of skeletal muscle relaxants. Most of this occurs through alterations in neurotransmission due to the inhibitory effects of γ-aminobutyric acid (GABA). In the limbic cortex, this creates reflex muscle relaxation in many patients. The benzodiazepines are most commonly prescribed but long-term use contraindicated because of the risk of development of dependence. Benzodiazepines are usually taken at bedtime because of their sedative effects. Diazepam is the most commonly used anxiolytic but because of its long elimination half-life, it should be prescribed with caution to older patients or to patients who cannot tolerate or function with residual sedation on the following day.

Skeletal Muscle Relaxants

These medications do not seem to have direct effect on myofascial trigger point pain. They do not work on the motor end plate but rather exert their influence on local circuits within the spinal cord and within the reticular activating system. Some of their analgesic effect may be due to sedation. Included in this group are the typical skeletal muscle relaxants (e.g., carisoprodol) and cyclobenzaprine. The $GABA_B$ agonist baclofen may also be employed.

With this class of medications, daytime sedation may reduce compliance with the prescribed medication regimen.

Antidepressant Medication

Antidepressants are better suited for longer-term use in the chronic myofascial pain patient. The therapeutic window for pain management generally requires dose amounts below those commonly used for behavioral therapy. In addition to their neurohumoral pain-reducing mechanisms, they also tend to improve sleep in chronic pain patients. Most often tricyclic antidepressant medications are employed, although clinicians may prescribe a selective serotonin reuptake inhibitor (SSRI). SSRIs may result in better patient compliance due to a reduced side effect profile when compared with tricyclic antidepressants, but studies as to their efficacy in managing myofascial pain are lacking.

Newer Medications

More recent pharmacologic approaches have included the use of the $alpha_2$ agonists (tizanidine) and the injection of botulinum toxin into the involved musculature. The clinical efficacy of these approaches for myofascial pain has yet to be defined and studies are needed.

Behavioral Modification

Behavioral approaches for patient management fall into two categories. The first concerns itself with the psychological manifestations of the patient's pain syndrome. Whether the problems are endogenous or reactive, functional difficulties due to behavioral input will affect the course of treatment and this level of care should be instituted when indicated.

The second approach involves the use of biofeedback training. As stated previously, oral parafunctional habits are common in patients with orofacial myofascial trigger points. A biofeedback therapist may be able to effect a reduction in these deleterious habits and educate the patient in self-modulation of facial muscle tension.

Summary

The complexities encountered in analyzing and managing masticatory myofascial pain create challenges to the practitioner because of the multiple areas of diagnosis and treatment that may have to be addressed. The clinician must be sure that facial myofascial trigger points are the primary disorder and are not associated with another pathologic process. Differential diagnosis should include appropriate studies along with medical and dental consultation. When perpetuating factors exist, there is often difficulty in long-term management of masticatory muscle problems owing to patient inability to control these aggravating issues. However, levels of improvement to allow for daily functional comfort are usually attainable. Careful diagnosis and adequate technique should provide pain management in an area of the human soma that is crucial to the day-to-day comfort and function of most individuals. Most importantly, the neurophysiology underlying muscular pain and the pathophysiology of myofascial trigger points are now only beginning to be understood, and future research will lead to new therapeutic approaches.

References

1. Bell WE: Temporomandibular Disorders: Classification Diagnosis, Management, 3rd ed. St Louis, Mosby-Year Book, 1990.

2. Clark G, Kiyoshi K, Brown P: Oral motor disorders in humans. California Dental Association Journal, January 1993, pp 19–30.
3. Dohrenwend B, Raphael K, Marbach J, Gallagher R: Why is depression comorbid with chronic myofascial face pain? A family study of alternative hypotheses. Pain 83:183–192, 1999.
4. Fricton JR, Kroening RJ, Hathaway KM: TMJ and Craniofacial Pain: Diagnosis and Management, 1st ed. St Louis, Ishiyaku EuroAmerica, 1988.
5. Gerwin RD: Differential diagnosis of myofascial pain syndrome and fibromyalgia. J Musculoskeletal Pain 7:209–216, 1999.
6. Gilman S, Newman S: Manter and Gatz's Essentials of Clinical Neuroanatomy and Physiology, 7th ed. Philadelphia, FA Davis, 1993.
7. Huffman K, Vernoy M, Vernoy J: Psychology in Action. Emigsville, PA, Progressive Information Technologies, 1997, p 507.
8. Knobler R (ed): Contemporary Approaches to Managing Pain: Emerging Concepts in Myofascial Pain. Secaucus, NJ, Physicians World Communications Group (Professional Post Graduate Services).
9. Mense S:Considerations concerning the neurobiological basis of muscle pain. Can J Physiol Pharmacol 69:612, 1990.
10. Pertes R, Cohen H: Clinical management of temporomandibular disorders: Part 2. Compendium Continuing Education Dent 12:270, 410, 1992.
11. Pertes R, Heir G: Chronic orofacial pain—a practical approach to differential diagnosis. Dent Clin North Am 35:30, 1991.
12. Raphael K, Marbach J, Klausner JM: Myofascial face pain—clinical characteristics of those with regional vs. widespread pain. J Am Dent Assoc 131:161–171, 2000.
13. Sigiura K, Robinson G, Stuart D: Illustrated guide to the Central Nervous System, St Louis, Ishiyaku EuroAmerica, 1989, p 114.
14. Sternbach RA: Chronic pain as a disease entity. Triangle 20:27–32, 1981.
15. Stohler C, Zhang X, Lund J: The effect of experimental jaw muscle pain on postural muscle activity. Pain 66:215–222, 1996.
16. Travell J, Simons D: Myofascial pain and dysfunction. The trigger point manual, Baltimore, Williams & Wilkins, 1983.
17. Wilson-Pauwels L, Akesson E, Stewart P: Cranial Nerves, Anatomy and Clinical Comments, Toronto, BC Decker, 1988, p 51.

Part II

Trigger Point Management

Chapter 9

Trigger Points

Edward S. Rachlin, MD

Epidemiology

Almost every person will experience some type of muscle pain over a lifetime. Chronic and recurrent muscle pain affects 10% to 20% of the U.S. population over 18 years of age,[50] a comparable statistic to other countries such as Israel, the United Kingdom, and Canada,[6] and is the second most common medical condition after upper respiratory illness.[37] Untreated myofascial pain syndromes can become chronic pain conditions. Chronic pain not only causes disability due to pain but can also be responsible for related conditions including depression, physical deconditioning due to lack of exercise, sleep disturbances, and other psychosocial and behavioral disturbances.[21, 59]

When individuals experience chronic pain, it affects not only the individuals but also their families and coworkers and their ability to function actively and positively in society. As medical providers learn how to treat *and educate patients to prevent* myofascial pain syndromes, much suffering in the population will be alleviated.

The incidence of myofascial pain syndromes is higher in women than men,[6, 51] and although trigger points (TrPs) have been diagnosed in children and young adults, they are most often seen in the age range of 31 to 50 years of age.[42, 79, 86]

Current literature cites myofascial pain due to TrPs as the cause of a multitude of chronic pain conditions including but not limited to work-related pain,[49] back pain, headaches, facial pain, herpes zoster pain, plantar fasciitis, pelvic pain, pain following surgery or failed surgery, and pain in animals as studied by veterinarians.[17]

A study by Skootsky and associates found that myofascial pain in the upper body was more common than in other areas of the body.[80] Sola and colleagues surveyed 200 asymptomatic young adults to determine the presence of asymptomatic (latent) TrPs in the shoulder girdle muscles.[86] Hypersensitive areas (TrPs) were found in 54% of female subjects and 45% of male subjects. Ninety-nine (49.5%) subjects had one or more TrPs. Referred pain was demonstrated in 12.5% of all subjects. Four muscles—the trapezius, levator scapulae, infraspinatus, and scalenus—accounted for 84.7% of the TrPs, those in the trapezius (34.7%) and the levator scapulae (19.7%) occurring most frequently.[86] Table 9–1 presents the epidemiology of trigger points.

It has been reported that 85% of back pain[75] and 54.6% of chronic headache and neck pain are due to myofascial pain.[15, 20]

There has probably been more research and publication on the prevalence and treatment of orofacial pain due to myofascial pain syndromes by the dental and orthodontial fields than by any other area of practice. A multidisciplinary pain center for management of temporomandibular disorders found that 90% of the patients had primary myofascial pain syndromes and no direct temporomandibular joint (TMJ) involvement.[16] In a study by Schiffman and coworkers of 269 subjects (of the "general"

Table 9–1.
Epidemiology of Trigger Points

Higher incidence in women than men
Most common in 30- to 50-year age range
Most commonly found in the following muscles: trapezius, levator scapulae, axial postural muscles
Chronic pain clinics study reported incidence of 85% of patients having myofascial pain syndrome
Asymptomatic shoulder girdle trigger points are found in 54% of females and 45% of males

female population 20–40 years of age), 50% had myofascial pain in the masticatory muscles, with 6% having symptoms severe enough to cause them to seek treatment.[66] Carlson and colleagues injected upper trapezius TrPs in 20 patients with ipsilateral masseter muscle pain and observed significant reduction in pain intensity of the masseter region and reduction in electromyographic (EMG) activity of the masseter muscle.[8]

Brazilian researchers found that 45 out of 54 patients with chronic postherpetic neuralgia had active or latent TrPs and that treatment of the TrPs significantly (and often completely) decreased neuropathic pain.[59] A paper on case studies by Chen and associates cited the alleviation of intercostal muscle pain secondary to herpes zoster infection by treating TrPs in the area with injections.[10]

Imamura and associates relieved pain in failed back surgery (with 150 days follow-up) by treating TrPs and taut bands in the muscles.[40] In a study of postthoracotomy pain in 27 patients, Hamada and coworkers found that myofascial pain was a significant factor that must be examined and treated.[29]

In a double-blind study with a 2-year follow-up, Imamura and colleagues found that treating TrPs in calf muscles resolved plantar fasciitis pain.[39]

The persistent and chronic nature of untreated myofascial pain syndromes explains the large numbers of myofascial pain patients seeking help at pain clinics. Understanding myofascial pain syndromes and fibromyalgia has become of major importance in pain management and eradication.

Etiology

Healthy muscles do not have symptomatic TrPs. Trigger points may occur in any skeletal muscle and arise from multiple causes (Fig. 9–1). Muscles become vulnerable when they are under acute or chronic stress.[1, 52, 100] Trigger points may develop after prolonged periods of spasm, tension, stress, fatigue, and chill.[44] Stress and tension are among the most common causes of TrPs.[45, 68, 81] McNulty and associates showed the influence of emotional stress on TrPs when 14 subjects with upper trapezius TrPs were studied. Findings showed psychological stress caused increased EMG activities in the TrPs, while the adjacent muscles remained electrically silent.[52] Trigger points occur most frequently in axial muscles used to maintain posture. This is due to the

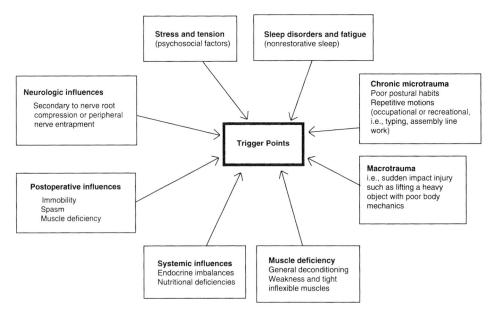

Figure 9–1. Trigger points—causes and contributing factors.

constant tension and microtrauma of poor postural habits, both in everyday living and in the workplace.[99] Occupational or recreational activities that require repeated stress or overload on a specific muscle or muscle group similarly cause chronic stress leading to TrPs.[99] Examples of predisposing activities include holding a telephone receiver between the ear and shoulder to free the arms, prolonged bending over a table, sitting in chairs with poor back support and improper height of armrests or none at all, poor sitting posture when typing or working at a computer for long periods, or loading heavy boxes using improper body mechanics (see Chapters 16 and 20).

Acute trauma can also result in TrPs, especially if the trauma leads to prolonged myofascial involvement as in the case of whiplash[23] and other motor vehicle–related injuries.

Physical deconditioning secondary to immobility following acute trauma, chronic illness, arthritic conditions, and lack of exercise in general may predispose patients to TrPs. (Deconditioned muscles are more easily stressed than muscles with good strength and flexibility.) This is probably one of the reasons that TrPs may develop in patients suffering from connective tissue disorders such as osteoarthritis, rheumatoid arthritis, and myositis.[14, 40, 64]

Preoperative and postoperative care in musculoskeletal surgery should include an examination for myofascial involvement and TrPs as sources of preoperative or postoperative pain. Unnecessary operative procedures may be avoided.[13, 61, 62, 65, 89, 97]

Trigger points are often overlooked in the treatment of athletic injuries. A common cause of failure in achieving therapeutic results in the management of tennis elbow is the lack of diagnosis and treatment of TrPs in the extensor and supinator muscles of the forearm.[62]

Joint malalignment (i.e., facet joint dysfunction) may contribute to TrP formation.[46, 79] When joints are out of alignment, they cause the attached and opposing muscle groups to be lengthened and/or shortened, and also compromise surrounding connective tissues and neuromuscular structures. Muscle spasm, tension, and increased sympathetic output ensue, resulting in muscle pain, shortening, and TrPs.

Nonrestorative sleep patterns (disturbance in stage 4 sleep) have been found by Moldofsky[55–57] to be a cause of muscular pain and the development of tender points associated with fibromyalgia as well as myofascial pain syndromes. Researchers in Norway conducted a study of 96 females with muscle pain and found that insufficient sleep correlated with a high index of pain.[95]

Trigger points may result in areas of pain due to nerve root compression from discogenic disease as well as peripheral nerve entrapment.[14, 36, 98] Postlaminectomy pain may be due to TrPs that were present prior to surgery or developed afterward.[29, 61, 62, 65]

Although vitamin and nutritional deficiencies may be found in patients with myofascial pain, the specific role of nutrition in the cause and treatment of myofascial pain syndrome requires further investigation. Good nutrition and vitamins are necessary for healthy neurologic functioning and oxygen metabolism. Adequate B vitamins such as thiamine, pyridoxine, niacin, and vitamin B_{12} are essential for healthy nerve function. Vitamin C is important for muscles and preventing capillary fragility. Nutritional deficiencies, including calcium, potassium, iron, and magnesium, may affect the irritability of myofascial TrPs.[79, 94] Controlled studies should be undertaken, not only to investigate the effect of nutritional deficiencies on muscle pain but also to investigate the effects of excesses of substances such as refined sugar and stimulants (e.g., coffee, cigarettes) and potential food and substance intolerances (e.g., drugs, dairy, and wheat) on muscle tension and pain.

Multiple TrPs may result from endocrine factors, e.g., estrogen levels[11] and hypothyroidism (see Chapter 4).

The Four Causes of Muscle Pain

Hans Kraus described four causes of muscle pain (which he called the four *types* of muscle pain): trigger points, muscle spasm, muscle tension, and muscle deficiency.

Correct diagnosis of the cause of muscle pain will determine the appropriate and most effective treatment.[81] The four causes of muscle pain are usually interrelated and must be managed comprehensively (see Chapter 15 and Fig. 10–1).

Muscle Spasm

Muscle spasm is the involuntary contraction of muscle caused by chronic or acute trauma, excessive tension, or organic disorders.[81] Muscle spasm may create shortening of muscles, limited motion, and pain. Untreated spasm and the "protective" immobility due to pain lead to decreased local blood flow in the muscles, causing more pain and contraction, resulting in a vicious cycle of muscle spasm and pain.

Muscle Tension

Kraus defined muscle tension as "prolonged contraction of a muscle or muscle groups beyond functional or postural need."[45] Muscle tension may have postural, emotional, or situational causes.[24, 51, 81] Postural tension occurs when a stressful position, such as holding the telephone between the shoulder and ear, or slouched sitting, is repeated frequently and for prolonged periods of time. Emotional tension can be triggered by negative emotional experiences (e.g., unresolved anger), and causes muscular tension when it is chronically present. Situational tension arises when one is forced to adjust to unpleasant circumstances, such as tension in the work atmosphere. EMG study[52] has shown that psychological stress causes increased electrical activity in upper trapezius TrPs, and Banks and coworkers showed that EMG activity of a TrP could be decreased or silenced with the use of relaxation training.[2]

Muscle Deficiency

Adequate muscular fitness is necessary to meet the requirements of activities of daily living such as walking, lifting, and bending. When muscles are weak or stiff, they are considered deficient. Muscle deficiencies make one prone to injury and can themselves be a source of pain. For example, weakening of abdominal muscles can bring on back pain, particularly during pregnancy. Premature ambulation following immobility of the lower extremity can cause pain by overstretching and overloading tight, weak muscles.

Definition and Types of Trigger Points

Myofascial TrPs are small circumscribed hyperirritable foci in muscles and fascia, often found within a firm or taut band of skeletal muscle.[5, 44, 47, 93] Trigger points may also occur in ligaments, tendons, joint capsule, skin, and periosteum. They have been described as tender nodes of degenerated muscle tissue that can cause local and radiating pain. Historically, they have been referred to as *Muskelhärten* (muscle hardening) or *Myogelosen* (myogelosis) hardenings by Lang,[47] as myalgic spots by Gutstein,[28] and were later described as TrPs by Steindler.[88] Travell and Simons have published extensively on TrPs and referred pain patterns.[79, 91, 94] In regional myofascial pain syndromes, TrPs may be limited to a single muscle or to several muscle groups.[47, 99] Palpating the TrP may elicit a local or referred pain pattern, or both, that is consistent and characteristic of the primary muscles involved.[5, 8, 28, 44, 47, 78, 79, 83, 93] The distant area of referred pain has been called the zone of reference.[83, 93] Referred pain patterns do not correspond to dermatomal, myotomal, or sclerotomal patterns. Kellgren[41] confirmed the specificity of muscular and ligamentous referred pain patterns by studying the effect of muscular injections using 0.1 to 0.3 mL of hypertonic saline. A more recent study that used hypertonic saline injection to observe its effect on referred pain also observed referred pain patterns elicited by intramuscular electrical stimulation.[1] Some referred pain patterns that have been reported lack universal

Table 9–2.
Myofascial Trigger Points: Symptoms and Physical Findings

Symptoms	Physical Findings
1. Local and referred pain patterns	1. Local tenderness
2. Pain with isometric/isotonic muscle contraction	2. Referred pain
3. Muscle stiffness and limited joint motion	3. Single or multiple muscle involvement
4. Muscle weakness	4. Palpable nodules ("knots")
5. Paresthesia and numbness	5. Firm or taut bands in muscle
6. Proprioceptive disturbances: loss of balance, dizziness, tinnitus	6. "Twitch response"
7. Symptoms of autonomic dysfunction: lacrimation, coryza, pilomotor activity	7. Jump sign
	8. Muscle shortening
	9. Limited joint motion
	10. Muscle weakness

agreement by clinical investigators.[58] Presenting symptoms may include pain; muscle weakness; decreased joint motion; paresthesia; and autonomic symptoms, including sweating, lacrimation, localized vasoconstriction, coryza, and pilomotor activity. Trigger points that are located in the head and neck may cause proprioceptive disturbances such as problems with balance, dizziness, and tinnitus (Table 9–2). Trigger points may be classified as primary, secondary, satellite, active, or latent[89, 90] (Fig. 9–2).

Primary trigger points develop independently and not as the result of TrP activity elsewhere.

Secondary trigger points may develop in antagonistic muscles and neighboring protective muscles as the result of stress and muscle spasm. It is common for patients to experience the pain of a secondary TrP once a primary TrP is eliminated.

Satellite trigger points can develop in the area of referred pain as the result of persistent resting motor unit activity in the muscle.[79, 94] Visceral organ diseases can refer pain to muscle (e.g., appendicitis) and can lead to satellite TrPs in those muscles.[1, 79]

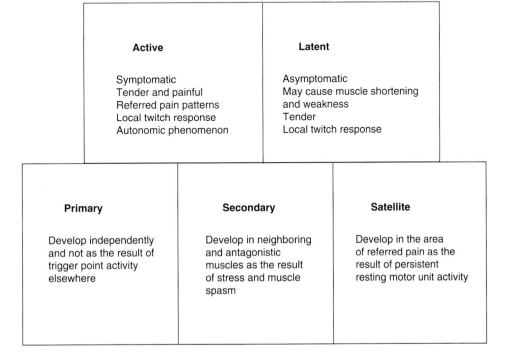

Figure 9–2. Types of trigger points.

Multiplication of TrPs results from the development of secondary and satellite TrPs. This chain reaction of TrP multiplication may be initiated by several factors, including muscle imbalances, muscle weakness, postural abnormalities, and tension (see Chapters 17 and 18).[46, 99] This combination of factors may, for example, explain the persistence of pain in the postlaminectomy patient, or "failed back syndrome."[61, 65] Patients may receive only partial or temporary relief from TrP management if treatment is limited to secondary or satellite TrPs; the primary TrP must also be addressed.

Active trigger points are always tender, painful, and symptomatic. Pain may be present at rest and during motion. Palpation of the TrP may cause a local or specific referred pain pattern, or both.[35] Hong and associates found that the greater the intensity of pain of an active TrP, the greater the occurrence of referred pain. This study also showed that referred pain was elicited more frequently by needling than by palpation.[35] Under experimental conditions, another study concluded that the size of referred pain corresponds to the intensity and duration of the ongoing local muscle pain.[1] Snapping palpation of a taut band of muscle fibers or needling of the TrP may cause a visible "local twitch response" of the muscle or skin, or both. A more common reaction to TrP palpation is the "jump response"[28, 75]: The patient tends to jump or suddenly move away from the examiner's palpating hand. Movement to avoid pain is often accompanied by a vocal reaction.

Referred pain patterns are specific for primary TrPs.[5, 26, 41, 44, 47, 84, 95] Specific knowledge and understanding of referred pain patterns are necessary to avoid the mistake of treating TrPs (satellite) in the referred pain areas and overlooking the primary TrP. The most common TrP locations are illustrated in Figure 10–4. Table 10–2 illustrates pain patterns frequently misdiagnosed as common orthopedic conditions.[61] See Appendix for diagrams of pain areas and common muscle TrPs that may be responsible for local or referred pain.

Latent trigger points are asymptomatic and do not require treatment unless they are activated. However, latent TrPs may predispose one to having an active TrP. Activation of latent TrPs can occur if the muscle is stressed by tension, mechanical overloading, or prolonged muscle shortening.[79] They are often found coincidentally on palpation. Latent TrPs are tender and may demonstrate a local twitch response and show lowered pressure pain threshold when using a pressure algometer.[31] Although latent TrPs do not cause pain, they may be a cause of muscle shortening and weakness. It is not uncommon to find latent TrPs on physical examination in patients who are asymptomatic.[79] Latent TrPs are found most frequently in the shoulder girdle muscles, the trapezius, and the levator scapulae.[83, 87]

Uncertainty in diagnosis can exist when differentiating the tender points found in fibromyalgia[70, 82, 101] from the findings of TrPs in myofascial pain syndromes.[22, 77, 78] Multiple symmetrical bilateral tender points occur in specific locations in fibromyalgia (see Chapters 1 and 2). Trigger points may occur in any skeletal muscle and may be singular or multiple. They may be found in the same locations as the tender points of fibromyalgia. When the findings of a palpable taut band, local twitch response, and referred pain pattern are present, the diagnosis of TrP is evident.[79] At this stage in our knowledge of TrP diagnosis and pathology, the significance of tender areas must be judged within the clinical context. It is not unusual for tender points and TrPs, as defined, to coexist in fibromyalgia,[22, 63, 96] both requiring an appropriate therapeutic approach.

Small tender lipomas, which may represent fat herniations, may be found in the sacroiliac area. These tender nodules should not be mistaken for TrPs. Episacroiliac lipomas may refer pain to the groin and lateral aspect of the thigh.[60] A local anesthetic and steroid may be injected into the tender area with good therapeutic results. If symptoms return, surgery may be indicated. This is not a frequent surgical indication. Clinical correlation should strongly support this diagnosis before surgery is considered.

Histopathology

Glogowski and Wallraff[25] described biopsy findings in palpable hardenings of hip and back muscles. They found waxy degeneration of muscle fibers, destruction of fibrils, agglomeration of nuclei, and fatty infiltration. No control groups were included for comparisons and the findings were nonspecific.[100] Miehlke and coworkers[54] carried out biopsies of the upper trapezius, dividing them into four groups, groups 1 to 4, differing in symptomatology and findings. Palpable hardenings were reported in groups 3 and 4. Biopsy of groups 3 and 4 demonstrated marked degeneration of the fibers as well as changes in the interstitial connective tissue. Yunus and colleagues[100] noted that muscle fiber changes in groups 3 and 4 were similar to those reported by Glogowski and Wallraff,[25] but both studies were uncontrolled. Group 1 had generalized pain without palpable findings; biopsy results in this group were normal. These studies indicate that TrPs may begin as a neuromuscular dysfunction and progress to a dystrophic pathologic state.

In a study conducted by Bengtsson and associates,[3] 77 biopsy specimens from 57 patients showed fibers that appeared "moth-eaten" in 35 of 57 patients and "ragged red fibers" in 15 of the 41 trapezius muscles.[19] Fassbender and Wegner[12] looked at biopsies of patients with probable myofascial pain syndromes of fibrositis. The majority of the biopsies were abnormal, initially showing swollen mitochondria and moth-eaten myofilaments, progressing to necrosis of myofilaments, irregularity of sarcomeres, and greatly reduced glycogen stores. The final stage examined demonstrated dissolution of contractile elements.[7] Other histologic studies of fibrositic tissue have confirmed the findings of Fassbender and Wegner, as well as changes in enzyme patterns and increased amounts of water, mucopolysaccharides, and ground substance.

Although abnormalities are reported, they are nonspecific and inconsistent. The significance of these findings in relation to hormonal and abnormal clinical states remains unclear and requires further study.[100]

The Pathophysiologic Development of the Trigger Point

The pathophysiology of the TrP is an area of much research and discussion. Previous hypotheses noted the fibrotic nodule resulting from decreased blood supply as the cause of TrPs. More recent concepts have been proposed by David Simons,[79] Hubbard and Berkoff,[37, 38] Gunn,[27] and Andrew Fischer (see Chapter 7).

The formation or activation of a TrP may be due to an acute injury or chronic microtrauma to the muscle (e.g., sustained muscle contraction due to tension and poor posture). This stress creates a disruption of the sarcoplasmic reticulum that causes the release of free calcium ions. In the presence of adenosine triphosphate (ATP), the free calcium stimulates actin and myosin interaction and increased metabolic activity.[92] The increased metabolic activity activates an increase in the release of serotonin, histamine, kinins, and prostaglandins. These substances raise the sensitivity and firing of groups III and IV muscle nociceptors, which converge with other visceral and somatic inputs, creating the perception of local and referred pain.[67, 71, 72] The pain, by way of the central nervous system, stimulates motor units, inducing muscle spasm and splinting. If the muscle spasm and secondary splinting go untreated, a vicious cycle of muscle pain and spasm is initiated, causing decreased local blood flow to the muscle and therefore decreased ATP and calcium pump action. This results in interaction of free calcium and ATP and increased contractile activity, perpetuating the pain-spasm cycle. Over time this cycle of events leads to sustained noxious metabolites in the area that build up in the connective tissue, eventually creating localized fibrosis. The pain caused by the fibrotic tissue stimulates more motor unit firing, leading back to the muscle spasm cycle. The cycle can be broken by restoring normal muscle length and addressing the cause and contributing factors (Fig. 9–3).

David Simons describes an "integrated hypothesis" of the pathophysiology of myofascial TrPs based on EMG and histologic findings.[76, 80] At the crux of this hypothesis is the idea of multiple dysfunctional motor end plates at the neuromuscular junction in the TrP region. Excessive release of the neurotransmitter acetylcholine (or possibly poor uptake of this substance) creates an abnormal environment and interruption of normal neuromuscular information and processing. EMG studies show spontaneous electrical activity (continuous low-amplitude action potentials, often accompanied by

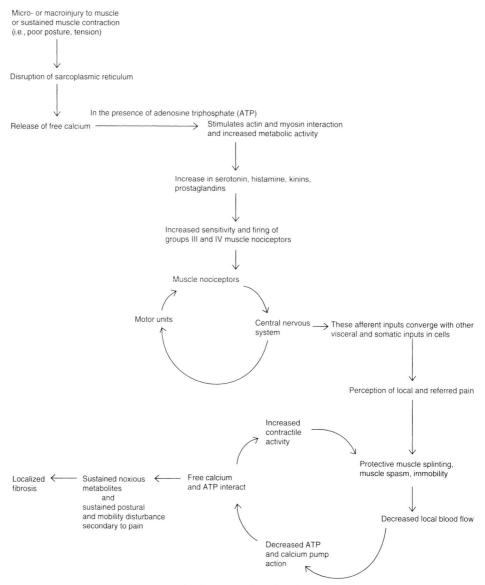

Figure 9–3. Pathophysiology of myofascial pain syndromes.

intermittent large amplitude spikes) in the TrP region that researchers believe is due to the excess acetylcholine release in the area.[76, 77]

Through a number of EMG studies on rabbits and humans, researchers found that there are multiple "sensitive loci"[33] throughout a muscle, most of which are concentrated in the TrP region.[9, 33, 34] When stimulated mechanically (e.g., by needling), sensitive loci in the TrP region can produce tenderness, referred pain, and a local twitch response; they are most likely nociceptors.[33]

"Active loci" are also described.[33, 76] The active locus is the dysfunctional motor end plate (at the neuromuscular junction), which shows spontaneous electrical activity and is associated with excessive release of acetylcholine. From his research in this field, Hong postulates that a TrP develops in a muscle when a sensitive locus and an active locus are in close proximity and form a TrP locus.[33]

The clinical changes palpated in the tissue associated with TrPs, i.e., the taut band, tender nodule, and attachment TrPs (the tender attachment regions of the taut band), have been explained histologically as the manifestations of multiple "contraction knots" in a TrP.[77, 79] The contraction knots within a TrP are located similarly to the active loci and also appear to be the result of the excessive acetylcholine at the dysfunctional motor end plate. In a longitudinal section of a TrP on which a biopsy has been performed, a contraction knot appears as a thickened portion of a muscle fiber (about the length of a motor end plate).[76] It is thickened because the sarcomeres are maximally shortened in that portion of the fiber (creating the nodule one can palpate in the tissue). The maximally contracted sarcomeres cause stretching of the sarcomeres on both sides, thereby creating increased tension of the fiber (palpated as the taut band).[76, 79] The continuous maximal contraction of these sarcomeres increases the local energy demand. Simultaneously, the tension due to the contracted sarcomeres constricts vascular structures and causes ischemia and hypoxia in the area, resulting in a decreased supply of energy. This energy crisis produces the release of neuroactive substances that can sensitize nociceptors and lead to local and referred pain.[76, 79]

"Muscle-Spindle Theory"

Hubbard and Berkoff[38] presented a pathophysiology of the TrP based on prolonged or chronic muscle-spindle tension.[37, 38] Hubbard wrote that EMG studies have shown that TrPs contain actively firing muscle fibers[37, 79] and that this EMG activity "arises from sympathetically mediated hyperactivity of the intrafusal muscle fibers of muscle spindles in the nidus of TrPs."[37] Muscle spindles are sensitive to both pain and pressure and are found throughout muscle tissue with high distribution in cervical and axial muscles (which harbor a high incidence of myofascial TrPs). The "muscle-spindle hypothesis" suggests that chronic muscle pain concurrent with TrPs originates with initial trauma or repetitive strain injury and becomes chronic through sympathetically mediated hyperactivity of muscle spindles (i.e., by α-adrenergic stimulation).[36] Emotional tension and stress have been shown to affect EMG data of TrPs, which suggests that these centrally mediated phenomena are probably significant perpetuating factors.[36, 48, 52]

Local Twitch Response

Studies performed by Hong and other researchers on rabbits and humans showed that the local twitch response (LTR) appears to be a spinal reflex that is not dependent on higher centers.[31]

Mechanisms of Referred Pain

Selzer and Spencer[69] postulated five neurologic mechanisms to explain referred pain: (1) convergence-projection, (2) peripheral branching of primary afferent nociceptors, (3) convergence-facilitation, (4) sympathetic nervous system activity, and (5) convergence or image projection at the supraspinal level.

Convergence-Projection

One nerve cell in the spinal cord may receive messages regarding pain from two different sources. The nerve may relay information about the internal organs and from nociceptors coming from the skin or muscles, or both. The brain has no mechanism for distinguishing whether the message comes from the skin, the muscles, or the visceral organs. When the brain interprets messages, it attributes the pain to the skin or muscles rather than internal visceral organs. Referred pain in TrPs may be pain that is "initiated by the muscle nociceptors but referred to the area served by other somatic receptors that converge on the spinothalamic tract cell."[74]

Peripheral Branching of Primary Afferent Nociceptors

A single neuron may serve several areas of the body by branching out. It is possible for the brain to interpret messages from one part of the body as coming from another.

In the case of a nerve that serves both the leg and the lower back, the message of pain in the back may be interpreted as coming from the leg.

Convergence-Facilitation

This hypothesis suggests that neural activity (somatic afferent impulses from the skin), which is generally below threshold, may be influenced in such a way by visceral impulses that it excites the spinothalamic tract fibers. This mechanism of pain production places the active myofascial TrP in the position of acting as a peripheral pain generator.[69, 74]

Sympathetic Nervous System Activity

Stimulation of sympathetic nerves may cause pain in the referred pain area by two mechanisms: (1) by restricting blood flow to vessels that serve sensory nerve fibers and (2) by releasing substances that sensitize primary afferent nerve endings in the area of referred pain. Mense conducted a series of experiments on rats through which he hypothesized that the sensation of radiating pain may be caused by the changes in the dorsal horn of the spinal cord due to the spread of excitability of adjacent neurons in the presence of muscle inflammation.[54]

Convergence or Image Projection at the Supraspinal Level

Pain pathways may converge at the thalamic or cortical level, causing image projection of a referred pain pattern.

Mechanism of Pain Relief Following Stretch and Spray

Vaporized coolant spray (vapocoolant spray) cools the skin by evaporating quickly. A sudden drop in skin temperature causes stimulation of skin afferent sensory fibers that affect polysynaptic reflexes in the spinal cord, closing the pain "gate" and preventing reflex hyperstimulation of muscle or the sensation of pain at higher centers. This temporary anesthesia then allows increased passive stretching of the muscle, which has a direct therapeutic effect on the TrP and restoration of normal muscle length[7] (Fig. 9–4).

When cold, in the form of ice or vaporized coolant spray, is applied to an area of the body, the metabolic rate and inflammation are decreased. Vasoconstriction causes a decreased blood flow in the area. The muscle can no longer contract once the metabolic rate drops. This cooling relieves muscle spasm. Nerve activity is also reduced. In the treatment of TrPs and muscle spasm, ice or vaporized coolant spray is used to relieve pain and muscle spasm. Ethyl chloride spray is especially effective because it combines (1) intense stimulation of a cold shock and rapid rate of change in skin temperature, (2) some degree of direct depression of cutaneous receptors by cooling, and (3) effects analogous to those produced by a light stroking massage[43, 90, 93] (see Chapter 11 for a discussion of Fluori-Methane and ethyl chloride vapocoolant spray).

Mechanisms of Pain Relief Following Trigger Point Injection

Several mechanisms have been suggested that, theoretically, may contribute to the inactivation of TrPs by injection.[94]

- Mechanical disruption of the trigger point by disrupting muscle elements or nerve endings
- Depolarization of nerve fibers due to the release of intracellular potassium that occurs with mechanical disruption of the muscle fibers

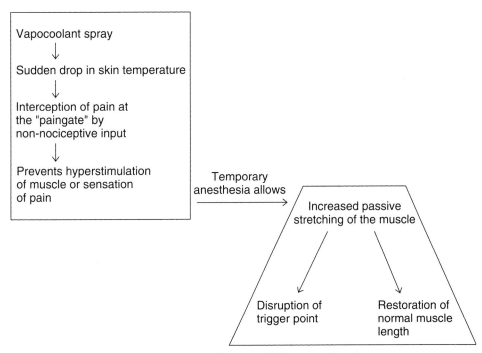

Figure 9–4. Mechanism of pain relief following stretch and spray.

- In contrast to dry needling, injected fluid, such as a local anesthetic or saline, dilutes nerve-sensitizing substances
- Local vasodilation effect of procaine increases the energy supply and removal of metabolites in the area
- Interruption of feedback mechanisms by local anesthetic
- Focal necrosis depending on which local anesthetic is injected, as noted in animal experimentation[4]

In addition to the aforementioned, pain relief may occur due to an increase in endogenous opioids (e.g., neurohormonal β-endorphins or somatospecific dorsal horn enkephalins).[30]

Electromyography

Electromyography has been used both to investigate and validate the location and behavior of TrPs and to quantify the effects of treatment on them.

Hubbard and Berkoff,[38] and later, Simons and Hong,[77, 79] found spontaneous EMG activity in TrPs that was not present in nearby muscle even 1 mm from the TrP. McNulty and colleagues[52] and Banks and coworkers[2] also conducted studies showing that TrPs are electrically active compared with surrounding tissues, and that that activity can be increased by psychological stress and decreased by the use of relaxation training.[2] Simons[71] noted increased motor unit action potentials associated with the visible signs of a local twitch response following a snapping palpation of taut muscle bands. The motor unit electrical activity of the muscular bands harboring TrPs was found to be significantly higher than that of normal muscles tested.[18] It has been suggested that satellite TrPs develop as the result of this constant resting motor unit activity.[94]

In a study by Carlson and associates, 20 patients with upper trapezius muscle TrPs and ipsilateral masseter muscle pain were given a TrP injection of 2% lidocaine solution in the upper trapezius muscle. Following the injection, there was both a significant reduction in pain intensity and EMG activity in the masseter muscle.[8]

Hubbard and Berkoff found that the TrP EMG mean amplitudes were significantly greater in the study groups with headaches and fibromyalgia than in the "normal" groups.[38]

References

1. Arendt-Nielsen L, Graven-Nielsen T, Svensson P: Assessment of muscle pain in humans—clinical and experimental aspects. J Musculoskeletal Pain 7(1/2):25–41, 1999.
2. Banks S, Jacobs D, Gevirtz R, Hubbard DR: Effects of autogenic relaxation training on electromyographic activity in active myofascial trigger points. J Musculoskeletal Pain 6(4):23–32, 1998.
3. Bengtsson A, Henriksson KG, Larsson J: Muscle biopsy in primary fibromyalgia: Light-microscopical and histochemical findings. Scand J Rheumatol 15:1–6, 1986.
4. Benoit PW: Effects of local anesthetics on skeletal muscle, Anat Rec 169:276–277, 1971.
5. Bonica JJ: Management of myofascial pain syndromes in general practice. JAMA 732–738, June 1957.
6. Buskila D, et al: The prevalence of pain complaints in a general population in Israel and its implications for utilization of health services. J Rheumatol 27(6):1521–1525, 2000.
7. Campbell SM, Bennett RM: Fibrositis. St Louis, Mosby-Year Book, 1986.
8. Carlson CR, Okenson JP, Falace DA, et al: Reduction of pain and EMG activity in the masseter region by trapezius trigger point injection. Pain 55(3):397–340, 1993.
9. Chang YC, Kao SF, Kuan TS, Hong CZ: Distribution of sensitive loci where localized twitch response can be elicited in rat skeletal muscle. J Rehab Med Assoc ROC 26(1):1–8, 1998.
10. Chen SM, Chen JT, Kuan TS, Hong CZ: Myofascial trigger points in intercostal muscles secondary to herpes zoster infection of the intercostal nerve. Arch Phys Med Rehabil 79:336–338, 1998.
11. Dao TT, Knight K, Ton-That V: Modulation of myofascial pain by the reproductive hormones: A preliminary report. J Prosthet Dent 79(6):663–670, 1998.
12. Fassbender HG, Wegner K: Morphologie und Pathogenese des Weichteilrheumatismus. Z Rheumaforsch 32:355–374, 1973.
13. Feinberg B, Feinberg R: Resistant pain after total knee arthroplasty: Treatment with manual therapy and trigger point injections. J Musculoskeletal Pain 6(4):85–95, 1998.
14. Fischer AA: Treatment of myofascial pain. J Musculoskeletal Pain 7(1/2):131–142, 1999.
15. Fishbain DA, Goldberg M, Steele R, et al: DSM-III diagnoses of patients with myofascial pain syndrome (fibrositis). Arch Phys Med Rehabil 70:433–438, 1989.
16. Foreman PA: The changing focus of chronic temporomandibular disorders: Management within a hospital-based, multidisciplinary pain centre. NZ Dent J 94:23–31, 1998.
17. Frank EM: Myofascial trigger point diagnostic criteria in the dog. J Musculoskeletal Pain 7(1/2):231–237, 1999.
18. Fricton JR, Auvinen MD, Dykstra D, et al: Myofascial pain syndrome: Electromyographic changes associated with local twitch response. Arch Phys Med Rehabil 66:314–317, 1985.
19. Fricton JR, Awad EA (eds): Advances in Pain Research and Therapy, vol 17. New York, Raven, 1990.
20. Fricton JR, Kroening R, Haley D, et al: Myofascial pain syndrome of the head and neck: A review of clinical characteristics of 164 patients. Oral Surg Oral Med Oral Pathol 60(6):615–623, 1985.
21. Fricton JR, Kroening R, Haley D, et al: Myofascial pain syndrome of the head and neck: A review of clinical characteristics of 164 patients. Oral Surg 60:615–623, 1985.
22. Gerwin RD: Myofascial pain syndromes (MPS) and fibromyalgia (FM): Misdiagnosis and mistreatment—challenge to the fibromyalgia community. Presentation at the Janet G. Travell Seminar Series—Focus on Pain '98, March 12–15, 1998, San Antonio, Texas.
23. Gerwin RD: Myofascial trigger points in chronic cervical whiplash syndrome [abstract]. J Musculoskeletal Pain 6(Suppl. 2):28, 1998.
24. Gil IA, Rizatti Barbosa CM, Moteiro Pedro V, et al: Multidisciplinary approach to chronic pain from myofascial pain dysfunction syndrome: A four year experience at a Brazilian center. Journal of Craniomandibular Practice 16(1):18–25, 1998.
25. Glogowski G, Wallraff J: Ein Beitrag zur Klinik und Histologie der Muskelhärten (Myogelosen). Z Orthop 80:237–268, 1951.
26. Good MG: Rheumatic myalgias. Practitioner 146:167–174, 1941.
27. Gunn CC: The Gunn approach to the treatment of chronic pain, intramuscular stimulation for myofascial pain of radiculopathic origin, 2nd ed. New York, Churchill Livingstone, 1996.
28. Gutstein M: Diagnosis and treatment of muscular rheumatism. Br J Phys Med 1:302–321, 1938.
29. Hamada H, Moriwaki K, Shiroyama K, et al: Myofascial pain in patients with postthoracotomy pain syndrome. Reg Anesth Pain Med 25(3):302–305, 2000.
30. Hameroff SR, Crago BR, Blitt CD, et al: Comparison of bupivacaine, etidocaine, and saline for trigger-point therapy. Anesth Analg 60:752–755, 1981.
31. Hong CZ: Pathophysiology of myofascial trigger point. J Formos Med Assoc 95(2):93–104, 1996.
32. Hong CZ: Algometry in evaluation of trigger points and referred pain. J Musculoskeletal Pain 6(1):47–59, 1998.

33. Hong CZ: Current research on myofascial trigger points: Pathophysiological studies. J Musculoskeletal Pain 7(1/2):121–129, 1999.
34. Hong CZ, Chen YN, Twehous D, Hong D: Pressure threshold for referred pain by compression on the trigger point and adjacent areas. J Musculoskeletal Pain 4(3):61–79, 1996.
35. Hong CZ, Kuan Ta-Shen, Chen JT, Chen SM: Referred pain elicited by palpation and needling of myofascial trigger points: A comparison. Arch Phys Med Rehabil 78:57–60, 1997.
36. Hsue TC, Yue S, Kuan TS, Hong CZ: Association of active myofascial trigger points and cervical disc lesions. J Formos Med Assoc 97(3):174–180, 1998.
37. Hubbard DR: Chronic and recurrent muscle pain: Pathophysiology, treatment, and review of pharmacologic studies. J Musculoskeletal Pain 4(1/2):123–143, 1996.
38. Hubbard DR, Berkoff GM: Myofascial trigger points show spontaneous needle EMG activity. Spine 18(13):1803–1807, 1993.
39. Imamura M, Fischer AA, Imamura ST, et al: Treatment of myofascial pain components in plantar fasciitis speeds up recovery. In Fischer AA (ed): Muscle Pain Syndrome and Fibromyalgia. New York, Haworth Medical, 1998.
40. Imamura ST, Riberto M, Fischer AA, Imamura M, et al: Successful pain relief by treatment of myofascial components in patients with hip pathology scheduled for total hip replacement. J Musculoskeletal Pain 6(1):73–89, 1998.
41. Kellgren JH: A preliminary account of referred pains arising from muscle. BMJ 2:325–327, 1938.
42. Kraft GH, Johnson EW, LaBan MM: The fibrositis syndrome. Arch Phys Med Rehabil 49:155–162, 1968.
43. Kraus H: The use of surface anesthesia in the treatment of painful motion. JAMA 116:2582–2583, 1941.
44. Kraus H: Clinical treatment of back and neck pain. New York, McGraw-Hill, 1970.
45. Kraus H (ed): Diagnosis and Treatment of Muscle Pain. Chicago, Quintessence, 1988.
46. Kuan TS, Wu CT, Chen SM, et al: Manipulation of the cervical spine to release pain and tightness caused by myofascial trigger points. Arch Phys Med Rehabil 78:1040–1041, 1997.
47. Lang M: Die Muskelhärten (Myogelosen). Munich, Lehmann, 1931.
48. Lewis C, Gevirtz R, Hubbard D, Berkoff G: Needle trigger point and surface frontal EMG measurements of psychophysiological responses in tension type headache patients. Biofeedback Self Regul 9(3):274–275, 1994.
49. Lin TY, Teixeira MY, Fischer AA, et al: Work related musculoskeletal disorders. Phys Med Rehabil Clin North Am 8(1):113–117, 1997.
50. Magni G: The epidemiology of musculoskeletal pain. In Voeroy H, Merskey H (eds): Progress in Fibromyalgia and Myofascial Pain. Amsterdam, Elsevier Science, 1993.
51. Marini I, Fairplay T, Vecchiet F, Checci L: The treatment of trigger points in the cervical and facial area. J Musculoskeletal Pain 7(1/2):239–245, 1999.
52. McNulty WH, Gevirtz RN, Hubbard DR, Berkoff GM: Needle electromyographic evaluation of trigger point response to a psychological stressor. Psychophysiology 31(3):313–316, 1994.
53. Mense S: Biochemical pathogenesis of myofascial pain. J Musculoskeletal Pain 4(1/2):145–162, 1996.
54. Miehlke K, Schulze G, Eger W: Clinical and experimental studies on the fibrositis syndrome. Z Rheumaforsch 19:310–330, 1960.
55. Moldofsky H (chairman): Workshop on sleep studies. Am J Med 81(Suppl. 3A):107–109, 1986.
56. Moldofsky H: Sleep and musculoskeletal pain. Am J Med 81(Suppl. 3A):85–89, 1986.
57. Moldofsky H, Scarisbrick P, England R, et al: Musculoskeletal symptoms and non-REM sleep disturbance in patients with "fibrositis syndrome" and healthy subjects. Psychosom Med 37:341–351, 1975.
58. Nice DA, Riddle DL, Lamb RL, et al: Intertester reliability of judgments of the presence of trigger points in patients with low back pain. Arch Phys Med Rehabil 73:893–898, 1992.
59. Okada M, Stump P, Lin TY, et al: The occurrence of latent and active myofascial trigger points in patients with post-herpetic neuralgia [abstract]. J Musculoskeletal Pain 6(Suppl. 2):29, 1998.
60. Pace JB: Commonly overlooked pain syndromes responsive to simple therapy. Postgrad Med 58:107–113, 1975.
61. Rachlin ES: Musculofascial pain syndromes. Medical Times, The Journal of Family Medicine, January 1984:34–37.
62. Rachlin ES: The importance of trigger point management in orthopedic practice. Phys Med Rehab Clin North Am 8(1):171–177, 1997.
63. Raphael KG, Marbach JJ, Klausner J: Myofascial face pain: Clinical characteristics of those with regional vs. widespread pain. J Am Dent Assoc 131(2):161–171, 2000.
64. Reynolds MD: Myofascial trigger point syndromes in the practice of rheumatology. Arch Phys Med Rehabil 62:111–114, 1981.
65. Rubin D: Myofascial trigger point syndromes: An approach to management. Arch Phys Med Rehabil 62:107–110, 1981.
66. Schiffman E, Fricton J, Haley D, et al: Prevalence and treatment needs of subjects with temporomandibular disorders, J Am Dent Assoc 120(3):295–303, 1990.
67. Schwartz RG, Gall NG, Grant AE: Abdominal pain in quadriparesis: Myofascial syndrome as unsuspected cause. Arch Phys Med Rehabil 65:44–46, 1984.
68. Sella GE: Surface EMG in the investigation and treatment of myofascitis. Presentation at the Janet G. Travell Seminar Series—Focus on Pain '98, March 12–15, 1998, San Antonio, Texas.
69. Selzer M, Spencer WA: Convergence of visceral and cutaneous afferent pathways in the lumbar spinal chord. Brain Res 14:331–348, 1969.

70. Simms RW, Goldenberg DL, Felson DT, et al: Tenderness in 75 anatomic sites. Arthritis Rheum 31:182–187, 1988.
71. Simons DG: Electrogenic nature of palpable bands and "jump sign" associated with myofascial trigger points. Adv Pain Res Ther 1:913–918, 1976.
72. Simons DG: Myofascial trigger points, a possible explanation. Pain 10:106–109, 1981.
73. Simons DG: Fibrositis/fibromyalgia: A form of myofascial trigger points? Am J Med 8(Suppl. 3A):93–98, 1986.
74. Simons DG: In Fricton JR, Awad EA (eds): Advances in Pain Research and Therapy, vol 17. New York, Raven, 1990.
75. Simons DG: Examining for myofascial trigger points. Arch Phys Med Rehabil 74:676, 1993.
76. Simons DG: Diagnostic criteria of myofascial pain caused by trigger points. J Musculoskeletal Pain 7(1/2):111–120, 1999.
77. Simons DG, Hong CZ, Simons LS: Comment to Dr. Baldry's dry needling technique. J Musculoskeletal Pain 3(4):81–85, 1995.
78. Simons DG, Travell JG: Myofascial origins of low back pain: 1. Principles of diagnosis and treatment. Postgrad Med 73:99–108, 1983.
79. Simons DG, Travell TG, Simons LS: Myofascial pain and dysfunction. The Trigger Point Manual, vol 1, 2nd ed. Baltimore, Williams & Wilkins, 1999.
80. Skootsky SA, Jaeger B, Oye RK: Prevalence of myofascial pain in general internal medicine practice. West J Med 151:157–160, 1989.
81. Skubick D: The upper quadrant myofascial syndrome from a biomechanical, ergonomic, and psychophysical perspective. Presentation at the Janet G. Travell Seminar Series—Focus on Pain '98, March 12–15, '98, San Antonio, Texas.
82. Smythe H: Referred pain and tender points. Am J Med 81(Suppl. 3A):90–92, 1986.
83. Sola AE: Treatment of myofascial pain syndromes. In Benedetti C, Chapman R, Moriocca R (eds): Advances in Pain Research and Therapy, vol 7. New York, Raven Press, 1984, pp 467–485.
84. Sola AE: Trigger point therapy. In Roberts JR, Hedges JR (eds): Clinical Procedures in Emergency Medicine. Philadelphia, WB Saunders, 1985, pp 674–686.
85. Sola AE, Kuitert JH: Myofascial trigger point pain in the neck and shoulder girdle. Northwest Med 54:980–984, 1955.
86. Sola AE, Rodenberger MS, Gettys BB: Incidence of hypersensitive areas in posterior shoulder muscles: A survey of two hundred young adults. Am J Phys Med 34:585–590, 1955.
87. Sola AE, Williams RL: Myofascial pain syndromes. Neurology 6:91–95, 1956.
88. Steindler A: Lectures on the Interpretation of Pain in Orthopedic Practice. Springfield, Ill, Charles C Thomas, 1959.
89. Teresa M, Jacob RJ, Jacob LG, et al: Myofascial pain impairing the results of carpal tunnel syndrome surgery [abstract]. J Musculoskeletal Pain 6(Suppl. 2):43, 1998.
90. Travell J: Ethyl chloride spray for painful muscle spasm, Arch Phys Med 33:291–298, 1952.
91. Travell J: Myofascial trigger points: Clinical view. In Bonica JJ, Albe-Fessard D (eds): Advances in Pain Research and Therapy, vol 1. New York, Raven Press, 1976, 919–926.
92. Travell J: Identification of myofascial trigger point syndromes: A case of atypical facial neuralgia. Arch Phys Med Rehabil 62:100–106, 1981.
93. Travell J, Rinzler SH: The myofascial genesis of pain. Postgrad Med 11:425–434, 1952.
94. Travell JG, Simons DG: Myofascial pain and dysfunction: The trigger point manual. Baltimore, Williams & Wilkins, 1983.
95. Ursin R, Endresen IM, Vaery H, Hjelmen AM: Relations among muscle pain, sleep variables, and depression. J Musculoskeletal Pain 7(3):59–72, 1999.
98. Wolfe F, Simons DG, Fricton J, et al: The fibromyalgia and myofascial pain syndromes: A preliminary study of tender points and trigger points in persons with fibromyalgia, myofascial pain syndrome and no disease. J Rheumatol 19:944–951, 1992.
97. Wreje U, Brorsson B: A multicenter randomized controlled trial of injections of sterile water and saline for chronic myofascial pain syndromes. Pain 61(3):441–444, 1995.
98. Wu C-M, Chen H-H, Hong C-Z: Inaction of myofascial trigger points associated with lumbar radiculopathy: Surgery versus physical therapy. Arch Phys Med Rehabil 78:1040–1041, 1997.
99. Yue SK: Compartment approach to the shoulder and pelvic girdles related pain syndrome. Presentation at the Janet G. Travell Seminar Series—Focus on Pain '98, March 12–15, 1998, San Antonio, Texas.
100. Yunus MB, Masi AT, Aldag JC: A controlled study of primary fibromyalgia syndrome: Clinical features and association with other functional syndromes. J Rheumatol 16:62–71, 1989.
101. Yunus MB, Masi AT, Calabro JJ, et al: Primary fibromyalgia (fibrositis): Clinical study of 50 patients with matched normal controls. Semin Arthritis Rheum 11:151–171, 1981.

Chapter 10

History and Physical Examination for Myofascial Pain Syndrome

Edward S. Rachlin, MD

Therapeutic results in the management of regional myofascial pain due to trigger points (TrPs) depends on an accurate diagnosis and total assessment of all factors related to muscle pain.[1, 22, 30, 48] Myofascial TrPs should not be evaluated as a single entity, but as one component of interrelated causes of muscle pain (muscle spasm, muscle tension, muscle deficiency, and TrPs) (Fig. 10–1; see Chapter 15). The necessity for a thorough history and physical examination cannot be overemphasized (Table 10–1).

The physician who treats patients with myofascial pain must be not only knowledgeable but interested in the patient as a human being. A proper history takes time and should not be rushed. All factors contributing to the pain must be investigated.[19, 21, 41, 50, 51, 67] A history of trauma and the finding of TrPs may not in themselves be sufficient to explain the occurrence of symptoms, the patient's progress, or the chronicity of symptoms.[16, 21, 37, 51] An episode of pain may be precipitated by emotional problems, tension, business strain, physical activities at work, or athletic activities to which the patient is unaccustomed.[30] Endocrine factors (e.g., hypothyroidism) may contribute to the development and prolongation of myofascial pain. A complete medical and surgical history should be obtained to rule out other causes of pain, followed by a history focused on myofascial pain.

History

The myofascial pain history emphasizes the patient's current complaints, the history of onset, characteristics of pain, referred pain patterns, and the factors that precipitate and prolong symptoms. Information is obtained concerning previous episodes of pain, treatment, and response to treatment.

Figure 10–1. The four causes of muscle pain.

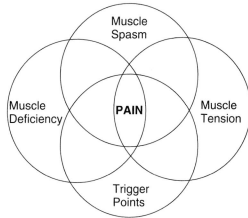

Table 10–1.
Patient Evaluation: History and Physical Examination for Myofascial Pain

A. History
  1. Medical and surgical history
     a. System review
     b. Trauma
     c. Previous medical conditions and treatment
     d. Surgical procedures
     e. Chronic debilitating disorders (e.g., arthritis)
     f. Endocrine disorders
     g. Dental problems
     h. Allergies
     i. Medications
  2. History related to myofascial pain
     a. Characteristics of pain
     b. History of onset: current and past episodes
     c. Occupational activities
     d. Athletic activities
     e. Sleep problems
     f. Psychological factors that contribute to tension
     g. Endocrine symptoms
     h. Temporomandibular joint symptoms

B. Physical examination
  1. Complete physical examination as indicated
  2. Observation of patient's posture and movement
  3. Postural examination
  4. Muscle evaluation
     a. Range of motion
     b. Flexibility of muscles
     c. Muscle strength
     d. Muscle spasm
     e. Muscle tension
     f. Trigger points
  5. Neurologic examination
C. Diagnostic studies (as indicated)
  1. Laboratory tests
     a. Blood chemistries, urinalysis
     b. CBC
     c. ESR
     d. T_3, T_4, RIA
  2. Radiologic studies
     a. CT scans
     b. MRI
     c. Myelogram
  3. Neurologic testing
     a. EMG and nerve conduction syndrome

CBC, complete blood count; ESR, erythrocyte sedimentation rate; T_3, triiodothyronine; T_4, thyroxine; RIA, radioimmunoassay; CT, computed tomography; MRI, magnetic resonance imaging; EMG, electromyography.

Current Complaints

Current complaints may include pain, stiffness, fatigue, deep tenderness, muscle weakness, restricted joint motion, a specific referred pattern of pain or numbness, autonomic symptoms (e.g., lacrimation, coryza), and proprioceptive disturbances (e.g., dizziness, poor balance).

Characteristics of Pain

Location and Type of Pain

Patients are asked to point to the area of pain with one finger. They may be given a body diagram and asked to describe the location and type of pain they are experiencing by noting it on the diagram (Fig. 10–2). If the patient complains of hip pain when referring to the back or speaks of a generalized pain, a drawing will help him or her to be more specific. The drawing can be completed by the patient or the examiner. Areas are marked using different symbols representing different types of sensations (e.g., pain, ache, burning, numbness, pins and needles). Referred pain patterns can be visualized. On the drawing, the patient can indicate precisely where the pain is located, indicating which area is most or least frequently painful. The sequence of the history of the symptoms can be noted. The drawing not only serves as a useful way to identify the presenting problem but also becomes a record for comparison with pain on later visits so that recovery can be observed. A series of such drawings represents a pictorial description of the patient's clinical course.

Patient's Rating of Pain

Patients are asked to rate their pain on a scale of 0 to 10 (0 = no pain, 10 = extreme pain). This number is written down or marked on the scale and may be used as a future indicator of the patient's progress (see Fig. 10–2). An additional body diagram can be used by the examiner to mark tender points and TrPs.

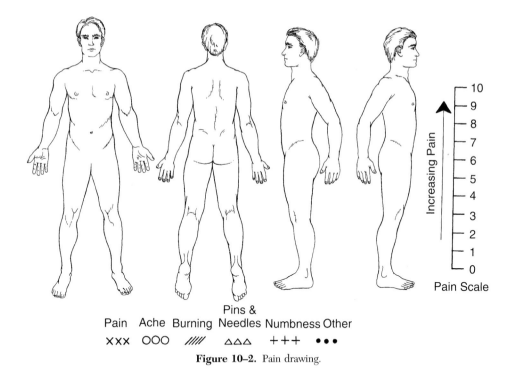

Pain   Ache   Burning   Pins & Needles   Numbness   Other

xxx   ooo   /////   △△△   +++   •••

Figure 10–2. Pain drawing.

Description of Pain

Patients are asked to describe their pain. Is the pain constant or intermittent? What is the type of pain (i.e., deep, dull, burning, shooting, localized, diffuse, radiating)?[31, 33] If the patient describes a referred pain typical of cervical and lumbar radiculopathy, disc involvement should be ruled out. Active TrPs in the lumbar, gluteal, trapezius, and levator scapulae areas may cause symptoms resembling nerve root compression.[40, 46] The referred pain may be felt close to the primary TrP or may be a distance away. Specific referred pain patterns are characteristic of myofascial TrPs. Referred pain patterns do not follow dermatomal, myotomal, or sclerotomal patterns (Table 10–2).

Effects of Rest and Activity

Is the pain relieved by rest or activity? Trigger points may cause pain at rest or can be aggravated by physical activity. Passive and active motion of shortened muscles harboring TrPs elicits pain. Pain after exertion may result from muscle weakness. Pain that occurs with the onset of movement following rest is typical of arthritis or muscle stiffness. Pain of sudden onset with "lightning" radiation and persistence may indicate nerve root involvement and must be differentiated from radiating pain due to TrPs. Pain may be caused by improper posture or tension. Pain of delayed onset after trauma is typical of muscle strain, and activation of TrPs (active or latent). Trigger point pain that occurs after inactivity can be relieved by short periods of joint range of motion. Trigger point pain that occurs after activity can be relieved with moist heat, slow, gentle stretching, and short periods of rest.

Pain Relief

What have patients found to be effective in relieving their pain? Patients may have treated themselves for some time by taking hot baths or applying hot packs or ice. They may have been treated previously by other health practitioners. Ask about the positive and negative effects of prescription and over-the-counter drugs that they have been or are taking. Ask if they have received physical therapy (modalities and manual)

Table 10–2.
Pain Patterns Frequently Misdiagnosed as Common Orthopedic Conditions

Locations of Muscular Trigger Points	Pain Pattern	Commonly Confused with Trigger Point Pain
Temporal, masseter, and occipital muscles	Radiation to head, headache, neck pain	Cervical arthritis, cervical syndrome
Sternocleidomastoid	Neck pain	Menière's disease, intracranial abnormality
Scalenus muscles, posterior neck muscles	Dizziness, numbness in 4th and 5th fingers, headaches	Peripheral nerve entrapment, cervical syndrome
Trapezius (upper)	Neck and shoulder pain	Cervical arthritis
Supraspinatus	Arm pain	Cervical disk, bicipital tendinitis
Infraspinatus	Arm pain	Cervical disk, bursitis of shoulder, bicipital tendinitis
Rhomboid (upper and lower)	Interscapular, scapular, and dorsal pain	Arthritis of dorsal spine, glenohumeral arthritis, radiculopathy
Pectoral	Arm pain	Bursitis (shoulder), cardiac pain, cervical radiculopathy
Deltoid	Upper back, neck, and arm pain	Cervical radiculopathy, bursitis (shoulder)
Forearm muscle group	Forearm and elbow pain	Epicondylitis
Sacrospinalis	Pain radiating downward to buttock	Sciatica, herniated disk
Tensor fascia, gluteus medius	Pain radiating to lateral aspect of thigh and leg	Herniated disk, bursitis
Piriformis	Sciatic radiation	Herniated disk
Adductor longus	Groin pain	Arthritis of hip, adductor muscle strain
Gastrocnemius	Calf and leg pain	Tennis leg, plantaris tendon, or gastrocnemius rupture
Soleus	Heel pain	Calcaneal bursitis, Achilles tendinitis
Adductor hallucis	Pain in metacarpophalangeal (MCP) joint area of big toe	Gout, arthritis of MCP joint of big toe
Tibialis anterior	Pain in front of leg and big toe	Herniated disk, anterior compartment syndrome
Vastus medialis, semimembranosus, sartorius	Knee pain	Chondromalacia, arthritis of knee
Peroneus longus	Ankle pain	Arthritis of ankle
Interossei of foot	Foot pain, radiating to toes	Morton's neuroma, metatarsalgia

From Rachlin ES: Musculofascial pain syndromes. Medical Times, The Journal of Family Medicine, January 1984: 34–47, with permission.

and what the effects of physical therapy were. Were they given an exercise program with proper supervision and instruction on how to perform the exercises? (See Chapter 15.)

History of Onset

When was the patient first aware of the pain? Is there a history of physical or emotional trauma?[22, 63] Did the pain occur suddenly or increase over a prolonged period of time? Was there a specific incident or activity that preceded it? Knowledge of the activity can give clues to which TrP may have been activated.

Patients with TrPs frequently have a history of pain in a specific muscle or muscle group that recurs following specific activities or situations. Symptoms may be of several years' duration. Patients may experience long periods of remission during which time TrPs may be asymptomatic and which are referred to as latent TrPs. Latent TrPs are found most frequently in shoulder girdle muscles.[70, 71]

Review of Contributing Causes

Prolonged Muscle Tension or Recurrent Spasm

Patients with TrPs often describe muscle spasms and tension. Muscle spasm occurs in muscles that have been shortened owing to prolonged inactivity. Pain may be most intense upon awakening because of the shortened position of the muscle during sleep. Any activity that requires the patient to remain in a fixed position for a length of time may have this effect.

Pain Related to Occupational Activities

Inquire about the patient's job and how the work is performed. Repetitive movements, poor postural attitudes at work, and poor body mechanics may give rise to TrPs or aggravate latent TrPs. Permanent relief of symptoms will require instruction in proper posture and body mechanics as well as an ergonomically correct work area and equipment for the individual.

Properly constructed chairs should be available for sedentary work. Does the patient sit in a chair of proper height, with a back support, and proper supportive armrests to prevent muscle tension and stress? Constant tightening and hunching of the shoulders is a common cause of cervical and trapezius pain in drivers and typists. Holding a telephone between the ear and shoulder to free both hands when talking for long periods is a frequent cause of neck pain. Muscle tension and strain during the workday owing to poor body mechanics or environmental conditions must be addressed if therapy is to succeed (see Chapter 20). Feelings of powerlessness at work, frustration with coworkers, or dissatisfaction with one's job lead to emotional stress (suppressed anger), which may be the primary cause or a contributing cause of muscle tension.

Athletic Activities

Does the patient exercise regularly? Do exercises include stretching and relaxation, warm-up, and cool-down? Most patients with regional myofascial pain syndrome and fibromyalgia will give a history of inactivity. Fibromyalgia patients will profit from an aerobic exercise program (see Chapter 2). Trigger points are frequent sequelae of athletic injuries resulting from microtrauma and macrotrauma. In taking an athletic history, details concerning the nature of the activity are necessary to determine the factors contributing to the onset and prolongation of symptoms. A knowledge of techniques unique to specific sports may be helpful in treating athletic injuries. Trigger points are a frequent cause of tennis elbow. This may result from faulty tennis equipment, poor stroke, or prolonged unaccustomed playing (overuse syndrome). Excessive repetitive movements such as practicing tennis serves or hitting a bucket of golf balls may produce or activate latent TrPs in the shoulder girdle muscles. Back pain in a tennis player may be caused by arching the back in performing an American twist serve. In this case treatment must be extended to correcting the serving technique.

Tension

Emotional stress and tension play a major role in muscle tension and TrP formation.[39, 61, 63] It is essential to take a psychosocial history to find out if the patient is suffering from business, personal, family, or marital problems.[22] Does the patient like his or her work? Is there constant stress in the workplace? Does the patient appear tense or angry? Is the patient receiving psychotherapy? Often unresolved stress (or anger) from earlier in life manifests as chronic tension and somatic symptoms in adulthood. Does the patient appear tense? It is important to prescribe ways of decreasing stress as part of the treatment programs. Examples of ways to decrease stress are:

- Hobbies (e.g., music, singing, artwork)
- Taking a walk

- Aerobic exercise
- Biofeedback[8, 39, 64]
- Deep relaxation techniques, meditation
- Psychological counseling
- Couples/family counseling
- Altering occupational circumstances, e.g., workload, personal interrelationships
- Drug therapy (if necessary, prescribed by a physician)

Fishbain and associates[17, 18] found a high incidence of depression, anxiety, and conversion (somatosensory disorders, alcohol and drug dependence, and personality disorders) among chronic pain patients. Fricton and colleagues found in two studies on masticatory myofascial pain that psychosocial factors such as depression were a primary predisposing factor to chronicity of the pain problem.[22] This does not imply that all people with pain suffer from these conditions but does imply that there is often a link between muscle pain, chronic pain, and mental and emotional issues and personality disorders.[17, 18, 63]

Stress and tension may manifest in the musculoskeletal system or in other physical conditions such as duodenal ulcer, ulcerative colitis, emotional depression, sleep disorder, or irritable colon.[63]

Arthritis

Does the patient have a history of joint pain and swelling? Pain, decreased joint mobility, weakness, and shortening of muscles predispose the surrounding muscles to the development of TrPs.[62] Muscles surrounding arthritic joints often harbor active TrPs that are overlooked as a source of pain and weakness in arthritic patients.[42] During examination for signs of myofascial disorders, Reynolds[62] found that the number of tender points and local twitch responses in women with rheumatoid arthritis was twice that found in women free of rheumatic illness. A study of 164 patients with head and neck myofascial pain syndromes showed that 42% of patients had a coexisting diagnosis of joint problems. It is suspected that the reflex muscle splinting, which occurs as a means to protect a painful joint from aggravating movement, contributes to the development of TrPs.[23] A similar process develops in patients who suffer from chronic debilitating diseases.

Trauma and Surgery

Is there a history of trauma or surgical procedures? Injuries and surgical procedures may lead to the formation of TrPs, causing repeated episodes of pain.[26, 28] Patients who have had back surgery are more likely to have TrPs than those who have not. Active or latent TrPs may be present prior to or may result from surgery.[60] Preoperative and postoperative evaluation for TrPs is necessary to prevent unnecessary surgery and improve postoperative results.[9, 60, 73, 79]

Endocrine Disorders

Myofascial pain and TrPs may be associated with hypothyroidism and estrogen imbalances.[5, 69, 72] Signs of hypothyroidism include brittle nails, dry skin, hair loss, constipation, depression, dry hair, difficulty losing weight, feeling cold, lethargy, and menstrual irregularity. Is the patient menopausal? Was menopause associated with hot flashes, vaginitis, or nervousness? Was estrogen given? Treatment of TrPs will not give lasting relief if endocrine problems contributing to muscle disorders are not treated. Endocrine problems should be treated prior to beginning TrP injections (see Chapter 4 for discussion of the endocrine aspects of myofascial pain).

Dental Problems

Grinding or clenching of the teeth often plays a role in headaches and facial, neck, and upper back pain.[22, 30] This can be related to mechanical disturbances involving the teeth and temporomandibular region as well as to tension (see Chapter 8).

Dentists and orthodontists have noted that bite difficulties, regardless of their origin (teeth, temporomandibular joint, emotional problems), often result in tension, and later in spasm and TrPs of the masticatory muscles.[47]

Sleep Problems

Sleep disturbance is frequently associated with both myofascial pain syndromes and fibromyalgia.[22] Patients report insomnia, waking in the night with inability to return to sleep, or inability to fall asleep. The diagnosis of fibromyalgia syndrome includes multiple bilateral tender points found in specific locations together with a frequent history of nonrestorative sleep (see Chapters 1 and 2). Does the patient wake up with pain or stiffness? Nonrestorative sleep as a cause of myofascial TrPs has been described by Moldofsky.[53-55] Is there a cause of sleeplessness (e.g., pain, sleep apnea, psychological stress)?

Neurologic Symptoms

Does the patient have symptoms of muscle weakness, sensory loss, or paresthesia? Symptoms related to proprioceptive disturbances include dizziness, tinnitus, and problems with balance (unsteady gait). Patients may complain of lacrimation or coryza due to autonomic dysfunction. Are there bladder or bowel irregularities? Trigger points may cause symptoms of nerve entrapment or referred pain patterns that may be mistaken for nerve root compression (e.g., disc herniation)[2, 46, 59] (see Table 10–2).

Joint (Articular) Dysfunction

David Simons names "articular dysfunctions that require manual mobilization" as one of the three major categories of musculoskeletal pain syndromes that are "often overlooked."[68] Naturally, the skeletal system must be in correct alignment to avoid muscular imbalance and stress. One can think of the muscles like the strings of a puppet; if a muscle is tight and harbors spasm or TrPs, it may pull the bone (e.g., a vertebra) out of alignment, causing joint dysfunction and stress to the neighboring neurovascular structures. Conversely, if a joint is malaligned, some attached muscles will be shortened while others are lengthened. A number of practitioners and researchers from allopathic, osteopathic, chiropractic, and physical therapy fields discuss the importance of treating both the articular dysfunction and the muscle dysfunction when necessary.[8, 68]

Routine Inquiries

Before treating a patient with a TrP injection, one must make several routine inquiries: Is the patient diabetic? Is there a history of allergy? Is the patient allergic to procaine or lidocaine? Is the patient on medications, particularly anticoagulants? Does the patient have a bleeding disorder? Does the patient have a history of fainting? Is pain experienced in other parts of the body (e.g., other joints or muscles)? Multiple areas of pain may indicate a systemic disease. Is the patient pregnant? Is there a history of recent and past infection (e.g., hepatitis, human immunodeficiency virus [HIV]-positive)? The presence of infection is a contraindication to TrP injection (see Chapter 11 for contraindications to TrP injections).

Physical Examination

A complete physical examination is performed as indicated. The physical examination should include observation of the patient's movement and posture; testing of range of motion, muscle strength, and neurologic integrity; palpation of muscles; and algometry, if available.

A general physical examination with appropriate laboratory testing is important whenever the possibility of a systemic disease is present and to rule out other causes of muscle pain. Emphasis of the examination will differ according to the nature of the patient's complaints. The examination will elicit information to evaluate muscle abnormalities (spasm, tension, muscle deficiency, TrPs), skeletal and postural abnormalities, and neurologic dysfunction.

Observation

Observe the patient's movement during the history taking. A person suffering from myofascial TrPs learns how to move in ways that are least painful. The patient may hold the neck stiff or walk with a shortened gait in order to limit movement that causes muscle pain. The practitioner who is sensitive to this will carefully observe the way the patient enters the room, the way the patient walks, sits, and holds his or her head. Does the patient lean to one side? This may be due to a disc lesion, facet joint impingement, or acute muscle spasm in the back due to muscle strain. It may also be a result of TrPs. Does the patient show signs of tension by maintaining the shoulders in an elevated posture during the interview and not relaxing the upper extremities?[261]

Postural Examination

Evaluate key postural muscles when appropriate. Structural measurements for skeletal abnormalities such as scoliosis, leg length measurements, and chest expansion are done. Poor postural habits, including forward head position, rounded shoulders, slouched sitting, and knee hyperextension, are noted.

Muscle Evaluation
Joint Mobility

Trigger points may cause shortening of muscles and limited joint motion. Pain may accompany any attempt to extend the joint. Some patients may not be aware of the restricted motion that may develop insidiously due to inactivity and lack of full use ("functional disuse"). Limited joint motion may also be a cause of TrPs (Fig. 10–3).

Muscle Strength

A muscle evaluation comparing the left and right sides is performed. Joint stiffness and muscle weakness may be the presenting symptoms. If the patient has complaints referable to the back, the Kraus-Weber test should be performed to evaluate muscle deficiencies (see Chapter 15). The Kraus-Weber test is not performed if the patient is in acute pain.

Muscle Tension

Muscle tension may be the cause of the patient's pain. Does the patient let go or tighten up when asked to perform certain motions? Reflexes that are difficult to obtain without distraction may be a sign of tension. Tension can be evaluated in the Kraus-

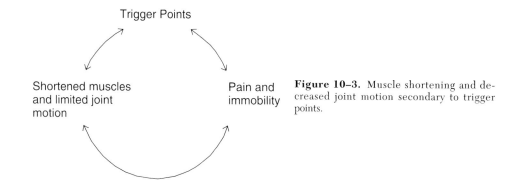

Figure 10–3. Muscle shortening and decreased joint motion secondary to trigger points.

Weber test when patients are asked to slowly reach toward the floor with their knees straight. The tense patient may reach farther on the second attempt when instructed to "relax and let go." Does the patient maintain his or her shoulder in a hunched position? Is the patient holding his or her breath or breathing fully? Shallow breathing and a clenched jaw are also indicative of tension.

Muscle Spasm

Muscles in spasm may be hard, rigid, and inflexible. Muscle spasm must be relieved before the examiner can palpate specific TrPs. Proper TrP examination requires the muscles to be relaxed. The patient should be reevaluated after muscle spasm has been successfully treated. (See Chapters 11, 16 and 19 for treatment of muscle spasm.)

Trigger Points

Trigger points can be diagnosed by palpation of the muscle.[2, 16, 24, 68] The patient may be able to direct the physician to the TrP and describe the area of local and referred pain.[57] Generally, the examiner uses the tips of the fingers with the hand relaxed and the fingers slightly bent. If the patient's muscles become tense, it is necessary to wait until they are relaxed again. As noted earlier, TrPs cannot be diagnosed if the muscle is in spasm. If the patient has normally firm muscles or excessive adipose tissue, the examiner may place one hand on top of the other to increase the strength of the palpating hand. Trigger point tenderness must be differentiated from the tenderness typical of fibrositis. In fibrositis, the subcutis is characterized by tenderness elicited by rolling and squeezing the skin.[47]

Trigger points may be identifiable to the examiner as tender, small hard knots or nodules, or a tender area in a firm, taut band of muscle fibers surrounded by normal muscle tissues.[29, 33, 57, 68] Trigger points may measure 2 to 5 mm in diameter.[20] The firm localized area may also be palpated when the muscle is gently stretched. The patient will report pain when the TrP is touched and may jump away from the examiner's hand, wince, or cry out (a reaction known as the "jump response").[33, 57] A local "twitch response" (muscle or skin twitch) may be visible as the TrP is palpated or touched with a needle.[36] A TrP will often refer pain to a distant area. Hong and associates found that in a study of 95 patients with TrPs, the greater the intensity of pain elicited in an active TrP, the more frequent the occurrence of referred pain.[36] Patterns of referred pain are specific and constant for individual muscles.[68] Familiarity with referred pain patterns is necessary to know where to look for the primary TrP that requires treatment. Lasting results are achieved only when the primary TrP is treated.[33, 48, 49, 74]

Trigger points occur most frequently in the muscles used to maintain posture (axial muscles) (Fig. 10–4). They may occur as a single muscle TrP or in multiple muscles. Neighboring muscles and the antagonists should be examined for secondary TrPs, which often become painful after the primary TrP is eliminated. The gluteal muscles should be included when the lumbar area is examined. A cervical examination should include the anterior cervical as well as the posterior muscles. The finding of local tenderness in a taut band of muscle fibers together with a local twitch response and referred pain has not been diagnosed with sufficient consistency by independent examiners in a controlled blind study to consider their presence as absolute requirements for the diagnosis of TrP.[38, 56, 78] However, a study by Gerwin and coworkers[29] showed that after examiners were given a training period on how to identify myofascial TrPs, interrater reliability was successfully established. They found that the interrater reliability in identifying a local twitch response was more difficult than that of a tender taut band, and that the identification of TrP features varied among different muscles.[29] David Simons has also written on the subject of the need for examiners to be trained in the skill of locating taut bands and local twitch responses and to practice this skill.[66] In a study by Wolfe and associates, taut muscle bands and muscle twitches were common and found equally in persons with fibromyalgia, myofascial pain, and no disease.[78] The clinical findings for the identification of TrPs, as described by Travell

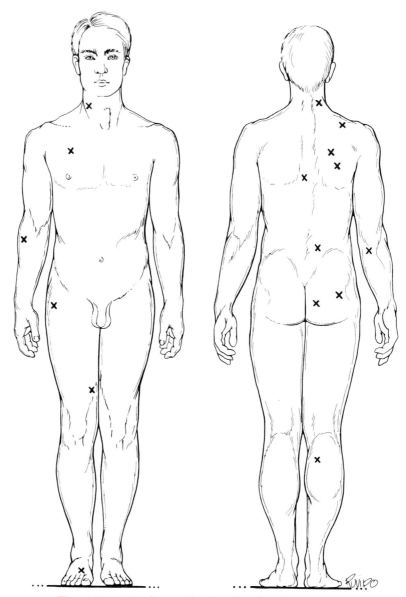

Figure 10–4. Most frequent locations of myofascial trigger points.

and Simons,[75] may not always be present in regional myofascial pain syndrome (MPS). The interpretation of the findings of tenderness depends on clinical correlation.

Tender Points

Tender points are subjective areas of tenderness, not accompanied by other signs of TrPs (Table 10–3). Multiple bilateral symmetrical tender points in specific areas are found in fibromyalgia (see Chapter 1). Agreement is lacking in deciding the actual number of tender points required for diagnosis.[65] Tender points and TrPs can occur simultaneously in fibromyalgia patients.[4, 25, 32] The American College of Rheumatology has established criteria for the classification of fibromyalgia in addition to empirical criteria suggested for the diagnosis of MPS (see Chapter 1). Diffuse multiple tender areas or multiple TrPs may indicate an endocrine problem that requires investigation. The significance of the finding of tenderness must be judged within the clinical

Table 10–3.
Trigger Points vs. Tender Points

Trigger Points	Tender Points
1. Local tenderness, taut band, local twitch response, jump sign	1. Local tenderness
2. Can be singular or multiple	2. Multiple
3. May occur in any skeletal muscle	3. Occur in specific locations and are symmetrically located
4. Specific referred pain pattern	4. Do *not* cause referred pain
5. May have autonomic and proprioceptive symptoms	

context.[27] Tenderness may not represent the tender points of fibromyalgia or the TrPs of MPS. The patient who is "tender all over" may represent a case of psychogenic rheumatism. Psychological factors, factors related to secondary pain, individual pain perception, and pain behavioral patterns must all be considered in evaluating the subjective complaint of tenderness.

Melzack and colleagues[52] noted a high degree of correspondence (71%) between the spatial distribution and associated pain patterns of TrPs and acupuncture points.

Neurologic Examination

A neurologic examination is performed for evidence of nerve root pressure, peripheral nerve entrapment, disc herniation, and neurologic disease. Trigger points may cause nerve entrapment. Examination includes testing for reflex loss, pathologic reflexes, sensory loss, and localized muscle weakness. Examination for referred pain patterns due to TrPs in the lumbar area includes straight leg raising tests in addition to testing for hip joint abnormalities. The clinician will also examine for findings of autonomic dysfunction, e.g., sweating, lacrimation, localized vasoconstriction, coryza, and pilomotor activity. Proprioceptive findings may include unsteadiness, poor balance, abnormal gait, or lack of dexterity.

Algometry

Algometry can be a valuable asset in the diagnosis of myofascial pain.[7, 15, 35, 58] Local tenderness can be assessed by using a pressure gauge devised by Fischer[10, 13, 14] (see Chapter 7). Tolerance to pressure is lower in areas where TrPs are present than in areas of normal muscle. The patient's sensitivity to pain is described by the pressure threshold, the minimum pressure or force that causes the patient discomfort, and by the pressure tolerance, the maximum pressure tolerated.[11, 12] Hong found that active TrPs show the lowest pain pressure threshold (PPT) and that latent TrPs and taut bands show lower PPT than normal muscle tissue.[35]

Tissue compliance is the consistency of the tissue with regard to its resistance to pressure.[10] The tissue compliance meter developed by Fischer enables a quantitative measurement of the softness or firmness of the muscle tissue. The meter is pressed against the skin and gauges the depth of penetration for a given amount of pressure (see Chapter 7). Algometry can be used before and after treatment as a quantitative measurement of improvement.[16]

Jaeger and Reeves[43] used the pressure algometer to quantify changes in myofascial TrP sensitivity following passive stretching. They found that the TrP sensitivity decreased in response to passive stretching and that intensity of referred pain is related to the sensitivity of the associated TrP.[43]

A high level of skill is necessary to obtain reliable information when using an algometer. Proper training, practice, and application is essential.[14, 68]

Pain Patterns Typical of Specific Myofascial Trigger Points

Referred pain patterns are characteristic of individual muscle TrPs° (see Chapter 12 and Appendix). The primary TrP may be distant from the area of complaint. A knowledge of pain patterns enables the physician to locate the primary TrP responsible for symptoms (see Table 10–2).

Figure 10–4 illustrates the most frequent locations of TrPs encountered in orthopedic practice (see Chapter 8 for common head and orofascial TrPs). The areas illustrated are:

- Posterior neck muscles
- Sternocleidomastoid and scalenus muscles
- Trapezius
- Infraspinatus
- Supraspinatus
- Levator scapula, rhomboid, thoracic paraspinalis
- Lumbar paraspinalis (sacrolumbar), quadratus lumborum
- Gluteal muscles (maximus, medius, minimus), tensor fasciae latae, piriformis
- Rectus femoris, vastus medialis
- Flexor and extensor muscles of the forearm
- Pectoral muscles (major, minor)
- Gastrocnemius muscle (medial)
- Foot muscles (interossei)

Trigger points causing referred pain patterns are often overlooked as the cause of symptoms and confused with common orthopedic diagnoses, e.g., cervical and lumbar disc herniations, bicipital tendinitis, bursitis, and arthritis.[19] Table 10–2 demonstrates referred pain patterns of TrPs that may be erroneously diagnosed as representing specific common orthopedic conditions. Preoperative muscle evaluation and treatment may avoid unnecessary surgery and will increase the success of surgery if it is necessary.[19]

After completion of the history and physical examination, appropriate laboratory work may be indicated, depending on the findings and the area of the body to be treated. Basic laboratory work-up may include blood chemistries, complete blood count (CBC), sedimentation rate, urinalysis, triiodothyronine (T_3) and thyroxine (T_4) radioimmunoassays, and serum levels of vitamins B_1, B_6, B_{12}, folic acid, and vitamin C if vitamin deficiency is suspected as a cause of TrPs.[76] Routine roentgenograms and further studies include computed tomography (CT) scans, magnetic resonance imaging, myelograms, or electrical diagnostic studies. Consultation may include neurologic, rheumatologic, psychological, orthopedic, and, less frequently, vascular when arterial disease must be ruled out (e.g., Leriche's syndrome as a cause of buttock and leg pain). There are no abnormal routine laboratory findings or radiographic studies diagnostic of regional MPS.

References

1. Avleciems LM: Myofascial pain syndrome: A multidisciplinary approach. Nurse Pract 20(4):18, 21–22, 24–28, 1995.
2. Borg-Stein J, Stein J: Trigger points and tender points: One and the same? Does injection help? 22(2):305–322, 1996.
3. Carlson CR, Okenson JP, Falace DA, et al: Reduction of pain and EMG activity in the masseter region by trapezius trigger point injection. Pain 55(3):337–340, 1993.
4. Cimino R, Michelotti A, Stadi R, Farinaro C: Comparison of clinical and psychologic features of fibromyalgia and masticatory myofascial pain. J Orofac Pain 12:35–41, 1998.

°See references 3, 6, 33, 34, 44, 45, 47, 49, 68, 74–77.

5. Dao TT, Knight K, Ton-That V: Modulation of myofascial pain by the reproductive hormones: a preliminary report. J Prosthet Dent 79(6):663–670, 1998.
6. DeJung B: Manual trigger point treatment in chronic lumbosacral pain. Schweiz Med Wochenschr Suppl 62:82–87, 1994.
7. Delany GA, McKee AC: Inter- and intra-rater reliability of the pressure threshold meter in measurement of myofascial trigger point sensitivity. Am J Phys Med Rehabil 72(3):136–139, 1993.
8. Donaldson CC, Nelson DV, Schulz R: Disinhibition in the gamma motoneuron circuitry: A neglected mechanism for understanding myofascial pain syndromes? Appl Psychophysiol Biofeedback 23(1):43–57, 1998.
9. Feinberg B, Feinberg R: Resistant pain after total knee arthroplasty: Treatment with manual therapy and trigger point injections. J Musculoskeletal Pain 6(4):85–95, 1998.
10. Fischer AA: Tissue compliance meter for objective, quantitative documentation of soft tissue consistency and pathology. Arch Phys Med Rehabil 68:122–124, 1987.
11. Fischer AA: Advances in documentation of pain and soft tissue pathology. Medical Times, The Journal of Family Medicine, December 1983, pp 24–31.
12. Fischer AA: Diagnosis and management of chronic pain in physical medicine and rehabilitation. In Ruskin AP (ed): Current Therapy in Physiatry: Physical Medicine and Rehabilitation. Philadelphia, WB Saunders, 1984.
13. Fischer AA: Myofascial pain and fibromyalgia, trigger point management. In Rachlin ES (ed): Myofascial Pain and Fibromyalgia. St. Louis, Mosby, 1994.
14. Fischer AA: Pressure algometry (dolorimetry) in the differential diagnosis of muscle pain. In Rachlin ES (ed): Myofascial Pain and Fibromyalgia. St. Louis, Mosby, 1994.
15. Fischer AA: Introduction: Pressure algometry in quantification of diagnosis and treatment outcomes. J Musculoskeletal Pain 6(1):1–29, 1998.
16. Fischer AA: Treatment of myofascial pain. J Musculoskeletal Pain 7(1/2):131–142, 1999.
17. Fishbain DA, Goldberg M, Meagher R, et al: Male and female chronic pain patients categorized by DSM-III psychiatric diagnostic criteria. Pain 26:181–197, 1986.
18. Fishbain DA, Goldberg M, Steele R, et al: DSM-III diagnoses of patients with myofascial pain syndrome (fibrositis). Arch Phys Med Rehabil 70:433–438, 1989.
19. Flax HJ: Myofascial pain syndrome—the great mimicker. Bol Asoc Med P R 87(10–12):167–170, 1995.
20. Fricton JR: Clinical care for myofascial pain. Dent Clin North Am 35:1–26, 1991.
21. Fricton JR: Myofascial pain. Baillieres Clin Rheumatol 8(4):857–880, 1994.
22. Fricton JR: Etiology and management of masticatory myofascial pain. J Musculoskeletal Pain 7(1/2):143–160, 1999.
23. Fricton JR, Awad EA (eds): Advances in Pain Research and Therapy, vol 17. New York, Raven, 1990.
24. Gerwin RD: Neurobiology of the myofascial trigger point. Baillieres Clin Rheumatol 8(4):747–762, 1994.
25. Gerwin RD: A study of 96 subjects examined both for fibromyalgia and myofascial pain. J Musculoskeletal Pain 3(Suppl. 1):121, 1995.
26. Gerwin RD: Myofascial pain syndrome in the upper extremity. J Hand Ther 10(2):130–136, 1997.
27. Gerwin RD: Myofascial pain syndromes (MPS) and fibromyalgia (FM):Misdiagnosis and mistreatment—challenge to the fibromyalgia community. Presentation at the Janet Travell Seminar Series—Focus on Pain '98, March 12–15, 1998, San Antonio, Texas.
28. Gerwin RD: Myofascial trigger points in chronic cervical whiplash syndrome [abstract]. J Musculoskeletal Pain 1998; 6(Suppl. 2):28, 1998.
29. Gerwin RD, Shannon S, Hong CZ, et al: Interater reliability in myofascial trigger point examination. Pain 69(1–2):65–73, 1997.
30. Gil IA, Rizatti Barbosa CM, Moteiro Pedro V, et al: Multidisciplinary approach to chronic pain from myofascial pain dysfunction syndrome: A four year experience at a Brazilian center. J Craniomandibular Practice 16(1):18–25, 1998.
31. Good MG: Rheumatic myalgias. Practitioner 146:167–174, 1941.
32. Granges G, Littlejohn G: Prevalence of myofascial pain syndrome in fibromyalgia syndrome and regional pain syndrome: A comparative study. J Musculoskeletal Pain 1(2):19–35, 1993.
33. Gutstein M: Diagnosis and treatment of muscular rheumatism. Br J Phys Med 1:302–321, 1938.
34. Hong CZ: Lidocaine injection versus dry needling to myofascial trigger point: The importance of the local twitch response. Am J Phys Med Rehabil 73(4):256–263, 1994.
35. Hong CZ: Algometry in evaluation of trigger points and referred pain. J Musculoskeletal Pain 6(1):47–59, 1998.
36. Hong CZ, Kuan Ta-Shen, Chen JT, Chen SM: Referred pain elicited by palpation and needling of myofascial trigger points: A comparison. Arch Phys Med Rehabil 78:57–60, 1997.
37. Hopwood MB, Abram SE: Factors associated with failure of trigger point injections. Clin J Pain 10(3):227–234, 1994.
38. Hsieh CY, et al: Interexaminer reliability of the palpation of trigger points in the trunk and lower limb muscles. Arch Phys Med Rehabil 81(3):258–264, 2000.
39. Hubbard DR: Getting tension. Biofeedback Winter:14–15, 21, 1996.
40. Hubbard DR: Chronic and recurrent muscle pain: Pathophysiology, treatment, and review of pharmacologic studies. J Musculoskeletal Pain 4(1/2):123–143, 1996.
41. Imamura ST, Fischer AA, Imamura M, et al: Pain management using myofascial approach when other treatments failed. Phys Med Rehabil Clin North Am 8:179–196, 1997.
42. Imamura ST, Riberto M, Fischer AA, et al: Successful pain relief by treatment of myofascial components

in patients with hip pathology scheduled for total hip replacement. J Musculoskeletal Pain 6(1):73–89, 1998.

43. Jaeger B, Reeves JL: Quantification of changes in myofascial trigger point sensitivity with the pressure algometer following passive stretch. Pain 27:203–210, 1986.

44. Kellgren JH: A preliminary account of referred pains arising from muscle. BMJ 2:325–327, 1938.

45. Kellgren JH: Observations on referred pain arising from muscle. Clin Sci 3:175–190, 1938.

46. Kraus H: Pseudo-disc. South Med J 60:416–418, 1967.

47. Kraus H: Clinical Treatment of Back and Neck Pain. New York, McGraw-Hill, 1970.

48. Kraus H (ed): Diagnosis and Treatment of Muscle Pain. Chicago, Quintessence, 1988.

49. Lang M: Die Muskelhärten (Myogelosen). Munich, Lehmann, 1931.

50. Ling FW, Slocumb JC: Use of trigger point injections in chronic pelvic pain. Obstet Gynecol Clin North Am 20(4):809–815, 1993.

51. Marini I, Fairplay T, Vecchiet F, Checci L: The treatment of trigger points in the cervical and facial area. J Musculoskeletal Pain 7(1/2):239–245, 1999.

52. Melzack R, Stillwell DM, Fox EJ: Trigger points and acupuncture points for pain: Correlations and implications. Pain 3:3–23, 1977.

53. Moldofsky H (chairman): Workshop on sleep studies. Am J Med 81(Suppl. 3A):107–109, 1986.

54. Moldofsky H: Sleep and musculoskeletal pain. Am J Med 81(Suppl. 3A):85–89, 1986.

55. Moldofsky H, Scarisbrick P, England R, et al: Musculoskeletal symptoms and non-REM sleep disturbance in patients with "fibrositis syndrome" and healthy subjects. Psychosom Med 37:341–351, 1975.

56. Nice DA, Riddle DL, Lamb RL, et al: Intertester reliability of judgments of the presence of trigger points in patients with low back pain. Arch Phys Med Rehabil 73:893–898, 1992.

57. Njoo KH, Van der Does E: The occurrence and inter-rater reliability of myofascial trigger points in the quadratus lumborum and gluteus medius: A prospective study in non-specific low back pain patients and controls in general practice. Pain 58(3):317–323, 1994.

58. Pontinen PJ: Reliability, validity, reproducability of algometry in diagnosis of acute and latent tender spots and trigger points. J Musculoskeletal Pain 6(1):61–71, 1998.

59. Rachlin ES: Musculofascial pain syndromes. Medical Times, The Journal of Family Medicine, January 1984:34–37.

60. Rachlin ES: The importance of trigger point management in orthopedic practice. Phys Med Rehabil Clin North Am 8(1):171–177, 1997.

61. Rachlin ES, Kraus H: Management of back pain. Intern Med 8:1987.

62. Reynolds MD: Myofascial trigger point syndromes in the practice of rheumatology. Arch Phys Med Rehabil 62:111–114, 1981.

63. Sarno J: The Mind Body Prescription: Healing the Body, Healing the Pain. New York: Warner Books, 1998.

64. Sella GE: Surface EMG in the investigation and treatment of myofascitis. Presentation at the Janet G. Travell Seminar Series—Focus on Pain '98, March 12–15, 1998, San Antonio, Texas.

65. Simons DG: Fibrositis/fibromyalgia: A form of myofascial trigger points? Am J Med 8(Suppl. 3A):93–98, 1986.

66. Simons DG: Examining for myofascial trigger points. Arch Phys Med Rehabil 74:676, 1993.

67. Simons DG: Myofascial trigger points: The critical experiment. J Musculoskeletal Pain 5(4):113–118, 1997.

68. Simons DG, Travell TG, Simons LS: Myofascial Pain and Dysfunction. The Trigger Point Manual, vol 1, 2nd ed. Baltimore, Williams & Wilkins, 1999.

69. Sola AE: Trigger point therapy. In Roberts JR, Hedges JR (eds): Clinical Procedures in Emergency Medicine. Philadelphia, WB Saunders, 1985, pp 674–686.

70. Sola AE, Kuitert JH: Myofascial trigger point pain in the neck and shoulder girdle. Northwest Med 54:980–984, 1955.

71. Sola AE, Rodenberger MS, Gettys BB: Incidence of hypersensitive areas in posterior shoulder muscles: A survey of two hundred young adults. Am J Phys Med 34:585–590, 1955.

72. Sonkin LS: Myofascial pain in metabolic disorders. In Kraus H (ed): Diagnosis and Treatment of Muscle Pain. Chicago, Quintessence, 1988, pp 91–95.

73. Teresa M, Jacob RJ, Jacob LG, et al: Myofascial pain impairing the results of carpal tunnel syndrome surgery [abstract]. J Musculoskeletal Pain 6(Suppl. 2):43, 1998.

74. Travell J, Rinzler SH: The myofascial genesis of pain. Postgrad Med 11:425–434, 1952.

75. Travell JG, Simons DG: Myofascial Pain and Dysfunction: The Trigger Point Manual. Baltimore, Williams & Wilkins, 1983.

76. Travell JG, Simons DG: Myofascial Pain and Dysfunction: The Trigger Point Manual, vol 2, The Lower Extremities. Baltimore, Williams & Wilkins, 1992.

77. Tschopp KP, Gysin C: Local injection therapy in 107 patients with myofascial pain syndrome of the head and neck. Otorhinolaryngol Relat Spec 58(6):306–310, 1996.

78. Wolfe F, Simons DG, Fricton J, et al: The fibromyalgia and myofascial pain syndromes: A preliminary study of tender points and trigger points in persons with fibromyalgia, myofascial pain syndrome and no disease. J Rheumatol 19:944–951, 1992.

79. Wreje U, Brorsson B: A multicenter randomized controlled trial of injections of sterile water and saline for chronic myofascial pain syndromes. Pain 61(3):441–444, 1995.

Chapter 11

Trigger Point Management

Edward S. Rachlin, MD ▪ Isabel Rachlin, PT

Indications for Trigger Point Injection

Not all trigger points (TrPs) require needling. Many active TrPs may respond to a physical therapy program (see Chapters 16–19). This is especially true in the early stages of TrP formation (the neuromuscular dysfunctional stage) prior to the development of fibrotic pathologic changes (the dystrophic stage) (Fig. 11–1). Trigger point injection and needling is the most effective and best treatment in cases of chronic TrPs with fibrotic scar formation. Trigger point injection is indicated in patients who have symptoms and findings consistent with active TrPs (TrPs causing symptoms).[31] Latent TrPs are asymptomatic and do not require treatment by injection. Latent TrPs may cause muscle stiffness and weakness, which often is not noticed by the patient. They are often found on routine examination in asymptomatic persons as incidental findings.[75] Latent TrPs may be addressed with massage, postural re-education, ergonomic correction, and exercise to help prevent them from becoming active TrPs.

To be considered for injection, TrPs should be reasonably limited in number and suitable for injection therapy. Multiple tender points and TrPs found in patients suffering from fibromyalgia or endocrine disturbances are not suitable for initial TrP injection therapy. Evaluation and treatment are indicated before considering TrP injection (see Chapter 10). After several weeks of endocrine therapy the patient is re-evaluated to determine which tender spots or TrPs remain. The finding of tenderness in itself is not an indication for TrP injection. The significance of tenderness requires an understanding of the total clinical context (see Chapter 9 under Definition and Types of Trigger Points). Patients with fibromyalgia may also have myofascial pain TrPs. It is not unusual to find both conditions coexisting. In a 1996 study, Hong and Hsueh compared the use of TrP injections for patients who had TrPs and fibromyalgia concurrently, and for those with only TrPs. They found that the TrP-only group had greater pain relief immediately following injections and that the group with fibromyalgia was likely to experience more postinjection soreness and for a longer duration.[33] In treating pain due to TrPs, it is not always necessary to require the finding of a taut band and local twitch response with a referred pain pattern on palpation to determine that injection is appropriate. (However, accurately palpating a taut band and TrP will increase the likelihood of successful treatment.) Depending on the total clinical context, the finding of tender points in the classic areas of TrP locations coinciding with the patient's complaints, together with a "jump sign," is sufficient to justify TrP injection. In cases of referred pain, it is not sufficient to inject only the TrP in the referred pain area (zone of reference). The primary TrP causing the pain must be found and treated to obtain a lasting result (see Fig. 10–4 and Table 10–2).

Active TrPs will usually require treatment before the patient is placed on an exercise program that engages the involved muscles. Exercise in the presence of TrPs may activate symptoms. However, pain-free movement including pain-free aerobic exercise is encouraged and can be helpful. A noninvasive therapeutic approach including physical therapy modalities (see Chapter 19), soft tissue mobilization techniques (see Chapters 16–18), an exercise program, and lifestyle changes may be tried prior to injection therapy. The post–TrP injection follow-up program described later is recommended as a conservative therapeutic treatment approach. Active exercise is a vital part of the treatment program to achieve therapeutic results and prevent recurrences.[22] The patient may respond favorably to any or all of the physical therapy

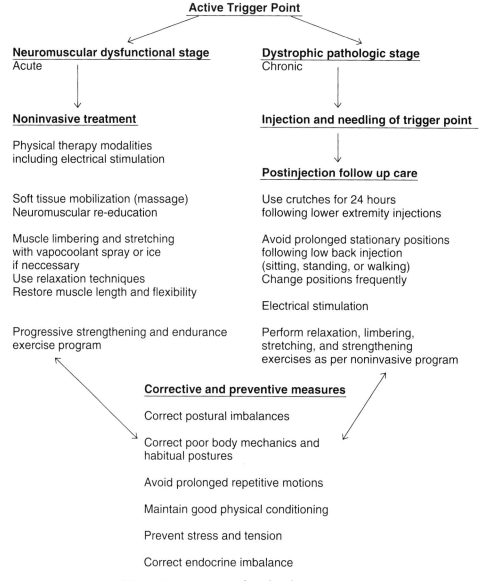

Figure 11–1. Treatment of myofascial trigger point.

techniques. *Injection and needling of TrPs is a beginning, not an end, to therapy.* It enables the patient to begin a therapeutic exercise program, which must be incorporated in a comprehensive treatment plan for the management of myofascial pain (Fig. 11–2).

To quote Hans Kraus from later in this text (Chapter 15), "It is obvious that injections alone will not help a person who has no physical outlet [for stress], exhibits weakness and stiffness of key postural muscles, and leads a tension-filled life." The practice of utilizing TrP injection techniques has become increasingly popular and is now common in pain clinics throughout the world. It appears that many and probably most of these physicians do not prescribe a sufficient follow-up program or address etiologic factors, particularly in the realm of stress, tension, and lifestyle. Without the attention to the whole person, results, at best, will be temporary. Physicians who intend to or already do TrP injections should read Chapter 15 in particular, as well as the other chapters in Part III of this book.

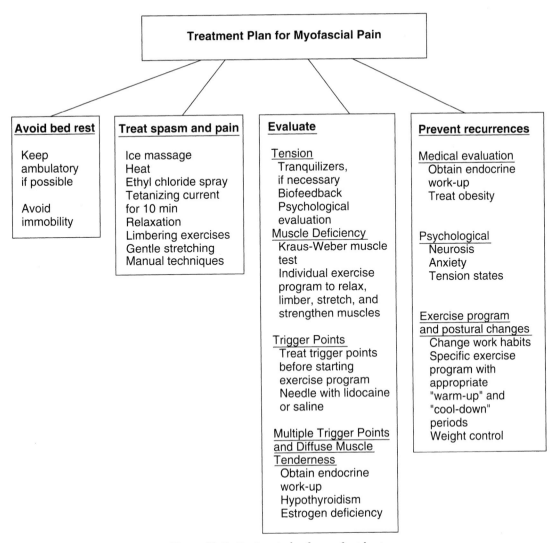

Figure 11–2. Treatment plan for myofascial pain.

Contraindications to Trigger Point Injection

- Do not inject in the presence of systemic or local infection.
- Do not inject patients with bleeding disorders or patients on anticoagulants without proper medical evaluation and control.
- Avoid injections in patients who are pregnant.
- Avoid injections in patients who appear to be or feel ill.

Reasons for Failure in Trigger Point Injection

- Success in TrP injection is optimized by the ability of the patient to receive proper postinjection follow-up care (see later discussion). Injection of ligamentous TrPs does not require the follow-up TrP injection program because ligamentous TrPs do not cause the muscle spasm that is often seen after muscular TrP injection.
- Patients with multiple TrPs due to endocrine disturbance (e.g., hypothyroidism [see Chapter 4] or fibromyalgia [see Chapters 1 and 2]) should receive appropriate

systemic care and be re-evaluated before any local injections to relieve symptoms are attempted.

- Do not inject while muscles are in spasm. Muscular TrPs cannot be properly diagnosed in the presence of muscle spasm. Muscle spasm must first be treated (see later discussion for follow-up management of TrP injections, and Chapters 16 and 19 for the treatment of muscle spasm). Palpation of TrPs becomes possible after muscle relaxation is achieved.
- Emotionally unstable patients do not respond well to surgically invasive procedures[44] and are also unpredictable. Some patients receive no relief whereas others become addicted to all forms of treatment and request repeated injections, always receiving some relief but never enough to discontinue treatment. This type of treatment requires both professional judgment and integrity as to whether to start treatment and how long to continue it. Decisions may sometimes be clearer after a short period of treatment. (Temporary relief in some patients may be explained by a placebo effect associated with all medical therapies, including TrP injection.)
- Patients with low pain thresholds will usually find the experience very tension-provoking and will not do well. Tranquilizers (diazepam [Valium]) may be tried prior to injection.
- When possible, do not inject more than one TrP area at a time. For example, inject the gluteal and lumbar areas on separate visits. Multiple site injections covering many areas may cause muscle spasm and irritation, which interfere with muscle rehabilitation.
- Tenderness in the referred pain area may represent secondary TrPs or satellite TrPs and not the primary TrPs causing the patient's symptoms. Limiting injections to TrPs in the referred pain area and omitting the primary TrP will give only temporary relief. Conversely, after the primary TrP has been treated, TrPs in neighboring muscle groups and antagonist muscle groups need to be addressed for total pain relief.
- Do not use procaine or lidocaine in patients who are allergic to these drugs. Avoid aspirin-like drugs 1 week prior to injections.
- Avoid inadequate medical work-up, e.g., omitting radiographs or other tests necessary for proper diagnosis.
- Avoid using needles that are too thin or too short to accomplish TrP needling.
- Patients who are involved in litigation may show poor results of treatment.
- Patients taking calcium channel blockers may not respond to TrP injections (although electrical stimulation, superficial heat, and massage may be useful). Further studies are needed on this subject.[72]
- Pre-existing factors that may significantly affect treatment outcome include lack of employment due to pain at the time of treatment, prolonged duration of pain, constant pain, lack of relief from analgesic medication, changes in social activity, and lower levels of coping ability.[34]

Trigger Point Injection Technique

Equipment

The basic equipment for TrP injection includes the following (Fig. 11–3):

- Povidone-iodine (Betadine).
- Sterile gauze pads, 4 × 4 in.
- Forceps.
- Clamp.
- Needles:
    16-gauge 1.5-in. for withdrawal of anesthetic solution.
    22- to 25-gauge 1.5-in. for scalenus and sternocleidomastoid muscles, and interossei.
    25-gauge 1.5-in. for temporomandibular joint muscles.
    22-gauge 1.5-in. for cervical and suboccipital areas, upper extremities, and ankle and foot.

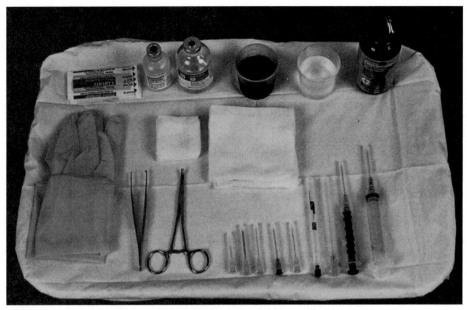

Figure 11–3. Basic equipment for trigger point injection includes sterile gloves, sterile gauze pads, forceps and clamp, povidone-iodine (alcohol may be used in addition), lidocaine, isotonic saline, vapocoolant spray, needles and syringes of various sizes, and Band-Aids. See text for details.

21-gauge 2.0-in. for extremities.

20- to 21-gauge 3-in. for lumbar and gluteal areas.

25-gauge 2.0-in. for gastrocnemius (a thinner gauge is used because of muscle sensitivity). If sterilization equipment is available, nondisposable needles and syringes may be used.

- A tray with sterile covering is used to hold syringes and needles of various sizes. These are determined depending on the muscle injected.
- Sterile gloves.
- Vaporized coolant spray (ethyl chloride or Fluori-Methane).
- Plastic strip bandages (Band-Aids).
- Solutions for injections: 0.5% procaine, 1% lidocaine, isotonic saline. Do not use epinephrine. Isotonic saline or dry needling may be used in patients who are allergic to local anesthetics. Steroids may be used for ligamentous TrPs.
- Procaine or lidocaine may be used for local anesthetic.

Procaine hydrochloride 0.5% (Novocain) exhibits the following characteristics:

1. Potent vasodilation.
2. Relatively high incidence of allergic reactions (typical of ester-type local anesthetics).
3. Short action.
4. Onset of action 6 to 10 minutes.
5. Lower systemic toxicity.

Lidocaine hydrochloride 1% (Xylocaine) exhibits the following characteristics:

1. Allergic reactions are virtually nonexistent (amide local anesthetic).
2. Rapid onset of action.
3. Longer duration than procaine.
4. Greater potency.
5. More profound anesthesia.

Long-acting anesthetics (e.g., bupivacaine) have also been used.

Dry Needling

The elimination of TrPs by needling depends mainly on the mechanical disruption of the TrP rather than the solution used during injection.[20] Dry needling is effective[11, 25, 50]; however, greater postinjection pain has been reported.[11, 32, 50, 56] The efficacy of treatment for both dry needling and injections has been found to be related to the intensity of pain produced at the trigger zone and the precision in needling the exact site of maximal tenderness.[11, 32] The immediate analgesia produced has been called the *needle effect*.[48]

Researchers have conducted studies in an attempt to find the most effective injection solution. In a 1996 study by Tschopp and Gysin comparing different types of injection solutions, they concluded that the type of solution was not significant and that pain relief was likely achieved by what they referred to as "reflex mechanisms" rather than by the pharmacologic agents injected.[79] In a study of 64 myofascial pain patients, 23 were injected with 5% dextrose water, 20 were injected with normal saline, and 21 were injected with 0.05% lidocaine.[41] At 7 days following injection, the dextrose water–injected group showed the best outcome. The researchers, Kim and associates, theorized that the effectiveness may be attributed to the glucose giving anaerobic metabolism in the area a boost, decreasing the local energy crisis, and possibly affecting uptake of excessive synaptic acetylcholine.[41] Based on a series of pharmacologic studies, Hubbard reported significant TrP pain reduction and elimination using noncompetitive alpha-blocker phenoxybenzamine. A study of 23 patients with TrP pain of head, neck, and shoulders found injections with 1% lidocaine significantly more effective than injections with saline solution or results in those receiving a sphenopalatine ganglion block.[19] Fischer considers needling combined with infiltration of a local anesthetic to be maximally effective and recommends that a pre-injection block be administered to desensitize the treated area to avoid causing the patient undue pain from the needling and injection treatment.[20] Fischer describes his technique of needling the entire taut band including its bony attachments. He observes that this method (with injection of anesthetic) produces immediate and long-term pain relief[20] (see Chapter 13).

A number of studies have shown botulinum toxin injection (botulinum neurotoxin type A) to be safe and effective with long-lasting positive results.[20, 64, 73, 83] Simons urges that the minimum amount necessary of this injection agent be used due to its ability to destroy normal end plates as well as dysfunctional TrP end plates.[74]

Steps in Injection Technique

The operator should communicate with the patient. Inform the patient that pain is to be expected when a TrP is encountered and explain the importance of indicating when pain is felt. The use of local anesthetic provides a short period of pain relief following the injection; it is not used to avoid the feeling of pain when the TrP is encountered. Although TrPs may sometimes be felt with the tip of the needle as hard nodules and fibrotic areas, we depend on the patient's reaction to confirm the contact with a TrP. A needle inserted into normal tissue will not normally cause complaints of pain. Patients readily learn to distinguish between the sensation in normal muscle and the pain felt when a TrP is encountered. Most of the time patients will tell their physician whether a TrP has been encountered. Pain may be experienced locally in addition to referred pain.

The patient is positioned comfortably. The position will depend on the muscle to be injected. It is best to do injections with the patient lying down. Vasodepressor syncope (fainting) can occur during or after local anesthetic injection. Advising the patient to take deep breaths in and out and to concentrate on breathing during the injection will help in decreasing pain sensation and promote relaxation. Communicate with the patient during the injection. In unusual cases, relaxation techniques, self-hypnosis, or tranquilizers (diazepam) to relax the patient sufficiently for TrP injection may be necessary.

Identify the primary TrP and bony landmarks. It is important to know the anatomy of the area to perform the injections properly and avoid complications. Distinguish between primary TrPs and TrPs in referred pain areas. Frequently, multiple TrPs are found involving neighboring muscles. The most symptomatic TrPs are injected first.

Trigger points in neighboring muscles may become symptomatic and require treatment after the primary TrP has been eliminated. When injecting more than one TrP or muscle group, a second TrP may be injected 2 days later while the patient is receiving follow-up care for the preceding TrP injection.

Trigger point injection is performed under sterile conditions. Sterile gloves are worn after surgical washing of the hands. Sterile gloves permit identification of TrPs by palpation after surgical preparation of the skin and immediately prior to injection. The ability to palpate the TrP avoids the necessity of scratching the skin with a needle to mark the TrP area. A sterile covered tray is used to receive instruments (clamps, syringes, needles, and sponges). An assistant opens the packages of sterile and selected syringes and needles and places them on the tray. Figure 11–4 shows the equipment used for TrP injection. When injection is performed, the sterile tray will contain only those needles and syringes that are to be used. It is best to keep syringes and needles out of the patient's sight. The skin is prepared with povidone-iodine using 4 × 4-in. gauze pads. The area of injection may be draped if necessary (Fig. 11–5). Be aware of the sterile area, which is demarcated by the povidone-iodine preparation. Do not violate sterility by touching the nonsterile surroundings.

The assistant holds the lidocaine bottle inverted; usually 10 mL of lidocaine is withdrawn (Fig. 11–6). Epinephrine should not be used.

Prior to injection, the assistant may spray a vaporized coolant sparingly on the site chosen for injection. An anesthetic spray decreases needle insertion pain, thereby decreasing the patient's anxiety and muscle tension prior to injection (Fig. 11–7). Avoid excessive use of the spray, which increases bleeding immediately following injection and may frost the skin. Fischer recommends the use of a pre-injection block to prevent pain caused by needle penetration and to improve long-term effect of the needle and injection treatment. He uses lidocaine (1%) and spreads it where the nerve enters the muscle along the taut band to be injected[20] (see Chapter 13). The use of sterile gloves permits palpation and the identification of TrPs immediately prior to injection and enables the physician to isolate the TrPs between two fingers (Fig. 11–8) or between the fingers and thumb (Fig. 11–9). A taut band may or may not be palpated. The patient is reminded to take slow, deep breaths and to inform the physician when pain is felt.

When a TrP is encountered, several milliliters of anesthetic are injected. Anesthetic should not be injected prior to the patient noting that a TrP has been encountered.

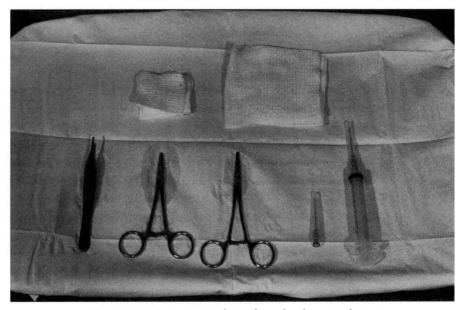

Figure 11–4. Instruments to be used are placed on a sterile tray.

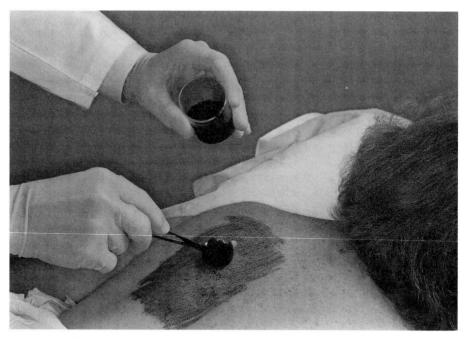

Figure 11–5. Skin is prepared with povidone-iodine using sterile technique. Provide a generous area of sterility.

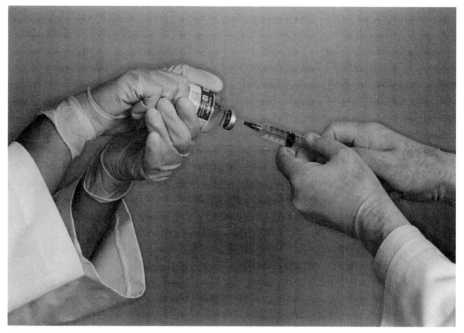

Figure 11–6. Assistant holds the lidocaine bottle inverted for aspiration of the anesthetic.

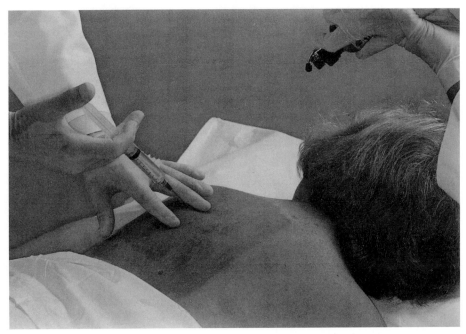

Figure 11–7. Application of a vapocoolant spray prior to injection decreases needle insertion pain.

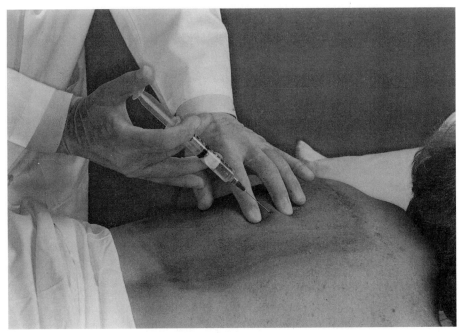

Figure 11–8. Injection of trigger point in the left rhomboids. Using sterile precautions, one may isolate the trigger point between the index and middle fingers.

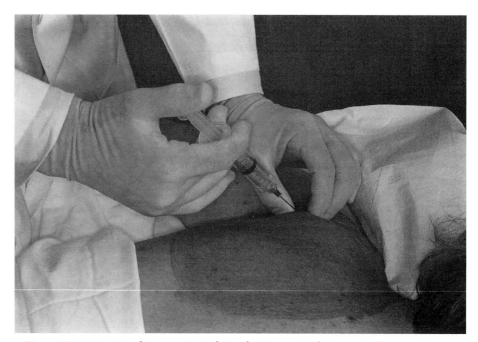

Figure 11–9. Injection of trigger point, isolating the trigger point between the fingers and thumb.

The patient may experience local or referred pain, or both. A muscle twitch is often seen when the TrP is struck. The trigger point may feel fibrotic. If the anesthetic is injected prematurely, TrPs will not be recognized. Palpation must be performed for additional areas of tenderness before concluding that all TrPs were found and injected. After injection and needling, the patient may quickly note relief of symptoms. When a "no-touch" sterile technique (no hand-to-skin contact) is used, two hands are required for injection. The stability of the syringe and needle is ensured by using forceps to hold the hub of the needle or syringe to control the depth and direction of needling. Sterility of the skin should not be violated (Fig. 11–10). The trigger point is marked with a needle scratch for identification prior to injection.

Technique of injection may include multiple entries into a single muscle using different entry points and/or using a single entry and withdrawing but not bringing the needle out of the skin, changing directions in a circular fan-like covering of the TrP area (Fig. 11–11). The needle is used in a probing fashion in search of additional TrPs. A combination of techniques can be used. Trigger points are most often found in the areas of origin and insertion (see Chapter 13 for Fischer's technique). The multiple dry needling technique resembles that used by Gunn[28] in treating muscle shortening and muscle spasm based on his theory of the neuropathic cause of myofascial pain. Gunn uses an acupuncture technique using acupuncture needles. Although the techniques appear to overlap, the concept and the objective are quite different.

Aspirate prior to injection. This is extremely important when the possibility of entering arteries and large veins or penetrating the chest cavity is present. The needle should be angled tangentially, not vertically, when injecting in the area of the chest wall to avoid entering the intercostal space (Fig. 11–12) (see later discussion of complications). A needle 1.0 to 1.5 in. long should be used when injecting the region of the chest wall. Do not inject if blood or bubbles are aspirated when injecting in the chest area. The needle depth should be well controlled and the syringe stabilized when injecting in the chest wall area. Stabilize the syringe by gently resting the hand holding the syringe on the patient. Hold the hub of the needle and syringe between the thumb and index finger while aspiration is performed. After aspiration, with the syringe and needle still stabilized in the same position, injection is performed. To avoid entering the chest cavity when injecting the trapezius, elevate the trapezius

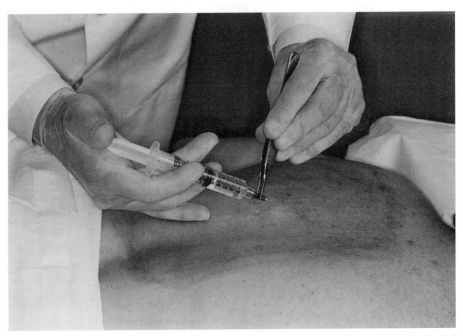

Figure 11–10. No-touch technique using forceps to control the stability, direction, and depth of the syringe and needle.

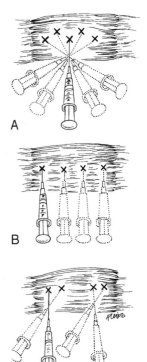

Figure 11–11. *A,* Single-entry injection using a circular fan-like covering of the trigger point area. *B,* Multiple separate needle entries for needling and injection. *C,* Combination of multiple needle entries and circular fan technique of individual trigger point area.

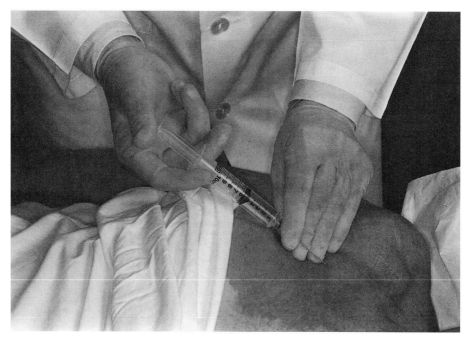

Figure 11–12. Injection of pectoralis muscles. Needle is directed tangentially in relationship to the chest cavity, avoiding the intercostal space. The syringe is stabilized with one hand to control the direction and depth of the needle once the trigger point is encountered. Aspirate prior to injection. Avoid pneumothorax.

muscle by grasping the muscle between the thumb, index, and middle fingers and gently lifting the muscle (Fig. 11–13). Aspirate prior to injections. The same technique is used for injection of the sternocleidomastoid muscle (Fig. 11–14). When one injects the quadratus lumborum and lumbosacral muscles, the needle should be directed parallel to the frontal plane of the patient or tangential to the patient (Fig. 11–15; see Fig. 12–1).

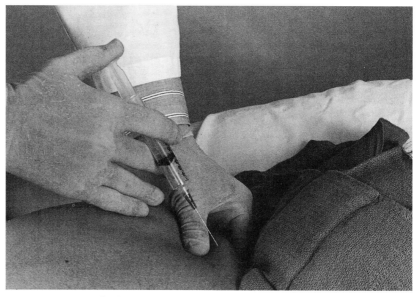

Figure 11–13. Injection of right trapezius muscle. Grasp the trapezius between the thumb and index finger, elevating the trapezius muscle to avoid puncturing the chest cavity (see Chapter 12).

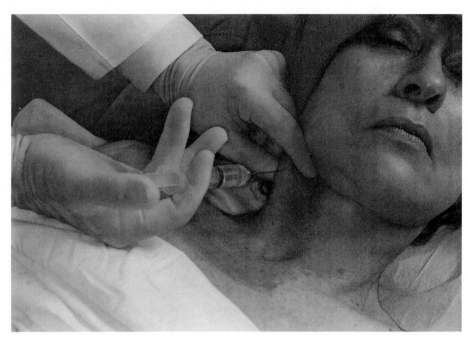

Figure 11–14. Injection of sternocleidomastoid muscle is performed by grasping the muscle between the thumb and index finger to localize the trigger point area and control localization of the needle. Aspirate prior to injection. Avoid the external jugular vein (see Chapter 12).

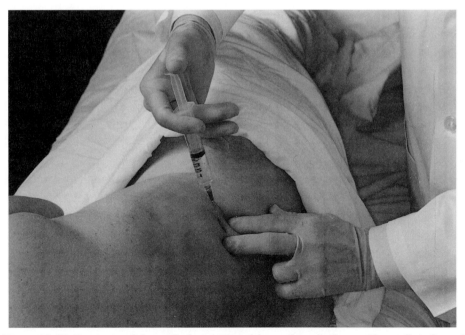

Figure 11–15. Positioning of the needle for injection of the quadratus lumborum. The needle is directed parallel or tangentially to the frontal plane of the patient.

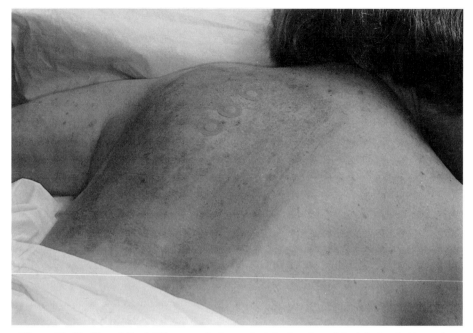

Figure 11–16. Shaped Band-Aids are applied over the injection sites of the left rhomboid muscles.

Do not inject if severe cramping pain is felt. Cramping pain is typical of radiculopathy and may represent a needle encountering a nerve.

If bleeding is encountered, remove the needle and apply pressure over the injected area to diminish hematoma formation.

Band-Aids are applied over each puncture area following the injection unless the patient is allergic to adhesives. Figure 11–16 shows a patient who has had TrP injections for the rhomboids.

Ice pack may be applied after injection to decrease needling pain and bleeding.

At this point inquire about unusual sensations, e.g., numbness, paresthesia, and muscle weakness, in the lower or upper extremities, depending on the injection given. The patient should remain on the treatment table for a few minutes following injection therapy.

For successful and lasting therapeutic results, the TrP injection is only the first step in relieving symptoms. The patient should be treated in physical therapy on 3 or 4 successive days following the TrP injection and adhere to the TrP follow-up program in its entirety (see later discussion).

The injection of muscle groups, rather than individual muscles, is usually performed; e.g., injection and needling of the gluteal area includes the gluteus maximus, minimus, and medius.

Injection for Ligamentous Trigger Points

Ligamentous TrP injections are given directly into the area of tenderness. Steroids are often used with a local anesthetic. The postinjection follow-up program is not necessary for ligamentous TrP injection. Although it is not usual to require physical therapy for muscle spasm following a ligamentous TrP injection, the conditioning of muscles and the use of physical therapy for both therapeutic purposes and prevention must not be overlooked.

Complications of Trigger Point Injections

Complications of TrP injections may be due to the side effects and reactions to local anesthetics or to injection technique.

Allergic Reaction to Local Anesthetics

The patient may develop hives, dermatitis, pruritus, bronchospasm, or anaphylaxis following the injection of local anesthetics. Most allergies are due to the *p*-aminobenzoic acid groups and the preservative methylparaben. The use of an amide-type local anesthetic without preservative, e.g., lidocaine, is recommended to avoid allergic reactions. Procaine is typical of an ester-type local anesthetic.[66]

Treatment

Treatment of an allergic reaction is as follows:

* Maintain ventilation and oxygenation.
* Give epinephrine 0.2 to 0.5 mL of 1:1,000 solution subcutaneously; a second injection may be needed.
* Epinephrine by intravenous (IV) infusion of 1:100,000 solution to treat hypotension.
* Antihistamine, e.g., diphenhydramine 50 to 80 mg intramuscularly (IM) or IV.
* Steroids.
* Atropine.

Prevention

The physician must take a history of any allergic condition. The history should include inquiries concerning allergy to local anesthetics and drugs, asthma, and food allergies. Perform a skin test if necessary. Use saline or dry needling technique if allergy is suspected.

Toxic Symptoms

Toxic symptoms are related to drug dose. Excessive local anesthetic cerebral blood levels may cause seizures. Toxic symptoms may include ringing in the ears and a feeling of tingling around the mouth and facial muscles. It is important to aspirate before injecting to avoid injecting into a vein or artery. Intravascular injection may be responsible for producing a toxic level of local anesthetic. The amount used in TrP injection should fall far below the maximum average dose for an adult. It is recommended that a maximum dose of lidocaine without epinephrine not exceed 300 mg. The dose should not exceed 2 mg/lb.[56] The average dose used for TrP injection is 5 to 10 mL.

Treatment

Seizures are treated by (1) maintaining ventilation and oxygenation, and (2) performing cardiopulmonary resuscitation if hypotension occurs.

Anaphylaxis

A systemic reaction due to hypersensitivity to local anesthetics may occur during the injection or moments afterward. The *symptoms* are urticaria, angioedema, wheezing, shortness of breath, hoarseness, tachycardia, and hypotension.

Treatment

Anaphylaxis is treated with:

* Epinephrine 0.2 to 0.5 mL of 1:1,000 solution subcutaneously with repeat doses at 3-minute intervals as necessary.
* Oxygen.
* IV fluids and volume expanders.
* Epinephrine IV 1:100,000 solution to treat hypotension.
* Aminophylline 0.25 to 0.5 g IV for bronchospasm.
* Corticosteroid IV.

Prevention

Prevention mandates careful history taking with respect to allergies, skin testing if necessary, and the use of saline or dry needling if there is a question of allergy.

Neuropathy

Neuropathic injuries may be due to local mechanical trauma from the needle or to a toxic reaction to injected medications. The nerve may be traumatized when nerve fibers are penetrated by the needle or when local anesthetics are injected intraneurally.[8] The paresthesia that may be obtained with TrP injection must be distinguished from the pattern of paresthesia of neural origin. Paresthesia due to TrPs is diffuse and nonspecific. In contrast, paresthesia or pain due to neural injury follows a specific nerve distribution; do not inject when these symptoms are present. A cramping pain may indicate injection into a nerve. If motor or sensory symptoms occur, obtain a baseline electromyography study, which will aid in determining a preexisting nerve abnormality. This can be compared with a study done after several weeks, if necessary.

Prevention

A knowledge of anatomy will prevent injecting of peripheral nerves. The risk of nerve injury is reduced if a short beveled needle is used instead of a standard long beveled needle.[66]

Hematoma Formation

Always aspirate before injections and when performing dry needling. Aspiration will alert the physician to an arterial or venous puncture. Do not inject if blood is withdrawn. Withdraw the needle and apply pressure to avoid bleeding. If an artery is punctured, apply only enough pressure to prevent bleeding without occluding the artery, so that the pulse can still be palpated. Maintain the pressure for 7 to 10 minutes. This will permit blood flow and enable the puncture wound to close. Complete occlusion of the artery will prevent blood flow, which is necessary for closure of the arterial puncture wound. Venous puncture wounds will close with compression that occludes the vein.

If a hematoma appears to be developing or is present, apply pressure to stop the bleeding and follow with ice and compression. If a large hematoma forms in the thigh with persistent swelling, follow-up radiographs should be taken after several weeks to determine if calcification of the hematoma has occurred.

Prevention

Needling should not be performed on patients who are on anticoagulants. A knowledge of anatomy is necessary to avoid arterial and venous structures.

Pneumothorax

Always aspirate prior to injection when injecting a TrP in the area of the chest wall. Aspiration of air bubbles into the syringe indicates a puncture of the pleural cavity. The syringe used, however, must have a tight-fitting, airtight attachment between the needle and the syringe. If air bubbles are encountered, injection is not performed.

Coughing or chest pain during the injection suggests that the pleura may have been punctured. An x-ray film should then be obtained. If a pneumothorax is present, it must be treated appropriately. Only a small number of pneumothorax cases require chest tube drainage. A small pneumothorax involving 10% to 25% of the pleural space may be asymptomatic and may not need treatment. In the case of a modest pneumothorax, the patient may develop tachycardia, restlessness, and diminished breath sounds on the affected side. Serial radiographs should be obtained to assess the progression of the pneumothorax. A tension pneumothorax may cause a collapsed lung and mediastinal shift. A tension pneumothorax may be life-threatening and requires emergency care, including chest tube insertion.

Although small pleural puncture wounds most often heal without specific treatment, recognition and observation are necessary to prevent extension of the opening in the pleura. The patient should avoid any strenuous activity.

Prevention

Always aspirate prior to injection. Observe if air bubbles are present in the syringe. Aspiration of blood will also indicate if the intercostal artery has been entered.

Angle the needle tangentially to the chest wall to avoid entering the intercostal space. Angle the needle in a caudal direction over the rib cage area to avoid injury to the intercostal artery as well as to the pleura. Do not direct the needle perpendicular to the chest wall (see Fig. 11–12 and earlier discussion of TrP injection technique).

Control the depth of the needle by holding the needle stationary with one hand resting on the patient's body for stability and injecting with the other (see Fig. 11–12). Debilitated patients present an additional risk. Patients who have thin chest walls are at high risk for pneumothorax; a small needle, e.g., a 22-gauge 1.5-in. short beveled needle, should be used in these patients.

Infection

Patients are instructed to report any signs of infection, including an increase in warmth, redness, swelling, and pain over the area of injection. Aspirate any collection of infected hematoma for culture and sensitivity prior to prescribing antibiotics. Incision and drainage of an abscess may be necessary.

Prevention

Avoid TrP injection in patients with systemic or local infections; use sterile technique; observe precautions in patients who are at high risk for infection, such as debilitated patients, patients on steroids, and diabetic patients.

Abdominal Puncture Wounds

Abdominal puncture wounds usually close without difficulties. Puncturing the rectosigmoid wall can cause infection. There is a risk of liver injury when injecting abdominal muscles, intercostal muscles, and the serratus posterior inferior muscle. There is a risk of kidney injury when injecting the quadratus lumborum muscle.

Needle Breakage

Do not insert the full length of the needle into the muscle when injecting. When probing for TrPs using a circular fanning technique (see Fig. 11–11), withdraw the needle to a more superficial plane without exiting the skin.

Patient Advice

Patients should be advised of the possible complications of TrP injection. The patient should be aware that although pain may be relieved almost immediately, more often pain and muscle soreness may persist for several days. Infection is a potential complication. The patient should be alerted to any signs of unusual swelling, progressive pain, and warmth and redness occurring in the area of the injection. These signs, together with temperature elevation, should alert the patient and physician to the possibility of infection. The patient should be reassured that areas of ecchymosis following injection are frequent and will be reabsorbed.

When more than one muscle or muscle group is to be injected, the next TrP may be injected 2 days later while the patient is receiving follow-up care for the preceding TrP injection. The patient is encouraged to increase vitamin C intake (by 500–1500 mg per day) for at least 3 days before and after injection to aid in tissue healing.

Physical Therapy Program for Follow-up Management of Trigger Point Injections (Noninvasive Therapy Program)

Therapeutic success following TrP injection depends on the ability to provide proper follow-up care,[6] and ultimate eradication of etiologic factors.[20, 23, 52, 74] The postinjection follow-up program and exercise regimen is based on the methodology of Dr. Hans Kraus.[44, 45] The physical therapy program outlined later is performed after injection and should be followed in its entirety. The same therapeutic program is used as a noninvasive treatment approach when TrP injection may not be necessary. Each injection should be followed by 3 to 4 successive days of physical therapy treatments to relax the muscles, avoid muscle spasm, and relieve postinjection pain. Therapy includes electrical stimulation, vaporized coolant spray and gentle limbering motions, and stretching techniques (active and passive) followed by an exercise program. Active motion is an important part of the stretching as well as the exercise program. Relaxation must be achieved prior to stretching.

The prevention and treatment of muscle spasm is a vital part of the physical therapy program and is the first objective to be addressed. The following principles should be observed[44]:

- Relief of pain.
- Gentle movements to achieve relaxation, flexibility, and normal muscle length.
- Do not pass the pain limit.
- Do not cause pain with movement.

Postinjection Physical Therapy Program

Electrical Stimulation

Electrical stimulation is given to relieve and prevent the muscle spasm that often follows TrP injection and needling. Electrical stimulation (sinusoidal current, surged, ramped) is administered for 15 minutes. If spasm is present when treating low back pain, precede the sinusoidal current with 10 minutes of tetanizing current to fatigue the muscle. Electrical stimulation also aids in treating postinjection hematoma and edema. Tetanizing current can enhance the production of β-endorphins for mild anesthesia in addition to muscle relaxation (see Chapter 19). Some patients find electrical stimulation uncomfortable, promoting tension rather than relaxation. These patients are best treated with moist heat. (Heat should be used with caution immediately after multiple TrP injections to prevent hematoma. Ice compresses may be used following TrP injection to prevent hematoma.) Electrical stimulation is used in preparation for exercise. Some practitioners have also found electrotherapy (electrical muscle stimulation and electrical nerve stimulation) to be a successful treatment of TrPs.[9]

Relaxation and Limbering

The patient is instructed to begin any exercise or stretching with relaxation. Deep, easy breathing and progressive relaxation techniques may be taught. Relaxation is followed by limbering movements which are simply gentle movements to warm up the muscles (i.e., active and active-assisted range of motion). Exercises are performed with or without the aid of vaporized coolant spray or ice to restore flexibility and range of motion. A coolant is sometimes necessary in the initial stage of therapeutic exercise and stretching. Moist heat may be applied beforehand for comfort.

Stretching

Progressive passive and active stretching is performed with or without vaporized coolant spray or ice to restore full muscle length and joint range of motion. Fischer and others also find the use of isometric contraction with reciprocal inhibition stretching helpful to achieve muscle relaxation for increased stretching.[20] Active and active-assisted stretching is an important part of the exercise program.

Spray and Stretch

Spray and stretch is an alternative noninvasive approach used in the treatment of TrPs and an excellent adjunct to follow-up care for TrP injection.[31, 43, 44, 79] A cold stimulus is used to provide hypoesthesia to a TrP area and an area of shortened muscle, thus allowing increased stretch with less pain. The spray and stretch is repeated until normal muscle length is attained. (Do not permit the area to become excessively cold.) It is the stretching rather than the coolant itself that directly helps to inactivate the TrP and obtain normal muscle length. Kraus[43] was the first to introduce the technique of vaporized coolant spray using ethyl chloride in muscle rehabilitation. He stressed the importance of exercise during and following the spray treatment ("spray and limbering").[46] Although ethyl chloride is the most effective vaporized coolant, it is not available in many institutions because of its flammable nature. The properties of the three most common coolants are summarized in Table 11–1. The procedure for the use of spray and stretch is as follows:

1. Assess the patient's movements and the direction of limited motion. Identify the shortened muscles and TrPs that are responsible for limitation in range of motion. Treat the primary TrPs and those in the referred pain area.

2. Position the patient so that he or she is comfortable with the body parts supported. The patient should be warm to avoid muscle spasm or tension due to chilling.

3. Stabilize one end of the muscle. One end of the muscle must be stabilized so that the other end can be both actively and passively stretched.

4. Apply the cold stimulus. Spray or ice should be applied over the length of the muscle at an even pace covering the entire muscle and referred pain areas while the muscle is passively and actively stretched to its end range within the patient's pain limit. Two to three layers of coolant may be applied. Continue steps 1 to 4 until normal muscle length has been reached, warming the area between applications. If ice is used, place plastic around the cube or "lollipop" to avoid dripping on the patient; wetness on the skin diffuses the cooling effect. Travell and Simons[78] provide specific instructions on how to apply vaporized coolant or ice. While the muscle is passively stretched, the coolant is administered in unidirectional parallel sweeps, applying it two to three times in the direction of the referred pain at a rate of 4 in./sec with the spray bottle held at a 30-degree angle 18 in. from the skin.[78] These exact details of application are not universally accepted. Most therapists will modify these guidelines. Full range of motion is achieved by encouraging active motion with the help of the spray beginning with limbering movements[46] in addition to passive stretch. Muscles

---

Table 11–1.
Common Coolants for Spray and Stretch Technique

Ethyl chloride
    1. Acts as a general anesthetic
    2. Colder than Fluori-Methane
    3. Flammable
    4. Potentially explosive when 4% to 15% of vapor is mixed with air
    5. Toxic vapor
Fluori-Methane
Not as cold as ethyl chloride
    1. Nonflammable
    2. Nonexplosive
    3. Contributes to the depletion of the ozone layer
Ice
    1. Nonflammable
    2. Nonexplosive
    3. Nontoxic
    4. More difficult to use correctly; can cause undesirable wetness on the skin

should be relaxed prior to stretching. Emphasis is placed on the patient's active movements.

Following the spray and stretch the patient should perform a few sets of five repetitions of active range-of-motion exercises with the treated part. The patient should also be instructed in stretching and active range-of-motion exercises to be done at home. At this stage some practitioners apply moist heat to increase muscle relaxation; others do not find this necessary.

The use of vaporized coolant or ice is contraindicated in the case of allergy or hypersensitivity to cold.

Joint Mobilization and Manipulation

If joint malalignment is contributing to myofascial pain, the joint should be manipulated to correct alignment.[47] Kuan and coworkers showed that manipulation of the cervical spine to treat facet joint dysfunction decreased associated TrPs.[47]

Massage

Massage and other manual physical therapy techniques are valuable modalities in the treatment of TrPs.[31, 65] These techniques are also used to facilitate muscle relaxation. Indications and techniques are described in Chapters 16–18.

Neuromuscular Re-education

Patients often suffer from myofascial pain and TrPs long after the precipitating cause is gone. The nervous system and unconscious are still guarding the area and still associating it with pain, maintaining a pain/tension cycle. The Trager® Approach of Psychophysical Integration and Mentastics® Movement Education[57, 76, 80] and the Feldenkrais Method and Awareness Through Movement®[18, 71] are two excellent approaches of neuromuscular re-education that may be utilized to interrupt recent or chronic patterns and re-educate the neuromuscular system to restore health.

Exercise Program

The following instructions outline the principles discussed in Chapter 15. The exercise program should be tailored to the individual patient's requirements. Test the patient for specific muscle weaknesses, flexibility, and signs of tension (Kraus-Weber exercises; see Chapter 15). Begin all exercise programs with relaxation and limbering of muscles prior to stretching and strengthening. Exercises must be done in a relaxed and unhurried manner. It is better to do fewer exercises unhurried than rush through the full exercise program.

Relaxation

Begin and end all therapy and exercise programs with relaxation. The patient should lie supine with pillows under the knees. Instruct the patient to close the eyes and take deep, slow breaths. The patient may rotate the head gently from side to side and then shrug the shoulders up while inhaling and let them drop while exhaling (see discussion of relaxation exercises in Chapter 15).

Exercises performed under tension will not promote the relaxation of muscles necessary for proper stretching. Each exercise is performed for only three to four repetitions. Excessive repetition promotes muscle stiffening and should be avoided. Exercises are added progressively. Do not give too many exercises in one session. Reverse the sequence of exercises so that all exercises are done for a total of six to eight repetitions, ending the exercise session with relaxation. Exercises are taught to the patient by the therapist and are performed with the help and guidance of the therapist during the physical therapy sessions. These exercises are to be performed and continued in a home program. The patient is not to be presented with a sheet of exercises without proper instruction on how they are to be performed. After the patient completes the exercise program and is symptom-free, he or she may progress to exercises promoting endurance and strength, which may include the use of free weights, Universal or Nautilus-type equipment, Pilates exercises, yoga, and so forth. The patient must be made aware that the ability to achieve relaxation and the performance of prescribed exercises are the most important aspect of the rehabilitation program. Exercises must be done regularly as described, beginning with warm-up exercises and ending with a cool-down. This is especially important prior to and after athletic activities to prevent injury and maintain the muscles in a relaxed, flexible, and normal length. Most athletic injuries occur as a result of muscle deficiency.

Corrective and Preventive Measures

The patient's education prior to discharge should include factors that precipitated and may continue to contribute to the patient's symptomatology.[20–22, 65, 74, 75] This may include adaptive changes in the workplace (see Chapter 20), changes in postural habits, and changes of a psychological and psychosocial nature (i.e., marital relationships, job dissatisfaction, depression or attitudinal factors) (see Chapters 5 and 6).[1, 23, 55] Corrective measures must be instituted to achieve therapeutic results and prevent recurrences (see Fig. 11–2).[36, 52, 75]

Frequency of Treatment

Trigger point injections may be given two times per week provided each injection can be followed by 3 to 4 successive days of physical therapy. Following the injection of all TrPs, the exercise program is continued until the patient can complete the full exercise program properly. A level of flexibility, strength, and endurance should be achieved prior to returning the patient to his or her occupation. This depends on the individual's requirements.

Patient Instructions

The patient is instructed as follows:

- Following injection for the lumbar and gluteal areas, the patient is instructed to avoid prolonged walking, sitting, or lying down. Positioning should be changed frequently after injections of TrPs. In the lower extremities, the patient should use crutches for 24 hours to avoid limping, pain, and muscle spasm. A sling may be used for the upper extremity.
- The patient should be aware that the immediate relief of pain may be temporary. Soreness may be present for 24 to 48 hours.
- The patient should be made aware of the possibility of infection following injection and is advised to report any unusual signs of infection such as pain, swelling, redness, or warmth.
- After TrP injection, other TrPs in neighboring muscles may become symptomatic. This appears as a "shifting-type pain," and is a common phenomenon. Secondary TrPs that produce symptoms require treatment.
- Patients should avoid traveling long distances to the treatment facility for follow-up physical therapy. Prolonged travel promotes muscle spasms and jeopardizes therapeutic results.
- The patient is to perform home exercises as directed.

The Use of Integrative Therapies in the Treatment and Prevention of Myofascial Pain and Chronic Pain Syndromes

With contributions by Mary F. Bezkor, MD, and Mathew H. M. Lee, MD

As physicians and health practitioners, it is our calling and responsibility to help alleviate people's suffering. Helping people feel better is what makes us feel good. Quite often the methods that we regard as "traditional" medicine do not meet the needs of our patients and they seek "alternative" therapies. It is estimated that the

Table 11–2.
Key Ingredients for Recovery and Health for Chronic Pain Patients

- Taking an active role in treatment and health maintenance.
- A healthy mental outlook and positive thinking.
- Necessary changes to:
  Behavior
  Habits
  Diet
  Surroundings
  that foster balance and health for that individual.
- Expression of emotions (i.e., through therapies, music, art, communication, etc.).
- Exercise—particularly aerobic exercise or disciplines that foster feelings of empowerment in one's body (i.e., martial arts, yoga, weight lifting, etc.).

number of visits to alternative medicine practitioners now exceeds those to conventional physicians.[42] A 1997 survey showed that 42.1% of Americans utilize therapies outside of mainstream medicine.[13, 17]

As a profession we can be eagerly learning about and utilizing all approaches that help our patients (i.e., injections, surgery, acupuncture, herbal medicine, and the like). Naturally, critical thinking should be used when evaluating alternative therapies, just as it should be when prescribing traditional treatments such as pharmaceuticals that may aid patients but can cause harm with long-term use.

The following sections discuss a number of modalities and topics that may be useful in the treatment and prevention of myofascial pain and chronic pain conditions.

Relaxation and Breathing

There are few things more beneficial to the body and mind than relaxation and full, expansive breathing.[4, 16] "Breathing patterns are a direct link to altering autonomic nervous system patterns, which in turn affect mood, feelings, and behavior."[24] It can be observed that most patients (and practitioners) do not breathe fully throughout the day. As we rush through the day, breathing may become shallow, and jaws and muscles may tighten. This type of everyday stress may eventually cause enough muscular tension to create pain (temporomandibular joint [TMJ] syndrome, headaches, TrPs) or to make one prone to injury. Encouraging our patients to take "breathe breaks" for a couple of minutes a few times a day helps to remind the nervous system to breathe more fully in general. It also reminds us, the practitioners, to do the same! A breathe break consists of a minute of deep breathing that allows the chest, ribs, abdomen, and back to expand fully (Fig. 11–17).

Relaxation prior to exercise is discussed earlier in this chapter, and Dr. Hans Kraus emphasizes the need for relaxation in healing the musculoskeletal system in Chapter 15. Numerous studies have documented the physiologic effects of relaxation and its efficacy in treating chronic pain.[4, 5, 16, 38]

Relaxation via recreation (fun) and vacation are vital to decrease stress and maintain health. Relaxation may also be derived through biofeedback, meditation, guided imagery and hypnosis, as well as exercise and expressive arts (see also Chapter 5).

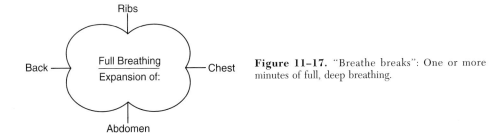

Figure 11–17. "Breathe breaks": One or more minutes of full, deep breathing.

Exercise

The physical and psychological benefits of exercise are well known, and the benefits to those with chronic muscle pain has been widely documented (see Chapters 2 and 16). Some of the benefits of exercise can include cardiovascular fitness, improved strength and flexibility, increased endurance for activities of daily living, improved self-esteem, improved relationship with spouse,[53] decreased depression, and weight management. Aerobic exercise can provide the release of endorphins. "Endorphins (endogenous morphine), through their connection to the hindbrain, are strong inhibitors of pain. Through their connection to the hypothalamus they may also have a calming effect on the overactive sympathetic nervous system [of those with fibromyalgia]. Vigorous exercise stimulates endorphin production within the central nervous system and in the periphery. The result is pain relief and a feeling of calm and relaxation."[40]* Aerobic exercise and disciplines that foster mind/body empowerment such as martial arts, Qi-gong, yoga, weight training, and core-conditioning may be particularly beneficial. The commitment to exercise and maintenance of exercise habits may be an essential component to wellness.

Diet/Food

It is essential for the neuromuscular system to have ample nutrition, including adequate vitamins, minerals, and protein. Lack of protein or other elements may cause fatigue, lethargy, and compromised immune response (e.g., to upper respiratory viruses).

Each individual responds differently to foods and has unique requirements. There is a growing awareness that many people suffer from food sensitivities and allergies that can cause or aggravate symptoms such as migraine headaches, muscle and joint pain and stiffness, fatigue, lethargy, and asthma.[7, 35, 44, 51, 58, 61] Wheat, chocolate, coffee, and dairy products are some of the foods to which there are common sensitivities. A diet containing refined sugar and many processed foods may also contribute to joint and muscle stiffness and fatigue.[7, 26, 58] It is hoped that more research will be done in this area so that physicians will be better educated to offer their patients insight into these factors.

To determine if a food is causing or increasing symptoms, a patient can simply omit that food from the diet (*completely*) for one or more weeks and then add it back in and observe the effects. This method is simple, cost-free, and has no side effects.[26, 35, 58] (Allergy testing is also available from specialists in environmental and food allergies.) The sensitivity to refined sugars and processed foods may be a significant factor for patients with fibromyalgia or complaints of stiffness and pain. To observe the effects of these foods, it is suggested that they be omitted from the diet for 2 weeks. Many patients may find they have increased energy and decreased symptoms when offending foods are removed from their diet.

Acupuncture and Chinese Herbal Medicine

Traditional Chinese medicine is the world's oldest continuous literal medical system. Although rooted in ancient texts, it is the result of several thousand years of clinical observation and testing.

Acupuncture is a technology for regulating the physiology of the human body. The placement of thin solid metal needles in specific locations in muscle tissue initiates a cascade of neuroendocrine effects.[12, 39, 63, 82, 84] Stimulation of acupuncture points has been demonstrated to change functional MR imaging in the associated brain areas. For example, stimulation of a point on the foot for improving vision increased glucose uptake in a precise location in the visual cortex of study subjects.[10]

Acupuncture is extremely useful for musculoskeletal pain syndromes because of its

---

*Contributions by Paul J. Kiell.

endorphin effects and ability to increase blood flow to myalgic muscle and fascia. Placement of acupuncture needles at the origin and insertion of muscles is a safe and painless way to eradicate TrPs and promote healing.

Chinese herbal medicine has several thousand years of written records documenting observation of clinical outcomes.[2] Plant, animal, and mineral substances are used in specific proportions to address the specific needs of the individual (as diagnosed by the Chinese medicine practitioner).

Chinese herbal remedies are widely used for the treatment of traumatic injuries and chronic pain syndromes, including fibromyalgia and arthritis. Several companies in the United States manufacture these formulations to high pharmaceutical standards that include testing for contamination by pesticides, bacteria, and heavy metals, and tableting by lot number for tracking. As herbal supplements have been more widely marketed, many herbs are available in health food and drug stores. These herbs are usually sold to consumers with little information on dosage or optimal interaction with other substances. Chinese herbal remedies are most appropriately prescribed by a practitioner with advanced training in this field.

Cupping is a fast, efficient, and painless method of alleviating muscle spasms used by Chinese medicine practitioners. Round glass cups are warmed and placed on the painful spasming muscles causing a small vacuum and "sucking" of the muscle at the mouth of the cup. This vacuum effect helps increase circulation in the muscles, ending the pain/spasm cycle. It is hoped that research will be conducted on this simple modality so that Western practitioners will become familiar with its use.

In most Asian countries today, effective traditional methods are used alongside Western technological advances, utilizing the best of both worlds to help patients.

Massage

Massage is not considered an alternative therapy in most parts of the world. In many European countries, massage is provided in orthopedic offices. (See Chapters 16–18 for detailed discussions of massage techniques.) Shiatsu and acupressure use manual pressure to stimulate points on the body that address the body through the Asian view of meridians (energy pathways in the body that, when out of balance, lead to illness and injury).

Manipulative Therapies

The fields of osteopathy, chiropractic, and physical therapy all utilize various manual techniques of spinal and extremity manipulation (also referred to as mobilization). Joint malalignment (e.g., facet joint impingement, shoulder subluxation) can cause muscle spasm, pain, TrPs, and increased sympathetic activity. Correction of articular dysfunction therefore corrects the underlying cause of the associated symptoms.[47, 54, 74]

Music Therapy

Most people can immediately relate to the therapeutic effects of music in their lives—the feeling of well-being that comes from listening to music or making music. Listening, singing, chanting, and playing an instrument can all contribute to relaxation, self-expression, and participation in a group. Manual dexterity, coordination, timing, and vocalizing are all therapeutic for many conditions. Music therapy[59, 67, 70, 81] has been employed for patients with neurologic or muscular conditions and is used during some medical and dental procedures.

Art Therapy

Art therapy also allows for creative and expressive release. It can be important to express feelings that may be difficult to describe or are suppressed. The use of different media allows for varied options in expression and manual execution. Music,

art, and dance allow for expression of the right side of the brain, which may access feelings and experiences in a different way than "left brain" activities such as speech and writing.

Dance Therapy

Dance combines movement, coordination, rhythm, timing, music, self-expression, and creativity.[15] It allows the patient to move in ways that can release tension from the body and mind and to release feelings of loss, anger, anxiety, and depression associated with chronic pain. Dance, and other expressive therapies, may also allow the expression of joy, which may be suppressed in people with chronic pain. Improved strength and flexibility may be outcomes of dance therapy.[62]

Pet Therapy

Pet therapy[14, 68] uses both domestic animals and helpers to deliver the therapeutic effects of companionship, love, and connection. Pets are helpful in relieving anxiety and loneliness that so often accompany the experience of chronic pain. An added benefit for dog owners is getting outdoors for a walk multiple times daily.

Horticulture Therapy

Planting, working the soil, and harvesting have been productive activities since the origin of agricultural-based society. Connection with the earth and feelings of accomplishment may have much to do with reports of pain relief found with this form of therapy. The process of growth is a positive image for recovery from the state of chronic pain.

Akin to horticulture therapy[30] (and environmental influences, see later discussion) are the benefits of being outdoors in nature. Many people respond positively to the beauty and serenity of the natural world. Being surrounded by the vibrancy of animals, plants, water, rocks, and sky is revitalizing. Getting outdoors regularly in the wintertime also exposes one to significantly increased quantities of light, which aids in the production of vitamin D, which helps calcium absorption and protection against osteoporosis, and may aid in decreasing depression related to lower light levels in the wintertime.

Environmental Influences

The effect of environment has long been recognized by corporations and institutions. The use of color, lighting, and air quality is often manipulated for increasing productivity and decreasing stress. Feng shui (wind and water) is the Chinese art that utilizes light, color, water, mirrors, and object placement to achieve tranquility, productivity, or other desired qualities. One does not necessarily need to use feng shui to notice that adjusting one's surroundings (e.g., adding windows, plants, changing wall color) can support positive moods and physical comfort. These factors can aid in alleviating muscular and mental tension.

Touch and Movement Therapies

There are dozens of named touch therapies including massage, craniosacral therapy, myofascial release, Rolfing, and so forth. Most of the these techniques emphasize treatment of the muscles and connective tissues. The physiologic effects of massage are described in Chapter 16.

Therapies that emphasize "energy work," such as Polarity, Reiki, and Therapeutic Touch (TT), are less researched and described in scientific terms. There are studies showing the positive effects of these therapies, which claim to heal through the use

of intentionally directed energy.[27, 54, 69] These techniques are popular in the culture and are increasingly used by nurses, physical therapists, and occupational therapists.

As described earlier in this chapter, therapies of movement re-education, such as the Trager® Approach, the Feldenkrais Method, and Aston Patterning, help to interrupt dysfunctional patterns in the neuromuscular system that facilitate postural imbalances, tension, and pain. Increased pain-free function and well-being can result from utilization of these approaches.

Each type of modality must be evaluated individually and, as with surgery or injection therapy, may only be as effective as the skill level of the practitioner employing the technique.

References

1. Arnoff GM: Myofascial syndrome and fibromyalgia: A critical assessment and alternative view. Clin J Pain 14:74–85, 1998.
2. Arnold MD, Thornbrough LM: Treatment of musculoskeletal pain with traditional Chinese herbal medicine. Phys Med Rehabil Clin North Am 10(3):663–672, 1999.
3. Avleciems LM: Myofascial pain syndrome: A multidisciplinary approach. Nurse Pract 20(4):18, 21–22, 24–28, 1995.
4. Benson H: Timeless Healing. New York, Scribner's, 1980.
5. Berman BM, Jonas W, Swyers: Issues in the use of complementary/alternative medical therapies for low back pain. Phys Med Rehab Clin North Am 9(2):497–511, 1998.
6. Borg-Stein J, Stein J: Trigger points and tender points: One and the same? Does injection help? 22(2):305–322, 1996.
7. Brosroff J, Callacombe SJ (eds): Food Allergy and Intolerance. Philadelphia, WB Saunders, 1987.
8. Carron H, Korbon GA, Rowlingson JC: Regional Anesthesia Techniques and Clinical Applications. Orlando, Fla, Grune & Stratton, 1984.
9. Cheng PT, Hsuen TC, Hong CZ: The immediate effectiveness of electrical muscle stimulation and electrical nerve stimulation on myofascial trigger points. Am J Phys Med Rehabil 76(2):162, 1997.
10. Cho ZH, Chuag SC, Jones JP, et al: New findings of the correlation between acupoints and corresponding brain cortices using functional MRI. Proc Natl Acad Sci USA 95(5):2670–2673, 1998.
11. Chu J: Does EMG (dryneedling) reduce myofascial pain syndromes due to cervical nerve root irritation? Electromyogr Clin Neurophysiol 37(5):259–272, 1997.
12. Coan R, Wong G, Coan PL: The acupuncture treatment of neck pain: A randomized controlled study. Am J Chin Med 9:326–332, 1982.
13. Comarow A: Going outside the medical mainstream: Can 42 percent of Americans be wrong? U.S. News & World Report November 23, 1998:83.
14. Connor K, Miller J: Animal-assisted therapy: An in-depth look. Dimens Crit Care Nurs 19(3):20–26, 2000.
15. Cotter AC: Western movement therapies. Phys Med Rehab Clin North Am 10(3):603–616, 1999.
16. Delmont MM: Biochemical indices associated with meditation practice: A literature review. Neurosci Biobehav Rev 9:557–561, 1985.
17. Eisenberg DM, Davis RB, Ettner SL, et al: Trends in alternative medicine use in the United States, 1990–1997. JAMA 280:1569–1575, 1998.
18. Feldenkrais M: Awareness Through Movement. New York, Harper & Row, 1977.
19. Ferran FM, Kaufman AG, Dunbar SA, et al: Sphenopalatine ganglion block for the treatment of myofascial pain of the head, neck, and shoulders. Pain Med 23(1):30–36, 1998.
20. Fischer AA: Treatment of myofascial pain. J Musculoskeletal Pain 7(1/2):131–142, 1999.
21. Flax HJ: Myofascial pain syndrome—the great mimicker. Bol Asoc Med P R 87(10–12):167–170, 1995.
22. Fricton JR: Myofascial pain. Baillieres Clin Rheumatol 8(4):857–880, 1994.
23. Fricton JR: Etiology and management of masticatory myofascial pain. J Musculoskeletal Pain 7(1/2):143–160, 1999.
24. Fritz S: Mosby's Fundamentals of Therapeutic Massage. St. Louis, Mosby, 2000.
25. Garvey TA, Marks MR, Wiesel SW: A prospective, randomized, double-blind evaluation of trigger-point injection therapy for low-back pain. Spine 14:962–964, 1989.
26. Golan R: Optimal Wellness. New York, Ballantine Books, 1995.
27. Gordon A, Merenstein JH, D'Amico F, et al: The effects of therapeutic touch on patients with osteoarthritis of the knee. J Fam Pract 47:271–277, 1998.
28. Gunn CC: Treating myofascial pain: Intramuscular stimulation (IMS) for myofascial pain syndromes of neuropathic origin. Seattle, University of Washington, 1989.
29. Gunn CC, Milbrandt WE: Tenderness at motor points: An aid in the diagnosis of pain in the shoulder referred from the cervical spine. J Am Osteopath Assoc 77:196–212, 1977.
30. Heliker D, Chadwick A, O'Connell J: The meaning of gardening and the effects on perceived well being of gardening project on diverse populations of elders. Activities, Adaptation & Aging 24(3):35–56, 2000.

31. Hong CZ: Considerations and recommendations regarding myofascial trigger point injection. J Musculoskeletal Pain 2(1):29–58, 1994.
32. Hong CZ: Lidocaine injection versus dry needling to myofascial trigger point: The importance of the local twitch response. Am J Phys Med Rehabil 73(4):256–263, 1994.
33. Hong CZ, Hsueh TC: Difference in pain relief after trigger point injections in myofascial patients with and without fibromyalgia. Arch Phys Med Rehabil 77(11):1161–1166, 1996.
34. Hopwood MB, Abram SE: Factors associated with failure of trigger point injections. Clin J Pain 10(3):227–234, 1994.
35. Hughes EC, Gott PS, Weinstein RC, Binggeli R: Migraine: a diagnosis test for etiology of food sensitivity by nutritionally supported fast and confirmed by long-term report. Ann Allergy 55:23–32, 1985.
36. Imamura ST, Fischer AA, Imamura M, et al: Pain management using myofascial approach when other treatments failed. Phys Med Rehab Clin North Am 8:179–196, 1997.
37. Jaeger B, Skootsky SA: Double blind, controlled study of different myofascial trigger point injection techniques [abstract]. Pain 31:S292, 1987.
38. Kabat-Zinn J, Lipworth L, Burney R: The clinical work of mindfulness—meditation for the self-regulation of chronic pain. Behav Med 8:163, 1985.
39. Kho HG, Robertson EN: The mechanisms of acupuncture analgesia: review and update. American Journal of Acupuncture 25(4):261–281, 1997.
40. Kiell PJ: Psychological benefits of exercise in the pain of fibromyalgia and myofascial pain disorders. Paper delivered to the American Association of Sports Medicine, July 22, 2000, New York.
41. Kim MY, Na YM, Kang SW, Moon JH: Myofascial trigger point therapy: Comparison of dextrose, water, saline, and lidocaine. Arch Phys Med Rehabil 78:1041, 1997.
42. Kraft GH: Foreword. Phys Med Rehab Clin North Am (10)3:xiii, 1999.
43. Kraus H: The use of surface anesthesia in the treatment of painful motion. JAMA 116:2582–2583, 1941.
44. Kraus H: Clinical Treatment of Back and Neck Pain. New York, McGraw-Hill, 1970.
45. Kraus H: Muscle deficiency. In Rachlin ES (ed): Myofascial Pain and Fibromyalgia. St. Louis, Mosby, 1994.
46. Kraus H, Fischer AA: Diagnosis and treatment of myofascial pain. Mt Sinai J Med 58:235–239, 1991.
47. Kuan TS, Wu CT, Chen SM, et al: Manipulation of the cervical spine to release pain and tightness caused by myofascial trigger points. Arch Phys Med Rehabil 78:1040–1041, 1997.
48. Lewit K: The needle effect in the relief of myofascial pain. Pain 6:83–90, 1979.
49. Little CH, Stewart AG, Fennessy MR: Platelet serotonin release in rheumatoid arthritis as studied in food intolerant patients. Lancet ii:297–299, 1983.
50. Malamed SF: Handbook of Local Anesthesia, ed 2. St Louis, Mosby-Year Book, 1986.
51. Mansfield LE, Vaughan ST, Walter, et al: Food allergy and adult migraine: Double-blind and mediator confirmation of an allergic etiology. Ann Allergy 55:126–129, 1985.
52. Marini I, Fairplay T, Vecchiet F, Checci L: The treatment of trigger points in the cervical and facial area. J Musculoskeletal Pain 7(1/2):239–245, 1999.
53. McCain G: Treatment of fibromyalgia and myofascial pain syndromes. In Rachlin ES (ed): Myofascial Pain and Fibromyalgia. St. Louis, Mosby, 1994.
54. McPartland J, Miller B: Bodywork therapy systems. Phys Med Rehab Clin North Am 10(3):583–602, 1999.
55. Monsein M: Disability evaluation and management of myofascial pain. In Rachlin ES (ed): Myofascial Pain and Fibromyalgia. St. Louis, Mosby, 1994.
56. Mulroy MF: Regional Anesthesia. Boston, Little, Brown, 1989.
57. Murphy J: Trager. Advance for Physical Therapists July 11, 1994:4.
58. Murray M, Pizzorno J: Encyclopedia of Natural Medicine, 2nd ed. Rocklin, CA, Prima Publishing, 1998.
59. Nagle JC, Lee MHM: On Music and Health. Brooklyn, NY, Elementary Media, 1999.
60. Nice DA, Riddle DL, Lamb RL, et al: Intertester reliability of judgments of the presence of trigger points in patients with low back pain. Arch Phys Med Rehabil 73:893–898, 1992.
61. Ortolani C: Atlas of mechanisms in adverse reaction to foods. Allergy 50(Suppl. 20):5–81, 1995.
62. Perlman SG, Connell KJ, Sinacore JM, et al: Dance-based aerobic exercise for rheumatoid arthritis. Arthritis Care and Research 3(1):29–35, 1990.
63. Pomeranz B: Scientific basics of acupuncture. In Stux G, Pomeranz B (eds): Acupuncture Textbook and Atlas. Berlin: Springer-Verlag, 1987.
64. Porta M, Valla P, Gamba M, Ferro MT: Muscle spasm, myofascial pain and treatment by botulinum toxin [abstract]. J Musculoskeletal Pain 2(Suppl.):54, 1998.
65. Rachlin I: Therapeutic massage in the treatment of myofascial pain syndromes and fibromyalgia. In Rachlin ES (ed): Myofascial Pain and Fibromyalgia. St. Louis, Mosby, 1994.
66. Raj PP: Handbook of Regional Anesthesia. New York, Churchill Livingstone, 1985.
67. Reilly CM: Relaxation: A concept analysis. Graduate Research Nursing 2(1):11, 2000.
68. Roenke L, Mulligan S: The therapeutic value of the human-animal connection. Occupational Therapy in Health Care 11(2):27–43, 1998.
69. Rosa L, Rosa E, Sarner L, et al: A close look at therapeutic touch. JAMA 279:1005–1010, 1998.
70. Schorr JA: Music and pattern change in chronic pain. ANS Adv Nurs Sci 15(4):27–36, 1993.
71. Shaeferman S: Awareness Heals: The Feldenkrais Method for Dynamic Health. Reading, Mass, Perseus Books, 1997.
72. Shenoi R, Willibald N: Trigger points related to calcium channel blockers. Muscle Nerve February 1996: 256.

73. Silberstein S, Mathew N, Saper J, Jenkins S: Botulinum toxin type A as a migraine preventive treatment. Headache 40(6):445–450, 2000.
74. Simons DG, Travell TG, Simons LS: Myofascial pain and dysfunction. The Trigger Point Manual, vol 1, 2nd ed. Baltimore, Williams & Wilkins, 1999.
75. Sola AE, Rodenberger MS, Gettys BB: Incidence of hypersensitive areas in posterior shoulder muscles: A survey of two hundred young adults. Am J Phys Med 34:585–590, 1955.
76. Trager M. Trager mentastics: Movement as a way to agelessness. Tarrytown, NY, Station Hill, 1989.
77. Travell J, Rinzler SH: The myofascial genesis of pain. Postgrad Med 11:425–434, 1952.
78. Travell JG, Simons DG: Myofascial Pain and Dysfunction: The Trigger Point Manual. Baltimore, Williams & Wilkins, 1983.
79. Tschopp KP, Gysin C: Local injection therapy in 107 patients with myofascial pain syndrome of the head and neck. Otorhinolaryngol Relat Spec 58(6):306–310, 1996.
80. Watrous IS: The Trager approach: An effective tool for physical therapy. Physical Therapy Forum April 10, 1992:22–25.
81. White JM: State of the science of music interventions: Critical care and perioperative practice. Critical Care Nursing Clinics of North America 12(2):219–225, 2000.
82. Wong JY, Rapson LM: Acupuncture in the management of pain of musculoskeletal and neurologic origin. Phys Med Rehabil Clin North Am (10)3:531–545, 1999.
83. Yue SK: Compartment approach to the shoulder and pelvic girdle related pain syndrome. Presentation at the Janet G. Travell Seminar Series—Focus on Pain '98, March 12–15, 1998, San Antonio, Texas.
84. Zashin SJ: Complementary and alternative therapies for arthritis: Science or fiction? J Musculoskeletal Med 17(6):330–340, 345, 2000.

Chapter 12

Injection of Specific Trigger Points

Edward S. Rachlin, MD

Muscles of the Trunk

Quadratus Lumborum

Symptoms and Pain Pattern

- Low back pain present at rest as well as with motion of the lumbar areas.
- Limited range of motion of the lumbosacral spine due to pain and muscle stiffness. Patient may feel immobilized.
- Coughing and sneezing can cause pain in the low back without radiation.
- Pain may radiate to the lower extremity or anteriorly to the inguinal region including the scrotum and testicles.[22, 24]
- Referred pain may be limited to the sacroiliac region and buttocks[51] (Fig. 12–1).
- Referred pain to the anterior abdominal wall.[42]

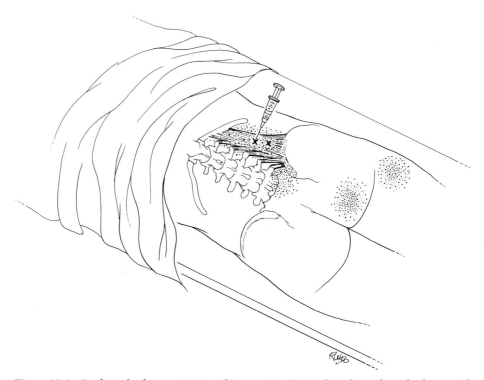

Figure 12–1. Quadratus lumborum. Injection of trigger points (*X's*) in the right quadratus lumborum with the patient in the prone position. Injection may also be performed with the patient lying on the uninvolved side. Trigger point pain pattern is shown by *stippling*. Direct the needle tangentially or parallel to the frontal plane of the patient.

Findings on Examination

- Palpation of trigger points (TrPs) may cause local as well as referred pain. With the patient in the prone position, palpate TrPs lateral and deep to the iliocostalis lumborum. It is sometimes helpful in palpating beneath the iliocostalis lumborum to have the patient lying on the uninvolved side with slight forward rotation of the upper body.
- Muscle spasm.
- Muscle spasm will prevent an adequate examination for TrPs. Muscle spasm should be treated and relieved prior to TrP evaluation. (See postinjection follow-up program in Chapter 11.)
- Functional scoliosis.
- Limited motion in the lumbar area.

Differential Diagnosis

- Kidney stone.
- Trochanteric bursitis.
- Herniated lumbar disc.
- Lumbosacral sprain.

Anatomy

Origin: the iliolumbar ligament and posterior iliac crest.
Insertion: 12th rib and transverse processes of L1–4.
Action: fixation of last two ribs; flexes the spine laterally.
Nerve supply: ventral primary divisions (T12 and L1–3 or L1–4).

Noninvasive Therapy

The post–TrP injection follow-up program described in Chapter 11 is recommended as a conservative therapeutic treatment approach. Noninvasive therapy can include:

- Physical therapy modalities (e.g., electrical stimulation and warm packs; see Chapter 19).
- Manual physical therapy techniques (e.g., massage, joint mobilization, and the Trager® Approach [neuromuscular re-education]; see Chapters 16–18 for additional manual techniques).
- Active and passive stretching and limbering of muscles with or without the use of vaporized coolant spray or ice. Active exercise is part of the stretch-and-spray technique. Limbering and relaxation of muscles are necessary prior to stretching. Contract–relax techniques may be used.
- Stretch and spray for the quadratus muscle: The patient should lie on the uninvolved side. Stretching of the quadratus lumborum is achieved by rotating the upper body forward and upward, opening the area between the 12th rib and pelvis. The right hip and pelvis are stabilized. Stretching is also achieved in the sitting position in the bend-rotation exercise by lateral rotation and flexion as described in back exercises in Chapter 15. Electrical stimulation, limbering of muscles, and warm packs should precede stretch and spray to relax muscles.
- Exercises and a home program for the low back are described in Chapter 15. Exercise programs include relaxation, limbering, stretching, and strengthening. When the patient is free of pain and full motion has been achieved, there should be progression to strength and endurance programs.

Injection Technique

Position patient in the prone or side-lying position on the uninvolved side. Trigger points are palpated lateral and deep to the border of the iliocostalis lumborum muscle.

Inject only the TrPs in the lower portion of the quadratus lumborum to avoid the diaphragm area. Direct the needle tangentially or parallel to the frontal plane of the patient (see Figs. 12–1 and 11–15); the injection technique is described in Chapter 11.

Needle size: 1.5, 2.0, 3.0 in., 20 gauge.
Solution: Any one of the following solutions may be used: 0.5% procaine; 1.0% lidocaine; saline and dry needling in case of allergy. Do not use epinephrine.

Precautions

- To avoid causing pneumothorax, do not inject the upper portion of the quadratus lumborum.
- Direct the needle tangentially or parallel to the frontal plane of the patient.

Postinjection Follow-up Physical Therapy Program

The patient should receive 3 to 4 consecutive days of treatment. Physical therapy should include electrical stimulation, relaxation, limbering, and stretching of the involved muscle using vaporized coolant spray or ice as needed combined with and followed by an exercise program. Active and active-assisted exercises are an integral part of the physical therapy program (see Chapter 11 for details).

Exercise and Home Program

Exercises for the quadratus lumborum and back muscles are prescribed. Exercises should at first be performed under the guidance of a therapist. When the patient is free of pain and full motion has been achieved, add strength and endurance programs. Begin and end exercise session with relaxation and stretching. (See Chapter 15 for exercise details.)

Corrective and Preventive Measures

- Failure to do warm-up exercises prior to athletic activities predisposes to the development of TrPs and the activation of latent TrPs. Continue the exercise program to avoid recurrence.
- Correct foot deformities, e.g., flatfoot. Prescribe orthoses as necessary.
- Correct leg length inequality with heel lifts.
- Recommend a buttock lift for small hemipelvis or scoliosis as indicated.[52]
- Proper chair design: backrest with lumbar support, armrests of proper height; feet should rest comfortably on the floor (see Chapter 20).
- Prescribe a lumbar roll if necessary.

Latissimus Dorsi and Teres Major

Symptoms and Pain Pattern

- Pain may be experienced over the midthoracic area, lower medial aspect of the scapula, anterior aspect of the shoulder, and in the posterior axillary region[27, 52] (Fig. 12–2).
- Pain may radiate to the medial aspect of the arm to the fourth and fifth fingers.
- Working for long periods with the arms elevated and forward may cause TrPs or aggravate latent TrPs.

Findings on Examination

- With the patient supine, the arm is abducted and externally rotated. The latissimus dorsi is grasped between the thumb and index finger to palpate for TrPs. Palpation may also be performed with the patient prone.

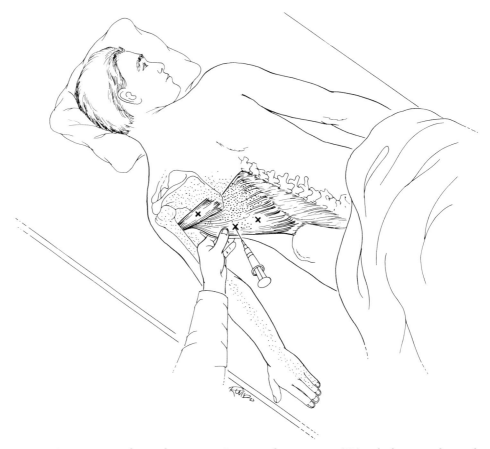

Figure 12–2. Latissimus dorsi and teres major. Injection of trigger points *(X's)* in the latissimus dorsi and teres major with the patient prone. Injection may also be performed with the patient supine. Anatomic landmarks are noted. Pain pattern *(stippling).* Area of trigger point is grasped between the thumb and fingers.

- Local and referred pain may be elicited.
- Range-of-motion assessment may reveal limitation in elevation and external rotation.

Differential Diagnosis

- Cervical disc herniation.
- Thoracic outlet syndrome.
- Intrathoracic disease.
- Dorsal sprain.

Anatomy

Latissimus Dorsi

Origin: spinous processes and supraspinous ligaments of the lower thoracic vertebrae, lumbar fascia, posterior part of the crest of the ilium, the four lower ribs, and from the angle of the scapula.

Insertion: the floor of the bicipital groove.

Action: adduction, medial rotation, and extension of the arm.

Nerve supply: thoracodorsal (C6, 7, 8).

Teres Major

Origin: back of the inferior angle and axillary border of the scapula.
Insertion: front of the humerus bicipital groove.
Action: medial rotator and adductor of arm.
Nerve supply: inferior subscapular (C5, 6).

The teres major is superior and adjacent to the latissimus dorsi. Anatomically, it is an extension of the latissimus dorsi and both are treated together.

Noninvasive Therapy

The post–trigger point injection follow-up program described in Chapter 11 is recommended as a conservative therapeutic treatment approach. Noninvasive therapy can include:

- Physical therapy modalities (e.g., electrical stimulation and warm packs; see Chapter 19).
- Manual physical therapy techniques (e.g., massage, joint mobilization, and the Trager® Approach [neuromuscular re-education]; see Chapters 16–18 for additional manual techniques).
- Active and passive stretching and limbering of muscles with or without the use of vapocoolant spray or ice. Active exercise is part of the stretch-and-spray technique. Limbering and relaxation are necessary prior to stretching. Contract-relax techniques may be used.
- Stretch and spray for the latissimus dorsi and teres major include the TrP and referred pain area. Use vaporized coolant or ice (see Chapter 11). Stretch in the direction of abduction, external rotation, and extension. Electrical stimulation, limbering of muscles, and warm packs should precede stretch and spray to relax muscles.
- Exercises and a home program for the shoulder are described in Chapter 15. Exercise programs include relaxation, limbering, stretching, and strengthening. When the patient is free of pain and full motion has been achieved, progress to strength and endurance programs.

Injection of Trigger Point

With the patient prone or supine the TrP is located and sometimes can be held between the thumb and index finger or isolated between the index and middle fingers. If the TrP cannot be held, the tender area may be injected. The needle should be directed tangentially or parallel to the thorax (see Fig. 12–2 and Chapter 11 for injection technique).

Needle size: 1.5 in., 22 gauge.
Solution: Any one of the following solutions may be used: 0.5% procaine; 1.0% lidocaine; saline and dry needling in case of allergy. Do not use epinephrine.

The teres major may also be injected over its scapular origin in addition to the posterior axillary area.

Precautions

Control the depth of the needle. Direct the needle tangentially or parallel to the chest wall to avoid pneumothorax (see Chapter 11 for complications). Maintain the TrP area between two fingers or the finger and thumb when possible.

Postinjection Follow-up Physical Therapy Program

The patient should receive 3 to 4 consecutive days of treatment. Physical therapy should include electrical stimulation, relaxation, limbering, and stretching of the involved muscle using vaporized coolant spray or ice as needed combined with and followed by an exercise program. Active and active-assisted exercises are an integral part of the physical therapy program (see Chapter 11 for details).

Exercise and Home Program

Exercises should at first be performed under the guidance of a therapist. When the patient is free of pain and full motion has been achieved, progress to strength and endurance programs. Begin and end the exercise session with relaxation and stretching. (See Chapter 15 for exercise details.)

Corrective and Preventive Measures

- Avoid working with the arms elevated and forward for long periods.
- Do warm-up exercises for the back and upper extremities before athletic activities (see Chapter 15).
- Patients who have walked with crutches for a prolonged period of time develop shortness of the latissimus dorsi, e.g., paraplegic patients. Encourage stretching and range-of-motion exercises for the upper extremities.

Thoracolumbar Paraspinal Muscles

Sacrospinalis, spinalis

Symptoms and Pain Pattern

- Thoracolumbar muscles, both superficial and deep, are treated as a group rather than individually.
- Injection is into the muscle group rather than to individual muscles. The sacrospinalis muscle or erector spinae consists of the iliocostalis, longissimus, and spinalis.
- These muscles may refer pain to the upper dorsal area, flank, and buttock[4, 7, 15, 16, 20, 22, 51] (Fig. 12–3).
- Trigger points in the dorsal musculature may cause radiating chest pain and pleurodynia.[7] The deep paraspinal muscles include the semispinalis thoracis, multifidi, and rotators.
- Trigger points found in the deep paraspinal muscle may give rise to thoracic pain and pain over the spinous processes, in addition to coccygodynia.[10, 51]
- Lumbar muscle TrPs may refer pain to the abdomen.[15, 16]

Findings on Examination

- Patients with thoracolumbar and low back pain demonstrate restricted spinal motion due to pain, muscle stiffness, muscle spasm, muscle shortening, and TrPs.
- Trigger point examination should be performed with the patient prone with a pillow under the abdomen as well as in the side-lying position.
- Trigger points causing local and referred pain to the buttocks or chest area may be palpable both superficially and deep.
- Neighboring muscle groups often develop TrPs (e.g., gluteal, tensor fasciae latae).

Differential Diagnosis

- Herniated disc.
- Lumbosacral sprain.
- Dorsal lumbar sprain.
- Kidney stones.
- Spinal fractures.
- Metastatic disease.

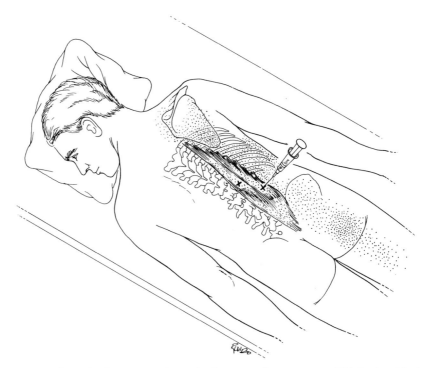

Figure 12–3. Thoracolumbar paraspinal muscle. Injection of trigger points *(X's)* in the right lumbar paraspinal muscles with the patient supine. Direct the needling tangentially in relation to the frontal plane of the patient. Anatomic landmarks are noted. Trigger point pain pattern is shown by *stippling.*

Anatomy

The sacrospinalis (erector spinae) includes the iliocostalis, longissimus, and spinalis. The three muscle groups have an extensive common origin. Three columns arise from the common origin.

Origin: sacral spines and transverse processes, lumbar and lower thoracic spinous processes, posterior part of crest of the ilium.

Outer Column
Iliocostalis Thoracis

Origin: upper border of angles of lower six ribs.
Insertion: upper borders of ribs 1–6, transverse process of C7.

Costalis

Origin: lower six ribs.
Insertion: upper six ribs.

Costocervicalis

Origin: upper three to six ribs.
Insertion: transverse processes of C4–6.

Intermediate Column
Longissimus Thoracis

Origin: sacral spines and transverse processes, lumbar and lower thoracic spinous processes, posterior part of crest of the ilium.
Insertion: transverse processes of all thoracic and lumbar vertebrae, lower 10 ribs.

Longissimus Cervicis

Origin: transverse processes of T1–5.
Insertion: transverse processes of C2–6.

Longissimus Capitis

Origin: transverse processes of T1–7, articular processes of C5–7.
Insertion: posterior margin of mastoid process.
Nerve supply: dorsal rami of the lower cervical, thoracic, and lumbar spinal nerves.

Medial Column

Spinalis

Origin: thoracic spines of T11 and L1–2.
Insertion: thoracic spines of T1–8.

Spinalis Cervicis

Origin: spinous processes of C7 and T1–2.
Insertion: spinous processes of C2–5.
Action: iliocostalis acts as extensor, lateral flexor, and rotator of the spine to the same side; longissimus thoracis and cervicis extend the spine and bend the spine to one side.
Nerve supply: dorsal rami of the cervical and thoracic spinal nerves.

Noninvasive Therapy

The post–trigger point injection follow-up program described in Chapter 11 is recommended as a conservative therapeutic treatment approach. Noninvasive therapy can include:

- Physical therapy modalities (e.g., electrical stimulation and warm packs; see Chapter 19).
- Manual physical therapy techniques (e.g., massage, joint mobilization, and the Trager® Approach [neuromuscular re-education]; see Chapters 16–18 for additional manual techniques).
- Active and passive stretching and limbering of muscles with or without the use of vaporized coolant spray or ice. Active exercise is part of the stretch-and-spray technique. Limbering and relaxation are necessary prior to stretching. Contract-relax techniques may be used.
- Stretch and spray: Stretching is performed in flexion, rotation of the spine, and lateral bending to the opposite side. The back exercise program (see Chapter 15) also includes stretching in the sitting position. Electrical stimulation, limbering of muscles, and warm packs should precede stretch and spray to relax muscles.
- Exercises and home program for the paraspinal muscles (see Chapter 15 for back exercise and see Chapters 16–18 for massage techniques). Exercise programs include relaxation, limbering, stretching, and strengthening. When the patient is free of pain and full motion has been achieved, progress to strength and endurance programs.

Injection Technique

See Figure 12–3.

The patient is placed in the prone position with a pillow under the abdomen. Identify TrPs. Injection is performed under sterile precautions. Injection is performed in the thoracolumbar area without specific anatomic differentiation of individual muscles. *The muscles are treated as a group* (see Fig. 12–3, and Chapter 11 for injection technique).

Needle size: 2.0, 3.0, 3.5 in., 20–22 gauge.
Solution: Any one of the following solutions may be used: 0.5% procaine; 1.0% lidocaine; saline and dry needling in case of allergy. Do not use epinephrine.

Multiple needle entries are required, in addition to approaching the TrP directly. Both superficial and deep TrPs are injected as a group. Multiple entries usually encounter TrPs that are missed on palpation. Injections should be performed with the needle directed tangentially in the lower lumbar area. The direction of the needle should be angled parallel or tangential to the frontal plane of the patient to avoid penetrating too deeply in the upper lumbar area. Lidocaine 10 mL is usually sufficient. To avoid entering the intervertebral space when injecting the deep paraspinalis (e.g., the multifidi), angle the needle in a caudal direction in relation to the laminae, which slant caudally, guarding the intercostal space. This is the same principle used in injecting in the area of the rib cage to avoid entering the intercostal space.

Postinjection Follow-up Physical Therapy Program

The patient should receive 3 to 4 consecutive days of treatment. Physical therapy should include electrical stimulation, relaxation, limbering, and stretching of the involved muscle using vaporized coolant spray or ice as needed combined with and followed by an exercise program. Active and active-assisted exercises are an integral part of the physical therapy program (see Chapter 11 for details).

Exercise and Home Program

Exercises for the low back are prescribed. Exercises should at first be performed under the guidance of a therapist. When the patient is free of pain and full motion has been achieved, progress to strength and endurance programs. Begin and end exercise sessions with stretching and relaxation (see Chapter 15 for exercise details).

Corrective and Preventive Measures

- Correct postural foot deformities (e.g., use orthoses for flatfeet). Use an appropriate heel lift in case of leg length discrepancy.
- Correct lumbar-pelvic asymmetry (e.g., sitting with an appropriate cushion under one buttock in case of scoliosis or small hemipelvis).[51]
- Correct faulty postural habits (e.g., improper sitting and standing). Use correct method of lifting at work (see Chapter 20).
- Eliminate stress and tension as a cause of back pain.
- The physician should instruct the patient in proper sleeping positions.
- Recommend a firm mattress and bed board.
- Recommend a properly designed chair and a lumbar roll (see Chapter 20).
- Recommend a lumbosacral support in acute pain for ambulation as a temporary measure.
- Recommend continuing exercise program to avoid recurrence.
- Eliminate metabolic causes of muscle pain.

Serratus Posterior Superior

Symptoms and Pain Pattern

- Pain over the scapula, most pronounced over the upper medial border.
- Pain may radiate to the posterior aspect of the shoulder, upper arm, forearm, and to the hand, and fifth finger.[51]
- Pain in the area of the medial scapula border may be difficult to distinguish from symptoms caused by the rhomboids or trapezius muscles.

Findings on Examination

- Palpation of TrPs may cause local and referred pain.
- The insertion of the serratus posterior superior muscle extends to the rib margins, which are covered by the medial border of the scapula. Palpation of this area is best accomplished by abducting the scapula. To move the scapula laterally, the arm can be brought around to the front of the chest or permitted to hang forward with the patient in the prone position. It is difficult to distinguish TrPs in the region of the origin and medial portion of the muscle because of the overlying rhomboids and trapezius muscles.

Differential Diagnosis

- Rhomboid and trapezius trigger points.
- Cervical radiculopathy.
- Subscapular bursitis.

Anatomy

Origin: spinous processes of C7, and T1–3.
Insertion: outer surfaces of ribs 2–5 lateral to the rib angles.
Action: elevator of the upper ribs.
Nerve supply: second, third, fourth, and fifth intercostal nerves.

Noninvasive Therapy

The post–trigger point injection follow-up program described in Chapter 11 is recommended as a conservative therapeutic treatment approach. Noninvasive therapy can include:

- Physical therapy modalities (e.g., electrical stimulation and warm packs; see Chapter 19).
- Manual physical therapy techniques (e.g., massage, joint mobilization, and the Trager® Approach [neuromuscular re-education]; see Chapters 16–18 for additional manual techniques).
- Stretching is minimally effective in treating the serratus posterior superior. Stretch and spray of neighboring muscles that harbor TrPs, such as the rhomboids and trapezius, would be effective. Flexing the upper thoracic spine does not accomplish the type of stretch that is therapeutically effective. Emphasis should be placed on massage techniques, which include ischemic compression, the use of electric modalities, and the treatment of neighboring muscles.

Injection of Trigger Point

The patient lies on the uninvolved side. The scapula is abducted and the TrP is specifically localized and held between two fingers. The needle is directed to the rib to avoid the intercostal space. Aspirate prior to injection. The needle is directed tangentially in relation to the chest wall to avoid causing pneumothorax (Fig. 12–4; see also Fig. 11–12 for injection technique when approaching the chest wall, e.g., the pectoralis muscle).

Needle size: 1.5, 2.0 in., 21 gauge.
Solution: Any one of the following solutions may be used: 0.5% procaine; 1.0% lidocaine; saline and dry needling in case of allergy. Do not use epinephrine.

Precautions

- Aspirate prior to injection.
- Angle the needle tangentially in relation to the chest wall.
- Avoid the intercostal space.

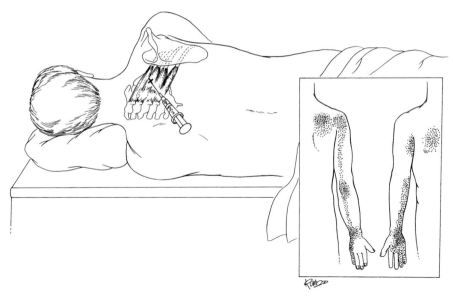

Figure 12–4. Serratus posterior superior. Injection of trigger point *(X)* in the right serratus posterior superior. Localize the trigger point by palpation and direct the needle in the direction of a rib and tangentially in relation to the chest wall to avoid entering the intercostal space. Aspirate prior to injection. Trigger points in the region of muscle insertion are more easily palpated with abduction of the right scapula. Observe precautions to prevent pneumothorax. *Inset,* trigger point pain pattern *(stippling).*

Postinjection Follow-up Physical Therapy Program

The patient should receive 3 to 4 consecutive days of treatment. Physical therapy should include electrical stimulation, relaxation, limbering, and stretching of the neighboring muscle using vaporized coolant spray or ice as needed combined with and followed by an exercise program. Active and active-assisted exercises are an integral part of the physical therapy program (see Chapter 11 for details).

Exercise and Home Program

Exercises should at first be performed under the guidance of a therapist. When the patient is free of pain and full motion has been achieved, progress to strength and endurance programs. Begin and end exercise sessions with stretching and relaxation (See Chapter 15 for exercise details.)

Corrective and Preventive Measures

Recommend correct sitting and standing postures for cervical, dorsal, and lumbosacral spine (e.g., avoid head-forward posture and round-shouldered posture, and use lumbar roll for sitting).

Serratus Posterior Inferior

Symptoms and Referred Pain Pattern

- Patients report pain in the upper lumbar and lower dorsal area (Fig. 12–5).
- Symptoms may be aggravated by activities requiring rotation of the torso.
- Patients can often put their finger on the tender spot.

Findings on Examination

- Local tenderness over TrPs.
- Trigger points are located over the rib area.
- Pain with rotation to the opposite side.

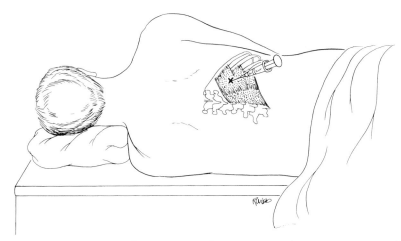

Figure 12–5. Serratus posterior inferior. Injection of trigger point in the serratus posterior inferior *(X)*. The trigger point should be well localized between the index and middle fingers or index finger and thumb. Avoid the intercostal space. The patient may be injected in the prone or side-lying position. Aspirate prior to injection. Direct the needle toward a rib pointing the needle in a caudal direction tangential to the chest wall. Pain pattern is shown by *stippling*.

Differential Diagnosis

- Kidney stone.
- Nephritis.
- Lumbar-dorsal sprain.
- Fracture of the rib.

Anatomy

Origin: spinous processes of T11, T12, L1, and L2.

Insertion: ribs 9–12; muscle fibers are directed upward and laterally to insert on the surfaces of the lower four ribs.

Action: maintains stability of the lower ribs; depressor of the lower ribs.

Nerve supply: ventral rami of the ninth, tenth, eleventh, and twelfth thoracic spinal nerves.

Noninvasive Therapy

The post–trigger point injection follow-up program described in Chapter 11 is recommended as a conservative therapeutic treatment approach. Noninvasive therapy can include:

- Physical therapy modalities (e.g., electrical stimulation and warm packs; see Chapter 19).
- Manual physical therapy techniques (e.g., massage, joint mobilization, and the Trager® Approach [neuromuscular re-education]; see Chapters 16–18 for additional manual techniques).
- Active and passive stretching and limbering of muscles with or without the use of vaporized coolant spray or ice. Active exercise is part of the stretch-and-spray technique. Limbering and relaxation are necessary prior to stretching. Contract-relax techniques may be used.
- Stretch and spray for the serratus posterior inferior is performed with the patient in the sitting position. Flex the thoracolumbar area with rotation to the opposite side. This exercise and stretch are a part of the low back exercise program described in Chapter 15. Electrical stimulation, limbering of muscles, and warm packs should precede stretch and spray to relax muscles.

- Exercises and a home program for the low back are described in Chapter 15. Exercise is done progressively. Exercises for flexion and rotation in the thoracolumbar area are included. Exercises include sitting with forward bending in flexion as well as with rotation. Exercise programs include relaxation, limbering, stretching, and strengthening. When the patient is free of pain and full motion has been achieved, progress to strength and endurance programs. Begin and end exercise sessions with relaxation and stretching.

Injection of Trigger Point

Position patient in prone or side-lying position on the uninvolved side. Trigger points are palpated and isolated between the index and middle fingers over the rib area. The needle is directed over the rib tangentially to avoid entering the intercostal space (see Fig. 12–5 and Chapter 11 for injection technique).

Needle size: 1.5 in., 20–22 gauge.
Solution: Any one of the following solutions may be used: 0.5% procaine; 1.0% lidocaine; saline and dry needling in case of allergy. Do not use epinephrine.

Precautions

- Avoid pneumothorax.
- Direct the needle tangentially over the rib.
- Avoid the intercostal space.
- Aspirate prior to injection.

Postinjection Follow-up Physical Therapy Program

The patient should receive 3 to 4 consecutive days of treatment. Physical therapy should include electrical stimulation, relaxation, limbering, and stretching of the involved muscle using vaporized coolant spray or ice as needed combined with and followed by an exercise program. Active and active-assisted exercises are an integral part of the physical therapy program (see Chapter 11 for details).

Exercise and Home Program

Exercises for the serratus posterior inferior include exercises for the back and thoracolumbar area (see Chapter 15 for back exercises). Exercises should at first be performed under the guidance of a therapist. When the patient is free of pain and full motion has been achieved, progress to strength and endurance programs. Begin and end exercise sessions with stretching and relaxation.

Corrective and Preventive Measures

- Avoid repetitive twisting of the torso or remaining in a rotated posture for prolonged periods. This may require correcting the working environment.
- Excessive repetitive hitting of golf balls (practice sessions) may cause or aggravate latent TrPs.
- Correct poor sitting posture, which may be due to pelvic asymmetry (e.g., use a cushion under one buttock as necessary).
- Correct leg length discrepancies (e.g., with a heel lift).

Serratus Anterior

Symptoms and Referred Pain Pattern

- Pain over the anterior, lateral, and posterolateral chest wall[54] (Fig. 12–6).
- Pain at rest and with movements of the rib cage.

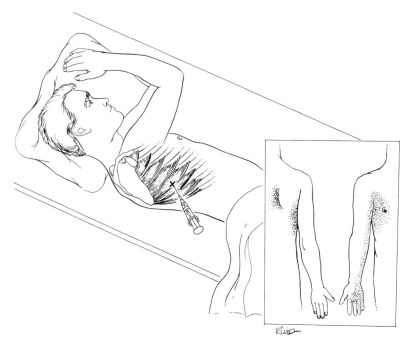

Figure 12–6. Serratus anterior. Injection of trigger point *(X)* in the right serratus anterior muscle in the midaxillary line. The patient is lying on the uninvolved side. Avoid entering the intercostal space. Aspirate prior to injection. *Inset,* pain pattern *(stippling).*

- Referred pain may be noted over the inner border of the arm radiating to the fourth and fifth fingers.[50]
- Pain may be aggravated with deep breathing.

Findings on Examination

- Local TrP tenderness is usually located in the midaxillary line between ribs 4 and 8.
- Referred pain pattern may be elicited with TrP palpation.

Differential Diagnosis

- Fracture of the rib.
- Cervical radiculopathy.
- Strain of serratus anterior muscle.
- Intercostal muscle trigger points.

Anatomy

Origin: outer surfaces of the upper eight ribs.
Insertion: ventral aspect of the whole length of the vertebral body of the scapula.
Action: holds the medial border of the scapula against the thorax; abducts the scapula, rotating it so that the glenoid cavity faces upward to support the arm when it is raised above the shoulder; may also act in forced inspiration.
Nerve supply: long thoracic (C5, 6, 7).

Noninvasive Therapy

The post–trigger point injection follow-up program described in Chapter 11 is recommended as a conservative therapeutic treatment approach. Noninvasive therapy can include:

- Physical therapy modalities (e.g., electrical stimulation and warm packs; see Chapter 19).
- Manual physical therapy techniques (e.g., massage, joint mobilization, and the Trager® Approach [neuromuscular re-education]; see Chapters 16–18 for additional manual techniques).
- Active and passive stretching and limbering of muscles with or without the use of vaporized coolant spray or ice. Active exercise is part of the stretch-and-spray technique. Limbering and relaxation are necessary prior to stretching. Contract-relax technique may be used.
- Stretch and spray for the serratus anterior is accomplished with the patient in the side-lying position lying on the uninvolved side. Stretching of the serratus anterior is achieved by actively and passively bringing the patient's arm backward and downward using a vaporized coolant spray or ice if needed. Electrical stimulation, limbering of muscles, and warm packs should precede stretch and spray to relax muscles.
- Exercises and a home program for the serratus anterior are described in Chapter 15 in the discussion of shoulder and upper extremity exercises. Exercise programs include relaxation, limbering, stretching, and strengthening. When the patient is free of pain and full motion has been achieved, progress to strength and endurance programs. Begin and end exercise programs with relaxation and stretching.

Injection of Trigger Point

Position the patient in the supine or side-lying position on the uninvolved side. Trigger points are palpated. The needle should be directed tangentially in relation to the chest wall, directing the needle over a rib to avoid the intercostal space (see Fig. 12–6). Isolate the TrP between the index and middle fingers. (See Chapter 11 for injection technique.)

Needle size: 1.5 in., 21 gauge.
Solution: Any one of the following solutions may be used: 0.5% procaine; 1.0% lidocaine; saline and dry needling in case of allergy. Do not use epinephrine.

Precautions

- Aspirate prior to injection.
- Avoid causing a pneumothorax.
- Direct the needle toward the rib to avoid the intercostal space.
- To control the position and depth of the needle, the needle and syringe may be stabilized with one hand while the other hand is used for injecting.
- Direct the needle tangentially in relation to the chest wall.

Postinjection Follow-up Physical Therapy Program

The patient should receive 3 to 4 consecutive days of treatment. Physical therapy should include electrical stimulation, relaxation, limbering, and stretching of the involved muscle using vapocoolant spray or ice as needed combined with and followed by an exercise program. Active and active-assisted exercises are an integral part of the physical therapy program (see Chapter 11 for details).

Exercise and Home Program

Exercises should first be performed under the guidance of a therapist. When the patient is free of pain and full motion has been achieved, progress to strength and endurance programs. Begin and end exercise sessions with stretching and relaxation. (See Chapter 15 for exercise details.)

Corrective and Preventive Measures

- Proper warm-up activities prior to performing exercises include push-ups and overhead weightlifting.
- Relaxation and stretching exercises prior to and after exercise sessions.

Rectus Abdominis and Obliquus

Symptoms and Pain Pattern

Sola,[40, 41] Kelly,[17] Kellgren,[15, 16] Lang,[24] Travell and Simons,[52] Melnick,[28] Ling and Slocumb,[25, 39] have reported referred pain patterns involving the abdominal muscles. Both somatovisceral and viscerosomatic interactions have been reported.

- Trigger points may cause abdominal pain, vomiting, diarrhea, urinary bladder symptoms, and referred pain to the lower back. Trigger point patterns have been reported in the obliquus, transverse abdominis, and rectus abdominis muscles. Trigger points in the rectus abdominis are a frequent result of muscle strains in athletic injuries (e.g., sit-ups). Often a history of a specific incident of trauma is lacking.
- Pain resulting from TrPs appears to persist long after an initial strain may have healed. Pain may be localized to the abdominal area (Fig. 12–7). Different symptoms have been attributed to the upper, mid-, and lower portions of the rectus abdominis.[51] The upper rectus abdominis refers pain to the midback in addition to producing abdominal symptoms characteristic of indigestion. The periumbilical area causes a colic-like pain. The lower rectus abdominis refers pain to the low back area in addition to simulating the pain of appendicitis when the TrP is on the right side.
- Melnick[28, 29] has described symptoms due to TrPs in the abdominal area: heartburn related to TrPs at the insertion of the abdominal muscles along the right costal margin from the xiphoid process to the angle of the ribs; abdominal fullness, nausea, and vomiting related to TrPs in the midline of the upper abdomen; and diarrhea resulting from TrPs in the left or right angle of the lower abdomen.

Findings on Examination

- Tenderness on palpation may cause local tenderness and referred pain patterns in addition to abdominal symptoms.

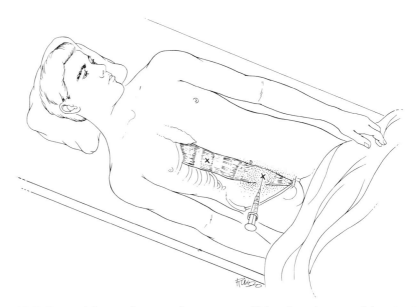

Figure 12–7. Rectus abdominis. Injection of trigger points (*X's*) in the right rectus abdominis with the patient supine. Anatomic landmarks are noted. Pain pattern is shown by *stippling*. Direct the needle tangentially to the abdominal wall.

- Placing the muscle under tension may produce characteristic pain (e.g., raising both legs, lifting both heels off the examining table, or performing sit-ups).

Differential Diagnosis

- Multiple causes of abdominal pain (e.g., appendicitis, gallbladder disease, diverticulitis).
- Abdominal muscle strain.

Anatomy

External Oblique

Origin: outer surfaces of the lower eight ribs.

Insertion: posterior fibers into the interior half of the iliac crest; the rest of the muscle inserts through the anterior superior iliac spine to the pubic tubercle and crest; the aponeurosis between these two points is thickened to form the inguinal ligament.

Nerve supply: intercostals (T8–12), iliohypogastric (T12, L1), ilioinguinal (L1).

Action: external oblique, internal oblique, and transversus compress the abdominal viscera, flex the trunk, and act as muscles of expiration.

Internal Oblique

Origin: transverse processes of the lumbar vertebrae.

Insertion: lower borders of the lower six costal cartilages by an aponeurotic sheet with the linea alba, to the pubic crest and iliopectineal line by the conjoined tendon.

Nerve supply: intercostals (T8–12), iliohypogastric (T12, L1), sometimes ilioinguinal (L1).

Action: external oblique, internal oblique, and transversus compress the abdominal viscera, flex the trunk, and act as muscles of expiration.

Transversus Abdominis

Origin: lower six costal cartilages of the transverse processes of the lumbar vertebrae.

Insertion: by an aponeurotic sheet to the midline attached to the xiphisternum, to the pubic crest and iliopectineal line.

Nerve supply: branches of thoracic nerves T8–12, iliohypogastric and ilioinguinal nerves.

Action: external oblique, internal oblique, and transversus compress the abdominal viscera, flex the trunk, and act as muscles of expiration.

Rectus Abdominis

Origin: medial head in front of the body of the pubis and the lateral head from the top of the crest of the pubis.

Insertion: the anterior aspect of the fifth, sixth, and seventh costal cartilages, and the lower border of the seventh.

Action: flexion of the pelvis on the trunk or the trunk on the pelvis.

Nerve supply: intercostal nerves (7–12).

Pyramidalis Muscle

Origin: a small triangular muscle inside the rectus sheath arising from the crest of the pubis.

Insertion: the linea alba.

Noninvasive Therapy

The post–trigger point injection follow-up program described in Chapter 11 is recommended as a conservative therapeutic treatment approach. Noninvasive therapy can include:

- Physical therapy modalities (e.g., electrical stimulation and warm packs; see Chapter 19).
- Manual physical therapy techniques (e.g., massage, joint mobilization, and the Trager® Approach [neuromuscular re-education]; see Chapters 16–18 for additional manual techniques).
- Active and passive stretching and limbering of muscles with or without the use of vaporized coolant spray or ice. Active exercise is part of the stretch-and-spray technique. Limbering and relaxation are necessary prior to stretching. Contract-relax techniques may be used.
- Stretch and spray for the rectus abdominis muscle is performed by arching the patient's back to achieve extension of the back. The legs may be supported by a stool off the examining table.[52] Spray is applied over the abdomen over the TrP area and referred pain area. Electrical stimulation, limbering of muscles, and warm packs to relax muscles should precede stretch and spray.
- Exercises and a home program for the abdominal muscles are described in Chapter 15. Exercise program includes relaxation, limbering, stretching, and strengthening. When the patient is free of pain and full motion has been achieved, progress to strength and endurance programs.

Injection of Trigger Point

Needle size: 1.5 and 2.0 in., 21 gauge.

Solution: Any one of the following solutions may be used: 0.5% procaine; 1.0% lidocaine; saline and dry needling may be used in case of allergy. Do not use epinephrine. Injection is performed with the patient supine (see Fig. 12–7).

Precautions

- Do not inject perpendicular to the patient.
- The needle should be directed tangential to the abdominal wall.
- Trigger points should be isolated between two fingers or between the thumb and index finger. Localizing the TrP and elevating it away from the abdominal cavity avoids puncturing the abdominal cavity.
- The needle should be well localized into the TrP area.

Postinjection Follow-up Physical Therapy Program

The patient should receive 3 to 4 consecutive days of treatment. Physical therapy should include electrical stimulation, relaxation, limbering, and stretching of the involved muscle using vaporized coolant spray or ice as needed combined with and followed by an exercise program. Active and active-assisted exercises are an integral part of the physical therapy program (see Chapter 11 for details).

Exercise and Home Program

Exercises are performed to strengthen the abdominal muscles. Exercises should at first be performed under the guidance of a therapist. When patients are free of pain and full motion has been achieved, they should progress to strength and endurance programs. Begin and end exercise sessions with stretching and relaxation (see Chapter 15).

Corrective and Preventive Measures

- Correct abdominal weakness with a progressive exercise program.
- Avoid excessive stress caused by poor body mechanics during gymnastics, athletic activities, and postural habits at work.

- Eliminate intra-abdominal pathologic conditions (visceral disease), which may be a cause of abdominal TrPs.
- Warm-up and cool-down exercises should be performed with all exercise and athletic activities.

Pectoral Muscles

Pectoralis Major, Pectoralis Minor

Symptoms and Pain Pattern

- A TrP in the pectoral muscle is often found to be the cause of pain in the upper arm.[22, 24]
- Pain may be noted over the pectoral area in front of the chest.[10, 54]
- Referred pain is noted over the deltoid area and may radiate to the upper and lower forearm or may be localized to the upper and lower forearm (Fig. 12–8).
- Radiation to the fourth and fifth fingers has been reported, in addition to cardiac arrhythmias due to TrPs between the fifth and sixth right ribs.[24, 50]
- Trigger points may develop in the chest wall from pain due to coronary artery disease.[50]
- Pectoral pain due to chest wall tenderness may resemble pain of cardiac origin.[5]

Findings on Examination

- Tender TrPs over the pectoral area may cause referred pain to the deltoid, and upper and lower arm.
- Active TrPs in the pectoralis minor that cause muscle shortening have been reported

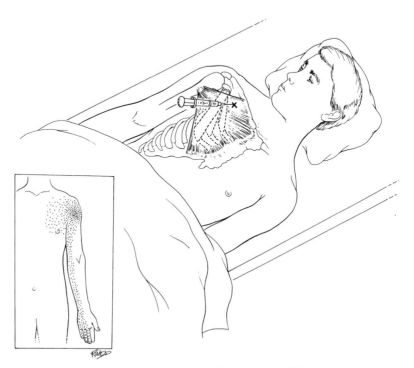

Figure 12–8. Pectoralis major and minor. Injection of trigger point (X) in the pectoral muscles. Direct the needle tangentially in relation to the chest wall to avoid puncturing the pleura. Aspirate prior to injection. Avoid the intercostal space. *Inset,* pain pattern *(stippling).*

to be responsible for a diminished radial pulse, in addition to arterial compression when the shoulder is abducted.[51]

Differential Diagnosis

- Cardiac pain.
- Costochondritis (Tietze's syndrome).
- Cervical radiculopathy.
- Subdeltoid bursitis.
- Intercostal muscle trigger points.

Anatomy

Pectoralis Major

Origin: medial half of anterior surface of the clavicle, the whole length of the front of the sternum, front of the upper six costal cartilages, and external rectus sheath.
Insertion: lateral lip of the bicipital groove of the humerus.
Action: adducts the arm, medially rotates and flexes the arm.
Nerve supply: medial and lateral pectoral (C5, 6, 7, 8, T1).

Pectoralis Minor

The pectoralis minor lies under the cover of the pectoralis major.
Origin: third, fourth, and fifth ribs near the costochondral junctions.
Insertion: medial border of the coracoid process.
Action: pulls the scapula forward and depresses the shoulder.
Nerve supply: medial pectoral nerve.

Noninvasive Therapy

The post–trigger point injection follow-up program described in Chapter 11 is recommended as a conservative therapeutic treatment approach. Noninvasive therapy can include:

- Physical therapy modalities (e.g., electrical stimulation and warm packs; see Chapter 19).
- Manual physical therapy techniques (e.g., massage, joint mobilization, and the Trager® Approach [neuromuscular re-education]; see Chapters 16–18 for additional manual techniques).
- Active and passive stretching and limbering of muscles with or without the use of vaporized coolant spray or ice. Active exercise is part of the stretch-and-spray technique. Limbering and relaxation are necessary prior to stretching. Contract-relax techniques may be used.
- *Pectoralis major:* Stretch and spray should be performed with abduction, external rotation, and extension of the arm, with the aid of vapocoolant spray or ice. Electrical stimulation, limbering of muscles, and warm packs may precede stretch and spray to relax the muscles.
- *Pectoralis minor:* Stretch and spray is performed by abducting and elevating the arm to pull the scapula back and elevate the shoulder.
- Exercises and a home program for the upper extremities are described in Chapter 15. Exercise programs include relaxation, limbering, stretching, and strengthening. When the patient is free of pain and full motion has been achieved, progress to strength and endurance programs can be made.

Injection of Trigger Point

The pectoralis minor is palpated through the pectoralis major. The pectoral muscles are most often treated together. With the patient in the supine position, TrPs are identified and local areas of tenderness are injected (see Figs. 12–8 and 11–12). Localize the TrPs between the index finger and middle finger or thumb. Avoid the intercostal space. (See Chapter 11 for injection technique.)

Needle size: 1.5 in., 21 gauge.
Solution: Any one of the following solutions may be used: 0.5% procaine; 1.0% lidocaine; saline and dry needling in case of allergy.

Precautions

- Direct the needle tangentially in relation to the chest wall to avoid puncturing the pleura and causing a pneumothorax.
- Aspirate before injecting or needling.
- See Chapter 11 for complications.

Postinjection Follow-up Physical Therapy Program

The patient should receive 3 to 4 consecutive days of treatment. Physical therapy should include electrical stimulation, relaxation, limbering, and stretching of the involved muscle using vaporized coolant spray or ice as needed combined with and followed by an exercise program. Active and active-assisted exercises are an integral part of the physical therapy program (see Chapter 11 for details).

Exercise and Home Program

Exercises for the upper extremity and pectoral muscles are prescribed. Exercises should at first be performed under the guidance of a therapist. When the patient is free of pain and full motion has been achieved, progress to strength and endurance programs can occur. Begin and end exercise sessions with relaxation and stretching. (See Chapter 15 for exercise details.)

Corrective and Preventive Measures

- Avoid activities that require holding the arms out in front of the body for long periods.
- Correct standing and sitting postures, e.g., use the proper height of chair armrests and a lumbar roll.

Sternalis

Symptoms and Pain Pattern

- Pain due to TrPs in the parasternal muscles is most often felt under the sternum[17, 30] (Fig. 12–9).
- Laterally located TrPs may refer pain to the scapula, upper extremities, and ulnar distribution of the forearm and hand.[24, 50]
- Symptoms may resemble angina or myocardial infarction.
- Chest pain resulting from myocardiac insufficiency may also be a cause of active TrPs involving the sternalis and pectoral muscles.[50]

Findings on Examination

- Local tender areas over the sternum refer pain to the arm, forearm, and hand. Look for TrPs in neighboring muscles (cervical and pectoral).

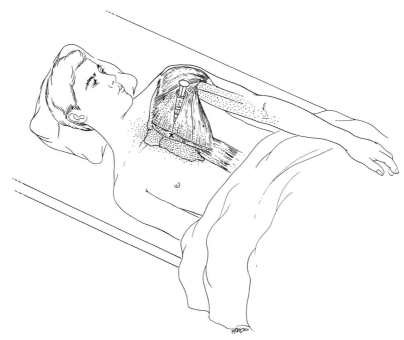

Figure 12–9. Sternalis. Injection of trigger point *(X)* in the sternalis with the patient supine. Observe precautions to avoid entering the chest cavity. Anatomic landmarks are noted. Pain pattern is shown by *stippling.*

Differential Diagnosis

- Costochondritis (Tietze's syndrome).
- Angina.
- Myocardial infarction.
- Pectoral muscle trigger points.
- Intercostal muscle trigger points.

Anatomy

Origin: deep aspect of the xiphoid and fifth, sixth, and seventh costal cartilages.
Insertion: posterior aspect of second to sixth costal cartilages.
Nerve supply: medial and lateral pectoral nerves (C7, 8, T1).

Noninvasive Therapy

The post–trigger point injection follow-up program described in Chapter 11 is recommended as a conservative therapeutic treatment approach. Noninvasive therapy can include:

- Physical therapy modalities (e.g., electrical stimulation and warm packs; see Chapter 19).
- Manual physical therapy techniques (e.g., massage, joint mobilization, and the Trager® Approach [neuromuscular re-education]; see Chapters 16–18 for additional manual techniques).
- Active and passive stretching and limbering of muscles when the pectoral muscles are involved, with or without the use of vaporized coolant spray or ice. Active exercise is part of the stretch-and-spray technique. Limbering and relaxation are necessary prior to stretching. Contract-relax techniques may be used.

Injection of Trigger Point

Needle size: 1.5 in., 22–25 gauge.

Solution: Any one of the following solutions may be used: 0.5% procaine; 1.0% lidocaine; saline and dry needling in case of allergy. Do not use epinephrine.

Precautions

- Direct needle tangentially.
- Avoid the intercostal space.
- Aspirate prior to injection (see Chapter 11 for pneumothorax complications).

Postinjection Follow-up Physical Therapy Program

The patient should receive 3 to 4 consecutive days of treatment (see Chapter 11). Physical therapy should include electrical stimulation and massage techniques. If neighboring muscles (pectoralis major and minor) are involved, appropriate therapy including exercises are prescribed (see discussion of exercises for the upper extremity, Chapter 15).

Corrective and Preventive Measures

- Sternalis TrPs may develop secondary to TrPs in the pectoralis major or minor.
- Treat medical and physical conditions that cause chest pain.

Muscles of the Lower Extremities

Gluteus Maximus

Symptoms and Pain Pattern

- Pain in the gluteal area is aggravated by walking or prolonged sitting and driving.
- Pain in the gluteal area at night.
- Pain usually remains localized in the gluteal area (Fig. 12–10).
- Referred pain may be felt as coccygodynia.[52]
- Sciatic-type pain radiation has been described by several authors.[8, 10, 22, 24]
- The gluteus maximus is active in raising the trunk from a bent-forward position and can be activated with such activities as raising the body's trunk after leaning over a sink, or getting up from a chair with the trunk in a bent-forward position.

Findings on Examination

- Trigger point examination may be performed with the patient lying on the unaffected side with the knee flexed or with the patient prone.
- On palpation, tender TrPs may be found next to the sacral attachments medially and distally as well as the region over the ischial tuberosity. Trigger points in the gluteal region can often be palpated as knots in the muscle, taut bands, or manifested only by the "jump sign." A jump sign is frequently elicited in this area (the patient quickly moves away when the painful TrP is palpated).
- Gluteus maximus muscle strength may be tested by placing the patient in the prone position with the knee flexed to 90 degrees, hyperextending the thigh at the hip against resistance.
- Trigger points are often found laterally over the gluteus medius. Trigger points involving the gluteus maximus, medius, minimus, paraspinal area, and hamstrings, as well as tensor fasciae latae, often occur together in patients with low back pain.
- Antagonistic muscles, such as the rectus femoris and iliopsoas, may develop TrPs and also may require treatment.

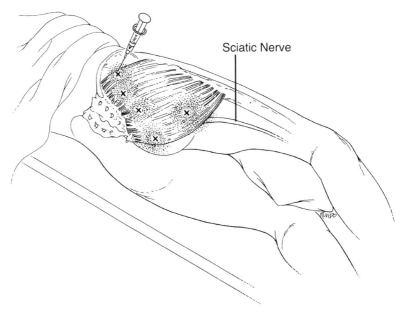

Figure 12–10. Gluteus maximus. Injection of trigger points *(X's)* in the gluteus maximus. Anatomic landmarks are noted. Avoid the sciatic nerve. Pain pattern is shown by *stippling.* Injection may be performed with the patient in the prone or side-lying position.

Differential Diagnosis

- Ischial bursitis.
- Coccygodynia.
- Herniated disc.
- Arthritis of the hip presenting as posterior buttock pain.

Anatomy

Origin: area on ilium above and behind the posterior gluteal line, the lateral mass of the sacrum, the sacrotuberous ligament.
Insertion: back of the sacrotuberous ligament.
Action: extensor and lateral rotator of thigh.
Nerve supply: inferior gluteal (L5, S1, 2).

Noninvasive Therapy

The post–trigger point injection follow-up program described in Chapter 11 is recommended as a conservative therapeutic treatment approach. Noninvasive therapy can include:

- Physical therapy modalities (e.g., electrical stimulation and warm packs; see Chapter 19).
- Manual physical therapy techniques (e.g., massage, joint mobilization, and the Trager® Approach [neuromuscular re-education]; see Chapters 16–18 for additional manual techniques).
- Active and passive stretching and limbering of muscles with or without the use of vaporized coolant spray or ice. Active exercise is part of the stretch-and-spray technique. Limbering and relaxation are necessary prior to stretching. Contract-relax techniques may be used.
- Stretch and spray for the gluteus maximus is performed with the patient lying on the uninvolved side. The hip is flexed bringing the knee to the abdomen. Use relaxation techniques to relax the gluteal muscles. Have the patient contract and

relax the buttocks. When contracting the gluteal muscles in the supine position, the patient should breathe in and exhale with release or letting go of the contraction. This may be accompanied by the use of vaporized coolant spray or ice if necessary. The therapist's hands should feel the contraction and relaxation of the muscle. The patient should be told that it is the relaxation ("letting go") of the muscle that is the most important part of the exercises. Electrical stimulation, limbering of muscles, and warm packs should precede stretch and spray to relax muscles.

- The exercise program for the hip and low back is described in Chapter 15. Include exercises that stretch the gluteus maximus area by bending forward in the sitting position. This should also be accompanied by appropriate relaxation and letting go. The patient should inhale when sitting up and exhale when bending forward. Movements should always be done slowly, smoothly, and with few repetitions (three to four).

Injection of Trigger Point

Trigger points may be palpated in the medial portion, lower midportion, and inferior portion of the gluteus maximus. A trigger point over the ischial bursa may be the cause of pain as well as TrPs below the crest of the ilium. Injection of TrPs should include multiple needle entries covering not only the area of the palpable tender TrP but a search for additional TrPs throughout the muscle (see Fig. 12–10). This would require injecting the four areas as noted in the figure. Trigger points over the area of the sciatic nerve should be well identified, isolated by palpation, and injected superficially, cautiously, and with avoidance of deep penetration. Injection may be performed with the patient prone with the pillow under the abdomen or in the side-lying position. (See Chapter 11 for injection technique.)

Needle size: Usually a 3-in., 21-gauge needle is necessary. For very thin persons a 1.5- to 2.0-in. needle may suffice.

Solution: Any one of the following solutions may be used: 0.5% procaine; 1.0% lidocaine; saline and dry needling in case of allergy. Do not use epinephrine.

Following injection apply pressure immediately. An ice compress may be used to prevent hematoma if excessive bleeding appears to be present or anticipated. The use of a moist heating pad or hot packs applied to the buttock for 5 to 10 minutes to reduce postinjection soreness should be done with caution. The use of hot packs after injection may encourage bleeding. Neither heat nor cold applications should be necessary following TrP injection.

Precautions

- Avoid the sciatic nerve, which lies at a midpoint between the ischial tuberosity and greater trochanter (as illustrated in Fig. 12–11).
- Tests for sciatic nerve involvement: Following injection the patient should not experience numbness, paresthesia in the lower extremity, or muscle weakness involving the foot.

Postinjection Follow-up Physical Therapy Program

The patient should receive 3 to 4 consecutive days of treatment. Physical therapy should include electrical stimulation, relaxation, limbering, and stretching of the involved muscle using vaporized coolant spray or ice as needed combined with and followed by an exercise program. Active and active-assisted exercises are an integral part of the physical therapy program (see Chapter 11 for details).

Exercise and Home Program

Exercises should at first be performed under the guidance of a therapist. Exercises include stretching of the gluteus maximus by flexing the hip and bringing the knee to the chest. This can be assisted and passively stretched by both the therapist and the patient at home. The patient must be given a home exercise program that includes active exercises as well as stretching. When the patient is free of pain and full motion has been achieved, there can be progress to strength and endurance programs. Begin and end exercise sessions with stretching and relaxation. Exercise programs include relaxation, limbering, stretching, and strengthening. When the patient is free of pain and full motion has been achieved, progress to strength and endurance programs (see Chapter 15 for details).

Corrective and Preventive Measures

- An unbalanced sitting posture for prolonged periods may produce TrPs in the gluteal muscles. Trigger points that are symptomatic may require a doughnut-like pillow designed to take weight off specific TrPs. Poor sitting posture may aggravate latent TrPs.
- Avoid improperly constructed seat cushions. Cushions that have prominences such as buttons may have an effect similar to carrying a wallet or other objects in the back pocket.
- Night pain may be helped by sleeping on the uninvolved side with a pillow between the thighs.
- Correct leg length discrepancies, e.g., with a heel lift.
- Correct foot abnormalities (flatfoot), e.g., with appropriate orthoses.

Gluteus Medius

Symptoms and Pain Pattern

- Pain occurs in the low back, buttock area, and lateral and posterior aspect of the thigh (Fig. 12–11).
- Pain may be sciatic in nature involving the posterior aspect of the lower extremity.[21, 24, 39, 41]

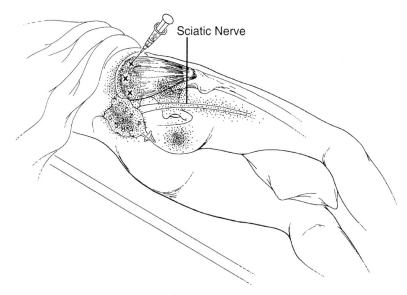

Figure 12–11. Gluteus medius. Injection of trigger points in the right gluteus medius. Multiple trigger points (*X's*) are noted. Anatomic skeletal landmarks are shown together with the sciatic nerve. The patient is positioned lying on the uninvolved side. Injection may also be performed with the patient prone. Pain pattern is noted by *stippled area.*

- Symptoms are similar to those found with TrPs in the gluteus maximus and often occur together with active TrPs in the gluteus maximus as well as in the lumbar and tensor fasciae latae muscles.
- Prolonged sitting, walking, or lying directly on the TrPs will cause localized pain that may radiate to the lower extremity.

Findings on Examination

- Tender TrPs noted on palpation in the gluteus medius just below the iliac crest posteriorly and anteriorly.
- A nodule or taut band of muscle fibers may be palpable. A jump sign is a frequent finding.
- Posteriorly, the gluteus medius is covered by the gluteus maximus. Most often a neighboring muscle or muscles will also harbor TrPs. Trigger points in the sacrospinalis, quadratus lumborum, and tensor fasciae latae will be found together with involvement of all the gluteal muscles. This is often the combination of multiple TrPs found in patients with low back pain.
- Contracture of the muscle may be present.
- Test for muscle weakness by having the patient lie on the uninvolved side. Pressure is exerted on the abducted hyperextended leg with the knee in extension. Depending on the degree of weakness, the patient may walk with a limp (gluteus medius limp). Slight weakness may cause postural changes such as scoliosis and pelvic tilt, which can give rise to TrPs in the lumbar area.

Differential Diagnosis

- Herniated lumbar disc.
- Sciatica.
- Trochanteric bursitis.
- Leriche's syndrome.
- Sacroilaic joint dysfunction.
- Sciatic neuritis due to arthritis or diabetes.

Anatomy

Origin: outer surface of the ilium between the posterior and medial gluteal line.
Insertion: outer aspect of the greater trochanter.
Action: abducts thigh; prevents opposite side of pelvis from dropping when walking.
Nerve supply: superior gluteal (L4, 5, S1).

Noninvasive Therapy

The post–trigger point injection follow-up program described in Chapter 11 is recommended as a conservative therapeutic approach. Noninvasive therapy can include:

- Physical therapy modalities (e.g., electrical stimulation and warm packs; see Chapter 19).
- Manual physical therapy techniques (e.g., massage, joint mobilization, and the Trager® Approach [neuromuscular re-education]; see Chapters 16–18 for additional manual techniques).
- Active and passive stretching and limbering of muscles with or without the use of vaporized coolant spray or ice. Active exercise is part of the stretch-and-spray technique. Limbering and relaxation are necessary prior to stretching. Contract-relax techniques may be used.
- Stretch and spray for the gluteus medius is performed in the side-lying position. Positioning may be improved by placing a flat pillow under the uninvolved hip. Stretching of the gluteus is performed by adduction of the thigh, bringing the leg

both posteriorly as well as anteriorly to stretch both portions of the gluteus medius posteriorly and anteriorly. The patient may be moved back toward the edge of the table with the leg partly off the table in extension supported by the therapist. The thigh is extended posteriorly, adducted, and externally rotated. The leg is also brought forward to the opposite side of the table, and the thigh extended, adducted, and internally rotated. Electrical stimulation, limbering of muscles, and warm packs may precede stretch and spray to relax the muscles. Stretching of muscle is also accomplished actively as well as with assistance during the exercise program. Active exercise is part of the stretch-and-spray technique. Use relaxation techniques (e.g., contract-relax). Electrical stimulation, limbering of muscles, and warm packs should precede stretch and spray to relax muscles.

- Exercise program: The exercise program for the gluteus medius is described in Chapter 15. Exercise programs include relaxation, limbering, stretching, and strengthening. When the patient is free of pain and full motion has been achieved, progress to strength and endurance programs.

Trigger Point Injection

Injection may be performed with the patient lying on the uninvolved side or prone (see Chapter 11 for technique). Tender TrPs are identified (see Fig. 12–11).

Needle size: 3 in., 22 gauge, is usually used for needling the gluteal area. In the case of thin persons, smaller needles of 1.5 to 2.0 in., 22 gauge, may be used.

Solution: Any one of the following solutions may be used: 0.5% procaine; 1.0% lidocaine; saline and dry needling in cases of allergy. Do not use epinephrine.

A small amount of vaporized coolant spray over the needle entry area prior to injection decreases the pain of needle entry. Many patients report that avoiding needle entry pain decreases the discomfort of the procedure appreciably and avoids tensing. This effect varies with the individual patient. Look for additional TrPs in addition to the local tender area. The gluteus medius should be palpated and explored using multiple needle entries as noted in Figure 12-11. Multiple TrPs involving the gluteus maximus, gluteus minimus, quadratus lumborum, and tensor fasciae latae may be present. Each muscle group must be treated individually. The low back muscles, such as the sacrospinalis and quadratus lumborum TrPs, may be treated separately or together.

Precautions

- Following the injection, the patient should not experience any paresthesia or muscle weakness in the lower extremity.
- Avoid injection in the area of the sciatic nerve, and avoid the greater sciatic notch area.
- Inject only one TrP area or muscle group at a time. Postinjection spasm after multiple muscle group injections may prevent a proper rehabilitation program.

Postinjection Follow-up Physical Therapy Program

The patient should receive 3 to 4 consecutive days of treatment. Physical therapy should include electrical stimulation, relaxation, limbering, and stretching of the involved muscle using vaporized coolant spray or ice as needed combined with and followed by an exercise program. Active-assisted and active exercises are an integral part of the physical therapy program (see Chapter 11 for details).

Exercise and Home Program

Exercises for the gluteus medius are prescribed. Exercises should at first be performed under the guidance of a therapist. When the patient is free of pain and full motion has been achieved, progress to strength and endurance programs. Begin and end the exercise sessions with stretching and relaxation. (See Chapter 15 for exercise details.)

Corrective and Preventive Measures

- Correct poor sitting and standing postures.
- Abnormalities of the pelvis such as a small hemipelvis may be corrected with a buttock lift.[51]
- Correct improper chair construction. Use a lumbar support to improve a car seat or chair.
- Remove objects from the back pocket, e.g., wallet.
- Correct leg length discrepancies, e.g., use a heel lift.
- Correct foot abnormalities such as flatfoot or Morton's foot. The physician should prescribe orthoses as necessary.

Gluteus Minimus

Symptoms and Pain Pattern

- The patient may experience pain over the buttock area in addition to sciatic referred-type pain radiating as far distally as the ankle (Fig. 12–12).
- Anterior TrPs refer pain along the lateral thigh, lower buttock, and lateral aspect of the ankle.
- Posterior TrPs refer pain to the buttock area and posterior upper thigh in addition to the calf.[22, 24] Travell and Simons[52] make a distinction between radiating pain patterns due to anterior and posterior fibers. Other authors[7, 15, 16, 23] are not as specific when attributing sciatic pain from the gluteal muscle area.

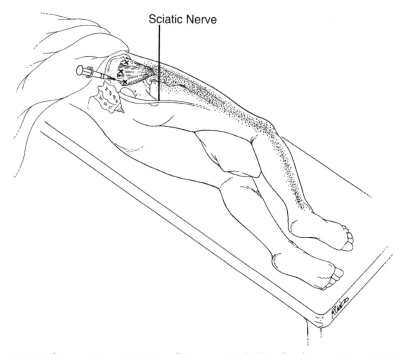

Figure 12–12. Gluteus minimus. Injection of trigger points *(X's)* in the gluteus minimus. Injection may be given with the patient in the prone or side-lying position. Anatomic landmarks and sciatic nerve are noted. Pain pattern *(stippling)* may extend to the ankle.

- A similar pattern of pain is experienced by patients with TrPs in the gluteus maximus and gluteus medius.[17, 24]
- Pain is noted with sitting and walking.
- Night pain occurs when lying on the TrP area.

Findings on Examination

- Trigger points may be found in the anterior and posterior portions of the muscle. Both may be palpated with the patient lying on the uninvolved side.
- Most often TrPs in the gluteus minimus are accompanied by TrPs in the surrounding muscles, e.g., the gluteus maximus, medius, piriformis, sacrospinalis, and latissimus dorsi.
- Referred pain may cause the development of TrPs in the posterior aspect of the thigh.
- Examination of the gluteus minimus may reveal weakness of abduction and shortening of the muscle.

Differential Diagnosis

- Sciatic radiculopathy.
- Herniated lumbar disc.
- Trochanteric bursitis.
- Arthritis of the hip.
- Lumbar facet joint arthritis.
- Sacroiliac joint dysfunction.

Anatomy

Origin: outer surface of the ilium between the middle and inferior gluteal lines.
Insertion: the greater trochanter of the femur.
Action: abductor and medial rotator of the femur.
Nerve supply: superior gluteal (L4, 5, S1).

Noninvasive Therapy

The post–trigger point injection follow-up program described in Chapter 11 is recommended as a conservative therapeutic treatment approach. Noninvasive therapy can include:

- Physical therapy modalities (e.g., electrical stimulation and warm packs; see Chapter 19).
- Manual physical therapy techniques (e.g., massage, joint mobilization, and the Trager® Approach [neuromuscular re-education]; see Chapters 16–18 for additional manual techniques).
- Active and passive stretching and limbering of muscles with or without the use of vaporized coolant spray or ice. Active exercise is part of the stretch-and-spray technique. Limbering and relaxation are necessary prior to stretching. Contract-relax techniques may be used.
- Stretch and spray may be performed with the patient lying on the uninvolved side. Positioning may be improved by placing a flat pillow under the uninvolved hip. Stretching of the gluteus minimus is performed by adduction of the thigh, bringing the leg both posteriorly as well as anteriorly to stretch both portions of the gluteus medius posteriorly and anteriorly. The patient may be moved back toward the edge of the table with the leg partly off the table in extension and supported by the therapist. The thigh is extended posteriorly, adducted, and externally rotated. The leg is also brought forward to the opposite side of the table, and the thigh extended, adducted, and internally rotated. Electrical stimulation, limbering of muscles, and warm packs should precede stretch and spray to relax the muscles. Stretching of

muscle is also accomplished actively as well as with assistance during the exercise program. Active exercise is part of the stretch-and-spray technique.

- Exercises and a home program for the gluteus minimus are described in Chapter 15. Exercise programs include relaxation, limbering, stretching, and strengthening. When the patient is free of pain and full motion has been achieved, progress to strength and endurance programs.

Injection of Trigger Point

Injection and needling may be performed with the patient lying on the uninvolved side (see Chapter 11 for technique). Tender TrPs are identified. In addition to local injection of the tender area, multiple needle entries may be necessary to probe for TrPs not felt on palpation. It is not unusual for the needle to penetrate the gluteus minimus and make contact with the ilium. Following injection, test for sciatic nerve symptoms and signs prior to permitting the patient to walk. The patient should remain on the table for a few minutes. Inquire about any abnormal sensation such as numbness or paresthesia in the lower extremity.

Needle size: 3 in., 22–20 gauge.
Solution: Any one of the following solutions may be used: 0.5% procaine; 1.0% lidocaine; saline and dry needling in case of allergy. Do not use epinephrine.

Postinjection Follow-up Physical Therapy Program

The patient should receive 3 to 4 consecutive days of treatment. Physical therapy should include electrical stimulation, relaxation, limbering, and stretching of the involved muscle using vaporized coolant spray or ice as needed combined with and followed by an exercise program. Active and active-assisted exercises are an integral part of the physical therapy program (see Chapter 11 for details).

Exercise and Home Program

Exercises include stretching for the gluteal and lumbar areas. Exercises should at first be performed under the guidance of a therapist. When the patient is free of pain and full motion has been achieved, progress to strength and endurance programs. Begin and end exercise sessions with stretching and relaxation. (See Chapter 15 for exercise details.)

Corrective and Preventive Measures

- Correct foot abnormalities (e.g., Morton's foot, flatfoot) and prescribe orthoses as indicated.
- Correct leg length discrepancy, e.g., prescribe an appropriate heel lift.
- Scoliosis due to small hemipelvis may be corrected by an ischial lift pad under the ischial area.[52]
- Correct postural stresses at work. Advise changing position frequently and using a footstool when standing and working at a table or sink. (See Chapter 20.)
- The patient should avoid poor sitting and standing postures.
- Chairs should be properly constructed and adjusted for individual needs, e.g., the height of armrests, the need for lumbar support.
- Advise removal of objects in the back pocket such as a wallet.[26]

Piriformis

Symptoms and Pain Pattern

- The patient may experience pain in the low back, buttock, and hip.
- Radiation of pain to the lower extremity involving the posterior thigh, calf, and foot (Fig. 12–13). This pain pattern is referred to by Kraus[21] as "pseudo-disc.")

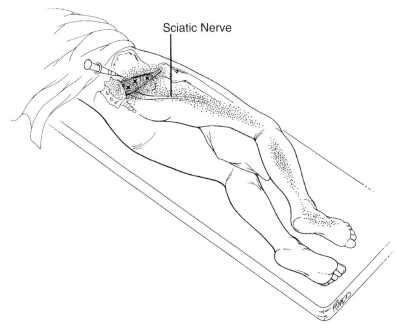

Figure 12–13. Piriformis. Injection of trigger points in the right piriformis muscle *(X's)*. The sciatic nerve is shown in addition to anatomic details. Injection is performed with the patient lying on the uninvolved side. A pillow is placed between the knees. The hip is flexed. Pain pattern is shown by *stippling*.

- Paresthesia may be experienced in the lower extremity.
- Pain may be noted after prolonged sitting or driving.[11]
- Pain occurs with prolonged stooping and squatting.[48]
- Sciatic pain may occur with symptoms of entrapment of the sciatic nerve.[19, 23, 33, 51]
- Pace and Nagle[31] have reported dyspareunia as a symptom of the piriformis syndrome.

Findings on Examination

- Piriformis syndrome[47] is seen more frequently in women than men, in a 6:1 ratio.
- Palpation may reveal tenderness of the piriformis muscle and is often noted in the sciatic notch.
- For the examiner to palpate the piriformis muscle, the patient should lie on the uninvolved side with the hip flexed and a pillow between the upper and lower legs.
- A taut band extending over the length of the piriformis (from the greater trochanter to the sacrum) may be found.
- Steiner and associates[46] found the most common trigger area to be located 3 cm caudal and lateral to the midpoint of the lateral border of the sacrum. The second TrP is located closer to its trochanteric insertion.[46]
- Piriformis tenderness with TrPs may also be palpated by rectal or intrapelvic examination.[1, 12, 31, 51] Coccygodynia is often caused by TrPs and spasm of the levator ani and coccygeus muscles.
- On palpation of a TrP a referred pattern of pain may be elicited.
- Diminished sensation in the lower extremity or depressed or absent ankle jerk with mild footdrop may represent neurologic findings resulting from TrPs in the piriformis.
- Restriction in internal rotation on the involved side occurs.
- A positive Trendelenburg's test is noted.
- There is pain and weakness on testing abduction strength in the seated position.
- Adduction may be limited and painful.

- The patient may maintain the leg in external rotation due to pain experienced with internal rotation.
- A leg length discrepancy may be noted in addition to asymmetry of the pelvis (e.g., hemipelvis).

Differential Diagnosis

The following conditions must be differentiated and are often mistaken for piriformis TrPs:
- Herniated intervertebral disc.
- Peripheral nerve entrapment can occur as a piriformis syndrome without TrPs.
- Sacroiliitis.
- Facet syndrome.

Anatomy

Origin: front of the middle three pieces of the sacrum.
Insertion: tip of greater trochanter.
Action: lateral rotation of the thigh, abduction of the thigh when the hip is flexed.
Nerve supply: branches from L5, S1, and S2.

Noninvasive Therapy

The post–trigger point injection follow-up program described in Chapter 11 is recommended as a conservative therapeutic treatment approach. Noninvasive therapy can include:

- Physical therapy modalities (e.g., electrical stimulation and warm packs; see Chapter 19).
- Manual physical therapy techniques (e.g., massage, joint mobilization, and the Trager® Approach [neuromuscular re-education]; see Chapters 16–18 for additional manual techniques).
- Active and passive stretching and limbering of muscles with or without the use of vaporized coolant spray or ice. Active exercise is part of the stretch-and-spray technique. Limbering and relaxation are necessary prior to stretching. Contract-relax techniques may be used.
- Stretch and spray for the piriformis is performed with the patient lying on the uninvolved side with the hip flexed to 90 degrees. Stretch is done in the direction of adduction and internal rotation. Electrical stimulation, limbering of muscles, and warm packs should precede stretch and spray to relax the muscles. Stretching of muscle is also accomplished actively as well as with assistance during the exercise program. Active exercise is part of the stretch-and-spray technique.
- Exercise and home program. Exercises include hip abduction with the limb in moderate external rotation. Piriformis muscle stretching is accomplished by adducting the thigh with the hip flexed. See Chapter 15 for hip and low back exercises. Exercise programs include relaxation, limbering, stretching, and strengthening. When the patient is free of pain and full motion has been achieved, progress to strength and endurance programs.

Injection of Trigger Point

Injection is accomplished with the patient lying on the unaffected side with the thigh flexed to approximately 60 to 45 degrees (see Fig. 12–13). The knee is dropped to the plinth. A pillow is placed between the knees. Identify the TrP by palpation. Several authors have recommended that injection of TrPs in the medial region of the muscle be performed bimanually. One finger palpates the TrP either by the rectal or vaginal approach and the other directs the needle externally in the direction of the intrapelvic palpating fingertip.[31, 52] (See Chapter 11 for injection technique.)

Needle size: 2, 3 in., 20 gauge.

Solution: Any one of the following solutions may be used: 0.5% procaine; 1.0% lidocaine; saline and dry needling in case of allergy. Do not use epinephrine.

Precautions

Postinjection complications: Test for sciatic nerve involvement following injection, including diminished sensation or muscle weakness. (See Chapter 11 for complications.)

Postinjection Follow-up Physical Therapy Program

After injection the patient is instructed not to sit, stand, or walk for prolonged periods. He or she is advised to change position often. The patient should receive 3 to 4 consecutive days of treatment. Therapy should include electrical stimulation, relaxation, limbering, and stretching of the involved muscle using vaporized coolant spray or ice as needed combined with and followed by an exercise program (see Chapter 11 for details).

Exercise and Home Program

Exercises should at first be performed under the guidance of a therapist. When the patient is free of pain and full motion has been achieved, there should be progress to strength and endurance programs. Begin and end exercise sessions with stretching and relaxation (see Chapter 15 for piriformis, hip, and low back exercise details). Advise the use of a pillow between the legs when sleeping on the side. Exercises should include stretching of the piriformis by adducting the thigh with the hip flexed and the pelvis stabilized (countertraction on the crest of the ilium).

Corrective and Preventive Measures

- Correct leg length inequality, e.g., with a heel lift.
- Postural corrections of small hemipelvis or scoliosis may require a buttock lift when sitting.[52]
- Correct foot deformities (e.g., flatfoot, Morton's foot) and prescribe orthoses.
- Patient must avoid prolonged unsupported lateral rotation of the leg on the accelerator when driving.
- Avoid sitting for long periods with the ankle crossed on the opposite knee.[50]

Tensor Fasciae Latae

Symptoms and Pain Pattern

- Pain over the lateral aspect of the hip[10] (Fig. 12–14).
- Referred pain may radiate to the greater trochanter area extending distally to the outer aspect of the thigh and below the knee. This pattern of referred pain may be mistaken for lumbar radiculopathy.[15, 16, 21, 24]
- Pressure on the TrP may cause pain when the patient lies on the involved side.
- Since TrPs in the gluteal muscles are frequently present together with those of the tensor fasciae latae, symptoms of gluteal muscle TrPs may also occur.
- Pain may be present with walking or running activities.

Findings on Examination

- Trigger points may be palpated along the tensor fasciae latae with the patient in the supine position or lying on the uninvolved side.
- The muscle extends laterally and inferiorly inserting into the iliotibial band.
- Tenderness may be found over the greater trochanter and in the area of referred pain.

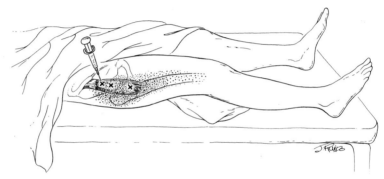

Figure 12–14. Tensor fasciae latae. Injection of trigger points in the right tensor fasciae latae *(X's)*. Anatomic landmarks are noted including the origin and insertion of the muscle. The patient is supine with a small pillow under the knee. Pain pattern is shown by *stippling*.

- Contracture of the tensor fasciae latae causes contracture of the iliotibial band, which can be demonstrated by a positive Ober's test. Ober's test for contraction of the iliotibial band is performed with the patient lying on the uninvolved side. The leg is abducted, the knee is flexed to 90 degrees, and the abducted leg is released. If the iliotibial tract is normal, the thigh should drop to the adducted position. In the presence of contracture of the fasciae latae or iliotibial band, the thigh remains abducted when the leg is released.[13] In less severe cases when a degree of tightness is present, limited adduction of the hip occurs.
- Palpation may cause a referred pain pattern to the outer aspect of the hip and lower extremity (see Fig. 12–14).

Differential Diagnosis

- Herniated disc.
- Trochanteric bursitis.
- Neuralgia paresthetica.[19]

Anatomy

Origin: outer surface of ilium, between the tubercle of the crest and the anterior superior iliac spine.
Insertion: iliotibial tract below the greater trochanter of the femur.
Action: assists gluteus maximus in tightening the iliotibial band.
Nerve supply: superior gluteal (L4, 5, S1).

Noninvasive Therapy

The post–trigger point injection follow-up program described in Chapter 11 is recommended as a conservative therapeutic treatment approach. Noninvasive therapy can include:

- Physical therapy modalities (e.g., electrical stimulation and warm packs; see Chapter 19).
- Manual physical therapy techniques (e.g., massage, joint mobilization, and the Trager® Approach [neuromuscular re-education]; see Chapters 16–18 for additional manual techniques).
- Active and passive stretching and limbering of muscles with or without the use of vaporized coolant spray or ice. Active exercise is part of the stretch-and-spray technique. Limbering and relaxation are necessary prior to stretching. Contract-relax techniques may be used.
- Stretch and spray for the tensor fasciae latae is performed with the patient side-

lying on the uninvolved side. Electrical stimulation, limbering of muscles, and warm packs should precede stretch and spray to relax the muscles. Begin stretch and spray with the knee extended to promote adduction, increasing knee flexion as adduction increases. As with all stretch movements about the hip, the pelvis must be stabilized. Follow with active stretching.

- Exercises and a home program for the hip and knee are described in Chapter 15. Exercise programs include relaxation, limbering, stretching, and strengthening. When the patient is free of pain and full motion has been achieved, progress to strength and endurance programs.

Injection of Trigger Point

The tensor fasciae latae may be palpated in the supine position or with the patient lying on the uninvolved side. Trigger point injection may be performed in the supine or side-lying position (see Fig. 12–14). A search for all TrPs is essential. Multiple entries and the use of a fanning, circular technique are necessary for proper TrP treatment. Injection of lidocaine is performed after the TrP is encountered. (See Chapter 11 for TrP injection technique.)

Needle size: 1.5 or 3.0 in., 21 gauge.
Solution: Any one of the following solutions may be used: 0.5% procaine; 1.0% lidocaine; saline and dry needling in case of allergy. Do not use epinephrine.

Postinjection Follow-up Physical Therapy Program

The patient should receive 3 to 4 consecutive days of treatment. Physical therapy should include electrical stimulation, relaxation, limbering, and stretching of the involved muscle using vaporized coolant spray or ice as needed combined with and followed by an exercise program. Active and active-assisted exercises are an integral part of the physical therapy program (see Chapter 11 for details).

Exercise and Home Program

Exercises include stretching of the tensor fascia latae. Stretch and spray with the patient in the side-lying position. Hip abduction is followed by adduction, permitting gravity to assist in the adduction maneuver. The stretch is first done with the leg extended, brought into the position of adduction. This progresses to performing the exercise with the knee flexed. The patient should be relaxed, permitting the flexed knee to fall assisted by gravity until it touches the plinth. The knee is then extended and the leg abducted. Exercises should at first be performed under the guidance of a therapist. When the patient is free of pain and full motion has been achieved, progress to strength and endurance programs. Begin and end exercise sessions with relaxation. (See Chapter 15 for exercise details.)

Corrective and Preventive Measures

- Correct leg length inequality, e.g., with a heel lift.
- Correct foot deformities: calcaneal valgus, flatfoot, Morton's foot. Prescribe orthoses as needed.

Hamstring Muscles

Semimembranosus, Semitendinosus, Biceps Femoris

Symptoms and Pain Pattern

- Pain from the hamstrings is noted in the gluteal region, lower thigh, and upper portion of the leg[17] (Fig. 12–15).

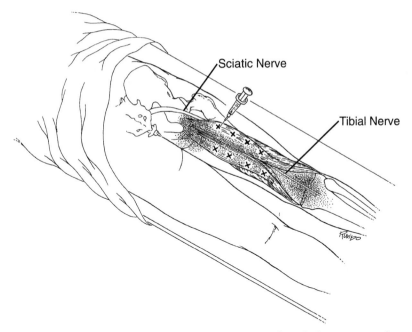

Figure 12–15. Hamstring muscles. Injection of trigger points in the right hamstring muscles with the patient prone. Injection of trigger points may be performed with the patient supine with the hip and knee in slight flexion and the leg externally rotated. It is preferable to do either the medial or lateral hamstring during one session. Injection of more than one muscle group promotes soreness and muscle spasm, which may interfere with rehabilitation. Anatomic landmarks are noted including the sciatic nerve. Pain patterns are noted by *stippling*.

- Pain may be referred by the biceps femoris to the lateral aspect of the knee posteriorly.[7, 9, 51]
- The semitendinosus or semimembranosus may refer pain to the medial side of the back of the knee.[10, 38]
- Symptoms may occur with walking or sitting.[32]
- Compression of TrPs will give rise to symptoms.

Findings on Examination
- Tender TrPs over the hamstrings may cause local or referred pain extending approximately to the gluteal area, distally to the posterior aspect of the thigh and the back of the knee.
- In cases of hamstring tightness and TrPs, the gluteal and lumbar areas should also be examined for TrPs.
- Limited straight leg raising with pain in the low back.
- Pain in the posterior aspect of the thigh and the back of the knee may be mistaken for a positive straight leg raising test owing to sciatic nerve irritation.

Differential Diagnosis
- Herniated lumbar disc.
- Peripheral neuritis.
- Knee disorders, e.g., osteoarthritis, torn posterior horn of meniscus.
- Ischial bursitis.

Anatomy
Biceps Femoris, Long Head
Origin: ischial tuberosity.
Insertion: head of fibula, lateral condyle of tibia.

Action: extends thigh, flexes leg.
Nerve supply: sciatic (tibial portion) (S1, 2, 3).

Biceps Femoris Short Head

Origin: linea aspera, intermuscular septum.
Insertion: lateral condyle of tibia.
Action: flexes leg.
Nerve supply: sciatic (common peroneal portion) (L5, S1, 2).

Semitendinosus

Origin: ischial tuberosity.
Insertion: medial body of the tibia behind the sartorius and inferior to the gracilis.
Action: extends thigh, flexes leg.
Nerve supply: sciatic (tibial portion) (L5, S1, 2, 3).

Semimembranosus

Origin: ischial tuberosity.
Insertion: posteromedial aspect of tibial condyle.
Action: extends thigh, flexes leg.
Nerve supply: sciatic (tibial portion) (L5, S1, 2).

Noninvasive Therapy

The post–trigger point injection follow-up program described in Chapter 11 is recommended as a conservative therapeutic treatment approach. Noninvasive therapy can include:

- Physical therapy modalities (e.g., electrical stimulation and warm packs; see Chapter 19).
- Manual physical therapy techniques (e.g., massage, joint mobilization, and the Trager® Approach [neuromuscular re-education]; see Chapters 16–18 for additional manual techniques).
- Active and passive stretching and limbering of muscles with or without the use of vaporized coolant spray or ice. Active exercise is part of the stretch-and-spray technique. Limbering and relaxation are necessary prior to stretching. Contract-relax techniques may be used.
- Stretch and spray: Electrical stimulation, limbering of muscles, and warm packs should precede stretch and spray to relax the muscles. Use vaporized coolant spray or ice to encourage flexion of the thigh and extension of the leg. Examine neighboring muscles for TrPs and muscle tightness. Lengthening neighboring muscles such as the adductor magnus followed by release of the gluteal muscles may be necessary prior to stretching the hamstring muscles.[54]
- Exercise and a home program for the hip and knee are described in Chapter 15. Exercise programs include relaxation, limbering, stretching, and strengthening. When the patient is free of pain and full motion has been achieved, progress to strength and endurance programs.

Injection of Trigger Point

The patient may be supine with the legs slightly externally rotated with the hip and knee in slight flexion. Injection may also be performed with the patient in the side-lying position or prone (see Fig. 12–15). It is preferable to do either the medial or lateral hamstring during one session. If more than one muscle group is injected, postinjection soreness and spasm may interfere with proper rehabilitation. It is essential to explore the length of the muscle by multiple needling in addition to any single TrP that is found on palpation. (See Chapter 11 for injection technique.)

Needle size: 1.5, 2.0, 3.0 in., 22 gauge.

Solution: Any one of the following solutions may be used: 0.5% procaine; 1.0% lidocaine; saline and dry needling in case of allergy. Do not use epinephrine.

Postinjection Follow-up Physical Therapy Program

The patient should receive 3 to 4 consecutive days of treatment. Physical therapy should include electrical stimulation, relaxation, limbering, and stretching of the involved muscle using vaporized coolant spray or ice as needed combined with and followed by an exercise program. Active and active-assisted exercises are an integral part of the physical therapy program. Crutches are used for 24 hours following injection to prevent pain, spasm, and limping. (See Chapter 11 for program details.)

Exercise and Home Program

Exercises for the hamstrings are prescribed. Exercises should at first be performed under the guidance of a therapist. When the patient is free of pain and full motion has been achieved, progress to strength and endurance programs. Begin and end exercise sessions with stretching and relaxation. (See Chapter 15 for exercise details.)

Precautions

- Avoid the sciatic nerve (see Fig. 12–15).

Corrective and Preventive Measures

- Avoid compression of the hamstrings by correction of poor sitting habits.
- Perform warm-up and cool-down exercises, which include hamstring stretches before and after athletic activity to prevent the development of TrPs and activation of latent TrPs.
- Continue home exercise program.

Quadriceps Femoris

Rectus Femoris, Vastus Intermedius, Vastus Medialis, Vastus Lateralis

Single muscle TrPs in the muscles of the quadriceps femoris commonly cause TrPs in neighboring muscles.

Rectus Femoris

Symptoms and Pain Pattern

- Trigger points in the rectus femoris refer pain to the lower thigh and anterior aspect of the knee.
- Pain at night occurring in front of the knee.[22, 24, 54]
- Feeling of weakness in the thigh.

Findings on Examination

- Tightness of the rectus femoris may be demonstrated in the side-lying position by extending the hip and flexing the knee. This can also be done with the patient lying in the supine position bringing the leg off the examination table and extending the hip and flexing the knee.
- Trigger points may be found on palpation along the entire length of the muscle. Most TrPs, however, are found in the regions of muscle origin and insertion. These areas are emphasized during examination for TrPs.[22]

- Quadriceps atrophy may be present due to disuse or symptomatic knee disorders.
- Chronic pain due to a knee abnormality may give rise to TrPs in the quadratus femoris muscles.

Differential Diagnosis

- Arthritis of the knee.
- Internal derangement of the knee.
- Chondromalacia.

Anatomy

Origin: the straight head from the anterior inferior iliac spine; the reflected head from the rim of the acetabulum.

Insertion: common tendon of quadriceps, upper border of patella, and through the patellar ligament to the tubercle of the tibia.

Action: extends leg, flexes thigh.

Nerve supply: femoral (L2, 3, 4).

Noninvasive Therapy

The post–trigger point injection follow-up program described in Chapter 11 is recommended as a conservative therapeutic treatment approach. Noninvasive therapy can include:

- Physical therapy modalities (e.g., electrical stimulation and warm packs; see Chapter 19).
- Manual physical therapy techniques (e.g., massage, joint mobilization, and the Trager® Approach [neuromuscular re-education]; see Chapters 16–18 for additional manual techniques).
- Active and passive stretching and limbering of muscles with or without the use of vaporized coolant spray or ice. Active exercise is part of the stretch-and-spray technique. Limbering and relaxation are necessary prior to stretching. Contract-relax techniques may be used.
- Stretch and spray for the rectus femoris is performed in the side-lying position with the help of vaporized coolant spray or ice. The hip is extended together with knee flexion. The TrP area and reference areas are sprayed as necessary to give pain relief. A self-stretch can be performed in the same manner with the patient in the standing position flexing the knee and pulling the heel toward the buttock, the opposite hand holding the table or wall for balance. Hold the stretch for 10 seconds. Relax and repeat. Electrical stimulation, limbering of muscles, and warm packs may precede stretch and spray to relax the muscles. Stretching of muscle is also accomplished actively as well as with assistance during the exercise program. Active exercise is part of the stretch-and-spray technique.
- Exercise and a home program for the rectus femoris are prescribed (see Chapter 15 for knee and hip exercises). Exercise programs include relaxation, limbering, stretching, and strengthening. When the patient is free of pain and full motion has been achieved, progress to strength and endurance programs.

Injection of Trigger Point

With the patient in the supine position, TrPs are identified and injected (see Chapter 11 for technique). Search for multiple TrPs emphasizing the area of origin and insertion (Fig. 12–16).

Postinjection Follow-up Physical Therapy Program

The patient should receive 3 to 4 consecutive days of treatment. Physical therapy should include electrical stimulation, relaxation, limbering, and stretching of the

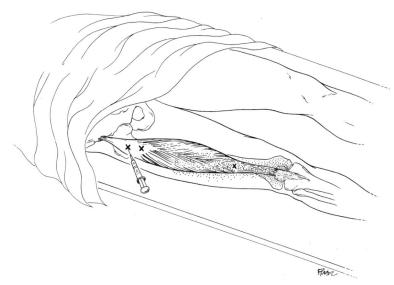

Figure 12–16. Rectus femoris. Injection of trigger points *(X's)* in the right rectus femoris. Note trigger points in the area of origin and distally toward the area of insertion. The patient is supine. The trigger point pain pattern is shown by *stippling*. Anatomic landmarks are noted.

involved muscle using vaporized coolant spray or ice as needed combined with and followed by an exercise program. Active and active-assisted exercises are an integral part of the physical therapy program.

Exercise and Home Program

Exercises for rectus femoris are prescribed. Exercises should at first be performed under the guidance of a therapist. When the patient is free of pain and full motion has been achieved, progress to strength and endurance programs. Begin and end exercise sessions with stretching and relaxation. (See Chapter 15 for exercise details.)

Corrective and Preventive Measures

- Avoid exercises that include deep squatting and knee bends greater than 90 degrees. Excessive squatting may damage a meniscus in addition to promotion of TrPs.
- Prolonged immobilization of the quadriceps can give rise to TrPs.

Vastus Medialis

Symptoms and Pain Pattern

- The vastus medialis may demonstrate atrophy in cases of knee abnormality and following surgery.
- Atrophy and TrPs may cause weakness, giving rise to feelings of giving way of the knee or buckling.
- Pain is located in the knee joint area and lower thigh[23, 24, 51] (Fig. 12–17).

Findings on Examination

- Tender TrPs in the vastus medialis.
- Atrophy of the vastus medialis.
- Weakness of the vastus medialis.

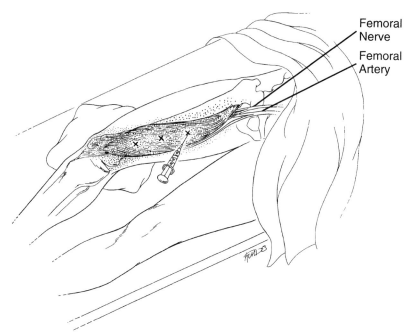

Figure 12–17. Vastus medialis. Injection of right vastus medialis trigger points *(X's)*. The patient is supine with a pillow under the knee. The leg is slightly externally rotated with flexion of the hip. Trigger point pain pattern is shown by *stippling*. Anatomic landmarks are noted including the femoral artery and nerve.

Differential Diagnosis

- Internal derangement of the knee.
- Chondromalacia.
- Arthritis of the knee.

Anatomy

Origin: intertrochanteric line, medial linea aspera.
Insertion: common tendon of the quadriceps to the medial side of the patella, through the patellar ligament to the tubercle of the tibia.
Action: extends leg.
Nerve supply: femoral (L2, 3, 4).

Noninvasive Therapy

The post–trigger point injection follow-up program described in Chapter 11 is recommended as a conservative therapeutic treatment approach. Noninvasive therapy can include:

- Physical therapy modalities (e.g., electrical stimulation and warm packs; see Chapter 19).
- Manual physical therapy techniques (e.g., massage, joint mobilization, and the Trager® Approach [neuromuscular re-education]; see Chapters 16–18 for additional manual techniques).
- Active and passive stretching and limbering of muscles with or without the use of vaporized coolant spray or ice. Active exercise is part of the stretch-and-spray technique. Limbering and relaxation are necessary prior to stretching. Contract-relax techniques may be used.
- Stretch and spray: Bring the knee into flexion using vaporized coolant spray or ice. Spray the TrP area and referred areas of pain. The extensor muscles are lengthened

by progressively flexing the knee. Electrical stimulation, limbering of muscles, and warm packs should precede stretch and spray to relax the muscles. Stretching of muscle is also accomplished actively and with assistance during the exercise program. Active exercise is part of the stretch-and-spray technique.

• Exercise and a home program for the lower extremity and knee and hip exercises are prescribed (see Chapter 15). Exercise programs include relaxation, limbering, stretching, and strengthening. When the patient is free of pain and full motion has been achieved, progress to strength and endurance programs.

Injection of Trigger Point

Injection may be given with the patient supine, with the leg outstretched or in slight flexion, abduction, and external rotation, depending on the findings, patient's comfort, and ease of the injection (see Fig. 12–17). Palpate all neighboring muscles for additional TrPs. Perform multiple needling to determine the presence of other TrPs that may not have been found with palpation.

Needle size: 1.5, 2.0, 3.0 in., 21 gauge. Length of needle depends on patient's size.
Solution: Any one of the following solutions may be used: 0.5% procaine; 1.0% lidocaine; saline and dry needling in case of allergy. Do not use epinephrine.

Precautions

• Avoid the femoral artery (see Fig. 12–17).
• Always aspirate before injecting.

Postinjection Physical Therapy Follow-up Program

Follow-up program requires 3 to 4 consecutive days of follow-up treatment. Physical therapy should include electrical stimulation, relaxation, limbering of muscles, and stretching of the involved muscles using vapocoolant spray or ice as needed combined with and followed by an exercise program. Active and active-assisted exercises are an integral part of the physical therapy program. When the lower extremities are injected, the patient should use crutches for 2 days to avoid full weight-bearing and prevent limping and muscle spasm. Following 3 to 4 days of physical therapy, the patient is then placed on a progressive exercise program (see Chapter 11 for details).

Exercise and Home Program

Exercises for the knee are prescribed. Exercises should at first be performed under the guidance of a therapist. When the patient is free of pain and full motion has been achieved, progress to strength and endurance programs. Begin and end exercise sessions with stretching and relaxation (see Chapter 15 for exercise details).

Corrective and Preventive Measures

• Check for malalignment of lower extremities, e.g., genu varus, genu valgus, or foot abnormalities (e.g., flatfoot).
• Prescribe orthoses as indicated.

Vastus Intermedius

Symptoms and Pain Pattern

• Pain in the thigh is noted with activity (Fig. 12–18).
• Pain may be present at rest.

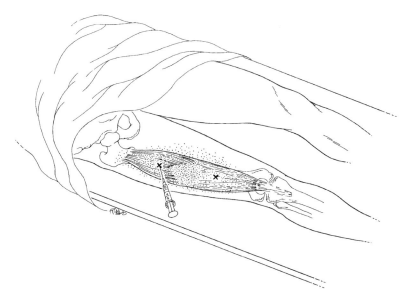

Figure 12–18. Vastus intermedius. Injection of trigger points *(X's)* in the right vastus intermedius with the patient supine. The leg is in neutral position. Trigger point pain is shown by *stippling*. Muscle origin and insertion are noted.

Findings on Examination

- Tender TrPs on palpation of the vastus intermedius together with vastus medialis, vastus lateralis, and femoris.
- Trigger points in these muscles cause shortening, which inhibits flexion of the knee.

Differential Diagnosis

- Osteoarthritis of the hip.
- Neuralgia paresthetica.
- Herniated lumbar disc.

Anatomy

Origin: upper anterior aspect of the shaft of the femur.
Insertion: common tendon of quadriceps through the patellar ligament to the tubercle of the tibia.
Action: extends leg.
Nerve supply: femoral (L2, 3, 4).

Injection of Trigger Point

With the patient in the supine position identify TrPs by palpation. Trigger points in a deep-lying muscle may be difficult to palpate. The vastus intermedius is covered by the rectus femoris. A needle that is long enough to penetrate the covering musculature should be used. Multiple needle entries along the length of the muscle are indicated in order to find all TrPs (see Fig. 12–17, and Chapter 11 for injection technique).

Needle size: 1.5–3.0 in., 21 gauge, depending on thigh musculature.
Solution: Any one of the following solutions may be used: 0.5% procaine; 1.0% lidocaine; saline and dry needling in case of allergy. Do not use epinephrine.

Noninvasive Therapy

The post–trigger point injection follow-up program described in Chapter 11 is recommended as a conservative therapeutic treatment approach. Noninvasive therapy can include:

- Physical therapy modalities (e.g., electrical stimulation and warm packs; see Chapter 19).
- Manual physical therapy techniques (e.g., massage, joint mobilization, and the Trager® Approach [neuromuscular re-education]; see Chapters 16–18 for additional manual techniques).
- Active and passive stretching and limbering of muscles with or without the use of vaporized coolant spray or ice. Active exercise is part of the stretch-and-spray technique. Limbering and relaxation are necessary prior to stretching. Contract-relax techniques may be used.
- Stretch and spray: Electrical stimulation, limbering of muscles, and warm packs should precede stretch and spray to relax the muscles prior to stretching. Flexion of the knee is performed passively and actively. The pelvis is stabilized. This can be performed both in the supine and sitting positions. Full range of motion of the knee is accomplished by stretching the extensors. Use vaporized coolant spray or ice as necessary. Stretching of the muscle is also accomplished actively and with assistance during the exercise program. Active exercise is part of the stretch-and-spray technique.
- Exercise and a home program for the hip and knee are prescribed (see Chapter 15). Exercise programs include relaxation, limbering, stretching, and strengthening. When the patient is free of pain and full motion has been achieved, progress to strength and endurance programs.

Injection of Trigger Point

With the patient in the supine position, identify TrPs by palpation. Trigger points in a deep-lying muscle may be difficult to palpate. The vastus intermedius is covered by the rectus femoris. A needle that is long enough to penetrate the covering musculature should be used. Multiple needle entries along the length of the muscle are indicated in order to find all TrPs (see Fig. 12–18, and Chapter 11 for injection technique).

Needle size: 1.5–3.0 in., 21 gauge, depending on thigh musculature.
Solution: Any one of the following solutions may be used: 0.5% procaine; 1.0% lidocaine; saline and dry needling in case of allergy. Do not use epinephrine.

Postinjection Follow-up Physical Therapy Program

Patient should receive 3 to 4 consecutive days of treatment. Physical therapy should include electrical stimulation, relaxation, limbering, and stretching of the involved muscle using vapocoolant spray or ice as needed combined with and followed by an exercise program. Active and active-assisted exercises are an integral part of the physical therapy program (see Chapter 11 for details).

Exercise and Home Program

Exercises for hip and knee are prescribed. Exercises should at first be performed under the guidance of a therapist. When the patient is free of pain and full motion has been achieved, progress to strength and endurance programs. Begin and end exercise sessions with stretching and relaxation. (See Chapter 15 for exercise details.)

Corrective and Preventive Measures

- Check for malalignment of the lower extremities, including genu varus or valgus.
- Check for foot abnormalities such as flatfoot.
- Prescribe orthoses as indicated.

Vastus Lateralis

Symptoms and Pain Pattern

- Pain over the lateral aspect of the thigh, which may radiate to the knee (Fig. 12–19).
- Pain when lying directly on the TrP.[7, 23]
- Myofascial TrPs in the distal end of the vastus lateralis can cause a completely locked patella, which will immobilize the knee joint.[54]

Findings on Examination

- Tenderness on palpating TrPs over the vastus lateralis.
- Pain may be limited to the area of palpation or may radiate distally to the knee.

Differential Diagnosis

- Neuralgia paresthetica.
- Trochanteric bursitis.
- Herniated lumbar disc.
- Internal derangement of the knee.

Anatomy

Origin: lateral lip of linea aspera, front of base of greater trochanter.
Insertion: common tendon of quadriceps, lateral part of patellar ligament to the tibial tubercle.
Action: extends leg.
Nerve supply: femoral (L2, 3, 4).

Noninvasive Therapy

The post–trigger point injection follow-up program described in Chapter 11 is recommended as a conservative therapeutic treatment approach. Noninvasive therapy can include:

- Physical therapy modalities (e.g., electrical stimulation and warm packs; see Chapter 19).
- Manual physical therapy techniques (e.g., massage, joint mobilization, and the Trager® Approach [neuromuscular re-education]; see Chapters 16–18 for additional manual techniques).

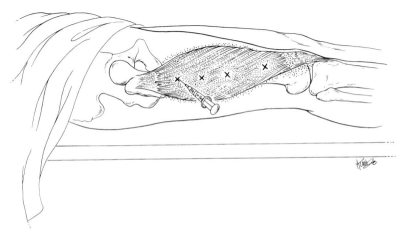

Figure 12–19. Vastus lateralis. Injection of trigger points *(X's)* in the right vastus lateralis with the patient supine. Trigger point pain pattern is shown by *stippling.* Muscle origin and insertion are noted.

- Active and passive stretching and limbering of muscles with or without the use of vaporized coolant spray or ice. Active exercise is part of the stretch-and-spray technique. Limbering and relaxation are necessary prior to stretching. Contract-relax techniques may be used.
- Stretch and spray: The knee is flexed to extend the shortened extensor muscle. The thigh extensors may be stretched in both the lying-down and sitting positions. Electrical stimulation, limbering of muscles, and warm packs may precede stretch and spray to relax the muscles. Stretching of the muscle is also accomplished actively and with assistance during the exercise program. Active exercise is part of the stretch-and-spray technique.
- Exercise and a home program for the vastus lateralis are prescribed (see Chapter 15 for exercises for the knee and hip). Exercise programs include relaxation, limbering, stretching, and strengthening. When the patient is free of pain and full motion has been achieved, progress to strength and endurance programs.

Injection of Trigger Point

In the supine position, palpation for TrPs is performed from the most proximal part of the muscle (area of greater trochanter) to its insertion in the patellar ligament. All tender TrPs are injected (see Chapter 11 for technique). Perform multiple needle entries over the entire length of the muscle. Multiple needling may encounter TrPs that were missed on palpation. Most TrPs are found in the areas of origin and insertion.

Needle size: 2, 3 in., 21 gauge. The length of needle depends on the patient's size.
Solution: Any one of the following solutions may be used: 0.5% procaine; 1.0% lidocaine; saline and dry needling in case of allergy. Do not use epinephrine.

Postinjection Follow-up Physical Therapy Program

The patient should use crutches for 24 hours to avoid pain and limping. The patient should receive 3 to 4 consecutive days of treatment. Physical therapy should include electrical stimulation, relaxation, limbering, and stretching of the involved muscle using vaporized coolant spray or ice as needed combined with and followed by an exercise program. Active and active-assisted exercises are an integral part of the physical therapy program (see Chapter 11 for details).

Exercise and Home Program

Exercises for the hip and knee are prescribed. Exercises should at first be performed under the guidance of a therapist. When the patient is free of pain and full motion has been achieved, progress to strength and endurance programs. Begin and end exercise session with stretching and relaxation (see Chapter 15 for exercise details).

Corrective and Preventive Measures

- Check for malalignment of the lower extremities, e.g., genu varus, genu valgus, or foot abnormalities such as flatfoot.
- Prescribe orthoses as indicated.

Gracilis

Symptoms and Pain Pattern

- Pain over the inner aspect of the thigh over the gracilis (Fig. 12–20).
- Pain may be described as hot or stinging.[22, 52]

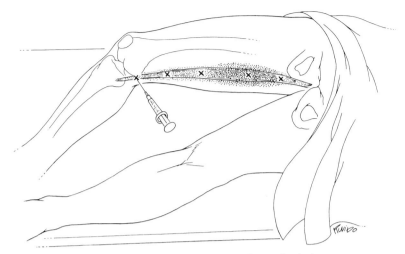

Figure 12–20. Gracilis. Injection of trigger points in the right gracilis *(X's)*. Note trigger points in the area of origin and insertion. The patient is in the supine position with the thigh in flexion, external rotation, and abduction. Trigger point pain pattern is shown by *stippling*.

Findings on Examination

- Tender TrPs along the gracilis, especially at its insertion at the medial upper aspect of the tibia.
- The patient demonstrates restriction in abduction of the thigh and knee extension.

Anatomy

Origin: lower symphysis pubis arch.
Insertion: upper medial tibia.
Action: adduction of the thigh, flexion of the knee.
Nerve supply: obturator (anterior division L3, 4).

Differential Diagnosis

- Pes anserinus bursitis.
- Osteitis pubis.
- Hip joint abnormality.

Noninvasive Therapy

The post–trigger point injection follow-up program described in Chapter 11 is recommended as a conservative therapeutic treatment approach. Noninvasive therapy can include:

- Physical therapy modalities (e.g., electrical stimulation and warm packs; see Chapter 19).
- Manual physical therapy techniques (e.g., massage, joint mobilization, and the Trager® Approach [neuromuscular re-education]; see Chapters 16–18 for additional manual techniques).
- Active and passive stretching and limbering of muscles with or without the use of vaporized coolant spray or ice. Active exercise is part of the stretch-and-spray technique. A self-stretch can be performed in the same manner with the patient in the standing position flexing the knee, and pulling the heel toward the buttock, while the opposite hand holds a table or the wall for balance. Hold the stretch for 10 seconds. Relax and repeat. Limbering and relaxation are necessary prior to stretching. Contract-relax techniques may be used.

- Stretch and spray: Use vaporized coolant spray or ice. Stretching should be performed by abducting the hip with the knee in extension. Spray the area of the gracilis muscle. Spray the trigger area and the length of the muscle. Follow stretch and spray with passive and active range-of-motion exercises as tolerated. Electrical stimulation, limbering of muscles, and warm packs should precede stretch and spray to relax muscles.
- Exercise and home program (see Chapter 15 for exercises for the hip and knee). Exercise programs include relaxation, limbering, stretching, and strengthening. When the patient is free of pain and full motion has been achieved, progress to strength and endurance programs.

Injection of Trigger Point

The gracilis muscle is superficial. In addition to the localized tender point, or TrP, the entire muscle body should be examined. Trigger points are most often found in the areas of origin and insertion. Injection is given with the patient in the supine position. The thigh is flexed, externally rotated, and abducted (see Fig. 12–20, and Chapter 11 for injection technique).

Needle size: 1.5–2.0 in., 21 gauge.
Solution: Any one of the following solutions may be used: 0.5% procaine; 1.0% lidocaine; saline and dry needling in case of allergy. Do not use epinephrine.

Postinjection Follow-up Physical Therapy Program

The patient should receive 3 to 4 consecutive days of treatment. Physical therapy should include electrical stimulation, relaxation, limbering, and stretching of the involved muscle using vaporized coolant spray or ice as needed combined with and followed by an exercise program. Active and active-assisted exercises are an integral part of the physical therapy program (see Chapter 11 for details).

Exercise and Home Program

Exercises for the hip and knee are prescribed. Exercises should at first be performed under the guidance of a therapist. When the patient is free of pain and full motion has been achieved, progress to strength and endurance programs. Begin and end exercise sessions with stretching and relaxation. (See Chapter 15 for exercise details.)

Corrective and Preventive Causes

- Avoid prolonged adduction and flexion of the thigh.

Sartorius

Symptoms and Pain Pattern

- Thigh pain extending medially along the course of the sartorius extending to the medial aspect of the knee[24] (Fig. 12–21).
- Symptoms of lateral femoral cutaneous entrapment consisting of pain and numbness over the anterolateral aspect of the thigh have been reported to be relieved by TrP injection. Injecting the TrP in the region of the nerve may have released muscle tension in the entrapment area.[19, 24, 54]

Findings on Examination

- Trigger point tenderness may be found in various areas extending from the origin to the insertion of the muscle.

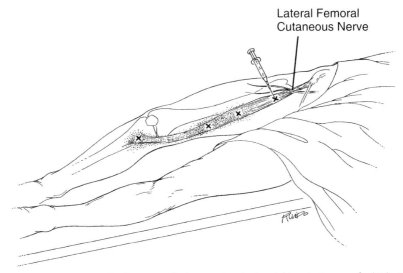

Lateral Femoral
Cutaneous Nerve

Figure 12–21. Sartorius muscle. Injection of trigger points in the right sartorius muscle *(X's)*. Anatomic landmarks are noted, including the lateral femoral cutaneous nerve. The patient is supine. Pain pattern is shown by *stippling*. Multiple trigger points are noted.

Differential Diagnosis

- Osteoarthritis of the hip.
- Knee joint abnormality.

Anatomy

Origin: anterior superior iliac spine.
Insertion: upper medial tibia.
Action: flexion, abduction, external rotation of thigh, flexion of the knee.
Nerve supply: femoral (L2, 3).

Noninvasive Therapy

The post–trigger point injection follow-up program described in Chapter 11 is recommended as a conservative therapeutic treatment approach. Noninvasive therapy can include:

- Physical therapy modalities (e.g., electrical stimulation and warm packs; see Chapter 19).
- Manual physical therapy techniques (e.g., massage, joint mobilization, and the Trager® Approach [neuromuscular re-education]; see Chapters 16–18 for additional manual techniques).
- Active and passive stretching and limbering of muscles with or without the use of vaporized coolant spray or ice. Active exercise is part of the stretch-and-spray technique. Limbering and relaxation are necessary prior to stretching. Contract-relax techniques may be used.
- Stretch and spray for the sartorius is performed by extension, adduction, and internal rotation of the hip and extension of the knee (see Chapter 11 for spray-and-stretch technique). The patient is moved forward to the edge of the foot of the table. The pelvis should be stabilized. The leg is held free and supported by the therapist off the examining table for the stretch maneuvers. Electrical stimulation, limbering of muscles, and warm packs should precede stretch and spray to relax the muscles prior to stretching. Stretching of muscle is also accomplished actively and with assistance during the exercise program. Active exercise is part of the stretch-and-spray technique.

- Exercises and a home program for the hip and knee are prescribed (see Chapter 15). Exercise programs include relaxation, limbering, stretching, and strengthening. When the patient is free of pain and full motion has been achieved, progress to strength and endurance programs.

Injection of Trigger Point

Injection is performed with the patient supine. Palpable tender areas are identified. Multiple needling along the length of the muscle is indicated. Needling is not limited to the initial area of tenderness. Look for additional TrPs along the muscle belly. Other neighboring thigh muscles such as the rectus femoris and vastus medialis may also have TrPs and should be carefully examined. The sartorius muscle is superficial. The needle may be angled and need not penetrate too deeply (see Fig. 12–21).

Needle size: One may use a 1.5- or 2.0-in. needle length, 21 gauge.
Solution: Any one of the following solutions may be used: 0.5% procaine; 1.0% lidocaine; saline and dry needling in case of allergy. Do not use epinephrine.

Postinjection Follow-up Physical Therapy Program

The patient should avoid prolonged sitting, walking, or standing. The patient should receive 3 to 4 consecutive days of treatment. Physical therapy should include electrical stimulation, relaxation, limbering, and stretching of the involved muscle using vaporized coolant spray or ice as needed combined with and followed by an exercise program. Active and active-assisted exercises are an integral part of the physical therapy program (see Chapter 11 for details).

Exercise and Home Program

Exercises for the hip and knee are prescribed. Exercises should at first be performed under the guidance of a therapist. When the patient is free of pain and full motion has been achieved, progress to strength and endurance programs. Begin and end exercise sessions with stretching and relaxation. (See Chapter 15 for exercise details.)

Corrective and Preventive Measures

- Correct leg length inequality, e.g., with a heel lift.
- Avoid sitting cross-legged with the knees flexed and hips externally rotated and abducted.

Adductor Magnus

Symptoms and Pain Pattern

- Patients may complain of pain in the groin in addition to the anteromedial aspect of the thigh (Fig. 12–22).[22, 24, 33]
- Intrapelvic referred pain has been reported (e.g., rectum or vagina).[52]
- Athletic activities frequently cause active TrPs in the adductor muscles, which are a cause of prolonged complaints when untreated.

Findings on Examination

- Trigger points are felt posteromedially in the region of the ischium as well as midthigh in the area of the muscle insertion.
- Limitation in lateral rotation, flexion, and adduction of the hips may be present and restriction in motion may be accompanied by pain.

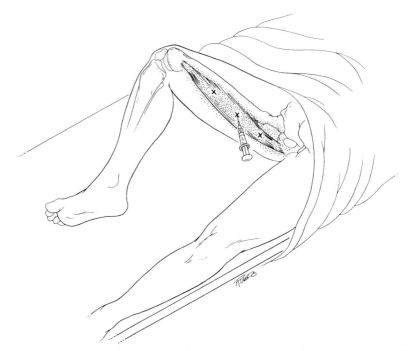

Figure 12–22. Adductor magnus. Injection of trigger points in the right adductor magnus *(X's)*. The patient is supine with slight flexion, abduction, and external rotation of the leg. Anatomic landmarks are noted. Pain pattern is shown by *stippling*.

- Look for TrPs in neighboring muscles (e.g., the adductor longus and adductor brevis).

Differential Diagnosis

- Hip joint abnormality.
- Intrapelvic disease.[51]

Anatomy

Origin: inferior ischiopubic rami, outer inferior ischial tuberosity.
Insertion: medial gluteal tuberosity, medial linea aspera.
Action: adduction and extension of hip joint; the ischial head acts as a hamstring muscle.
Nerve supply: obturator (posterior division L3, L4), branch from sciatic (common peroneal division L3, 4).

Noninvasive Therapy

The post–trigger point injection follow-up program described in Chapter 11 is recommended as a conservative therapeutic treatment approach. Noninvasive therapy can include:

- Physical therapy modalities (e.g., electrical stimulation and warm packs; see Chapter 19).
- Manual physical therapy techniques (e.g., massage, joint mobilization, and the Trager® Approach [neuromuscular re-education]; see Chapters 16–18 for additional manual techniques).
- Active and passive stretching and limbering of muscles with or without the use of

vaporized coolant spray or ice. Active exercise is part of the stretch-and-spray technique. Contract-relax techniques may be used.

- Stretch and spray for the adductor magnus is performed by stretching in hip abduction and flexion. Limbering and relaxation is necessary prior to stretching. Electrical stimulation, limbering of muscles, and warm packs should precede stretch and spray to relax muscles.
- Exercise and a home program for the adductor magnus are prescribed (see Chapter 15 for exercises for the hip). Exercise programs include relaxation, limbering, stretching, and strengthening. When the patient is free of pain and full motion has been achieved, progress to strength and endurance programs.

Injection of Trigger Point

With the patient supine the length of the muscle is best examined for TrPs with the thigh in flexion, abduction, and external rotation (see Fig. 12–22). Multiple needle entries are performed along the length of the muscle in addition to specific tender areas. Multiple needling may identify TrPs that are not found on palpation (see Fig. 12–22). Palpate neighboring muscles for TrPs. Most TrPs are found in the region of origin (ischial area).

Needle size: 2.0, 3.0 in., 21 gauge.
Solution: Any one of the following solutions may be used: 0.5% procaine; 1.0% lidocaine; saline and dry needling in case of allergy. Do not use epinephrine.

Postinjection Follow-up Physical Therapy Program

The patient should receive 3 to 4 consecutive days of treatment. Physical therapy should include electrical stimulation, relaxation, limbering, and stretching of the involved muscle using vaporized coolant spray or ice as needed combined with and followed by an exercise program. Active and active-assisted exercises are an integral part of the physical therapy program.

Exercise and Home Program

Exercises for the hip are prescribed (see Chapter 15). Exercises should at first be performed under the guidance of a therapist. When the patient is free of pain and full motion has been achieved, progress to strength and endurance programs. Begin and end exercise sessions with stretching and relaxation.

Corrective and Preventive Measures

- Correct leg length inequalities (e.g., with a shoe lift).
- Avoid prolonged adduction and flexion of the thigh.
- Avoid overstretch of adductors (e.g., athletic injury). Emphasize the importance of proper stretching before and after athletic activities.

Adductor Longus and Adductor Brevis

Symptoms and Pain Pattern

- Pain in the groin may radiate to the medial thigh and knee and leg (Fig. 12–23).[23, 24, 34, 52]
- Trigger points in the adductor muscles are frequently caused by athletic injuries and remain a source of prolonged complaints when left untreated.

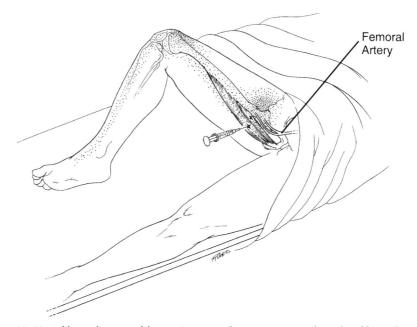

Figure 12–23. Adductor longus and brevis. Injection of trigger points in the right adductor longus and brevis *(X's)*. The femoral artery lies deep to the sartorius and is lateral to the long and short adductor muscles. The patient is positioned with the hip and knee flexed. The leg is externally rotated with slight abduction. Pain pattern is noted by *stippling*.

Findings on Examination

- Trigger point tenderness is found on palpation of the adductor longus.
- Pain of the TrP may cause the pain to radiate to the lower portion of the thigh to the knee.
- Pain and tightness of the adductor muscles may limit lateral rotation and abduction.
- The Faber test is often painful and of limited value.
- The adductor brevis muscle, which is under the adductor longus, demonstrates the same clinical picture.

Differential Diagnosis

- Hip disease (e.g., arthritis of the hip).
- Herniated disc L3–4.
- Strain of the adductor muscles.
- Osteitis pubis.

Anatomy

Adductor Longus

Origin: front of pubis.
Insertion: linea aspera.
Action: adduction and medial rotation of the thigh.
Nerve supply: obturator (anterior division L3, 4).

Adductor Brevis

Origin: inferior pubic ramus.
Insertion: linea aspera.
Action: adduction and flexion of the hip.
Nerve supply: obturator (anterior division L3, 4).

Noninvasive Therapy

The post–trigger point injection follow-up program described in Chapter 11 is recommended as a conservative therapeutic treatment approach. Noninvasive therapy can include:

- Physical therapy modalities (e.g., electrical stimulation and warm packs; see Chapter 19).
- Manual physical therapy techniques (e.g., massage, joint mobilization, and the Trager® Approach [neuromuscular re-education]; see Chapters 16–18 for additional manual techniques).
- Active and passive stretching and limbering of muscles with or without the use of vaporized coolant spray or ice. Active exercise is part of the stretch-and-spray technique by stretching in hip abduction and flexion. Electrical stimulation, limbering of muscles, and warm packs should precede stretch and spray to relax muscles. Limbering and relaxation are necessary prior to stretching. Contract-relax techniques may be used.
- Stretch and spray is performed with the leg in extension using gentle abduction. Add flexion, abduction, and external rotation as performed in the Faber test. Increase abduction and external rotation. Use relaxation techniques. Follow with passive and active range-of-motion exercises as tolerated. Electrical stimulation, limbering of muscles, and warm packs should precede stretch and spray to relax muscles.
- Exercise and a home program for the hip and knee are prescribed (see Chapter 15). Exercise programs include relaxation, limbering, stretching, and strengthening. When the patient is free of pain and full motion has been achieved, progress to strength and endurance programs.

Injection of Trigger Point

Trigger points are best palpated with the hip and knee in flexion, the hip abducted and externally rotated (Faber position) (see Fig. 12–23). Examine the adductor longus for TrPs beginning at its origin in the groin and progressing along the inner side of the thigh. The adductor longus is superficial to the adductor brevis. Look for multiple TrP areas by palpation and multiple needling. Most frequently TrPs will be found proximally at the adductor longus origin. Neighboring muscles, such as the adductor brevis, adductor magnus, pectineus, and gracilis, may demonstrate TrPs.

Needle size: 1.5, 2.0, 3.0 in., 22 gauge.
Solution: Any one of the following solutions may be used: 0.5% procaine; 1.0% lidocaine; saline and dry needling in case of allergy. Do not use epinephrine.

Precautions

Identify and avoid the femoral artery (see Fig. 12–23). The femoral artery lies lateral to the adductor muscle in the thigh.
Aspirate prior to injection.

Postinjection Follow-up Physical Therapy Program

The patient is advised to avoid prolonged standing, sitting, or walking, and to use crutches for 2 days. The patient should receive 3 to 4 consecutive days of treatment. Physical therapy should include electrical stimulation, relaxation, limbering, and stretching of the involved muscle using vaporized coolant spray or ice as needed combined with and followed by an exercise program. Active and active-assisted exercises are an integral part of the physical therapy program (see Chapter 11 for details).

Exercise and Home Program

Exercises for the adductor muscles are prescribed. Exercises should at first be performed under the guidance of a therapist. When the patient is free of pain and full motion has been achieved, progress to strength and endurance programs. Begin and end exercise sessions with stretching and relaxation. (See Chapter 15 for exercise details.)

Corrective and Preventive Measures

- Avoid prolonged adduction and flexion of the thigh.
- Emphasize proper warm-up prior to athletic activities to avoid muscle injury. Proper warm-up prior to athletic activities will prevent strains and sprains leading to TrP formation or activation of latent TrPs. Close athletic activities with stretching and relaxation.

Pectineus

Symptoms and Pain Pattern

- Patients with pectineus muscle TrPs may complain of pain in the hip joint, groin area, or over the medial aspect of the upper thigh (Fig. 12–24).
- The patient may experience pain and limitation in the groin area with abduction of the hip.
- Pain may radiate from the groin down the inner side of the thigh.[52]

Findings on Examination

- Tenderness on palpation of the pectineus. The pectineus is best palpated with the leg in abduction. Palpate the femoral artery. The pectineus is medial to the artery and lateral to the adductor brevis and adductor longus.
- Neighboring groups of muscles (e.g., adductors) should be examined for TrPs.

Differential Diagnosis

- Arthritis of the hip.
- Osteitis pubis.
- Obturator nerve entrapment.[19]

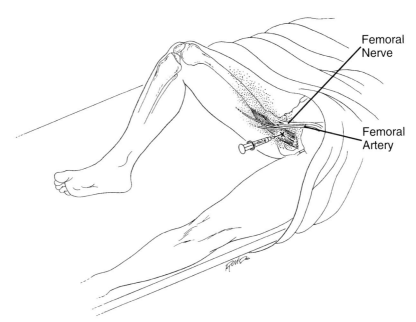

Figure 12–24. Pectineus. Injection of trigger point (X) in the right pectineus. Patient is supine, the thigh in slight flexion, abduction, and external rotation. Avoid the femoral artery. Anatomic landmarks, including the femoral artery and nerve, are noted. Trigger point pain pattern is shown by *stippling*.

Anatomy

Origin: superior ramus of the pubis.
Insertion: upper portion of the pectineal line below the lesser trochanter.
Action: flexes thigh, adducts and laterally rotates thigh.
Nerve supply: femoral (L2, 3, 4 and accessory obturator).

Noninvasive Therapy

The post–trigger point injection follow-up program described in Chapter 11 is recommended as a conservative therapeutic treatment approach. Noninvasive therapy can include:

- Physical therapy modalities (e.g., electrical stimulation and warm packs; see Chapter 19).
- Manual physical therapy techniques (e.g., massage, joint mobilization, and the Trager® Approach [neuromuscular re-education]; see Chapters 16–18 for additional manual techniques).
- Active and passive stretching and limbering of muscles with or without the use of vaporized coolant spray or ice. Active exercise is part of the stretch-and-spray technique. Limbering and relaxation are necessary prior to stretching. Contract-relax techniques may be used.
- Stretch and spray: Stretching should include abduction and extension of the hip. Neighboring muscles of similar function must be evaluated and often will require treatment (see Chapter 9). Electrical stimulation, limbering of muscles, and warm packs should precede stretch and spray to relax the muscles prior to stretching. Stretching of muscle is also accomplished actively and with assistance during the exercise program.
- Exercise and a home program for the pectineus and adductors are prescribed (see Chapter 15). Exercise programs include relaxation, limbering, stretching, and strengthening. When the patient is free of pain and full motion has been achieved, progress to strength and endurance programs.

Injection of Trigger Point

Trigger points in the pectineus are best injected with the patient supine, the thigh in slight flexion, abduction, and external rotation with flexion of the knee (see Chapter 11 for injection technique). Palpate the femoral artery, which lies over the pectineus, and direct the needle medial to the artery. Aspirate before injection (see Fig. 12–24). If the artery is entered, remove the needle and apply compression.

Needle size: 1.5, 2.0 in., 21 gauge.
Solution: Any one of the following solutions may be used: 0.5% procaine; 1.0% lidocaine; saline and dry needling in case of allergy. Do not use epinephrine.

Precautions

- Avoid the femoral artery.

Postinjection Follow-up Physical Therapy Program

The patient should receive 3 to 4 consecutive days of treatment. Physical therapy should include electrical stimulation, relaxation, limbering, and stretching of the involved muscle using vaporized coolant spray or ice as needed combined with and followed by an exercise program. Active and active-assisted exercises are an integral part of the physical therapy program (see Chapter 11 for details).

Exercise and Home Program

Exercises should at first be performed under the guidance of a therapist. When the patient is free of pain and full motion has been achieved, progress to strength and endurance programs. Begin and end exercise sessions with stretching and relaxation. (See Chapter 15 for exercise details.)

Corrective and Preventive Measures

- Avoid prolonged flexion and adduction of the hip.
- Correct leg length inequality. Use a heel lift if necessary.
- Correct pelvic asymmetry, e.g., a patient with a small hemipelvis or scoliosis may require a buttock lift (cushion) to improve alignment.

Iliopsoas

Psoas Major, Iliacus

Symptoms and Pain Pattern

Patients complain of pain in the low back, groin, and thigh. Symptoms may be aggravated by activity and relieved with rest (Fig. 12–25). A vertically oriented pattern of pain has been described in the low back in addition to pain in the front of the thigh.[51]

Findings on Examination

- Shortening of the iliopsoas muscle causes inability to extend the hip, increasing lordosis. To test for iliopsoas shortening, the patient flexes the uninvolved hip, flattening the lumbar spine. The involved hip will remain in flexion with the knee in flexion, indicating involvement of both one joint and two joint hip flexors. If the knee joint is permitted to extend and the hip extends normally, the one joint hip

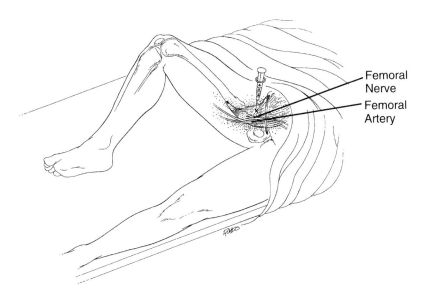

Femoral
Nerve
Femoral
Artery

Figure 12–25. Iliopsoas. Injection of trigger point *(X)* in the right iliopsoas. The patient is supine with the thigh flexed, abducted, and externally rotated. Anatomic landmarks are noted, including the inguinal ligament, femoral artery, and femoral nerve. Trigger point pain pattern is shown by *stippling*.

flexor muscle of the iliopsoas is normal, but the rectus femoris and probably the tensor fasciae latae are shortened.[18]
- Trigger points may be found in the area of the insertion at the lesser trochanter area of the femur, the medial wall of the femoral triangle, and behind the anterior superior iliac spine behind the brim of the pelvis. TrPs may also be found on palpation of the abdomen below the umbilicus lateral to the rectus abdominis.

Anatomy

Psoas Major

Origin: transverse processes of L1–5, and vertebral bodies of T12–L5.
Insertion: lesser trochanter.
Action: flexes thigh, rotates thigh laterally, flexor of the spine and lateral bending.
Nerve supply: ventral primary divisions (L2, 3).

Iliacus

Origin: iliac fossa, iliac crest, anterior sacroiliac ligaments at base of sacrum.
Insertion: tendon of psoas major into lesser trochanter.
Action: flexes and laterally rotates thigh.
Nerve supply: femoral (L2, 3).

Differential Diagnosis

- Kidney abnormality.
- Iliopsoas bursitis.
- Neuralgia paresthetica.
- Low back syndrome.

Noninvasive Therapy

The post–trigger point injection follow-up program described in Chapter 11 is recommended as a conservative therapeutic treatment approach. Noninvasive therapy can include:

- Physical therapy modalities (e.g., electrical stimulation and warm packs; see Chapter 19).
- Manual physical therapy techniques (e.g., massage, joint mobilization, and the Trager® Approach [neuromuscular re-education]; see Chapters 16–18 for additional manual techniques).
- Active and passive stretching and limbering of muscles with or without the use of vaporized coolant spray or ice. Active exercise is part of the stretch-and-spray technique. Electrical stimulation, limbering of muscles, and warm packs should precede stretch and spray to relax muscles. Limbering and relaxation are necessary prior to stretching. Contract-relax techniques may be used.
- Stretch and spray (see Chapter 11): Extend and medially rotate the hip area. Spray includes abdomen, groin, lower back, and area of referred pain as necessary.
- Exercise and a home program for low back pain and the hip are described in Chapter 15. Exercise program includes relaxation, limbering, stretching, and strengthening. When the patient is free of pain and full motion has been achieved, progress to strength and endurance programs.

Trigger Point Injection

With the patient in the supine position the right hip is abducted, flexed, and externally rotated. Palpate the femoral artery. Inject lateral to the femoral artery (see Fig. 12–25, and Chapter 11 for injection technique).

Needle size: 3 in., 20 gauge.

Solution: Any one of the following solutions may be used: 0.5% procaine; 1.0% lidocaine; saline and dry needling in case of allergy. Do not use epinephrine.

Precautions

- Note neurovascular structures found in the femoral triangle.
- Avoid femoral artery and nerve.
- Aspirate prior to injection.
- Inject lateral to the artery.

Postinjection Follow-up Physical Therapy Program

The patient should receive 3 to 4 consecutive days of treatment. Physical therapy should include electrical stimulation, relaxation, limbering, and stretching of the involved muscle using vaporized coolant spray or ice as needed combined with and followed by an exercise program. Active and active-assisted exercises are an integral part of the physical therapy program (see Chapter 11 for details).

Exercises and Home Program

Stretching the iliopsoas muscle requires hip extension. Prescribe McKenzie-type extension exercises for the low back, reminding the patient to keep the pelvis flat on the exercise mat. The patient lifts the upper body by extending the arms. Lumbar extension will stretch the iliopsoas. This should not be done if pain in the low back is aggravated. Home stretching and exercise programs are prescribed. Exercises should at first be performed under the guidance of a therapist. When the patient is free of pain and full motion has been achieved, progress to strength and endurance programs. Begin and end exercise sessions with relaxation (see Chapter 15 for details).

Corrective and Preventive Measures

Avoid prolonged sitting or lying with the hip in flexion. This can result from prolonged sitting in a wheelchair or from bed rest.

Tibialis Anterior

Symptoms and Pain Pattern

- Pain over the front of the leg along the path of the anterior tibial muscle[15, 16] (Fig. 12–26).
- Pain may be aggravated with activity.
- Weakness in dorsiflexion of the ankle.
- Tenderness over the tibialis anterior with local pain. Pain may radiate to the anteromedial side of the leg and big toe.[40, 50, 52]
- Symptoms are aggravated by walking or running.

Findings on Examination

- Examination may reveal tender TrPs in the tibialis anterior in addition to a referred pain pattern.
- A degree of dorsiflexion weakness and limitation in plantarflexion may be present.

Differential Diagnosis

- Anterior compartment syndrome.
- Lumbar radiculopathy.
- Shin splints.
- Tibial stress fracture.

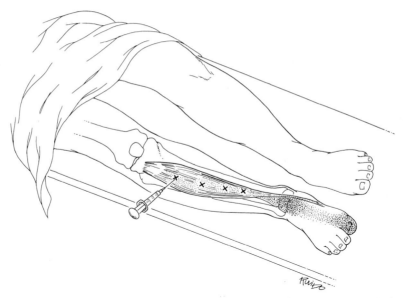

Figure 12–26. Tibialis anterior. Injection of trigger points in the right tibialis anterior with the patient supine. Multiple trigger points (*X's*) are noted. Anatomic landmarks are noted. Trigger point pain pattern is shown by *stippling*.

Anatomy

Origin: lateral tibial condyle, lateral tibia interosseous membrane.
Insertion: medial side of the first cuneiform, base of the first metatarsal.
Action: dorsiflexes foot, inverts foot.
Nerve supply: deep peroneal (L4, 5, S1).

Noninvasive Therapy

The post–trigger point injection follow-up program described in Chapter 11 is recommended as a conservative therapeutic treatment approach. Noninvasive therapy can include:

- Physical therapy modalities (e.g., electrical stimulation and warm packs; see Chapter 19).
- Manual physical therapy techniques (e.g., massage, joint mobilization, and the Trager® Approach [neuromuscular re-education]; see Chapters 16–18 for additional manual techniques).
- Active and passive stretching and limbering of muscles with or without the use of vaporized coolant spray or ice. Active exercise is part of the stretch-and-spray technique. Limbering and relaxation are necessary prior to stretching. May use contract-relax technique.
- Stretch-and-spray technique: Plantarflex the ankle and pronate the foot. Electrical stimulation, limbering of muscles, and warm packs should precede stretch and spray to relax the muscles prior to stretching. Stretching of the muscle is also accomplished actively as well as with assistance during the exercise program. Active exercise is part of the stretch-and-spray technique (see Chapter 11).
- Exercise and home program for the ankle are prescribed (see Chapter 15). Exercise programs include relaxation, limbering, stretching, and strengthening. When the patient is free of pain and full motion has been achieved, progress to strength and endurance programs.

Injection of Trigger Point

Trigger points are identified. Injection is performed with the patient in the supine position. Use multiple injection and needling technique (see Chapter 11). Look for additional TrPs over the length of the anterior tibial muscle by means of palpation and needle probing (see Fig. 12–26).

Needle size: 1.5, 2.0 in., 21 gauge.
Solution: Any one of the following solutions may be used: 0.5% procaine; 1.0% lidocaine; saline and dry needling in case of allergy. Do not use epinephrine.

Precautions

- Aspirate before injection.
- Avoid anterior tibial artery and deep peroneal nerve.

Postinjection Follow-up Physical Therapy Program

The patient is to use crutches to avoid full weight-bearing for 24 hours. The patient should receive 3 to 4 consecutive days of treatment. Physical therapy should include electrical stimulation, relaxation, limbering, and stretching of the involved muscle using vaporized coolant spray or ice as needed combined with and followed by an exercise program. Active and active-assisted exercises are an integral part of the physical therapy program (see Chapter 11 for details).

Exercise and Home Program

Home program: Continue exercises and stretching. Encourage plantarflexion and pronation. Exercises should at first be performed under the guidance of a therapist. When the patient is free of pain and full motion has been achieved, progress to strength and endurance programs. Begin and end exercise sessions with stretching and relaxation (see Chapter 15 for exercise details).

Corrective and Preventive Measures

- Avoid overuse syndromes (e.g., unaccustomed prolonged walking or running).
- Avoid walking on uneven surfaces for prolonged periods.
- Advise correction of foot abnormalities, e.g., flatfoot, Morton's foot.
- Prescribe orthoses as needed.

Peroneal Muscles

Peroneus Longus, Peroneus Brevis, Peroneus Tertius

Symptoms and Referred Pain Pattern

- Pain over the lateral aspect of the ankle and lateral dorsum of the foot[24] (Fig. 12–27).
- Muscle weakness of the ankle.[22, 50]

Findings on Examination

- Tenderness on palpation of peroneal muscles.
- Tightness of the peroneal muscles will restrict inversion.
- The peroneus tertius is a dorsiflexor. Shortening of the peroneus tertius will limit plantarflexion.
- Muscle testing may reveal a weakness in plantarflexion, dorsiflexion, and eversion.

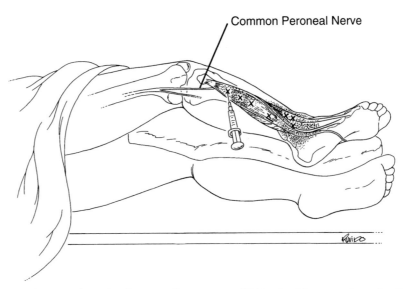

Common Peroneal Nerve

Figure 12–27. Peroneal muscles. Injection of trigger points *(X's)* in the right peroneal muscles. Patient is positioned lying on the uninvolved side. Anatomic landmarks are noted. Avoid the common peroneal nerve. Pain pattern is shown by *stippling*. Multiple trigger points are noted.

- Palpation of TrP may elicit distal referred pain over the lateral aspect of the ankle and lateral dorsum of the foot.

Differential Diagnosis

- Lumbar herniated disc.
- Common peroneal nerve entrapment.
- Peroneal muscle spasm due to foot abnormalities (flatfoot).
- Arthritis of the ankle.

Anatomy

Peroneus Longus

Origin: fibular head and proximal two thirds of fibula.
Insertion: base of first metatarsal and first cuneiform.
Action: plantarflexion and eversion of the foot.
Nerve supply: superficial peroneal (L4, 5, S1).

Peroneus Brevis

Origin: middle lateral aspect of the fibula.
Insertion: dorsal surface of fifth metatarsal.
Action: plantarflexion and eversion of the foot.
Nerve supply: superficial peroneal (L4, 5, S1).

Peroneus Tertius

Origin: distal fibula.
Insertion: base of fifth metatarsal.
Action: dorsiflexion of the foot.
Nerve supply: deep peroneal (L5, S1).

Noninvasive Therapy

The post–trigger point injection follow-up program described in Chapter 11 is recommended as a conservative therapeutic treatment approach. Noninvasive therapy can include:

- Physical therapy modalities (e.g., electrical stimulation and warm packs; see Chapter 19).
- Manual physical therapy techniques (e.g., massage, joint mobilization, and the Trager® Approach [neuromuscular re-education]; see Chapters 16–18 for additional manual techniques).
- Active and passive stretching and limbering of muscles with or without the use of vaporized coolant spray or ice. Active exercise is part of the stretch-and-spray technique. Limbering and relaxation are necessary prior to stretching. Contract-relax techniques may be used.
- Stretch and spray with vaporized coolant or ice. Stretch of the peroneus longus and brevis requires inversion and dorsiflexion. To stretch the peroneus tertius, plantarflexion is performed. Electrical stimulation, limbering of muscles, and warm packs should precede stretch and spray to relax the muscles. Stretching of muscle is also accomplished actively and with assistance during the exercise program.
- Exercise and a home program for the ankle are prescribed (see Chapter 15). Exercise programs include relaxation, limbering, stretching, and strengthening. When the patient is free of pain and full motion has been achieved, progress to strength and endurance programs.

Trigger Point Injection Technique

Trigger points are identified with the patient supine or lying on the uninvolved side. Multiple needling entry sites are usually necessary to locate additional TrPs that are not found on palpation (see Fig. 12–27; see Chapter 11 for technique).

Needle size: 1.5 in., 22 gauge.
Solution: Any one of the following solutions may be used: 0.5% procaine; 1.0% lidocaine; saline and dry needling in case of allergy. Do not use epinephrine.

Precautions

- Avoid the common peroneal nerve.[19]

Postinjection Follow-up Physical Therapy Program

The patient should receive 3 to 4 consecutive days of treatment. Therapy should include electrical stimulation, relaxation, limbering, and stretching of the involved muscle using vaporized coolant spray or ice as needed combined with and followed by an exercise program.

Exercise and Home Program

Exercises for the foot and ankle are prescribed (see Chapter 15). Instruct the patient on a daily exercise program for the foot and ankle. Exercise programs include relaxation, limbering, stretching, and strengthening. When the patient is free of pain and full motion has been achieved, progress to strength and endurance programs. Begin and end exercise sessions with relaxation and stretching.

Corrective and Preventive Measures

- Correct foot abnormalities such as flatfoot and Morton's foot. Prescribe orthoses as indicated.
- Avoid running on uneven surfaces.

Gastrocnemius Muscle Group

Gastrocnemius, Medial, and Gastrocnemius, Lateral

Symptoms and Pain Pattern

- Pain in the calf and back of the knee, which may radiate to the lower thigh[22, 33] (Fig. 12–28).
- Trigger points in the medial gastrocnemius may also refer pain to the plantar surface of the foot,[7, 52] Achilles tendon, and the heel.[39, 41]
- Trigger points have been reported as a frequent cause of nocturnal calf cramp and intermittent claudication.[39, 41, 52]
- Trigger points in the medial gastrocnemius may contribute to plantar fasciitis.[14]

Findings on Examination

- With the patient prone or sitting, tender TrPs are best palpated with the knee flexed and the ankle plantarflexed.
- Palpate the entire length of the medial and lateral gastrocnemius muscle. Local tenderness and referred pain may be elicited.
- Trigger points may be found frequently in both the medial and lateral heads of the gastrocnemius as well as along the midline.

Differential Diagnosis

- Tennis leg (plantaris tendon rupture, gastrocnemius rupture).
- Herniated lumbar disc.
- Phlebitis.
- Spinal stenosis.
- Intermittent claudication.

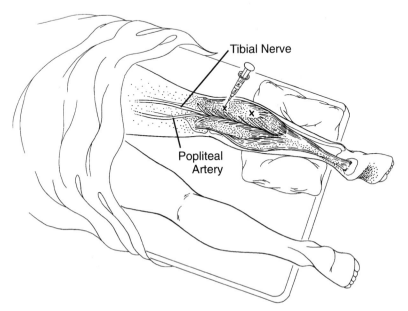

Figure 12–28. Gastrocnemius. Injection of trigger points *(X's)* in the lateral head of the right gastrocnemius. Trigger point pain pattern *stippling* is characteristic of both medial and lateral head trigger points. Only one side of the gastrocnemius is injected at a time when both are involved. The popliteal artery and tibial nerve are noted.

Anatomy

Gastrocnemius, Medial

Origin: medial femoral condyle.
Insertion: on the calcaneus as part of the Achilles tendon.
Action: flexes the leg, plantarflexes the foot.
Nerve supply: tibial (S1, 2).

Gastrocnemius, Lateral

Origin: lateral femoral condyle.
Insertion: on the calcaneus as part of the Achilles tendon.
Action: flexes the leg, plantarflexes the foot.
Nerve supply: tibial (S1, 2).

Noninvasive Therapy

The post–trigger point injection follow-up program described in Chapter 11 is recommended as a conservative therapeutic treatment approach. Noninvasive therapy can include:

- Physical therapy modalities (e.g., electrical stimulation and warm packs; see Chapter 19).
- Manual physical therapy techniques (e.g., massage, joint mobilization, and the Trager® Approach [neuromuscular re-education]; see Chapters 16–18 for additional manual techniques).
- Active and passive stretching and limbering of muscles with or without the use of vaporized coolant spray or ice. Active exercise is part of the stretch-and-spray technique. Limbering and relaxation are necessary prior to stretching. Contract-relax techniques may be used.
- Stretch and spray (see Chapter 11): Extend the knee and dorsiflex the foot with the help of vaporized coolant spray or ice, as needed, to regain full muscle length. Stretch is performed with the patient in the prone position with the feet off the examining table, as well as in the supine position. Electrical stimulation, limbering of muscles, and warm packs may precede stretch and spray to relax the muscles. Relaxation is accomplished prior to stretching. Stretching of the muscle is also accomplished actively as well as with assistance during the exercise program. Active exercise is part of the stretch-and-spray technique.
- Exercise and home program for the knee and ankle (see Chapter 15). Exercise programs include relaxation, limbering, stretching, and strengthening. When the patient is free of pain and full motion has been achieved, progress to strength and endurance programs. Begin and end exercise sessions with relaxation and stretching.

Injection of Trigger Point

If TrPs are found in both gastrocnemius muscles they should be injected on separate occasions 2 or 3 days apart. Multiple injections cause muscle soreness and spasm. Injection may be performed with the patient in the prone or side-lying position. The knee is relaxed. Trigger points are identified by palpation and needling. Use a multiple needling technique covering the length of the muscle (see Fig. 12–28 and Chapter 11 for injection technique).

Needle size: 1.5, 2.0 in., 22 gauge.
Solution: Any one of the following solutions may be used: 0.5% procaine; 1.0% lidocaine (approximately 2–10 mL); saline and dry needling in case of allergy. Do not use epinephrine.

Precautions

- Avoid the popliteal artery when injecting in the popliteal region. Aspirate prior to injection.

Postinjection Follow-up Physical Therapy Program

Crutches are used for 24 hours following the injection to avoid pain, muscle spasm, and limping. The patient should receive 3 to 4 consecutive days of treatment. Physical therapy should include electrical stimulation, relaxation, limbering, and stretching of the involved muscle using vaporized coolant spray or ice as needed combined with and followed by an exercise program. Active and active-assisted exercises are an integral part of the physical therapy program (see Chapter 11 for details).

Exercise and Home Program

Exercises for the ankle and knee are prescribed. Exercises should at first be performed under the guidance of a therapist. When the patient is free of pain and full motion has been achieved, progress to strength and endurance programs. Begin and end exercise session with relaxation (see Chapter 15 for exercise details).

Corrective and Preventive Measures

- Avoid overuse syndrome, e.g., unaccustomed prolonged walking and athletic activity.
- Correct foot deformities, e.g., flatfoot. Prescribe orthoses as necessary.
- Avoid walking or running for prolonged periods on uneven surfaces.
- Short gastrocnemius muscles are frequently found in women associated with prolonged wearing of high heels.
- Relaxation and stretching exercises prior to and after athletic activities.

Plantaris

Symptoms and Referred Pain Pattern

- Symptoms may present as pain in the back of the knee and upper calf.
- Pain is aggravated by walking and running.

Findings on Examination

- Anatomically, TrPs are difficult to diagnose. Findings and symptoms may resemble those related to the soleus and gastrocnemius muscles.
- Pain may be aggravated with dorsiflexion of the foot.

Differential Diagnosis

- Tear of gastrocnemius muscle.
- Rupture of the plantaris tendon (tennis leg).
- Trigger points may result from rupture of the plantaris tendon.

Anatomy

Origin: lateral supracondylar line of the femur, popliteal ligament.
Insertion: calcaneal tendon, medial side and posterior part of the calcaneus.
Action: the plantaris muscle crosses two joints; therefore, it flexes the knee and plantarflexes the foot.
Nerve supply: tibial (L4, 5, S1).

Noninvasive Therapy

The post–trigger point injection follow-up program described in Chapter 11 is recommended as a conservative therapeutic treatment approach. Noninvasive therapy can include:

- Physical therapy modalities (e.g., electrical stimulation and warm packs; see Chapter 19).
- Manual physical therapy techniques (e.g., massage, joint mobilization, and the Trager® Approach [neuromuscular re-education]; see Chapters 16–18 for additional manual techniques).
- Active and passive stretching and limbering of muscles with or without the use of vaporized coolant spray or ice. Active exercise is part of the stretch-and-spray technique. Limbering and relaxation are necessary prior to stretching. Contract-relax techniques may be used.
- Stretch and spray: Extend the knee and dorsiflex the foot with the help of vaporized coolant spray or ice. Electrical stimulation, limbering of muscles, and warm packs should precede stretch and spray to relax the muscles. Stretching of muscle is also accomplished actively and with assistance during the exercise program. Active exercise is part of the stretch-and-spray technique.
- Exercise and home program: Exercises for heel cord stretching and exercises for the ankle and foot are prescribed (see Chapter 15). Exercise programs include relaxation, limbering, stretching, and strengthening. When the patient is free of pain and full motion has been achieved, progress to strength and endurance programs.

Injection of Trigger Point

Trigger points are treated similarly to treatment of the lateral head of the gastrocnemius (see Fig. 12–28) and soleus (see Fig. 12–29).

Needle size: 1.5 or 2.0 in., 22 gauge.
Solution: Any one of the following solutions may be used: 0.5% procaine; 1.0% lidocaine; saline and dry needling in case of allergy. Do not use epinephrine.

Postinjection Follow-up Program

The patient should receive 3 to 4 consecutive days of treatment. Physical therapy should include electrical stimulation, relaxation, limbering, and stretching of the involved muscle using vaporized coolant spray or ice as needed combined with and followed by an exercise program. Active and active-assisted exercises are an integral part of the physical therapy program (see Chapter 11 for details).

Exercise and Home Program

Heel cord stretching, range-of-motion exercises for the knee and ankle, and exercises for the plantaris muscle are prescribed. Exercises should at first be performed under the guidance of a therapist. When the patient is free of pain and full motion has been achieved, progress to strength and endurance programs. Begin and end exercise sessions with relaxation (see Chapter 15 for exercise details).

Corrective and Preventive Measures

- Relaxation and stretching exercises prior to and after athletic activities will prevent plantaris and gastrocnemius muscle tears as well as TrP formation and activation of latent TrPs.

Soleus

Symptoms and Pain Pattern

- Pain in the calf and posterior aspect of the ankle (Fig. 12–29).
- Pain may be referred to the plantar aspect of the heel[14] and to the area of the sacroiliac joint.[52]
- Pain is aggravated with weight-bearing.
- May contribute to plantar fasciitis.[14]
- Heel pain may be mistaken for heel bursitis.

Findings on Examination

- The patient may be examined in the prone or side-lying position.
- The gastrocnemius muscle covers the soleus, making palpation of the soleus difficult.
- Relax the gastrocnemius by flexing the knee.
- It may be difficult to distinguish between TrPs in the gastrocnemius and soleus.
- Shortening of the soleus together with the gastrocnemius may cause a restriction in full dorsiflexion.
- To test for triceps surae strength, which would include the gastrocnemius and soleus muscles, ask the patient to stand on one leg while holding on to an object for balance and to lift his or her body weight by raising up on the toes by plantarflexing the foot. Difficulty rising on the toes indicates weakness of the triceps surae.
- In the standing position, weakness of the soleus and gastrocnemius can be differentiated. If the soleus is weak, the knee joint will flex and the ankle joints will dorsiflex. If the gastrocnemius is weak, the knee joints will tend to hyperextend and the ankle joints will plantarflex.[18]
- With the patient prone, ask the patient to hold the foot plantarflexed with the knee flexed. Place pressure against the calcaneus, pulling the heel plantarward. The patient will not be able to hold the foot in plantarflexion against resistance when the muscles are weak.[18]

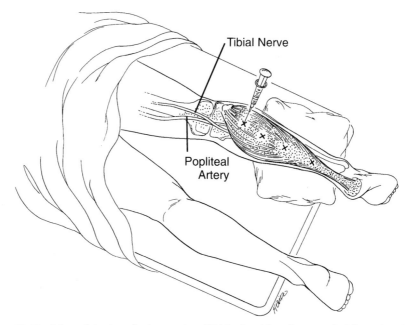

Figure 12–29. Soleus. Injection of trigger points (*X's*) in the right soleus muscle. The patient is in the prone position with a pillow under the leg for slight knee flexion. All trigger points are injected. Trigger point pain pattern is shown by *stippling*. The popliteal artery and tibial nerve are noted. Aspirate prior to injection.

Differential Diagnosis

- Thrombophlebitis.
- Heel bursitis, heel spur.
- Herniated lumbar disc (lumbar radiculopathy).
- Tennis leg (tear of gastrocnemius or plantaris).
- Achilles tendinitis.

Anatomy

Origin: head and upper fibula, upper midtibia.
Insertion: through the Achilles tendon to the calcaneus bone.
Action: plantarflexes the foot.
Nerve supply: tibial (L5, S1).

Noninvasive Therapy

The post–trigger point injection follow-up program described in Chapter 11 is recommended as a conservative therapeutic treatment approach. Noninvasive therapy can include:

- Physical therapy modalities (e.g., electrical stimulation and warm packs; see Chapter 19).
- Manual physical therapy techniques (e.g., massage, joint mobilization, and the Trager® Approach [neuromuscular re-education]; see Chapters 16–18 for additional manual techniques).
- Active and passive stretching and limbering of muscles with or without the use of vaporized coolant spray or ice. Active exercise is part of the stretch-and-spray technique. Limbering and relaxation are necessary prior to stretching. Contract-relax techniques may be used.
- Stretch and spray: Dorsiflex the foot and ankle with the knee in flexion using vaporized coolant spray or ice, as needed. Electrical stimulation, limbering of muscles, and warm packs may precede stretch and spray to relax the muscles. Stretching of muscle is also accomplished actively with assistance during the exercise program. Active exercise is part of the stretch-and-spray technique.
- Exercises and a home program for the knee and ankle are prescribed (see Chapter 15). Exercise programs include relaxation, limbering, stretching, and strengthening. When the patient is free of pain and full motion has been achieved, progress to strength and endurance programs. Begin and end exercise sessions with relaxation and stretching.

Injection of Trigger Point

The patient should be prone or side-lying with the knee flexed. Identify TrPs. Use sterile technique (see Chapter 11 for injection technique). In the lower half of the calf the soleus is covered by the gastrocnemius. The medial and lateral aspects are more accessible to injection than the covered midportion of the muscle (see Fig. 12–29).

Needle size: 1.5, 2.0 in., 22 gauge (3 in., 21 gauge may be necessary).
Solution: Any one of the following solutions may be used: 0.5% procaine; 1.0% lidocaine; saline and dry needling in case of allergy. Do not use epinephrine.

Precautions

- Aspirate before injection.
- Avoid posterior tibial artery and nerve, which lie deep to the soleus muscle.

Postinjection Follow-up Physical Therapy Program

The patient should receive 3 to 4 consecutive days of treatment. Physical therapy should include electrical stimulation, relaxation, limbering, and stretching of the involved muscle using vaporized coolant spray or ice as needed combined with and followed by an exercise program. Active and active-assisted exercises are an integral part of the physical therapy program (see Chapter 11 for details).

Exercise and Home Program

Exercises for the lower extremity include the knee, ankle, and foot. Exercises for heel cord stretching are prescribed. Exercises should at first be performed under the guidance of a therapist. When the patient is free of pain and full motion has been achieved, progress to strength and endurance programs. Begin and end exercise session with relaxation and stretching (see Chapter 15 for exercise details).

Corrective and Preventive Measures

- Avoid overuse syndrome (e.g., unaccustomed prolonged walking and running).
- Prevent prolonged plantarflexion (e.g., use of high heels).
- Avoid direct pressure on the calf muscles.
- Avoid running on uneven surfaces.
- Correct foot deformities (e.g., flatfoot, Morton's foot).
- The physician should prescribe orthoses as necessary.
- Perform relaxation and stretching exercises prior to and after athletic activities.

Tibialis Posterior

Symptoms and Referred Pain Pattern

- Patient may complain of localized calf pain.
- Pain may be referred to the Achilles tendon, extending to the sole of the foot and toes[52] (Fig. 12–30).
- Trigger points may contribute to plantar fasciitis.[14]
- Symptoms are aggravated by prolonged walking and running.

Findings on Examination

- Shortening of the tibialis posterior or spasm promotes limitation in pronation, abduction, and eversion of the foot.
- Tenderness may be palpated through the overlying muscles.
- In areas of deep tenderness it is difficult to distinguish between gastrocnemius or soleus muscle TrPs.

Differential Diagnosis

- Phlebitis.
- Lumbar radiculopathy.
- Achilles tendinitis.
- Pain due to structural foot deficiencies, e.g., flatfoot, Morton's foot.
- Heel bursitis.
- Posterior tibial tendinitis.

Anatomy

Origin: the interosseous membrane, posterior surface of the body of the tibia, upper two thirds of the medial surface of the fibula.

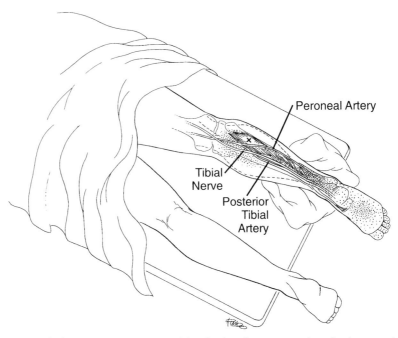

Figure 12–30. Tibialis posterior. Trigger point *(X)* and referred pain pattern *(stippling)* are noted. Trigger point injection is not recommended. Anatomic relations of the tibialis posterior and neurovascular structures (posterior tibial artery and tibial nerve) are noted.

Insertion: tuberosity of the navicula, sustentaculum tali, cuneiforms, cuboid, bases of metatarsals 2 and 3.
Action: plantarflexes, adducts, and inverts foot.
Nerve supply: tibial (L5, S1).

Noninvasive Therapy

The post–trigger point injection follow-up program described in Chapter 11 is recommended as a conservative therapeutic treatment approach. Noninvasive therapy can include:

- Physical therapy modalities (e.g., electrical stimulation and warm packs; see Chapter 19).
- Manual physical therapy techniques (e.g., massage, joint mobilization, and the Trager® Approach [neuromuscular re-education]; see Chapters 16–18 for additional manual techniques).
- Active and passive stretching and limbering of muscles with or without the use of vaporized coolant spray or ice. Active exercise is part of the stretch-and-spray technique. Limbering and relaxation are necessary prior to stretching. Contract-relax techniques may be used.
- Stretch and spray: Assess limitation in motion. With the foot everted and dorsiflexed, spray the TrP area and referred pain area including the heel and foot (see Chapter 11). Electrical stimulation, limbering of muscles, and warm packs should precede stretch and spray to relax muscles.
- Exercises and a home program for the lower extremities and ankle are described in Chapter 15. Exercise programs include relaxation, limbering, stretching, and strengthening. When the patient is free of pain and full motion has been achieved, progress to strength and endurance programs. Begin and end exercise sessions with stretching and relaxation.

Injection of Trigger Point

The surrounding muscle and bone make the precise localization of TrPs unlikely. This uncertainty in diagnosis coupled with the danger of injuring neurovascular structures in the area makes injection therapy an unwise approach; the risk of vascular injury outweighs the chance of benefiting from the TrP injection. Injection therapy is therefore not described (see Fig. 12–30). I agree with Travell and Simons, who do not recommend injecting the tibialis posterior.[52] Although a physician can attempt the TrP injection, a description of the injection technique is omitted to discourage this temptation. Steroid injections are commonly given for posterior tibial tendinitis in the area of the ankle and foot. Tendon rupture, however, can result from steroid injection.

Exercise and Home Program

Exercises for the lower extremity include the knee, ankle, and foot. Exercises for heel cord stretching are prescribed. Exercises should at first be performed under the guidance of a therapist. When the patient is free of pain and full motion has been achieved, progress to strength and endurance programs. Begin and end exercise sessions with relaxation and stretching (see Chapter 15 for exercise details).

Corrective and Preventive Measures

- Correction of foot deformities, e.g., flatfoot, Morton's foot. Prescribe orthoses as necessary.
- Avoid running on uneven surfaces (e.g., beach running).
- Avoid overuse syndrome (e.g., unaccustomed prolonged walking or running).
- Relaxation and stretching exercises prior to and after athletic activities.

Popliteus

Symptoms and Pain Pattern

- Pain in the back of the knee aggravated by activities such as walking or running (Fig. 12–31).

Findings on Examination

- Trigger points are difficult to palpate in view of the overlying muscles; the gastrocnemius must be relaxed. The popliteus is more easily examined with the knee in flexion. The popliteus may be palpated medial to the lateral gastrocnemius on the lateral side. The semimembranosus and semitendinosus must be relaxed in order to palpate the medial aspect of the popliteus.
- Shortening of the popliteus results in some restriction in lateral rotation of the tibia on the femur. This is noted with flexion of the knee.
- Shortening of the popliteus will also limit extension of the knee.

Differential Diagnosis

- Popliteal tendinitis.
- Tear of posterior horn of the lateral meniscus.
- Baker's cyst.

Anatomy

Origin: popliteal surface of tibia above the soleal line.
Insertion: lateral femoral condyle, the medial half of the muscle into the lateral meniscus.
Action: rotates knee (femur laterally or tibia medially), flexes the leg.
Nerve supply: tibial (L4, 5, S1).

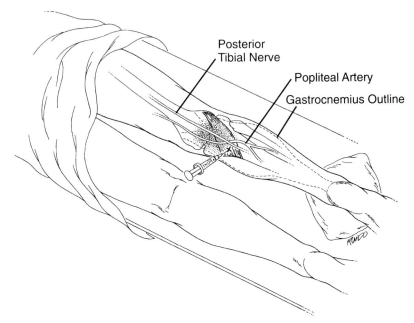

Figure 12–31. Popliteus. Injection of popliteal muscle trigger point *(X)*. The patient is prone with slight flexion of the knee to relax structures in the popliteal area. The popliteal muscle is covered by the gastrocnemius. Aspirate prior to injection. The patient may be prone or side-lying. Trigger point pain pattern is noted by *stippling. Dashed line* represents the gastrocnemius.

Noninvasive Therapy

The post–trigger point injection follow-up program described in Chapter 11 is recommended as a conservative therapeutic treatment approach. Noninvasive therapy can include:

- Physical therapy modalities (e.g., electrical stimulation and warm packs; see Chapter 19).
- Manual physical therapy techniques (e.g., massage, joint mobilization, and the Trager® Approach [neuromuscular re-education]; see Chapters 16–18 for additional manual techniques).
- Active and passive stretching and limbering of muscles with or without the use of vaporized coolant spray or ice. Active exercise is part of the stretch-and-spray technique. Limbering and relaxation are necessary prior to stretching. Contract-relax techniques may be used.
- Stretch and spray for the popliteus is performed by laterally rotating the knee while the joint is relaxed in flexion. Follow with spray and stretch in medial rotation and extension of the knee. Use vaporized coolant spray or ice as indicated. Electrical stimulation, limbering of muscles, and warm packs should precede stretch and spray to relax muscles.
- Exercise and a home program for the knee are described in Chapter 15. Exercise programs include relaxation, limbering, stretching, and strengthening. When the patient is free of pain and full motion has been achieved, progress to strength and endurance programs.

Injection of Trigger Point

Palpate TrPs with the patient in the prone position and the knee slightly flexed to relax the popliteal region. Palpate the popliteal artery (see Fig. 12–31).

Needle size: 1.5–2.0 in., 21 gauge.

Solution: Any one of the following solutions may be used: 0.5% procaine; 1.0% lidocaine; saline and dry needling in case of allergy. Do not use epinephrine.

Precautions

- Avoid the popliteal artery and vein and tibial nerve (see Fig. 12–31).
- Aspirate prior to injection.

Postinjection Follow-up Physical Therapy Program

The patient should receive 3 to 4 consecutive days of treatment. Physical therapy should include electrical stimulation, relaxation, limbering, and stretching of the involved muscle using vaporized coolant spray or ice as needed combined with and followed by an exercise program (see Chapter 11). Active and active-assisted exercises are an integral part of the physical therapy program. Crutches are used for 24 hours following the injection to avoid pain, muscle spasm, and limping.

Exercise and Home Program

Exercises should at first be performed under the guidance of a therapist. When the patient is free of pain and full motion has been achieved, progress to strength and endurance programs. Begin and end exercise sessions with stretching and relaxation (see Chapter 15 for exercise details).

Long Extensors of the Toes

Extensor Digitorum Longus, Extensor Hallucis Longus

Symptoms and Pain Patterns

- Pain is experienced over the lower third of the leg, both laterally and anteriorly. Pain may radiate distally to the foot.[22]
- Referred pain to the dorsum of the foot and middle three toes by the extensor digitorum longus. The extensor hallucis longus refers pain to the dorsum of the foot and metatarsophalangeal joint area of the big toe to the tip of the big toe[27, 50] (Fig. 12–32).
- Weakness of extension of the toes may occur with TrPs.
- Marked weakness may occur with entrapment of the deep peroneal nerve.

Findings on Examination

- Tenderness on palpation of TrPs with referred pain patterns involving the foot and toes.
- Weakness on testing dorsiflexors of the ankle and toes.

Differential Diagnosis

- Herniated lumbar disc.
- Morton's neuroma.
- Gout.

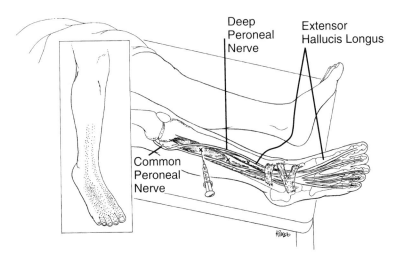

Figure 12–32. Long extensors of the toes. Injection of trigger points (*X's*) in the right extensor digitorum longus with the patient supine. Anatomic landmarks are noted, including the deep peroneal nerve. Aspirate prior to injection. Avoid the deep peroneal nerve and anterior tibial vessels. Localize trigger points by means of palpation prior to injection. Do not use multiple probing. *Inset,* trigger point pain pattern (*stippling).*

Anatomy

Extensor Digitorum Longus

Origin: lateral condyle of the tibia, proximal three fourths of the fibula, interosseous membrane.
Insertion: dorsum of the middle and the distal phalanx of the four lateral toes.
Action: extends toes, dorsiflexes the foot, everts the foot.
Nerve supply: deep peroneal (L4, 5, S1).

Extensor Hallucis Longus

Origin: middle anterior aspect of the fibula and interosseous membrane.
Insertion: base of distal phalanx of the big toe.
Action: extends the big toe, everts the foot.
Nerve supply: deep peroneal (L4, 5, S1).

Noninvasive Therapy

The post–trigger point injection follow-up program described in Chapter 11 is recommended as a conservative therapeutic treatment approach. Noninvasive therapy can include:

- Physical therapy modalities (e.g., electrical stimulation and warm packs; see Chapter 19).
- Manual physical therapy techniques (e.g., massage, joint mobilization, and the Trager® Approach [neuromuscular re-education]; see Chapters 16–18 for additional manual techniques).
- Active and passive stretching and limbering of muscles with or without the use of vaporized coolant spray or ice. Active exercise is part of the stretch-and-spray technique. Limbering and relaxation is necessary prior to stretching. Contract-relax techniques may be used.
- Stretch and spray is performed by plantarflexing the ankle, inverting the foot, and flexing the toes. Use vaporized coolant or ice as necessary. Electrical stimulation, limbering of muscles, and warm packs may precede stretch and spray to relax the muscles. Stretching of muscle is also accomplished actively and with assistance

during the exercise program. Active exercise is part of the stretch-and-spray technique.

- Exercises and a home program for the ankle, foot, and toes are prescribed (see Chapter 15). Exercise program includes relaxation, limbering, stretching, and strengthening. When the patient is free of pain and full motion has been achieved, progress to strength and endurance programs.

Injection of Trigger Point

With the patient supine, TrPs are identified. Injection is performed for well-localized TrPs (see Chapter 11). Multiple needling is not used (see Fig. 12–32).

Needle size: 1.5–2.0 in., 21 gauge.

Solution: Any one of the following solutions may be used: 0.5% procaine; 1.0% lidocaine; saline and dry needling may be used in case of allergy. Do not use epinephrine.

Precautions

- Avoid multiple needling because of neurovascular structures.
- Aspirate before injection.
- Avoid the deep peroneal nerve and anterior tibial vessels.

Postinjection Follow-up Physical Therapy Program

The patient should receive 3 to 4 consecutive days of treatment. Physical therapy should include electrical stimulation, relaxation, limbering, and stretching of the involved muscle using vaporized coolant spray or ice as needed combined with and followed by an exercise program. Use crutches (partial weight-bearing) for 24 hours to avoid limping, pain, and muscle spasm.

Exercise and Home Program

Exercises for the ankle, foot, and toes are prescribed. Exercises should at first be performed under the guidance of a therapist. When the patient is free of pain and full motion has been achieved, progress to strength and endurance programs. Begin and end exercise sessions with relaxation and stretching (see Chapter 15 for exercise details).

Corrective and Preventive Measures

- Avoid overuse syndromes, e.g., unaccustomed prolonged walking or jogging.
- Avoid jogging on uneven surfaces.
- Avoid positions of prolonged dorsiflexion of the foot and toes.
- Prescribe orthoses for flatfoot and Morton's foot as indicated.
- Continue home program for exercises for ankle, foot, and toes.

Long Flexor Muscles of the Toes

Flexor Digitorum Longus, Flexor Hallucis Longus

Symptoms and Pain Pattern

- Calf pain with walking or running.[23]
- Referred pain to the bottom of the foot and toes by the flexor digitorum longus[52] (Fig. 12–33).

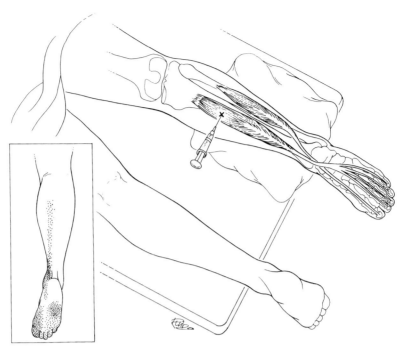

Figure 12–33. Long flexors of the toes. Injection of trigger point *(X)* in the flexor digitorum longus. Anatomic landmarks are noted for the flexor digitorum longus and flexor hallucis longus. Inject directly into the palpated trigger point. Insert needle just posterior to the medial border of the tibia for the flexor digitorum longus. *Inset,* trigger point pain pattern *(stippling).*

- Referred pain to the plantar aspect of the big toe and metatarsal head area by the flexor hallucis longus.[27, 52]

Findings on Examination
- Trigger points are found by palpating the flexor digitorum longus on the medial side of the leg, anteromedial to the medial gastrocnemius.
- The flexor hallucis longus is palpated on the lateral side of the middle lower portion of the leg.
- Overlying muscles make palpation of the long flexor muscles of the toes difficult.
- Look for local pain and referred pain pattern.

Differential Diagnosis
- Phlebitis.
- Tennis leg (plantaris tendon rupture, gastrocnemius rupture).
- Radiating pain of tarsal tunnel syndrome.
- Plantar fasciitis.
- Peripheral neuropathy.

Anatomy

Flexor Digitorum Longus

Origin: posterior tibia.
Insertion: base of distal phalanx, and second, third, fourth, and fifth toes.
Action: flexes the toes, plantarflexes the foot, inverts the foot.
Nerve supply: tibial (L5, S1).

Flexor Hallucis Longus

Origin: posterior fibula, interroseous membrane.
Insertion: base of distal phalanx of big toe.
Action: flexes the distal phalanx, plantarflexes the foot, inverts the foot.
Nerve supply: tibial (L5, S1, 2).

Noninvasive Therapy

The post–trigger point injection follow-up program described in Chapter 11 is recommended as a conservative therapeutic treatment approach. Noninvasive therapy can include:

- Physical therapy modalities (e.g., electrical stimulation and warm packs; see Chapter 19).
- Manual physical therapy techniques (e.g., massage, joint mobilization, and the Trager® Approach [neuromuscular re-education]; see Chapters 16–18 for additional manual techniques).
- Active and passive stretching and limbering of muscles with or without the use of vaporized coolant spray or ice. Active exercise is part of the stretch-and-spray technique. Limbering and relaxation are necessary prior to stretching. Contract-relax techniques may be used.
- Stretch and spray for the long flexors of the toes is performed with the toes dorsiflexed and the foot everted. Use vapocoolant spray or ice as indicated.
- Exercises and a home program for the toes and ankle are described in Chapter 15. Exercise programs include relaxation, limbering, stretching, and strengthening.

Injection of Trigger Point

With the patient in the prone position, identify TrPs. Trigger points are usually found in the upper lateral aspect of the leg for the flexor digitorum longus and over the medial aspect of the lower third of the leg for the flexor hallucis longus. In performing the injection the needle should be placed directly into the area of the TrP. Palpate the medial edge of the midshaft of the tibia, inserting the needle just posterior to the medial edge. The needle will then enter the flexor digitorum longus (see Fig. 12–33). (See Chapter 11 for injection technique.)

Needle size: 1.5, 2.0, 3.0 in., 21 gauge.
Solution: Any one of the following solutions may be used: 0.5% procaine; 1.0% lidocaine; saline and dry needling in case of allergy. Do not use epinephrine.

Precautions

- Inject isolated, well-localized TrPs.
- Do not use a fanning, circular technique or multiple needling techniques.
- Aspirate prior to injecting. The posterior tibial artery, vein, and tibial nerve and peroneal vessels lie between the long flexor muscles.

Postinjection Follow-up Physical Therapy Program

The patient should receive 3 to 4 consecutive days of treatment. Physical therapy should include electrical stimulation, relaxation, limbering, and stretching of the involved muscle using vaporized coolant spray or ice as needed combined with and followed by an exercise program. Active and active-assisted exercises are an integral part of the physical therapy program. Use crutches (partial weight-bearing) for 24 hours to avoid limping, pain, and muscle spasm. (See Chapter 11 for program details.)

Exercise and Home Program

Exercises should at first be performed under the guidance of a therapist. When the patient is free of pain and full motion has been achieved, progress to strength and endurance programs. Begin and end exercise sessions with relaxation and stretching (see Chapter 15 for exercise details).

Corrective and Preventive Measures

- Orthoses for foot abnormalities, e.g., flatfoot, Morton's foot.
- Avoid running on uneven surfaces.

Superficial Intrinsic Foot Muscles

Extensor Digitorum Brevis, Extensor Hallucis Brevis, Abductor Hallucis Longus, Flexor Digitorum Brevis, Abductor Digiti Minimi

Symptoms and Pain Pattern

- Trigger points in the muscles of the foot may cause pain on the sole or dorsum of the foot, or both. The following referred pain patterns have been described[52] (Fig. 12–34).
- The extensor hallucis brevis and extensor digitorum brevis refer pain to the dorsum of the foot.[17]
- The abductor hallucis longus refers pain to the medial side of the heel and instep.
- The abductor digiti minimi refers pain to the plantar aspect of the fifth metatarsal head.
- The flexor digitorum brevis refers pain to the heads of the second, third, fourth, and fifth metatarsals.

Findings on Examination

- Local tenderness over the muscles located above.
- Examination may find foot abnormalities that contribute to the development of TrPs, e.g., Morton's foot, flatfoot, calcaneovalgus.

Differential Diagnosis

- Ligamentous foot strain.
- Plantar fasciitis.
- Flatfoot.
- Metatarsalgia.
- Tarsal tunnel syndrome.

Anatomy

Abductor Digiti Quinti (Minimi)

Origin: lateral and medial process of the tuberosity of the calcaneus.
Insertion: lateral surface of the proximal phalanx of the small toe.
Action: flexes and abducts the proximal phalanx of the small toe.

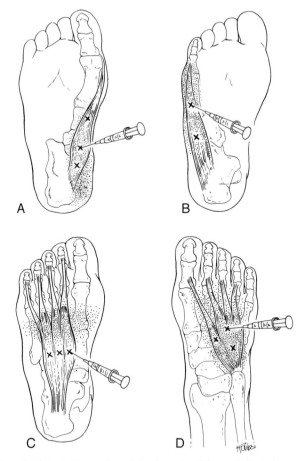

Figure 12–34. Superficial intrinsic muscles of the foot. *A,* Abductor hallucis longus; *B,* Abductor digiti quinti minimi; *C,* Flexor digitorum brevis; *D,* Extensor hallucis brevis and extensor digitorum brevis. Trigger points *(X's)* are identified. Needling is performed directly into the trigger point area. Trigger point pain patterns are shown by *stippling.*

Abductor Hallucis Longus

Origin: medial tuberosity of the calcaneus.
Insertion: medial side and base of the proximal phalanx of the big toe.
Action: flexes and abducts the big toe.

Flexor Digitorum Brevis

Origin: medial tubercle of the calcaneus, plantar aponeurosis.
Insertion: plantar surface of base of the middle phalanx of the second, third, fourth, and fifth toes.
Action: flexes toes.

Extensor Digitorum Brevis

Origin: upper lateral surface of the calcaneus.
Insertion: proximal phalanx of the great toe and tendon of the extensor digitorum longus of the second, third, and fourth toes.
Action: extends big toe, second, third, and fourth toes.

Extensor Hallucis Brevis

Origin: anterior fibula and interosseous membrane.
Insertion: base of the distal phalanx of the big toe.
Action: extends the big toe, everts the foot.

Noninvasive Therapy

The post–trigger point injection follow-up program described in Chapter 11 is recommended as a conservative therapeutic treatment approach. Noninvasive therapy can include:

- Physical therapy modalities (e.g., electrical stimulation and warm packs; see Chapter 19).
- Manual physical therapy techniques (e.g., massage, joint mobilization, and the Trager® Approach [neuromuscular re-education]; see Chapters 16–18 for additional manual techniques).
- Active and passive stretching and limbering of muscles with or without the use of vaporized coolant spray or ice. Active exercise is part of the stretch-and-spray technique. Limbering and relaxation are necessary prior to stretching. Contract-relax techniques may be used.
- Stretch and spray: Stretch opposite the direction of muscle function. Stretch the extensors by flexing the toes and inverting the foot. Flexor muscles are stretched in the direction of extension. (See Chapter 11 for stretch-and-spray technique.) Electrical stimulation, limbering of muscles, and warm packs may precede stretch and spray to relax the muscles. Stretching of muscles is also accomplished actively and with assistance during the exercise program. Active exercise is part of the stretch-and-spray technique.
- Exercise and a home program to increase strength and flexibility of toe extensors are described in Chapter 15. Exercise program includes relaxation, limbering, stretching, and strengthening.

Injection of Trigger Point

With the patient in the supine position TrPs are identified. Use multiple needling or fanning technique to find all TrPs in the area of the muscles involved (see Chapter 11). Figure 12–34 demonstrates TrP areas, muscular attachments, and pain patterns.

Needle size: 1.5, 2.0 in., 22–25 gauge.
Solution: Any one of the following solutions may be used: 0.5% procaine; 1.0% lidocaine; saline and dry needling in case of allergy. Do not use epinephrine.

Postinjection Follow-up Physical Therapy Program

The patient should receive 3 to 4 consecutive days of treatment. Physical therapy should include electrical stimulation, relaxation, limbering, and stretching of the involved muscle using vaporized coolant spray or ice as needed combined with and followed by an exercise program. Active and active-assisted exercises are an integral part of the physical therapy program (see Chapter 11 for details).

Exercise and Home Program

Exercises to increase strength and flexibility of the toes are prescribed (see Chapter 15). Exercises should at first be performed under the guidance of a therapist.

Corrective and Preventive Measures

- If foot deformities are present (e.g., Morton's foot, flatfoot, calcaneovalgus), prescribe orthoses as indicated.
- Treat metatarsalgia with metatarsal bars or orthoses.
- Correct source of foot pain, e.g., hammer toes, plantar callosities.
- Lower extremity casts should be applied so that free range of motion of the toes is possible to avoid muscle TrPs and joint stiffness.

- The patient should avoid running on uneven surfaces.
- The patient should wear properly sized shoes.

Deep Intrinsic Foot Muscles

Quadratus Plantae; Lumbricals, Second, Third, and Fourth; Adductor Hallucis, Oblique Head; Adductor Hallucis, Transverse Head; Flexor Hallucis Brevis; Interossei

Symptoms and Pain Pattern

- Pain on the sole and dorsum of the foot with weight-bearing.
- Patterns of numbness in the toes due to interossei TrPs that may be mistaken for Morton's neuroma.
- The quadratus plantae and lumbricals refer pain to the plantar surface of the heel.
- The adductor hallucis, oblique and transverse heads, refers pain to the plantar surface of the forefoot.[52]
- The flexor hallucis brevis refers pain to the head of the first metatarsal, and the medial and plantar aspects of the first and second toes.[17, 51]
- The interossei may refer pain and numbness to the side of the toe and dorsum of the foot.[22]
- The quadratus plantae refers pain to the bottom of the heel[51] (Fig. 12–35).

Findings on Examination

- Tender TrPs cause local and referred pain patterns. Examination may reveal foot abnormalities, e.g., flatfoot, Morton's foot, and calcaneovalgus, which contribute to the formation of TrPs and symptoms.

Differential Diagnosis

- Morton's neuroma.
- Heel bursitis.
- Metatarsalgia due to foot deformity.
- Foot strain.
- Stress fracture.

Anatomy

Quadratus Plantae

Origin: calcaneus.
Insertion: lateral border of the long flexor tendons.
Action: flexes toes.
Nerve supply: lateral plantar (S1, 2).

Lumbrical, First

Origin: medial side of the first long flexor tendon.
Insertion: proximal phalanx and extensor tendons of the second toe.
Action: flexes the proximal phalanx, extends the distal phalanx.
Nerve supply: medial plantar (L4, 5).

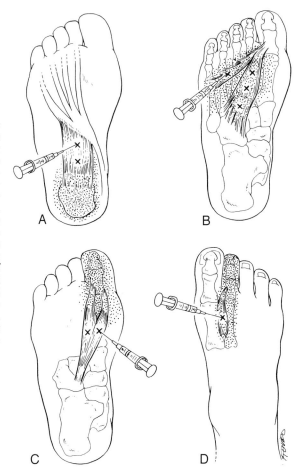

Figure 12–35. Deep intrinsic foot muscles. A, Injection of trigger points *(X's)* in the quadratus plantae. The foot may be dorsiflexed or turned to the side. The needle may be directed perpendicular to the quadratus plantae or tangentially. B, Injection of trigger points *(X's)* in the adductor hallucis, transverse and oblique heads. Injection is given into the plantar surface. C, Injection of trigger points *(X's)* in the flexor hallucis brevis. Injection is given into the plantar space. D, Injection of trigger point *(X)* in the right first dorsal interosseus. Injection is performed through the dorsum of the foot between the first and second metatarsals. The foot is in neutral position or slight plantarflexion. *A–D, stippling* shows pain patterns.

Lumbricals, Second, Third, and Fourth

Origin: long flexor tendons (second, third, and fourth).
Insertion: proximal phalanx and extensor tendons (third, fourth, and fifth).
Action: flexes the proximal phalanx, extends the distal phalanx.
Nerve supply: lateral plantar (S1, 2)

Adductor Hallucis, Oblique Head

Origin: peroneus longus sheath; base of second, third, and fourth metatarsals.
Insertion: lateral aspect of the base of the proximal phalanx of the big toe.
Nerve supply: lateral plantar (S1, 2 or S2, 3).

Adductor Hallucis, Transverse Head

Origin: capsules of third, fourth, and fifth metatarsophalangeal joints.
Insertion: lateral aspect of the base of the proximal phalanx of the big toe.
Action: adducts and flexes the proximal phalanx of the big toe.
Nerve supply: lateral plantar (S1, 2 or S2, 3).

Flexor Hallucis Brevis

Origin: cuboid and lateral cuneiform.
Insertion: medial and lateral sides or proximal phalanx of the great toe.
Action: flexes the proximal phalanx of the big toe.
Nerve supply: lateral plantar (S1, 2).

Interossei

Origin: three plantar interossei from the base and medial sides of the third, fourth, and fifth metatarsal bones; four dorsal interossei each arise by two heads from adjacent sides of metatarsal bones.

Insertion: base of proximal phalanges and dorsal digital expansions to the second, third, fourth, and fifth toes.

Action: adducts toes, flexes the proximal phalanx, extends the distal phalanx of the third, fourth, and fifth toes.

Nerve supply: lateral plantar (S2, 3), except muscles in the fourth interosseous space, which are supplied by the superficial branch of the same nerve. The first dorsal interosseous often receives a filament from the deep peroneal nerve, and the second a twig from the lateral branch of the same nerve.

Noninvasive Therapy

The post–trigger point injection follow-up program described in Chapter 11 is recommended as a conservative therapeutic treatment approach. Noninvasive therapy can include:

- Physical therapy modalities (e.g., electrical stimulation and warm packs; see Chapter 19).
- Manual physical therapy techniques (e.g., massage, joint mobilization, and the Trager® Approach [neuromuscular re-education]; see Chapters 16–18 for additional manual techniques).
- Active and passive stretching and limbering of muscles with or without the use of vaporized coolant spray or ice. Active exercise is part of the stretch-and-spray technique. Limbering and relaxation are necessary prior to stretching. Contract-relax techniques may be used.
- Stretch and spray (see Chapter 11): Vaporized coolant spray or ice may be used to aid in extension and abduction of toes. Movements should be both active and passive. Heat, massage, and ischemic pressure can be used. Electrical stimulation, limbering of muscles, and warm packs should precede stretch and spray to relax muscles.
- Exercises and a home program for flexion and extension of the toes are described in Chapter 15. Exercise program includes relaxation, limbering, stretching, and strengthening. When the patient is free of pain and full motion has been achieved, progress to strength and endurance programs.

Injection of Trigger Point

With the patient in the supine position TrPs are identified. Trigger points may be found both locally and in the referred pain area. Injections may be given with the patient supine with the foot in dorsiflexion or in the side-lying position (see Fig. 12–35).

Needle size: 1.5 in., 22 gauge.

Solution: Any one of the following solutions may be used: 0.5% procaine; 1.0% lidocaine; saline and dry needling in case of allergy. Do not use epinephrine.

Postinjection Follow-up Program

The patient should receive 3 to 4 consecutive days of treatment. Physical therapy should include electrical stimulation, relaxation, limbering, and stretching of the involved muscle using vaporized coolant spray or ice as needed combined with and followed by an exercise program.

Exercise and Home Program

Exercises to encourage toe flexion are prescribed. Exercises should at first be performed under the guidance of a therapist. When the patient is free of pain and full motion has been achieved, progress to strength and endurance programs. Begin and end exercise sessions with stretching and relaxation (see Chapter 15 for exercise details).

Corrective and Preventive Measures

- Correct foot deformities such as flatfoot and calcaneovalgus.
- Prescribe orthoses if necessary.
- The patient should be aware of his or her proper shoe size and avoid tight shoes.
- The patient should avoid unaccustomed prolonged walking or running, i.e., the overuse syndrome.
- He or she should avoid running on uneven surfaces.
- Lower extremity casts should be applied so that full range of motion of the toes is possible.

Cervical and Upper Dorsal Muscles

Sternocleidomastoid

Symptoms and Pain Pattern

- The sternocleidomastoid muscle consists of a more superficial sternal division and a deeper clavicular division (Fig. 12–36).
- The sternal portion of the muscle may refer pain to the cheek, temporomandibular joint area, supraorbital ridge, occipital area, and orbit. Autonomic symptoms such as lacrimation and coryza may occur on the same side as the TrPs.[24, 50, 54]
- The clavicular component may refer pain to the occipital area and across the forehead.[50]
- Symptoms may include dizziness, vertigo, and problems with equilibrium.
- Eye symptoms may include blurred vision.[51]
- Referred pain may involve the ear, jaw, and neck area.[6, 7]

Findings on Examination

- Tender TrPs on palpation of the sternocleidomastoid causing local or referred pain patterns, or both.
- May be a cause of torticollis with muscle shortening.
- Lacrimation, rhinitis may be present.

Differential Diagnosis

- Tension headache.
- Atypical facial neuralgia.
- Ménière's disease.
- Temporomandibular joint dysfunction.

Anatomy

Origin: sternum and clavicle.
Insertion: mastoid process.
Action: bends the head to the same side, rotates head and raises the chin to the opposite side; both right and left sternocleidomastoid muscles working together bend the head forward and also elevate the chin.
Nerve supply: spiral accessory (Cr 11) and ventral primary divisions (C2, 3).

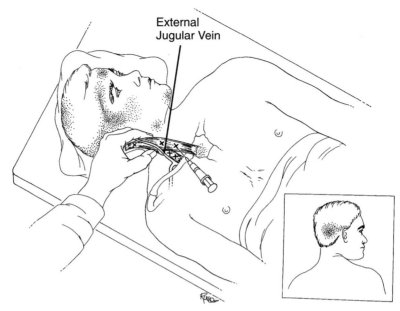

Figure 12–36. Sternocleidomastoid. Injection of right sternocleidomastoid trigger points (*X's*). The patient is supine, the head tilted toward the same side, the chin directed to the opposite shoulder. The muscle is grasped between the thumb, index, and middle fingers. Anatomic landmarks are noted. Avoid the jugular vein. Avoid deep penetration in the area of the clavicle. Pain pattern is shown by *stippling*.

Noninvasive Therapy

The post–trigger point injection follow-up program described in Chapter 11 is recommended as a conservative therapeutic treatment approach. Noninvasive therapy can include:

- Physical therapy modalities (e.g., electrical stimulation and warm packs; see Chapter 19).
- Manual physical therapy techniques (e.g., massage, joint mobilization, and the Trager® Approach [neuromuscular re-education]; see Chapters 16–18 for additional manual techniques).
- Active and passive stretching and limbering of muscles with or without the use of vaporized coolant spray or ice. Active exercise is part of the stretch-and-spray technique. Limbering and relaxation of muscles are necessary prior to stretching. Contract-relax techniques may be used.
- Stretch and spray: Bend head to the opposite side, raising the chin to the same side. Include rotation, raising the chin on the shoulder, flexion, and extension of the head. Treat both sides to achieve full range of motion.
- Exercises and a home program for the cervical area are described in Chapter 15 (exercises for the neck). Exercise program includes relaxation, limbering, stretching, and strengthening. When the patient is free of pain and full motion has been achieved, progress to strength and endurance programs.

Injection of Trigger Point

With the patient supine, tilt the chin to the opposite side and bend the head toward the side to be injected. The muscle is grasped between the thumb and index finger. All TrPs are injected and needled. Look for TrPs in the areas of origin and insertion. Avoid deep penetration in the area of the clavicle to avoid a pneumothorax. (See Chapter 11 for injection technique.)

Needle size: 1.5 in., 22–25 gauge.

Solution: Any one of the following solutions may be used: 0.5% procaine; 1.0% lidocaine; saline and dry needling in case of allergy. Do not use epinephrine.

Precautions

- Avoid the external jugular vein; aspirate prior to injection.
- Avoid deep penetration in the area of the clavicle to prevent puncturing the lung apex.

Postinjection Follow-up Physical Therapy Program

The patient should receive 3 to 4 consecutive days of treatment. Physical therapy should include electrical stimulation, relaxation, limbering, and stretching of the involved muscle using vaporized coolant spray or ice as needed combined with and followed by an exercise program. Active and active-assisted exercises are an integral part of the physical therapy program (see Chapter 11 for details).

Exercise and Home Program

Exercises should at first be performed under the guidance of a therapist. Begin and end exercise sessions with relaxation and stretching. (See Chapter 15 for exercise details.)

Corrective and Preventive Measures

- Avoid maintaining rotational positions of the neck for long periods, e.g., sitting in an airplane engaged in prolonged conversations with the head turned.
- Correct faulty posture, e.g., head-forward posture (see Chapters 16–18).
- Correct poor work postural attitudes, e.g., holding the telephone between the ear and shoulder to free both hands; avoid poor sitting and standing postures (see Chapter 20).

Scalene Muscle Group

Scalenus Anterior, Scalenus Medius, Scalenus Posterior

Symptoms and Pain Pattern

- Pain in the upper arm radiating to the forearm and hand (Fig. 12–37).
- Referred pain to the interscapular area, medial scapular border, upper back, upper chest, and radial side of the hand.[22, 50, 54]
- Symptoms of neurovascular entrapment indicative of thoracic outlet syndrome may include numbness in the fourth and fifth fingers.[33]

Findings on Examination

- On examination, tenderness over the scalene muscles producing local pain or referred pain patterns, or both.
- If TrPs cause neurovascular entrapment, Adson's sign may be positive in addition to diminished sensation of the fourth and fifth fingers and swelling of the hand.

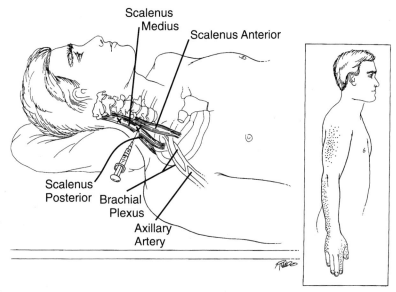

Figure 12–37. Scalene muscles. Injection of the scalenus medius muscle trigger points *(X's)*. The patient is supine, the head turned away from the area of pain. Anatomic landmarks are noted, including axillary artery and lateral chord. Referred pain pattern is shown by *stippling*.

Anatomy

Scalenus Anterior

Origin: tubercles of the transverse processes of C3–6.
Insertion: scalene tubercle on inner border of the first rib.
Action: flexion and lateral flexion of the neck, elevation of first rib.
Nerve supply: branches of cervical spinal nerves (C4–6).

Scalenus Medius

Origin: transverse processes of C2–6.
Insertion: upper surface of the first rib.
Action: lateral flexor of the neck and elevator of the first rib.
Nerve supply: branches of cervical spinal nerves (C3–8).

Scalenus Posterior

Origin: transverse processes of C5–7.
Insertion: outer surface of second rib.
Action: lateral flexor of the neck and elevator of second rib.
Nerve supply: branches of cervical spinal nerves (C6–8). The brachial plexus and
    subclavian artery exit between the scalenus anterior and scalenus medius.

Differential Diagnosis

- Thoracic outlet syndrome.
- Cervical herniated disc.
- Carpal tunnel syndrome.
- Cervical sprain.

Noninvasive Therapy

The post–trigger point injection follow-up program described in Chapter 11 is recommended as a conservative therapeutic treatment approach. Noninvasive therapy can include:

- Physical therapy modalities (e.g., electrical stimulation and warm packs; see Chapter 19).
- Manual physical therapy techniques (e.g., massage, joint mobilization, and the Trager® Approach [neuromuscular re-education]; see Chapters 16–18 for additional manual techniques).
- Active and passive stretching and limbering of muscles with or without the use of vaporized coolant spray or ice. Active exercise is part of the stretch-and-spray technique. Limbering and relaxation of muscles are necessary prior to stretching. Contract-relax techniques may be used.
- Stretch and spray: Use vaporized coolant or ice. Stretch by extending the neck and tilting the neck to the opposite side. Electrical stimulation, limbering of muscles, and warm packs may precede stretch and spray to relax the muscles. Stretching of muscle is also accomplished actively and with assistance during the exercise program. Active exercise is part of the stretch-and-spray technique.
- Exercise and a home program for the neck are prescribed (see Chapter 15). Exercise programs include relaxation, limbering, stretching, and strengthening.

Injection of Trigger Point

Identify the anterior border of the levator scapulae and the posterior border of the sternocleidomastoid. TrPs are palpated with the patient supine (see Fig. 12–37). The head is turned away from the area of pain. The TrP is isolated between two fingers. Maintain a distance of more than 1.5 in. above the clavicle to avoid the apex of the lung. The scalenus posterior is approached with the patient lying on the uninvolved side.

Needle size: Small-sized needles are used (1.0–1.5 in., 23–25 gauge).
Solution: Any one of the following solutions may be used: 0.5% procaine; 1.0% lidocaine; saline and dry needling in case of allergy. Do not use epinephrine.

Precautions

- Avoid the brachial plexus by isolating the TrPs between two fingers while controlling needle direction.
- Transient numbness and weakness may occur following injection.
- An injection performed too deeply may cause a stellate ganglion block.

Postinjection Follow-up Physical Therapy Program

The patient should receive 3 to 4 consecutive days of treatment. Physical therapy should include electrical stimulation, relaxation, limbering, and stretching of the involved muscle using vaporized coolant spray or ice as needed combined with and followed by an exercise program. Active and active-assisted exercises are an integral part of the physical therapy program (see Chapter 11 for details).

Exercise and Home Program

Exercises for the cervical spine are prescribed. Exercises should at first be performed under the guidance of a therapist. When the patient is free of pain and full motion has been achieved, progress to strength and endurance programs. Begin and end exercise sessions with stretching and relaxation (see Chapter 15 for exercise details).

Corrective and Preventive Measures

- Postural correction, e.g., correct forward head position.
- Correct poor reading habits, e.g., reading in bed holding a book with outstretched arms, and tilting the neck owing to poor lighting (see Chapter 20).

- Avoid holding the telephone between the ear and shoulder, which may cause and activate TrPs.
- Avoid paradoxical respiration, which has been noted as a cause of scalene overload.[52]

Trapezius

Upper Trapezius, Middle Trapezius, Lower Part of Trapezius

Symptoms and Pain Pattern

- The trapezius muscle is the most common muscle in the body to harbor TrPs. They are often found incidentally in asymptomatic persons.[43, 44]
- Upper trapezius TrPs may involve pain in the cervical area in addition to referred pain to the ear region, face, and frontal area.[2] Headaches may be noted in the temporal area. Patients may present with symptoms of dizziness and vertigo[9] in addition to pilomotor activity involving the upper arm.[51]
- Trapezius TrPs in the area of the midscapula may cause symptoms of brachial neuralgia and subdeltoid bursitis.[10, 17]
- Symptoms referable to the lower trapezius TrPs may refer pain to the paradorsal, high cervical area, medial border of the scapula, and acromion[7, 15, 17, 23, 30, 33, 51] (Fig. 12–38).

Findings on Examination

- Local tenderness over TrPs. Trigger points are most commonly located in the upper two thirds of the muscle.[41]

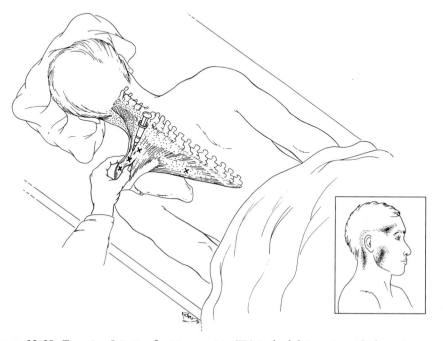

Figure 12–38. Trapezius. Injection for trigger points *(X's)* in the left trapezius with the patient prone. The upper portion of the left trapezius is grasped between the thumb, index, and middle fingers and elevated to avoid penetrating the apex of the lung. Several entries are usually necessary to treat all trigger points that are present. Aspirate prior to injection. Pain pattern is shown by *stippling*.

- Limitation in range of motion of the cervical spine.
- Pain with cervical rotation, flexion, and with shoulder shrug.
- Elevation of the arms and abduction may be limited by muscle shortening and pain.
- Trigger point palpation may give rise to referred pain patterns.

Differential Diagnosis

- Cervical disc.
- Temporomandibular joint dysfunction.
- Trapezius muscle sprain.

Anatomy

Upper Trapezius

Origin: occipital bone (ligamentum nuchae).
Insertion: outer one third of the clavicle.
Action: upper fibers elevate the shoulder (shrugging), rotates scapula, draws head to the same side, turns face to the opposite side; both trapezius muscles working together extend the head.
Nerve supply: accessory (spinal portion Cr 11).

Middle Trapezius

Origin: spinous processes of C7 and C8 and upper thoracic vertebrae.
Insertion: spine of the scapula and acromion.
Action: adduction of the scapula.
Nerve supply: accessory (spinal portion Cr 11).

Lower Part of Trapezius

Origin: spinous processes of lower thoracic vertebra.
Insertion: spine of the scapula.
Action: lowers and pulls the scapula down.
Nerve supply: accessory (spinal portion Cr 11).

Noninvasive Therapy

The post–trigger point injection follow-up program described in Chapter 11 is recommended as a conservative therapeutic treatment approach. Noninvasive therapy can include:

- Physical therapy modalities (e.g., electrical stimulation and warm packs; see Chapter 19).
- Manual physical therapy techniques (e.g., massage, joint mobilization, and the Trager® Approach [neuromuscular re-education]; see Chapters 16–18 for additional manual techniques).
- Active and passive stretching and limbering of muscles with or without the use of vaporized coolant spray or ice. Limbering and relaxation of muscles are necessary prior to stretching. Contract-relax techniques may be used for muscle lengthening.
- Stretch and spray: Stretch in the opposite direction of the muscle pull. Stretch the head gently toward the opposite side for stretch of the upper trapezius fibers. Adduct the arms across the chest, with flexion of the cervical area and upper back to stretch the mid- and lower portion of the trapezius. Trapezius muscle TrPs are often accompanied by neighboring TrPs found in the infraspinatus, supraspinatus, and levator scapulae.
- Exercise program: Exercises for the neck and shoulder (see Chapter 15) include relaxation, limbering, stretching, and strengthening. When the patient is free of pain and full motion has been achieved, progress to strength and endurance programs.

Injection of Trigger Point

With the patient in the supine position, TrPs are identified and injected under sterile precautions (see Chapter 11 for TrP injection technique). The upper trapezius is held between the thumb, index, and middle fingers and lifted slightly (see Figs 12–38 and 11–13). This helps control the depth of needle penetration to avoid the apex of the lung. Trigger points in the middle and lower fibers may sometimes be palpated best with the patient in the side-lying position. Trigger points should be well localized and held between two fingers during injection and needling in the chest wall area. Care must be taken that the direction of injection and needling is tangential to the thorax. The needle should avoid the intercostal space. Injections in the thoracic area are best given with the needle caudally directed to avoid entering the intercostal spaces.

Needle size: 1.5, 2.0 in., 21 gauge.

Solution: Any one of the following solutions may be used: 0.5% procaine; 1.0% lidocaine; saline and dry needling in case of allergy. Do not use epinephrine.

Precautions

- Elevate muscle to avoid puncturing the pleura (pneumothorax) (see complications in Chapter 11).
- Aspirate prior to injection and needling.

Postinjection Follow-up Physical Therapy Program

The patient should receive 3 to 4 consecutive days of treatment. Physical therapy should include electrical stimulation, relaxation, limbering, and stretching of the involved muscle using vaporized coolant spray or ice as needed, combined with and followed by an exercise program. Active and active-assisted exercises are an integral part of the physical therapy program (see Chapter 11 for details).

Exercise and Home Program

Exercises for neck and shoulder are prescribed. Exercises should at first be performed under the guidance of a therapist. When the patient is free of pain and full motion has been achieved, progress to strength and endurance programs. Begin and end exercise sessions with stretching and relaxation (see Chapter 15 for exercise details).

Corrective and Preventive Measures

- Avoid maintaining rotational positions of the cervical region for long periods, e.g., sitting in an airplane engaged in prolonged conversations with the head turned.
- Avoid holding the telephone between the ear and shoulder to free the arms; this is a common cause of neck pain.
- Avoid sitting in chairs with no armrests; patients with short arms require elevation of the arms to a proper height to avoid stress on the trapezius area. Correct sitting posture (see Chapter 20).
- Avoid reading and watching television in bed.
- Do not use a firm pillow. The pillow should be soft (e.g., stuffed with feathers) so that it contours to the neck area.

Splenius Capitis and Splenius Cervicis

Symptoms and Pain Pattern

- Patient may complain of headache.
- Pain in the posterior cervical area (Fig. 12–39).

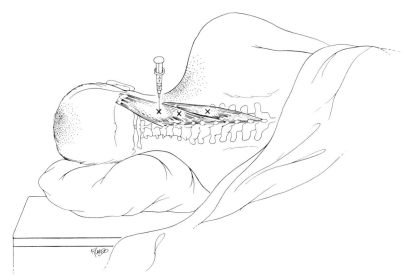

Figure 12–39. Splenius capitis and splenius cervicis. Injection of trigger points *(X's)* in the right splenius capitis and cervicis with the patient lying on the uninvolved side. Avoid the vertebral artery. Aspirate prior to injection. Anatomic landmarks are noted. Trigger point pain pattern is shown by *stippling.*

- Pain in the head and face.[41]
- The splenius capitis may refer pain to the top of the head (vertex), with blurring of vision on the same side.[54]
- The splenius cervicis refers pain to the occiput and back of the eye on the same side.[50, 51]

Findings on Examination

- Pain in the cervical area with rotation and flexion of the spine.
- Limitation in range of motion with rotation to the same side.
- Tender TrPs may cause local and referred pain.
- The splenius capitis can be palpated between the trapezius, which is behind the muscle, and the sternocleidomastoid in front.
- The splenius cervicis is palpated between the upper trapezius and levator scapulae.
- Neighboring TrPs (both active and latent) occur frequently with all neck muscles, e.g., the upper trapezius, levator scapulae.

Differential Diagnosis

- Cervical arthritis.
- Cervical disc herniation.
- Additional causes of headaches, e.g., tension, tumor.

Anatomy

Splenius Capitis

Origin: ligamentum nuchae and spinous processes of C7, T1–3.
Insertion: lateral part of occipital bone, and mastoid of the temporal bone.
Nerve supply: dorsal primary divisions (C4–8).

Splenius Cervicis

Origin: spinous processes of T3–6.
Insertion: transverse processes of C1–3.

Action: the splenius capitis and cervicis extend the head, bend the head laterally, and rotate the face to the same side.
Nerve supply: dorsal primary divisions (C4–8).

Noninvasive Therapy

The post–trigger point injection follow-up program described in Chapter 11 is recommended as a conservative therapeutic treatment approach. Noninvasive therapy can include:

- Physical therapy modalities (e.g., electrical stimulation and warm packs; see Chapter 19).
- Manual physical therapy techniques (e.g., massage, joint mobilization, and the Trager® Approach [neuromuscular re-education]; see Chapters 16–18 for additional manual techniques).
- Active and passive stretching and limbering of muscles with or without the use of vaporized coolant spray or ice. Active exercise is part of the stretch-and-spray technique. Limbering and relaxation of muscles are necessary prior to stretching. Contract-relax techniques may be used.
- Stretch and spray: Stretching is accomplished by flexion of the head, bending the head laterally to the opposite side, and rotating the face to the opposite side. Stretches are done with the patient in the sitting position. Electrical stimulation, limbering of muscles, and warm packs should precede stretch and spray to relax muscles.
- Exercises and home program for the splenius muscles (see Chapter 15 for neck exercises). Exercise programs include relaxation, limbering, stretching, and strengthening. When the patient is free of pain and full motion has been achieved, progress to strength and endurance programs.

Injection of Trigger Point

With the patient in the side-lying position, the TrP is well localized (see Chapter 11 for technique). Awareness of the posterior occipital triangle is necessary to avoid injecting in the area of the vertebral artery (see Posterior Cervical Muscles, next page).

Needle size: 1.5 in., 22–25 gauge.
Solution: Any one of the following solutions may be used: 0.5% procaine; 1.0% lidocaine; saline and dry needling in case of allergy. Do not use epinephrine.

Precautions

- Aspirate prior to injection.
- Avoid the vertebral artery.
- Avoid area of the posterior occipital triangle.

Postinjection Follow-up Physical Therapy Program

The patient should receive 3 to 4 consecutive days of treatment. Physical therapy should include electrical stimulation, relaxation, limbering, and stretching of the involved muscle using vaporized coolant spray or ice as needed combined with and followed by an exercise program. Active and active-assisted exercises are an integral part of the physical therapy program (see Chapter 11 for details).

Exercise and Home Program

Exercises for the cervical area are described in Chapter 15. Exercises should at first be performed under the guidance of a therapist. When the patient is free of pain and full motion has been achieved, progress to strength and endurance programs. Begin and end exercise sessions with stretching and relaxation.

Corrective and Preventive Measures

- Correct poor posture (forward head and neck position).
- Avoid occupational neck strain, e.g., place a computer screen and work activities and tools properly to avoid constant rotation of the cervical area (see Chapter 20).
- Use a soft pillow for sleeping (i.e., one that will contour to the neck). The physician should prescribe a cervical pillow if necessary.
- Use proper prescription of bifocal eyeglasses to avoid head-forward posture.
- Avoid chilling of the neck area, e.g., as often caused by an air conditioner directly above the patient.
- Continue the home exercise program.

Posterior Cervical Muscles

Semispinalis Capitis, Semispinalis Cervicis, Multifidi

Symptoms and Pain Pattern

- Trigger points in the posterior cervical muscles cause pain in the posterior cervical area.[23, 33]
- Different pain patterns have been described depending on the position of TrPs.
- Three TrP locations were described with individual pain patterns.[50, 51]
- The more distal TrPs, which lie in the deeper muscles, refer pain to the occipital area, neck, and vertebral body of the scapula.
- More proximal and superficial TrPs refer pain to the occipital area extending around the skull to the forehead and above the eye.
- Occipital nerve entrapment may occur causing symptoms of occipital neuralgia and headaches (Fig. 12–40).

Findings on Examination

- Tender TrPs cause local or referred pain.
- Restricted cervical spine motion is limited, mostly in flexion and extension.
- All motions may be restricted, especially with involvement of neighboring muscles.

Differential Diagnosis

- Cervical sprain.
- Cervical radiculopathy.
- Other causes of headache.

Anatomy

Semispinalis Capitis

Origin: transverse processes of C7–T7, articular processes of C4–6.
Insertion: occipital bone.
Action: extends the head, rotates the head and face to the opposite side.
Nerve supply: dorsal rami of cervical nerves.

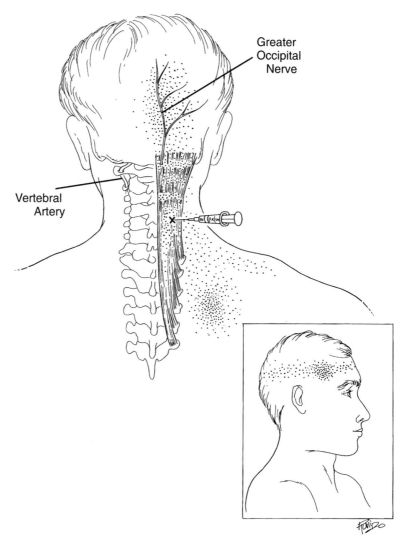

Figure 12–40. Posterior cervical muscles (semispinalis and multifidi). Injection of trigger point in the right posterior cervical muscle *(X)*. The greater occipital nerve is visualized. Anatomic landmarks are noted in addition to visualization of the left vertebral artery. Avoid the vertebral artery by injecting above or below the vertebral artery area. Aspirate prior to injection. Pain pattern is shown by *stippling*.

Semispinalis Cervicis

Origin: transverse processes of T1–6.
Insertion: spinous processes of C2–5.
Action: extends the vertebral column and rotates the cervical spine to the opposite side.
Nerve supply: dorsal rami of thoracic and cervical spinal nerves.

Multifidi (Cervical)

Origin: articular processes of C4–7.
Insertion: fibers of the multifidi pass up and into the sides of the spines of the vertebrae above, skipping two to four vertebrae.
Action: the multifidus muscle rotates the spine, flexes the vertebral column laterally, and rotates it to the opposite side; when acting together the multifidi extend the cervical dorsal area.
Nerve supply: dorsal rami of spinal nerves.

Noninvasive Therapy

The post–trigger point injection follow-up program described in Chapter 11 is recommended as a conservative therapeutic treatment approach. Noninvasive therapy can include:

- Physical therapy modalities (e.g., electrical stimulation and warm packs; see Chapter 19).
- Manual physical therapy techniques (e.g., massage, joint mobilization, and the Trager® Approach [neuromuscular re-education]; see Chapters 16–18 for additional manual techniques).
- Active and passive stretching and limbering of muscles with or without the use of vaporized coolant spray or ice. Active exercise is part of the stretch-and-spray technique. Limbering and relaxation of muscles are necessary prior to stretching. Contract-relax techniques may be used.
- Stretch and spray: Stretching of restricted range of motion is accomplished by flexing the head and rotating the head and face to the same side. If lateral flexion is restricted, stretch and spray is performed by stretching the cervical area to the opposite side. Vaporized coolant is applied to the TrP and referred pain area.
- Exercises and a home program for the cervical area are described in Chapter 15. Exercise programs include relaxation, limbering, stretching, and strengthening.

Injection of Trigger Point

The patient may be injected in the prone or side-lying position. Be aware of the location of the vertebral artery. The injection may be given above or below the area of the vertebral artery (suboccipital) (see Fig. 12–40). (See Chapter 11 for injection technique.)

Needle size: 1.5–2.0 in., 22–25 gauge.
Solution: Any one of the following solutions may be used: 0.5% procaine; 1.0% lidocaine; saline and dry needling in case of allergy. Do not use epinephrine.

Precautions

- Inject TrPs above and below the area of the vertebral artery to avoid puncturing the artery or causing vertebral artery spasm (see Fig. 12–39).
- Aspirate prior to injection.

Postinjection Follow-up Physical Therapy Program

The patient should receive 3 to 4 consecutive days of treatment. Physical therapy should include electrical stimulation, relaxation, limbering, and stretching of the involved muscle using vaporized coolant spray or ice as needed combined with and followed by an exercise program. Active and active-assisted exercises are an integral part of the physical therapy program (see Chapter 11 for details).

Exercise and Home Program

Exercises should at first be performed under the guidance of a therapist. Begin and end exercise sessions with relaxation and stretching. (See Chapter 15 for details.)

Corrective and Preventive Measures

- Avoid flexion, extension, and rotation of the cervical area for long periods.
- Do not use a firm pillow. The pillow should be soft (e.g., stuffed with feathers) so that it can contour to the neck area.
- Avoid reading and viewing television in bed.
- Correct poor postural habits, e.g., the head-forward posture (see Chapter 20).

Suboccipital Muscles

Obliquus Capitis Inferior, Obliquus Capitis Superior, Rectus Capitis Posterior Major, Rectus Capitis Posterior Minor, Suboccipital Triangle

Symptoms and Pain Pattern

- Trigger points in the suboccipital muscles are a frequent cause of headaches in addition to neck pain.[15, 16]
- Pain may be referred from the occiput to the forehead, including the area of the orbit[51] (Fig. 12–41).

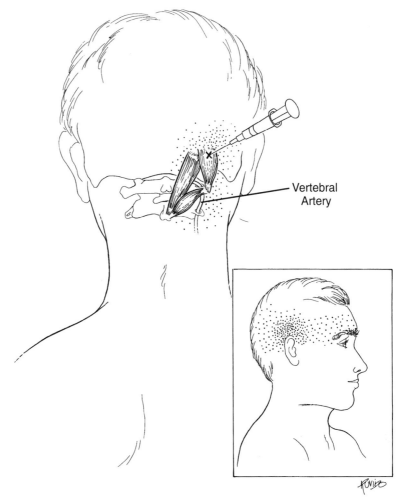

Figure 12–41. Suboccipital muscle. Injection of trigger point *(X)* in the obliquus capitis superior muscle with the patient in the prone position. Injection is localized directly over the trigger point and the superior portion of the occipital area to avoid the vertebral artery. The occipital triangle and vertebral artery are noted. Pain pattern is shown by *stippling*.

Findings on Examination

- Local tenderness in the suboccipital region.
- Patients are often able to identify the TrP.
- Trigger points may be well isolated and respond well to injection and needling.
- Trigger points occur frequently in neighboring muscles (e.g., the posterior cervical muscles).
- Pain in the upper cervical area with flexion, extension, and rotation movements.
- Restricted motion in flexion and rotation.

Differential Diagnosis

- Cervical sprain.
- Headaches due to other causes.

Anatomy

Obliquus Capitis Inferior

Origin: spinous process of the axis.
Insertion: back of the transverse process of the atlas.
Action: rotates the skull, turning the face to the same side.
Nerve supply: (C1) branches suboccipital.

Obliquus Capitis Superior

Origin: transverse process of the atlas.
Insertion: occipital bone between the superior and inferior nuchal lines.
Action: extends the head, pulls the head to the same side.
Nerve supply: (C1) branches suboccipital.

Rectus Capitis Posterior Major

Origin: spinous process of the axis.
Insertion: occipital bone below the inferior nuchal line.
Action: extends the head.
Nerve supply: (C1) branches suboccipital.

Rectus Capitis Posterior Minor

Origin: posterior tubercle on the arch of the atlas.
Insertion: medial area of the occipital bone below the inferior nuchal line.
Action: extends the head.
Nerve supply: (C1) branches suboccipital.

Suboccipital Triangle

The three sides of the suboccipital triangle are made up of the rectus capitis posterior major, obliquus capitis superior, and obliquus capitis inferior muscles. The floor of the triangle contains the posterior arch of the atlas and the vertebral artery. The greater occipital nerve crosses over the suboccipital triangle (see Figs. 12–40 and 12–41).

Noninvasive Therapy

The post–trigger point injection follow-up program described in Chapter 11 is recommended as a conservative therapeutic treatment approach. Noninvasive therapy can include:

- Physical therapy modalities (e.g., electrical stimulation and warm packs; see Chapter 19).
- Manual physical therapy techniques (e.g., massage, joint mobilization, and the

Trager® Approach [neuromuscular re-education]; see Chapters 16–18 for additional manual techniques).
- Active and passive stretching and limbering of muscles with or without the use of vaporized coolant spray or ice. Active exercise is part of the stretch-and-spray technique. Limbering and relaxation of muscles are necessary prior to stretching. Contract-relax techniques may be used.
- Stretch and spray for the suboccipital muscles is performed. Stretching is performed opposite the pull of shortened muscles. Stretch will usually be performed in the direction of flexion and rotation to the opposite side.
- Exercises and a home program for the cervical area are prescribed (see Chapter 15). Exercise program includes relaxation, limbering, stretching, and strengthening.

Injection of Trigger Point

With the patient in the prone position the TrP is carefully identified. Injection is localized directly over the TrP in the superior portion of the occipital area to avoid the vertebral artery (see Fig. 12–41). (See Chapter 11 for injection technique.)

Needle size: 1.5 in., 25 gauge.
Solution: Any one of the following solutions may be used: 0.5% procaine; 1.0% lidocaine; saline and dry needling in case of allergy. Do not use epinephrine.

Precautions

- Avoid the vertebral artery. Spasm of the vertebral artery may cause cerebral ischemia.
- Aspirate prior to injection.

Postinjection Follow-up Physical Therapy Program

The patient should receive 3 to 4 consecutive days of treatment. Physical therapy should include electrical stimulation, relaxation, limbering, and stretching of the involved muscle using vaporized coolant spray or ice as needed combined with and followed by an exercise program. Active and active-assisted exercises are an integral part of the physical therapy program (see Chapter 11 for details).

Exercise and Home Program

Exercises for the suboccipital muscles are prescribed. Exercise should at first be performed under the guidance of a therapist. Begin and end exercise sessions with stretching and relaxation (see Chapter 15 for details).

Corrective and Preventive Measures

- Avoid flexion, extension, and rotation of the cervical area for prolonged periods.
- Do not use a firm pillow. The pillow should be soft (e.g., stuffed with feathers) so that it can contour to the neck area.
- Avoid reading and viewing television in bed (see Chapter 20).
- Correct poor sitting and standing postures, e.g., the head-forward position.

Rhomboid Major and Rhomboid Minor

Symptoms and Pain Pattern

- Pain in the dorsal region between the vertebral body of the scapula and paraspinal muscles[22, 33] (Fig. 12–42).
- Pain may be present at rest.
- Pain may be aggravated with motions of the shoulder.
- Trigger points may result from a dorsal sprain or prolonged strain due to chronic

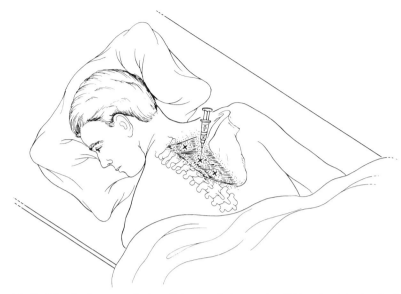

Figure 12–42. Rhomboid major and minor. Injection of trigger points *(X's)* in the right rhomboid muscles. Direct the needle tangentially and caudally to avoid entering the intercostal space. Anatomic landmarks are noted. Pain pattern is shown by *stippling*.

tension related to poor posture (e.g., the round-shouldered position with prolonged reading).

Findings on Examination

- Palpation may be performed with the patient sitting, standing, or in the prone position.
- Tender TrPs are found medial to the vertebral body of the scapula.
- Pain may be aggravated with motions of the shoulder.

Anatomy

Rhomboid Major

Origin: spinous processes of T2–5.
Insertion: vertebral border of the scapula, between the spine and inferior angle.
Action: adducts and rotates the scapula.
Nerve supply: dorsal scapular (C5).

Rhomboid Minor

Origin: lower part of ligamentum nuchae, spinous processes of C7 and T1.
Insertion: vertebral border of scapula opposite the root of the spine.
Action: the rhomboid muscles brace the back of the shoulder holding the scapula to the chest, and raise the scapula tilting the lower inferior angle medially.
Nerve supply: dorsal scapular (C5).

Differential Diagnosis

- Dorsal sprain.
- Intrathoracic disease.
- Cervical disc herniation.

Noninvasive Therapy

The post–trigger point injection follow-up program described in Chapter 11 is recommended as a conservative therapeutic treatment approach. Noninvasive therapy can include:

- Physical therapy modalities (e.g., electrical stimulation and warm packs; see Chapter 19).
- Manual physical therapy techniques (e.g., massage, joint mobilization, and the Trager® Approach [neuromuscular re-education]; see Chapters 16–18 for additional manual techniques).
- Active and passive stretching and limbering of muscles with or without the use of vaporized coolant spray or ice. Active exercise is part of the stretch-and-spray technique. Limbering and relaxation of muscles are necessary prior to stretching. Contract-relax techniques may be used.
- Stretch and spray (see Chapter 11): The scapula must be brought forward. This is best done with the patient sitting. The bend-sitting exercise position is appropriate for stretch and spray. Vaporized coolant or ice over the TrP areas and referred pain area are used as needed. The patient should perform bending with the arms between the knees as well as side-to-side bending as illustrated for active stretch (see Chapter 15). Electrical stimulation, limbering of muscles, and warm packs may precede stretch and spray to relax the muscles. Stretching of muscle is also accomplished actively and with assistance during the exercise program. Active exercise is part of the stretch-and-spray technique.
- Exercises and a home program for the shoulders and cervical and dorsal areas are described in Chapter 15. Instruct the patient in correct posture. Exercise programs include relaxation, limbering, stretching, and strengthening. When the patient is free of pain and full motion has been achieved, progress to strength and endurance programs.

Injection of Trigger Point

With the patient prone TrPs are identified. Identify bony landmarks. Palpate the entire muscle for multiple TrPs. Use multiple needle entries along the muscle belly. Angle the needle tangentially. Use sterile precaution. (See Chapter 11 for injection technique.)

Needle size: 1.5 in., 21 gauge.
Solution: Any one of the following solutions may be used: 0.5% procaine; 1.0% lidocaine; saline and dry needling may be used in case of allergy. Do not use epinephrine.

Precautions

- Angle the needle tangentially to avoid entering the chest cavity.
- Aspirate prior to injection.

Postinjection Follow-up Physical Therapy Program

The patient should receive 3 to 4 consecutive days of treatment. Physical therapy should include electrical stimulation, relaxation, limbering, and stretching of the involved muscle using vaporized coolant spray or ice as needed combined with and followed by an exercise program. Active and active-assisted exercises are an integral part of the physical therapy program (see Chapter 11 for details).

Exercise and Home Program

Instruct the patient in correct posture and use of lumbar supports to improve spinal alignment and decrease stress in the intrascapular area. Exercises for the shoulders and cervical and dorsal area are described in Chapter 15. Exercises should at first be performed under the guidance of a therapist. When the patient is free of pain and full motion has been achieved, progress to strength and endurance programs. Begin and end exercise sessions with relaxation.

Corrective and Preventive Measures

- Eliminate causes related to posture and tension, e.g., correct poor sitting posture. Chairs should have proper back supports and armrests (see Chapter 20).
- Change position often.
- Instruct the patient in a daily program of exercise and stretching.

Levator Scapulae

Symptoms and Pain Pattern

- Pain over the medial border of the scapula extending upward to the base of the occiput[30, 43] (Fig. 12–43).
- Generalized headaches.
- Pain may radiate to the head and shoulder.[22, 50]
- Pain may be noted around the ear.[41]
- Levator scapulae muscle pain is often involved in chronic cervical conditions.[41]
- Patients complain of limitation in rotation of the neck.

Findings on Examination

- Trigger points are most frequently found at the attachment of the muscle on the upper medial border of the scapula (the greatest point of mechanical stress).[44]
- In 200 asymptomatic persons examined for shoulder girdle muscle TrPs (100 male, 100 female), the levator scapulae was implicated in 19.7% of the patients, second in frequency to the trapezius (34.7%). The TrPs found most frequently in symptomatic persons were in the levator scapulae and infraspinatus. The trapezius was not

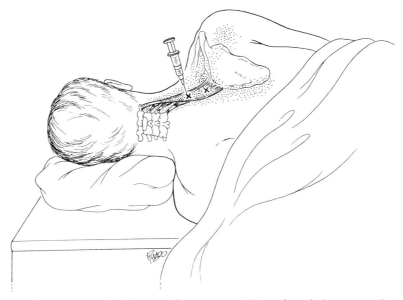

Figure 12–43. Levator scapulae. Injection of trigger points *(X's)* in the right levator scapulae. Aspirate prior to injection. Avoid the intercostal space and direct the needle tangentially to the frontal plane of the patient. Trigger point pain pattern is shown by *stippling*.

implicated as often in symptomatic patients (2% vs. 55% for the levator scapulae, and 31% for the infraspinatus).[44]
- Trigger points may be palpated in the upper portion of the levator scapulae at the base of the neck. Palpation is more easily achieved when the anterior border of the trapezius can be relaxed and retracted medially.
- Tenderness and referred pain may be produced on palpation of TrPs.
- Limited rotation of the neck to the opposite side. Limitation in lateral flexion to the opposite side.

Differential Diagnosis

- Cervical disc herniation.
- Scapulocostal syndrome.
- Cervical sprain.
- Neck and shoulder pain due to TrPs in neighboring muscles (e.g., trapezius, supraspinatus, rhomboids).

Anatomy

Origin: transverse processes of C1–4.

Insertion: medial border of the scapulae between the superior angle and root of the spine.

Action: with the origin fixed, the levator scapulae elevates the scapulae and rotates the glenoid cavity caudally; with the insertion fixed, acting unilaterally, the levator scapulae flexes and rotates the cervical vertebrae to the same side; acting bilaterally, the muscle acts as an extensor of the cervical spine.

Nerve supply: (C3, 4) and often branch from dorsal scapular (C5).

Noninvasive Therapy

The post–trigger point injection follow-up program described in Chapter 11 is recommended as a conservative therapeutic treatment approach. Noninvasive therapy can include:

- Physical therapy modalities (e.g., electrical stimulation and warm packs; see Chapter 19).
- Manual physical therapy techniques (e.g., massage, joint mobilization, and the Trager® Approach [neuromuscular re-education]; see Chapters 16–18 for additional manual techniques).
- Active and passive stretching and limbering of muscles with or without the use of vaporized coolant spray or ice. Active exercise is part of the stretch-and-spray technique. Limbering and relaxation of muscles are necessary prior to stretching. Contract-relax techniques may be used.
- Stretch and spray is performed by means of flexion, lateral stretch, and rotation to the opposite side of the symptoms. Electrical stimulation, limbering of muscles, and warm packs should precede stretch and spray to relax muscles. Limbering and relaxation of muscles are necessary prior to stretching.
- Exercises and a home program for the cervical area are described in Chapter 15. The exercise program includes relaxation, limbering, stretching, and strengthening. When the patient is free of pain and full motion has been achieved, progress to strength and endurance programs.
- Prevention and correction of contributing factors.

Injection of Trigger Point

Injection of TrPs is accomplished with the patent lying on the uninvolved side (see Fig. 12–43). Palpate for both upper and lower TrPs. Relaxation of the upper border of the trapezius permits better exposure of the levator scapulae. (See Chapter 11 for injection technique.)

Needle size: 1.5–2.0 in., 22–24 gauge.

Solution: Any one of the following solutions may be used: 0.5% procaine; 1.0% lidocaine; saline and dry needling in case of allergy. Do not use epinephrine.

Precautions

- Aspirate prior to injection.
- Avoid entering the chest cavity.
- The angle of the needle should be directed tangentially when in the region of the scapulae and chest cavity.

Postinjection Follow-up Physical Therapy Program

The patient should receive 3 to 4 consecutive days of treatment. Physical therapy should include electrical stimulation, relaxation, limbering, and stretching of the involved muscle using vaporized coolant spray or ice as needed combined with and followed by an exercise program. Active and active-assisted exercises are an integral part of the physical therapy program (see Chapter 11 for details).

Exercise and Home Program

Exercises for the cervical area are prescribed. Exercises should at first be performed under the guidance of a therapist. When the patient is free of pain and full motion has been achieved, progress to strength and endurance programs. Begin and end exercise sessions with stretching and relaxation (see Chapter 15 for details).

Corrective and Preventive Measures

- Avoid maintaining the cervical area in rotated postures for prolonged periods of time (e.g., as in conversation on an airplane with the head turned toward the interlocutor; improper placement of work tools necessitating the head and neck to be repeatedly rotated; see Chapter 20).
- Chairs should have armrests high enough to permit relaxation and support of the cervical and shoulder muscles.
- The patient should continue exercises, stressing relaxation, flexibility, and stretching.
- Avoid cervical strain by wearing proper eyeglasses.
- Avoid reading and viewing television in bed.
- The pillow used at night should be soft to contour to the neck area. Avoid the use of two pillows, which encourages cervical strain and a head-forward neck posture.
- The physician should prescribe a cervical pillow if necessary.

Muscles of the Upper Extremities

Deltoid

Symptoms and Pain Pattern

- Pain over the shoulder, either the anterior or posterior aspect, or both[7, 35] (Fig. 12–44).
- Pain in the upper back, neck, and arm.[33]
- Pain with abduction, forward flexion, and elevation of the shoulder.

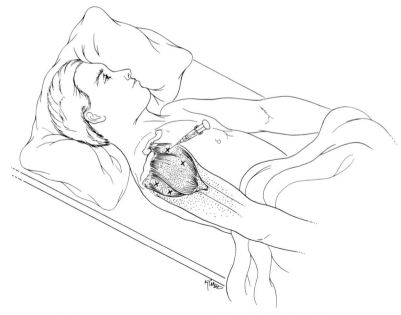

Figure 12–44. Deltoid. Injection of trigger points in the right deltoid muscle. Trigger points *(X's)* are noted in the posterior and anterior deltoid. Patient is in the side-lying position. Anatomic landmarks are noted. Pain pattern is shown by *stippling.*

Findings on Examination

- Tender TrPs may be found over the anterior, middle, or posterior aspect of the deltoid.
- Limitation in shoulder point motion.
- Pain with abduction and elevation.

Anatomy

Origin: anterior border of the clavicle, outer border of the acromion, lower edge of the spine of the scapula.

Insertion: outer side of the humerus.

Action: abducts the arm to the horizontal position, anterior fibers flex the shoulder, posterior fibers extend the arm at the shoulder joint.

Nerve supply: axillary (C5, 6).

Differential Diagnosis

- Cervical radiculopathy.
- Shoulder bursitis.
- Bicipital tendinitis.
- Rotator cuff injury.

Noninvasive Therapy

The post–trigger point injection follow-up program described in Chapter 11 is recommended as a conservative therapeutic treatment approach. Noninvasive therapy can include:

- Physical therapy modalities (e.g., electrical stimulation and warm packs; see Chapter 19).
- Manual physical therapy techniques (e.g., massage, joint mobilization, and the

Trager® Approach [neuromuscular re-education]; see Chapters 16–18 for additional manual techniques).
- Active and passive stretching and limbering of muscles with or without the use of vaporized coolant spray or ice. Active exercise is part of the stretch-and-spray technique. Limbering and relaxation are necessary prior to stretching. Contract-relax techniques may be used.
- Stretch and spray for the deltoid muscle is performed with the aid of vaporized coolant or ice. For anterior fibers, abduct and extend the arm. For posterior fibers, flex the shoulder and adduct the arm across the chest (see Chapter 11). Electrical stimulation, limbering of muscles, and warm packs may precede stretch and spray to relax the muscles. Stretching of muscle is also accomplished actively and with assistance during the exercise program. Active exercise is part of the stretch-and-spray technique.
- Exercises and a home program for the shoulder muscles are prescribed (see Chapter 15). The exercise program includes relaxation, limbering, stretching, and strengthening. When the patient is free of pain and full motion has been achieved, progress to strength and endurance programs.

Injection of Trigger Point

The patient may be injected for the anterior and middle deltoid in the supine position. The side-lying position can expose both the anterior and posterior aspects of the deltoid (see Fig. 12–44). All palpable TrPs are injected. Multiple needle entries are important to find those TrPs that are not recognized by palpation.

Needle size: 1.5 or 2.0 in., 21 gauge.
Solution: Any one of the following solutions may be used: 0.5% procaine; 1.0% lidocaine; saline and dry needling in case of allergy. Do not use epinephrine.

Postinjection Follow-up Physical Therapy Program

The patient should receive 3 to 4 consecutive days of treatment. Physical therapy should include electrical stimulation, relaxation, limbering, and stretching of the involved muscle using vaporized coolant spray or ice as needed combined with and followed by an exercise program. Active and active-assisted exercises are an integral part of the physical therapy program (see Chapter 11 for details).

Exercise and Home Program

Exercises for the shoulder are prescribed. Exercises should at first be performed under the guidance of a therapist. When the patient is free of pain and full motion has been achieved, progress to strength and endurance programs. Begin and end exercise sessions with relaxation and stretching. (See Chapter 15 for exercise details.)

Corrective and Preventive Measures

- Avoid repetitive activities involving shoulder joint motion, e.g., practicing tennis serves.
- Continue daily stretching activities.
- Do warm-up exercises before activities that stress the shoulder joint area.

Supraspinatus

Symptoms and Pain Pattern

- Pain with abduction and elevation of the arm.
- Pain is noted over the posterior aspect of the shoulder and referred to the deltoid region, upper arm, lateral epicondyle, and forearm[15, 16, 33, 50, 52, 54] (Fig. 12–45).

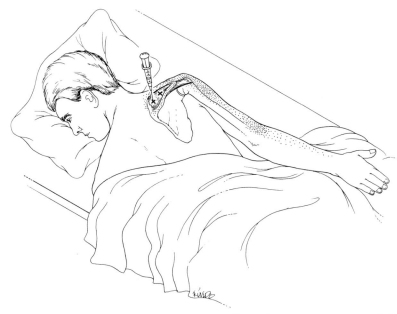

Figure 12–45. Supraspinatus. Injection of trigger points *(X's)* in the right supraspinatus with the patient prone. The needle is directed directly over the supraspinous fossa of the scapula to avoid penetrating the rib cage. Anatomic landmarks are noted. Pain pattern is shown by *stippling*.

Findings on Examination

- Local TrP tenderness or referred pain pattern to the upper extremity.
- Limited range of motion of the shoulders.
- Often accompanied by TrPs in neighboring muscles, e.g., the trapezius and infraspinatus.

Differential Diagnosis

- Deltoid bursitis.
- Cervical herniated disc.
- Cervical radiculopathy.
- Bicipital tendinitis.

Anatomy

Origin: supraspinous fossa.
Insertion: greater tuberosity of the humerus; the supraspinatus tendon is aligned with the lateral part of the upper part of the capsule of the shoulder joint.
Action: abductor and lateral rotator, helps as a fixator of the shoulder joint.
Nerve supply: suprascapular (C5).

Noninvasive Therapy

The post–trigger point injection follow-up program described in Chapter 11 is recommended as a conservative therapeutic treatment approach. Noninvasive therapy can include:

- Physical therapy modalities (e.g., electrical stimulation and warm packs; see Chapter 19).
- Manual physical therapy techniques (e.g., massage, joint mobilization, and the Trager® Approach [neuromuscular re-education]; see Chapters 16–18 for additional manual techniques).

- Active and passive stretching and limbering of muscles with or without the use of vaporized coolant spray or ice. Active exercise is part of the stretch-and-spray technique. Limbering and relaxation are necessary prior to stretching. May use contract-relax techniques.
- Stretch and spray for the supraspinatus muscle: Stretch in the direction of shoulder internal rotation and adduction using vaporized coolant or ice as needed. Electrical stimulation, limbering of muscles, and warm packs should precede stretch and spray to relax the muscles. Stretching of muscle is also accomplished actively as well as with assistance during the exercise program. Active exercise is part of the stretch-and-spray technique.
- Exercises and a home program for the shoulder are prescribed (see Chapter 15). Exercises for the shoulder begin with relaxation, limbering, and stretching. Stretch in the direction of elevation, adduction, and internal rotation. Begin strengthening exercises as symptoms decrease. When the patient is free of pain and full motion has been achieved, progress to strength and endurance programs.

Injection of Trigger Point

Injection may be performed with the patient in the prone or side-lying position (see Fig. 12–45). It is important that the needle be introduced directly over the supraspinous fossa of the scapula to avoid penetrating the rib cage. Injecting at the muscle insertion, directing the needle under the acromion, may be necessary in addition to multiple needling involving the area of the supraspinous fossa.

Needle size: 1.5 in., 21 gauge.
Solution: Any one of the following solutions may be used: 0.5% procaine; 1.0% lidocaine; saline and dry needling in case of allergy. Do not use epinephrine.

Precautions

- Identify anatomic landmarks prior to injection.
- Inject over the scapular area to avoid a pneumothorax.
- Insert the needle tangentially to avoid entering the chest wall.

Postinjection Follow-up Physical Therapy Program

The patient should receive 3 to 4 consecutive days of treatment. Physical therapy should include electrical stimulation, relaxation, limbering, and stretching of the involved muscle using vaporized coolant spray or ice as needed combined with and followed by an exercise program. Active and active-assisted exercises are an integral part of the physical therapy program.

Exercise and Home Program

Exercises for the shoulder are prescribed. Exercises should at first be performed under the guidance of a therapist. When the patient is free of pain and full motion has been achieved, progress to strength and endurance programs. Begin and end exercise sessions with relaxation and stretching. (See Chapter 15 for exercise details.)

Corrective and Preventive Measures

- Avoid overuse syndromes, e.g., prolonged activities involving elevation of the arms, overhead movements, or excessively repetitive motions such as practicing a tennis serve or throwing a ball.
- Perform warm-up exercises prior to activities that use repetitive shoulder motions, e.g., painting or tennis.

Infraspinatus and Teres Minor

Symptoms and Pain Pattern

- Pain over the posterior aspect of the shoulder and upper dorsal and cervical area.
- Referred pain pattern to the front of the shoulder, radiating pain to the front and lateral aspect of the arm and forearm extending to the radial aspect of the hand[30, 45, 52, 54] (Fig. 12–46).
- Referred pain may be noted over the lateral anterior aspect of the shoulder and anterior chest, together with sympathetic hyperactivity, which may contribute to dystrophy-like syndromes—shoulder girdle fatigue, weakness of grip, hyperhidrosis, and skin temperature changes.[45]
- Limited motion in activities that require placing the hand behind the back (internal rotation) and forward flexion.

Findings on Examination

- Local tenderness from TrPs occur most frequently along the lateral border of the scapula.[43, 44]
- Restriction in internal rotation may be present.
- Palpation of the TrPs may elicit a referred pain pattern.
- Pain as well as muscle shortening may restrict elevation of the shoulder and internal rotation.
- On examination for TrPs, the teres minor muscle appears anatomically as an extension of the infraspinatus. The teres minor is inferior to the infraspinatus. Because of their proximity they are treated together and are difficult to distinguish when one palpates the lateral aspect of the infraspinatus (see Fig. 12–46).

Differential Diagnosis

- Deltoid bursitis.
- Frozen shoulder (adhesive capsulitis).
- Cervical radiculopathy.

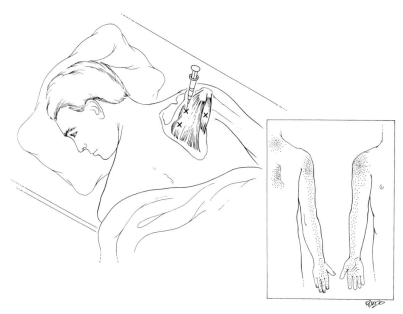

Figure 12–46. Infraspinatus and teres minor. Injection of trigger points (*X's*) in the right infraspinatus and teres minor. The patient is in the prone position. Anatomic landmarks are noted. *Inset,* pain pattern (*stippling*). Observe precautions to avoid entering the chest cavity.

Anatomy

Infraspinatus

Origin: infraspinous fossa.
Insertion: greater tuberosity of humerus.
Action: lateral rotator and stabilizes the head of the humerus in the glenoid cavity during movements of the shoulder joint.
Nerve supply: suprascapular (C5, 6).

Teres Minor

Origin: upper part of dorsal aspect of the axillary border of the scapula.
Insertion: greater tuberosity.
Action: lateral rotator and fixator, stabilizes the head of the humerus in the glenoid cavity during movements of the shoulder joint.
Nerve supply: axillary (C5).

Noninvasive Therapy

The post–trigger point injection follow-up program described in Chapter 11 is recommended as a conservative therapeutic treatment approach. Noninvasive therapy can include:

- Physical therapy modalities (e.g., electrical stimulation and warm packs; see Chapter 19).
- Manual physical therapy techniques (e.g., massage, joint mobilization, and the Trager Approach® [neuromuscular re-education]; see Chapters 16–18 for additional manual techniques).
- Active and passive stretching and limbering of muscles with or without the use of vaporized coolant spray or ice. Active exercise is part of the stretch-and-spray technique. Limbering and relaxation are necessary prior to stretching. Contract-relax techniques may be used.
- Stretch and spray for the infraspinatus and teres minor is performed by stretching in the direction of shoulder internal rotation and adduction.
- Exercises and a home program for the shoulder are prescribed (see Chapter 15). The exercise program includes relaxation, limbering, stretching, and strengthening. When the patient is free of pain and full motion has been achieved, progress to strength and endurance programs.

Injection of Trigger Point

With the patient in the prone or side-lying position, TrPs are identified and isolated between two fingers for injection. Further palpation of the muscle throughout its length is done to explore for additional TrPs. Multiple needling should be performed to identify those TrPs not found on palpation (see Fig. 12–46; see Chapter 11 for injection technique).

Needle size: 1.5 in., 21 gauge.
Solution: Any one of the following solutions may be used: 0.5% procaine; 1.0% lidocaine; saline and dry needling in case of allergy. Do not use epinephrine.

Precautions

- Identify bony landmarks.
- Aspirate prior to injection and needling.
- With needling stay within the borders of the scapula over the infraspinatus to avoid penetrating the thorax. Angle the needle tangentially when injecting and needling to avoid entering the chest wall (see Chapter 11 for complications).

Postinjection Follow-up Physical Therapy Program

The patient should receive 3 to 4 consecutive days of treatment. Physical therapy should include electrical stimulation, relaxation, limbering, and stretching of the involved muscle using vaporized coolant spray or ice as needed combined with and followed by an exercise program. Active and active-assisted exercises are an integral part of the physical therapy program (see Chapter 11 for details).

Exercise and Home Program

Exercises for the shoulder are prescribed. Exercises should at first be performed under the guidance of a therapist. When the patient is free of pain and full motion has been achieved, progress to strength and endurance programs. Begin and end exercise session with stretching and relaxation (see Chapter 15 for exercise details).

Corrective and Preventive Measures

- Avoid repetitive shoulder motions.
- Do warm-up exercises to include relaxation and stretching prior to activities involving shoulder motion, e.g., painting or tennis.
- Relaxation and stretching after athletic activities.
- Correct poor working habits, e.g., use a stool for overhead activities (see Chapter 20).

Subscapularis

Symptoms and Pain Pattern

- Pain in the shoulder area is most pronounced over the posterior deltoid with referred pain to the upper arm (Fig. 12–47).
- Pain may be felt in the wrist.[24, 50]
- Patients complain of pain with motions that require external rotation and abduction.
- Limited motion in abduction and lateral rotation.

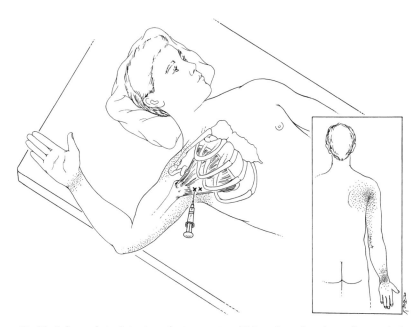

Figure 12–47. Subscapularis. Injection of trigger points (*X's*) in the right subscapularis with the patient supine. The arm is abducted. The axillary border of the scapula is palpated. Trigger points should be well localized by palpation prior to injection. The needle is directed into the trigger point area away from the chest wall to avoid puncturing the pleura. Pain pattern is shown by *stippling.*

Findings on Examination

- Palpate TrPs with the patient in the supine position. Abduct the arm and extend the examining finger anterior to the latissimus dorsi to palpate the axillary border of the scapula.
- Patients may complain of local and referred pain.
- Range of motion assessment may demonstrate limitation in abduction and lateral rotation.

Differential Diagnosis

- Cervical radiculopathy.
- Cervical spondylosis.
- Cervical disc herniation.
- Periadhesive capsulitis (frozen shoulder).

Anatomy

- *Origin:* subscapular fossa.
- *Insertion:* lesser tuberosity of humerus and shaft.
- *Action:* medial rotator and shoulder fixator.
- *Nerve supply:* superior and inferior subscapular (C5, 6).

Noninvasive Therapy

The post–trigger point injection follow-up program described in Chapter 11 is recommended as a conservative therapeutic treatment approach. Noninvasive therapy can include:

- Physical therapy modalities (e.g., electrical stimulation and warm packs; see Chapter 19).
- Manual physical therapy techniques (e.g., massage, joint mobilization, and the Trager® Approach [neuromuscular re-education]; see Chapters 16–18 for additional manual techniques).
- Active and passive stretching and limbering of muscles with or without the use of vaporized coolant spray or ice. Active exercise is part of the stretch-and-spray technique. Limbering and relaxation are necessary prior to relaxation. May use contract-relax technique.
- Stretch and spray: Stretching is performed in the direction of external rotation, abduction, and elevation. Use vaporized coolant spray or ice as needed. Electrical stimulation, limbering of muscles, and warm packs may precede stretch and spray to relax the muscles. Stretching of muscle is also accomplished actively and with assistance during the exercise program.
- Exercises and home program. Exercises for the shoulder and neck are described in Chapter 15. Exercise programs include relaxation, limbering, stretching, and strengthening. When the patient is free of pain and full motion has been achieved, progress to strength and endurance programs.

Injection of Trigger Point

With the patient in the supine position the arm is abducted (see Fig. 12–47). Palpate the axillary border of the scapula by abducting and elevating the arm. Inject those TrPs that can be palpated and localized. Observe precautions. (See Chapter 11 for injection technique.)

Needle size: 1.5–2.0 in., 21 gauge.
Solution: Any one of the following solutions may be used: 0.5% procaine; 1.0% lidocaine; saline and dry needling in case of allergy. Do not use epinephrine.

Precautions

- The needle should be directed tangentially and away from the chest wall to avoid pneumothorax. Inject only those TrPs that are palpated. The needle should be placed directly into the TrPs. Do not use the needle to explore for TrPs.
- Aspirate prior to injection.

Postinjection Follow-up Physical Therapy Program

The patient should receive 3 to 4 consecutive days of treatment. Physical therapy should include electrical stimulation, relaxation, limbering, and stretching of the involved muscle using vaporized coolant spray or ice as needed combined with and followed by an exercise program. Active and active-assisted exercises are an integral part of the physical therapy program (see Chapter 11 for details).

Exercise and Home Program

Exercises for the shoulder and neck are prescribed. Exercises should at first be performed under the guidance of a therapist. When the patient is free of pain and full motion has been achieved, progress to strength and endurance programs. Begin and end exercise sessions with stretching and relaxation (see Chapter 15 for details).

Corrective and Preventive Measures

- Avoid prolonged positions of adduction.
- Stretching exercises should be performed prior to and after athletic activities.
- Prevent the development of joint adhesions, muscle shortening, and TrPs by maintaining active and passive range of motion in patients who have injuries and paralysis of the upper extremity, e.g., stroke patients.

Biceps Brachii

Symptoms and Pain Pattern

- Pain in the front of the shoulder, upper arm, and suprascapular region[10, 37] (Fig. 12–48).
- Pain at rest as well as with abduction and elevation of the shoulder.

Findings on Examination

- Tenderness along the biceps extending from the upper portion to the elbow.
- Pain in the upper arm with flexion and supination of the forearm.
- Painful limited adduction and elevation of the shoulder.
- Limitation in extension and pronation of the elbow.

Differential Diagnosis

- Bicipital tendinitis.
- Cervical radiculopathy.

Anatomy

Origin: short head of the biceps from the tip of the coracoid process, long head from the supraglenoid tubercle of the scapula; the two heads join together about the middle of the upper arm.

Insertion: back of the tuberosity of the radius, the bicipital aponeurosis to the subcutaneous border of the ulna.

Action: supinates forearm, flexes elbow and shoulder.

Nerve supply: musculocutaneus (C5, 6).

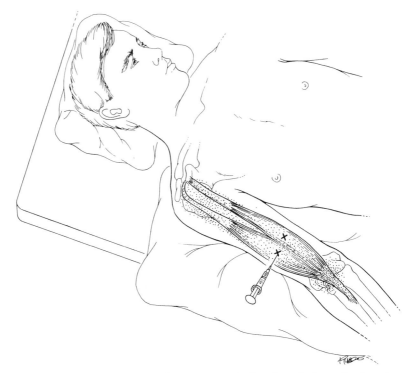

Figure 12–48. Biceps brachii. Injection of trigger points *(X's)* in the right biceps brachii. The patient is supine with slight abduction of the arm. Anatomic landmarks are noted. Pain pattern is shown by *stippling*.

Noninvasive Therapy

The post–trigger point injection follow-up program described in Chapter 11 is recommended as a conservative therapeutic treatment approach. Noninvasive therapy can include:

- Physical therapy modalities (e.g., electrical stimulation and warm packs; see Chapter 19).
- Manual physical therapy techniques (e.g., massage, joint mobilization, and the Trager® Approach [neuromuscular re-education]; see Chapters 16–18 for additional manual techniques).
- Active and passive stretching and limbering of muscles with or without the use of vaporized coolant spray or ice. Active exercise is part of the stretch-and-spray technique. Limbering and relaxation are necessary prior to stretching. Contract-relax technique may be used.
- Stretch and spray for the biceps brachii is performed with the elbow extended and pronated and the shoulder abducted and extended. The area of TrP and referred pain is sprayed with vaporized coolant (see Chapter 11). Electrical stimulation, limbering of muscles, and warm packs should precede stretch and spray to relax muscles.
- Exercise and a home program for the shoulder and elbow are prescribed (see Chapter 15). Exercise programs include relaxation, limbering, stretching, and strengthening. When the patient is free of pain and full motion has been achieved, progress to strength and endurance programs.

Injection of Trigger Point

Position the patient in the supine position (see Fig. 12–48). Trigger points are identified. As much of the muscle as possible is palpated for TrPs. Multiple needling along the body of the biceps brachii is usually required. Multiple needling may find TrPs not found on palpation. Trigger points may be held between the thumb and index finger or isolated between the index and middle fingers. (See Chapter 11 for injection technique.)

Needle size: 1.5, 2.0 in., 21 gauge.

Solution: Any one of the following solutions may be used: 0.5% procaine; 1.0% lidocaine; saline and dry needling in case of allergy. Do not use epinephrine.

Precautions

- Avoid median and radial nerves.

Postinjection Follow-up Physical Therapy Program

The patient should receive 3 to 4 consecutive days of treatment. Physical therapy should include electrical stimulation, relaxation, limbering, and stretching of the involved muscle using vaporized coolant spray or ice as needed combined with and followed by an exercise program. Active and active-assisted exercises are an integral part of the physical therapy program (see Chapter 11 for details).

Exercise and Home Program

Exercises for the shoulder and elbow are prescribed. Exercises should at first be performed under the guidance of a therapist. When the patient is free of pain and full motion has been achieved, progress to strength and endurance programs. Begin and end exercise sessions with stretching and relaxation (see Chapter 15 for details).

Corrective and Preventive Measures

- Home exercise program for shoulder and elbow.
- Relaxation and stretching exercises prior to and after strenuous activities, e.g., athletics, work activities requiring upper extremity effort.

Coracobrachialis

Symptoms and Pain Pattern

- Pain over the anterior aspect of the shoulder (Fig. 12–49).
- Referred pain to the posterior part of the arm, forearm, and dorsum of the hand.[51]
- Pain with abduction, extension, and elevation of the arms.

Findings on Examination

- Local TrP tenderness, especially over the area of muscle insertion and origin.
- Limitation in abduction and elevation.
- Pain with abduction, internal rotation, and elevation.
- Referred pain pattern may be elicited on palpation.
- Weakness in shoulder forward flexion may be noted in movements requiring simultaneous elbow flexion and supination, e.g., hair combing.[18]

Differential Diagnosis

- Cervical radiculopathy.
- Subdeltoid bursitis.

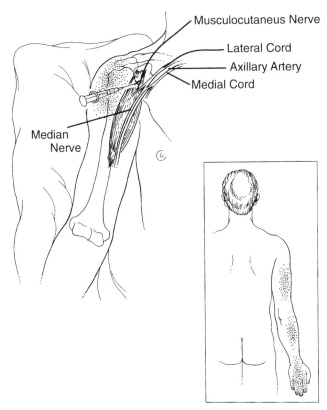

Figure 12–49. Coracobrachialis. Injection of trigger point (*X*) in the right coracobrachialis with the patient supine, the arm slightly externally rotated and abducted. Anatomic landmarks are noted including neurovascular structures and the musculocutaneus nerve. Pain pattern is shown by *stippling*.

Anatomy

Origin: apex of the coracoid of the scapula.

Insertion: medial aspect of the humerus, at the level of the middle of the humerus shaft.

Action: flexes and adducts the arm.

Nerve supply: musculocutaneus (C6, 7).

Noninvasive Therapy

The post–trigger point injection follow-up program described in Chapter 11 is recommended as a conservative therapeutic treatment approach. Noninvasive therapy can include:

- Physical therapy modalities (e.g., electrical stimulation and warm packs; see Chapter 19).
- Manual physical therapy techniques (e.g., massage, joint mobilization, and the Trager® Approach [neuromuscular re-education]; see Chapters 16–18 for additional manual techniques).
- Active and passive stretching and limbering of muscles with or without the use of vaporized coolant spray or ice. Active exercise is part of the stretch-and-spray technique. Limbering and relaxation are necessary prior to stretching. Contract-relax techniques may be used.
- Stretch and spray for the coracobrachialis is performed with the shoulder in abduction and elevation. Electrical stimulation, limbering of muscles, and warm packs should precede stretch and spray to relax muscles.

- Exercises and a home program for the shoulder are prescribed (see Chapter 15). The exercise program includes relaxation, limbering, stretching, and strengthening. When the patient is free of pain and full motion has been achieved, progress to strength and endurance programs.

Injection of Trigger Point

Trigger points are often found near the origin of the coracobrachialis at the coracoid process. Note the proximity of the musculocutaneus nerve (see Fig. 12–49). The coracoid process and coracobrachialis muscle are covered by the anterior deltoid. The lower portion of the coracobrachialis is covered by the pectoralis major. With the patient supine identify the TrP. This may require the arm to be slightly externally rotated and abducted. The TrP is maintained between two fingertips and the needle is inserted directly into the area of maximum tenderness. (See Chapter 11 for injection technique.)

Needle size: 1.5 in., 21 gauge.
Solution: Any one of the following solutions may be used: 0.5% procaine; 1.0% lidocaine; saline and dry needling may be used in case of allergy. Do not use epinephrine.

Precautions

- The musculocutaneus nerve at first lies medial to the coracobrachialis on the lateral side of the axillary artery. Aspirate prior to injection. Infiltration of the nerve may cause temporary weakness of the coracobrachialis, biceps, and brachialis, and anesthesia of the ball of the thumb and lower third of the back of the forearm.

Postinjection Follow-up Physical Therapy Program

The patient should receive 3 to 4 consecutive days of treatment. Physical therapy should include electrical stimulation, relaxation, limbering, and stretching of the involved muscle using vaporized coolant spray or ice as needed combined with and followed by an exercise program. Active and active-assisted exercises are an integral part of the physical therapy program (see Chapter 11 for details).

Exercise and Home Program

Exercises for the shoulder are prescribed. Exercises should at first be performed under the guidance of a therapist. When the patient is free of pain and full motion has been achieved, progress to strength and endurance programs. Begin and end exercise sessions with stretching and relaxation (see Chapter 15 for exercise details).

Corrective and Preventive Measures

- Relaxation and stretching exercises prior to and after athletic activities involving the upper extremities.
- Continue home exercise programs.
- Avoid repetitive activities involving the shoulder area, e.g., prolonged practicing of one's tennis serve.

Brachialis

Symptoms and Pain Pattern

- Pain due to TrPs in the brachialis muscle may be experienced in the upper arm and front of the elbow. Referred pain may include the base of the thumb and dorsum of the web space between the thumb and index finger[38] (Fig. 12–50).

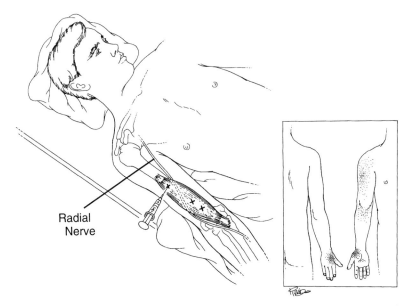

Radial
Nerve

Figure 12–50. Brachialis. Injection of trigger points in the right brachialis muscle *(X's)* with the patient supine. Anatomic landmarks, including the radial nerve, are noted. Exposure of the brachialis is best obtained if the biceps is shifted medially. *Inset,* pain pattern *(stippling).*

- Pain is noted with flexion and extension of the elbow.
- Paresthesia over the dorsum of the thumb has been reported due to entrapment of the sensory branch of the radial nerve[52] (see Fig. 12–50).

Findings on Examination

- Palpate TrPs by flexing the elbow and relax the biceps muscle, which covers the brachialis.
- Trigger points may cause local pain as well as referred pain to the elbow and base of the thumb.
- Flexion and extension of the elbow both actively and passively may cause pain.
- Hypoesthesia of the dorsum of the thumb.

Anatomy

Origin: front of the lower half of the shaft of the humerus and intermuscular septum.
Insertion: coronoid process and tuberosity of the ulna.
Action: flexes the elbow.
Nerve supply: musculocutaneus (C5, 6) and usually filament from radial.

Differential Diagnosis

- Cervical radiculopathy.
- Radial nerve entrapment.
- Muscle strain, e.g., acute or overuse syndrome.

Noninvasive Therapy

The post–trigger point injection follow-up program described in Chapter 11 is recommended as a conservative therapeutic treatment approach. Noninvasive therapy can include:

- Physical therapy modalities (e.g., electrical stimulation and warm packs; see Chapter 19).
- Manual physical therapy techniques (e.g., massage, joint mobilization, and the Trager® Approach [neuromuscular re-education]; see Chapters 16–18 for additional manual techniques).
- Active and passive stretching and limbering of muscles with or without the use of vaporized coolant spray or ice. Active exercise is part of the stretch-and-spray technique. Limbering and relaxation are necessary prior to stretching. Contract-relax techniques may be used.
- Stretch and spray for the brachialis muscle using vaporized coolant or ice is performed in the direction of elbow extension. Electrical stimulation, limbering of muscles, and warm packs should precede stretch and spray to relax muscles.
- Exercises and a home program for the shoulder and elbow are prescribed (see Chapter 15). Exercise programs include relaxation, limbering, stretching, and strengthening. When the patient is free of pain and full motion has been achieved, progress to strength and endurance programs.

Injection of Trigger Point

Injection is performed with the patient supine. The TrP is injected under sterile technique (see Fig. 12–50). Greater exposure of the brachialis is obtained by moving the biceps medially (see Chapter 11 for injection technique).

Needle size: 1.5, 2.0 in., 21 gauge.
Solution: Any one of the following solutions may be used: 0.5% procaine; 1.0% lidocaine; saline and dry needling in case of allergy. Do not use epinephrine.

Precautions

Avoid the radial nerve, which is superficial in the area of the brachialis as it passes to the front of the lateral epicondyle between the brachialis medially and the brachioradialis laterally (see Fig. 12–50).

Postinjection Follow-up Physical Therapy Program

The patient should receive 3 to 4 consecutive days of treatment. Physical therapy should include electrical stimulation, relaxation, limbering, and stretching of the involved muscle using vaporized coolant spray or ice as needed combined with and followed by an exercise program. Active and active-assisted exercises are an integral part of the physical therapy program (see Chapter 11 for details).

Exercise and Home Program

Exercises for the elbow are prescribed. Exercises should at first be performed under the guidance of a therapist. When the patient is free of pain and full motion has been achieved, progress to strength and endurance programs. Begin and end exercise sessions with stretching and relaxation. (See Chapter 15 for exercise details.)

Corrective and Preventive Measures

- Do not maintain the elbow in flexion for prolonged periods. Learn to change position and relax the extremity.
- Instruct the patient in relaxation and stretching exercises.
- All neighboring muscles should be examined for TrPs.

Supinator

Symptoms and Pain Pattern

- Pain over the outer aspect of the elbow, upper forearm, and lateral epicondyle[1, 17, 33] (Fig. 12–51).
- Radiation of pain to the dorsal web space of the thumb.[38]
- Pain resulting from TrPs is noted with flexion and extension of the fingers, handshaking, and is classically associated with tennis elbow related to poor tennis technique, and overuse syndromes related to work and athletic activities.
- Muscle weakness may result from entrapment of the deep radial nerve due to TrPs.[19, 51]

Findings on Examination

- Tenderness over the lateral epicondyle, typical of tennis elbow.
- Tenderness over the lateral upper forearm involving the extensor muscles.
- Limitation in full elbow extension.
- Pain with wrist extension and supination.

Differential Diagnosis

- Tendinitis involving the extensor forearm muscles.
- Lateral epicondylitis.
- Muscle strain of supinator and extensor muscles of the forearm.

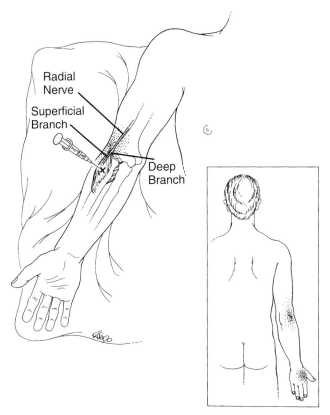

Figure 12–51. Supinator. Injection of trigger point (X) in the right supinator. The forearm is supinated with slight elbow flexion to relax the forearm muscles. Anatomic landmarks, including the deep branch of the radial nerve, are noted. Pain pattern is shown by *stippling*.

Anatomy

Origin: deep fibers from the supinator crest just below the radial notch of the ulna; oblique fibers more superficial from the back of the lateral epicondyle, lateral ligament of elbow, and annular ligament.

Insertion: neck and shaft of the radius.

Action: supination of the radius.

Nerve supply: radial (deep branch) (C6).

Noninvasive Therapy

The post–trigger point injection follow-up program described in Chapter 11 is recommended as a conservative therapeutic treatment approach. Noninvasive therapy can include:

- Physical therapy modalities (e.g., electrical stimulation and warm packs; see Chapter 19).
- Manual physical therapy techniques (e.g., massage, joint mobilization, and the Trager® Approach [neuromuscular re-education]; see Chapters 16–18 for additional manual techniques).
- Active and passive stretching and limbering of muscles with or without the use of vaporized coolant spray or ice. Active exercise is part of the stretch-and-spray technique. Limbering and relaxation are necessary prior to stretching. Contract-relax techniques may be used.
- Stretch and spray for the supinator muscle: Bring the wrist into pronation with elbow extension. Use vaporized coolant as needed. Electrical stimulation, limbering of muscles, and warm packs may precede stretch and spray to relax the muscles. Stretching of muscle is also accomplished actively as well as with assistance during the exercise program. Active exercise is part of the stretch-and-spray technique.
- Exercise and home program. Exercises for the shoulder, elbow, and wrist are described in Chapter 15. Exercise programs include relaxation, limbering, stretching, and strengthening. When the patient is free of pain and full motion has been achieved, progress to strength and endurance programs.

Injection of Trigger Point

Injection is performed with the patient supine. The forearm is supinated with slight elbow flexion to relax the forearm muscles. Identify the TrP. Inject medial to the brachioradialis (see Fig. 12–51). (See Chapter 11 for injection technique.)

Needle size: 1.5 in., 21 gauge.

Solution: Any one of the following solutions may be used: 0.5% procaine; 1.0% lidocaine; saline and dry needling in case of allergy. Do not use epinephrine.

Precautions

- Avoid the radial nerve when injecting the TrP (see Fig. 12–51).

Postinjection Follow-up Physical Therapy Program

The patient should receive 3 to 4 consecutive days of treatment. Physical therapy should include electrical stimulation, relaxation, limbering, and stretching of the involved muscle using vaporized coolant spray or ice as needed combined with and followed by an exercise program. Active and active-assisted exercises are an integral part of the physical therapy program (see Chapter 11 for details).

Exercise and Home Program

Increase flexibility, range of motion, and strengthening. After full range is obtained, strengthen the forearm muscles by means of isotonic exercise beginning with light weights (1 or 2 lb) and progressing gradually without overstressing the muscle. Dorsiflexion, volarflexion, pronation, and supination of the wrist are performed with the elbow stabilized in flexion.

The patient is placed on a home exercise program. Exercises should at first be performed under the guidance of a therapist. When the patient is free of pain and full motion has been achieved, progress to strength and endurance programs. Begin and end exercise sessions with stretching and relaxation (see Chapter 15 for exercise details).

Corrective and Preventive Measures

- Avoid overuse syndromes, whether athletic or occupational.
- Correct tennis technique. This will usually concern one's backhand and serve. Proper athletic equipment is essential. The patient may require a lighter, more flexible racquet with a proper grip. Tennis handle grips that are too small contribute to the development of tennis elbow. Physical therapy or surgery will not solve the tennis elbow problem if technique and athletic equipment are not corrected.
- Perform warm-up relaxation and stretching exercises (shoulder, elbow, wrist) prior to playing, and stretching and relaxation after exercise.

Palmaris Longus and Pronator Teres

Palmaris Longus

Symptoms and Pain Pattern

- Pain is produced by gripping any firm object in the palm.
- Referred pain pattern includes characteristic prickling and needling pain over the palm referred from a TrP in the upper midforearm in the palmaris longus[51] (Fig. 12–52).
- Local tenderness resulting from TrPs in the palm.

Findings on Examination

- Tenderness in the palm.
- Tender TrPs in the midportion of the palmaris longus and the palm.
- Contracture of the palmar fascia.[51]

Anatomy

Origin: common flexor origin.
Insertion: proximal end of palmar aponeurosis.
Action: flexes the wrist.
Nerve supply: median (C7, 8).

The palmaris longus may be absent in 10% of patients.

Differential Diagnosis

- Strain of forearm muscles.
- Palmar fibrosis.

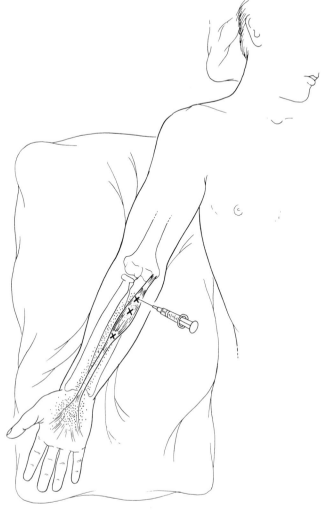

Figure 12–52. Palmaris longus. Injection of trigger points *(X's)* in the right palmaris longus. The patient is supine with the forearm supinated. Trigger point pain pattern is shown by *stippling*.

Pronator Teres

Symptoms and Pain Pattern
- Pain in the upper forearm at rest and with forearm motion.
- Pain radiating to the forearm and wrist.

Findings on Examination
- Tenderness in upper forearm.
- Pain with restriction in supination.

Differential Diagnosis
- Strain in forearm muscles

Anatomy
Origin: common flexor origin, front of medial epicondyle of the humerus, medial aspect of the coronoid process of the ulna.

Insertion: middle aspect of radius.
Action: flexion and pronation of the forearm.
Nerve supply: median (C6, 7).

Noninvasive Therapy

The post–trigger point injection follow-up program described in Chapter 11 is recommended as a conservative therapeutic treatment approach. Noninvasive therapy can include:

- Physical therapy modalities (e.g., electrical stimulation and warm packs; see Chapter 19).
- Manual physical therapy techniques (e.g., massage, joint mobilization, and the Trager® Approach [neuromuscular re-education]; see Chapters 16–18 for additional manual techniques).
- Active and passive stretching and limbering of muscles with or without the use of vaporized coolant spray or ice. Active exercise is part of the stretch-and-spray technique. Limbering and relaxation are necessary prior to stretching. Contract-relax techniques may be used.
- Stretch-and-spray techniques using vaporized coolant spray or ice: Stretching of the palmaris longus is performed by extending the wrist and fingers with the elbow extended. Stretch for pronator TrPs is performed by supination with the elbow extended. Electrical stimulation, limbering of muscles, and warm packs may precede stretch and spray to relax the muscles. Stretching of muscle is also accomplished actively as well as with assistance during the exercise program. Active exercise is part of the stretch-and-spray technique.
- Exercises and a home program for the elbow, wrist, and fingers are prescribed (see Chapter 15). Exercise programs include relaxation, limbering, stretching, and strengthening. When the patient is free of pain and full motion has been achieved, progress to strength and endurance programs.

Injection of Trigger Point

With the patient positioned comfortably in the supine position, the arm is supinated. The TrP in the palmaris longus is identified (see Fig. 12–52). Multiple needling should be performed over the muscle area to identify TrPs not diagnosed by palpation.

Needle size: 1.5 in., 21 gauge.
Solution: Any one of the following solutions may be used: 0.5% procaine; 1.0% lidocaine; saline and dry needling in case of allergy. Do not use epinephrine.

Postinjection Follow-up Physical Therapy Program

The patient should receive 3 to 4 consecutive days of treatment. Physical therapy should include electrical stimulation, relaxation, limbering, and stretching of the involved muscle using vaporized coolant spray or ice as needed combined with and followed by an exercise program. Active and active-assisted exercises are an integral part of the physical therapy program (see Chapter 11 for details).

Exercise and Home Program

Exercises for the elbow, wrist, and fingers are described in Chapter 15. Exercises should at first be performed under the guidance of a therapist. When the patient is free of pain and full motion has been achieved, progress to strength and endurance programs. Begin and end exercise sessions with relaxation and stretching.

Corrective and Preventive Measures
- Instruct patient in home exercise program and stretching.
- Avoid grasping firm objects in the palm for prolonged periods, e.g., a screwdriver, hedge clippers.
- Edges of casts applied for fractures should be well padded to avoid pressure areas in the palm and forearm. Casts should be trimmed to allow full range of motion of the fingers and thumb.
- Avoid prolonged repetitive pronation, occupational or athletic (excessive topspin stroke in tennis).

Wrist, Hand, and Finger Flexors

Flexor Carpi Ulnaris, Flexor Carpi Radialis, Flexor Digitorum Superficialis, Flexor Digitorum Profundus, Flexor Pollicis Longus

Symptoms and Pain Pattern
- Wrist flexors refer pain to the lower aspect of the wrist.[7]
- Trigger points in the wrist and finger flexors may refer pain to the medial aspect of the elbow ("medial tennis elbow"). Muscle weakness in the forearm and hand together with symptoms of numbness or paresthesia in the hand and fingers may be due to TrPs in muscles that originate in the flexor region of the medial epicondyle as well as from TrPs originating in extensor forearm muscles from the lateral epicondyle.
- Pain in the fingers and wrists may be due to myofascial TrPs in the flexor carpi radialis, flexor carpi ulnaris, flexor digitorum superficialis (Fig. 12–53), flexor digitorum profundus, flexor pollicis longus, and pronator teres. Finger flexors refer pain to their respective fingers; the flexor pollicis longus refers pain to the thumb.[51]
- Myofascial TrPs in the region of the medial epicondyle may be a cause of ulnar nerve entrapment, a mechanism similar to the radial nerve entrapment seen on the lateral aspect of the elbow.[19, 51]

Findings on Examination
- Local tenderness over the muscle belly with or without referred pain.
- Trigger points may be primary or secondary.
- Look for TrPs in neighboring muscles.
- Pain with active and passive motion of involved muscles.

Differential Diagnosis
- Forearm muscle strain.
- Carpal tunnel syndrome.
- Ulnar nerve entrapment.
- Cervical radiculopathy.

Anatomy
Flexor Carpi Radialis
Origin: medial epicondyle.
Insertion: base of second and third metacarpals.
Action: abductor and flexor of the wrist, wrist stabilizer.
Nerve supply: median (C6, 7).

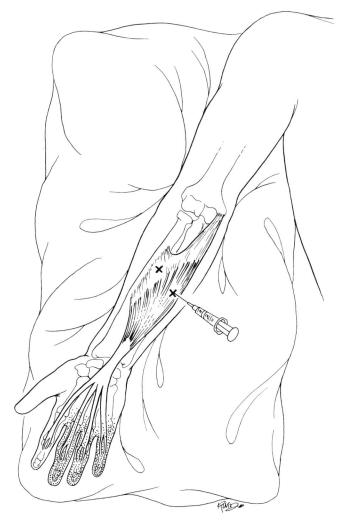

Figure 12–53. Injection of trigger points *(X's)* in the right flexor digitorum superficialis. The forearm is supinated and extended for easy access. Anatomic landmarks are noted. Pain pattern is shown by *stippling*.

Flexor Carpi Ulnaris

Origin: common flexor origin, upper two thirds of the border of the ulna.
Insertion: piriform bone, hook of hamate, fifth metacarpal.
Action: ulnar flexion and adduction of the wrist, wrist stabilizer.
Nerve supply: ulnar (C8, T1).

Flexor Digitorum Supeficialis

Origin: common flexor origin, coronoid process, anterior surface shaft of the radius.
Insertion: the sides of the middle phalanx of each finger.
Action: flexor of the middle phalanx and secondarily of the wrist.
Nerve supply: median (C7, 8, T1).

Flexor Digitorum Profundus

Origin: front and medial surface of shaft of the ulna and olecranon.
Insertion: terminal phalanges of the finger.
Action: flexor of terminal phalanx, secondarily flexion of other joints and fingers and wrist.
Nerve supply: ulnar (C8, T1) and median (palmar interosseus branch C8, T1).

Flexor Pollicis Longus

Origin: anterior aspect of shaft of the radius.
Insertion: front of base of the terminal phalanx of the thumb.
Action: flexion of the thumb.
Nerve supply: median (palmar interosseus branch C8, T1).

Noninvasive Therapy

The post–trigger point injection follow-up program described in Chapter 11 is recommended as a conservative therapeutic treatment approach. Noninvasive therapy can include:

- Physical therapy modalities (e.g., electrical stimulation and warm packs; see Chapter 19).
- Manual physical therapy techniques (e.g., massage, joint mobilization, and the Trager Approach [neuromuscular re-education]; see Chapters 16–18 for additional manual techniques).
- Active and passive stretching and limbering of muscles with or without the use of vaporized coolant spray or ice. Active exercise is part of the stretch-and-spray technique. Limbering and relaxation are necessary prior to stretching. Contract-relax techniques may be used.
- Stretch and spray for the finger flexors is performed by extending the fingers and wrist with the help of vaporized coolant spray or ice. Passive stretching as well as active motion should be performed. Electrical stimulation, limbering of muscles, and warm packs should precede stretch and spray to relax the muscles. Stretching of muscle is also accomplished actively as well as with assistance during the exercise program. Active exercise is part of the stretch-and-spray technique (see Chapter 11).
- Exercises and a home program for the wrist and finger flexors are described in Chapter 15. The exercise program includes relaxation, limbering, stretching, and strengthening.

Injection of Trigger Point

Identify TrPs in the forearm. Trigger points are injected with the patient supine, and the forearm supinated. The position may be changed according to the muscle to be injected. Figure 12–53 demonstrates TrPs in the flexor digitorum superficialis. (See Chapter 11 for injection technique.)

Needle size: 1.5 in., 22 gauge.
Solution: Any one of the following solutions may be used: 0.5% procaine; 1.0% lidocaine; saline and dry needling in case of allergy. Do not use epinephrine.

Postinjection Follow-up Program

The patient should receive 3 to 4 consecutive days of physical therapy. Therapy should include electrical stimulation, relaxation, limbering, and stretching of the involved muscle using vaporized coolant spray or ice as needed combined with and followed by an exercise program.

Exercise and Home Program

Exercises for wrist and fingers are described in Chapter 15. Exercises should at first be performed under the guidance of a therapist. Begin and end exercise sessions with stretching and relaxation.

Corrective and Preventive Measures

- Avoid overuse syndrome related to excessive flexion of the fingers, e.g., using scissors, gardening shears, excessive writing.
- Avoid repetitive occupational tasks requiring wrist flexion.

Triceps

Symptoms and Referred Pain Pattern

- Pain due to TrPs may be present over the posterior aspect of the upper arm and forearm in addition to pain over the shoulder, scapula, and trapezius area (Fig. 12–54).
- Pain over the medial and lateral aspect of the elbow with radiation to the fourth and fifth fingers.[37]

Findings on Examination

- Tenderness on palpation of the medial, long, or lateral head of the triceps.
- Lack of full extension of the elbow, shoulder, or both.
- Lack of full extension of the elbow is noted in patients with a long history of tennis elbow. All neighboring muscles surrounding the elbow contribute to the condition of tennis elbow, e.g., TrPs in the anconeus muscle, which arises from the posterior surface of the lateral epicondyle of the humerus, may contribute to lateral tennis elbow.

Differential Diagnosis

- Cervical radiculopathy.
- Medial or lateral epicondylitis.
- Thoracic outlet syndrome.

Anatomy

Origin: the long head from the infraglenoid tubercle of the scapula; the medial head from the posterior surface of the humerus below the spiral groove from the medial

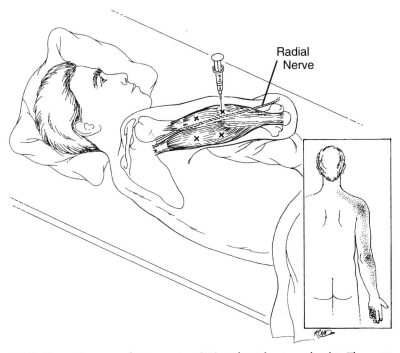

Figure 12–54. Triceps. Injection of trigger points *(X's)* in the right triceps brachii. The position of the patient is determined by the position of the trigger point to be injected. Pain pattern is noted by *stippling.* The radial nerve may be encountered with deep probing of the needle.

and lateral intermuscular septa; the lateral head from the ridge on back of the humerus above the musculospiral groove.

Insertion: by means of a conjoint tendon into the olecranon process of the ulna.

Action: extension of the elbow; the long head stabilizes the shoulder joint in abduction.

Nerve supply: radial (C7, 8).

Noninvasive Therapy

The post–trigger point injection follow-up program described in Chapter 11 is recommended as a conservative therapeutic treatment approach. Noninvasive therapy can include:

- Physical therapy modalities (e.g., electrical stimulation and warm packs; see Chapter 19).
- Manual physical therapy techniques (e.g., massage, joint mobilization, and the Trager® Approach [neuromuscular re-education]; see Chapters 16–18 for additional manual techniques).
- Active and passive stretching and limbering of muscles with or without the use of vaporized coolant spray or ice. Active exercise is part of the stretch-and-spray technique. Limbering and relaxation are necessary prior to stretching. Contract-relax techniques may be used.
- Stretch-and-spray techniques using vaporized coolant spray or ice in the direction of flexion of the elbow and extension of the shoulder. Spray is used in the TrP and referred pain areas. Electrical stimulation, limbering of muscles, and warm packs may precede stretch and spray to relax the muscles. Stretching of muscle is also accomplished actively as well as with assistance during the exercise program. Active exercise is part of the stretch-and-spray technique.
- Exercises and a home program for the elbow and shoulder are prescribed (see Chapter 15). Exercise programs include relaxation, limbering, stretching, and strengthening. When the patient is free of pain and full motion has been achieved, progress to strength and endurance programs.

Injection of Trigger Point

The position of the patient on the table is determined by the site of the TrP to be injected. Trigger points may involve the lateral head, medial head, or long head. They may be positioned for easy access to the individual TrP areas. This could require internally rotating or externally rotating the arm. Injection is not limited to the area of tenderness. Multiple insertions along the muscle belly of the triceps are necessary to localize TrPs that may be missed on palpation (see Fig. 12–54). (See Chapter 11 for injection technique.)

Needle size: 1.5, 2.0 in., 21 gauge

Solution: Any one of the following solutions may be used: 0.5% procaine; 1.0% lidocaine; saline or dry needling in case of allergy. Do not use epinephrine.

Precautions

- The radial nerve, which is found between the long head and the medial head of the triceps passing deep to the lateral head of the triceps and descending in the spiral groove behind the humerus, may be encountered with deep probing of the needle.

Postinjection Follow-up Physical Therapy Program

The patient should receive 3 to 4 consecutive days of treatment. Physical therapy should include electrical stimulation, relaxation, limbering, and stretching of the involved muscle using vaporized coolant spray or ice as needed combined with and followed by an exercise program. Active and active-assisted exercises are an integral part of the physical therapy program. (See Chapter 11 for program details.)

Exercise and Home Program

Exercises should at first be performed under the guidance of a therapist. When the patient is free of pain and full motion has been achieved, progress to strength and endurance programs. Begin and end exercise sessions with relaxation and stretching. (See Chapter 15 for exercise details.)

Corrective and Preventive Measures

- Avoid overuse syndromes, e.g., overzealous athletic activity for which the patient is not prepared.
- Encourage the patient to continue the exercise program.
- Relaxation and stretching exercises prior to and after athletic and strenuous work activities.

Extensor Muscles of the Wrist and Brachioradialis

Extensor Carpi Ulnaris, Extensor Carpi Radialis Longus, Extensor Carpi Radialis Brevis, Brachioradialis

Symptoms and Pain Pattern

- Pain in the upper forearm and lateral epicondyle. Trigger points in this area are frequently overlooked as a cause of tennis elbow symptoms[22] (Fig. 12–55).
- Trigger points in the extensor carpi radialis may refer pain to the lateral epicondyle and dorsum of the hand.[50] This muscle, together with the brachioradialis and supinator (see above), contributes to the pain experienced over the lateral epicondyle area diagnosed frequently in patients as tennis elbow. Omitting TrP management and directing treatment only to the area of the lateral epicondyle often results in poor therapeutic results.
- Pain may be experienced over the dorsum of the forearm, hand, and wrist.[9, 10, 17]
- Inhibition of grip strength due to pain (e.g., difficulty with grasp and handshaking).
- Pain is referred to the ulnar aspect of the wrist by the extensor carpi ulnaris, to the radial side by muscles on the radial side of the forearm. The brachioradialis refers pain to the wrist and base of the thumb and web space.[10, 50, 51]
- Trigger points may cause a tightening of the fibrous edge of the extensor carpi radialis brevis and supinator. When the extensor origin tightens it can compress both the deep radial nerve and its recurrent epicondylar branch. The mechanism of this nerve entrapment caused by supination, dorsiflexion, or radial deviation against resistance has been recognized as a possible cause of tennis elbow pain.[19]

Findings on Examination

- Local tenderness and referred pain on TrP palpation of the forearm muscles.
- When TrPs are in neighboring fingers the patient may experience pain with extension and flexion of the fingers (e.g., handshaking, repeated gripping).
- Pain with active wrist extension and when maintaining extension against resistance.
- Pain with supination, dorsiflexion.

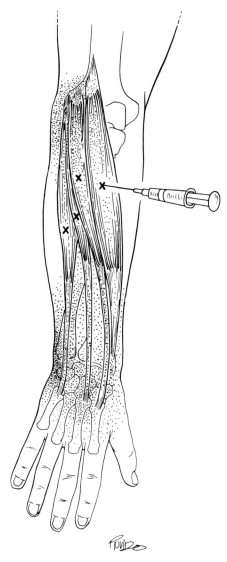

Figure 12–55. Extensor muscles of the wrist and the brachioradialis. Injection of a trigger point *(needle X)* in the brachioradialis. Trigger points in the extensor carpi radialis longus and brevis and extensor carpi ulnaris *(X's)* are shown also. The forearm is pronated. Anatomic landmarks are noted. Trigger point pain pattern is shown by *stippling*.

- Local tenderness over the lateral epicondyle area as well as the extensor forearm muscles.

Differential Diagnosis

- Tenosynovitis of extensor forearm muscles.
- de Quervain's disease.
- Arthritis of the wrist.
- Arthritis of the carpometacarpal joint of the thumb.
- Strain of extensor forearm muscles.
- Lateral epicondylitis.

Anatomy

Extensor Carpi Radialis Longus

Origin: lower one third of the lateral supracondylar ridge.
Insertion: back of the second metacarpal bone.

Action: extensor of the wrist and fixator of the wrist joint.
Nerve supply: radial (C6, 7).

Extensor Carpi Radialis Brevis

Origin: common extensor origin
Insertion: styloid process of base of the third metacarpal.
Action: extensor of the wrist and fixator of the wrist.
Nerve supply: radial (C6, 7).

Extensor Carpi Ulnaris

Origin: common extensor origin, and aponeurosis attached to the subcutaneous border of the ulna.
Insertion: dorsal aspect of the base of the fifth metacarpal.
Action: extension and adduction of the hand; fixator of the wrist.
Nerve supply: deep radial (C6, 7, 8).

Brachioradialis

Origin: upper two thirds of the lateral supracondylar ridge of the humerus.
Insertion: outer side of the base of the radial styloid process.
Action: flexion of the elbow when the forearm is midway between supination and pronation.
Nerve supply: radial (C5, 6).

Noninvasive Therapy

The post–trigger point injection follow-up program described in Chapter 11 is recommended as a conservative therapeutic treatment approach. Noninvasive therapy can include:

- Physical therapy modalities (e.g., electrical stimulation and warm packs; see Chapter 19).
- Manual physical therapy techniques (e.g., massage, joint mobilization, and the Trager® Approach [neuromuscular re-education]; see Chapters 16–18 for additional manual techniques).
- Active and passive stretching and limbering of muscles with or without the use of vaporized coolant spray or ice. Active exercise is part of the stretch-and-spray technique. Limbering and relaxation are necessary prior to stretching. Contract-relax techniques may be used.
- Stretch and spray is accomplished by flexing the wrists, thereby stretching the extensors. Muscles that cross the elbow joint (extensor carpi radialis longus, brachioradialis) require the elbow to be extended when the wrist is flexed. Stretching of the extensor carpi ulnaris may be accomplished with the elbow in flexion. Brachioradialis stretch includes extension of the elbow and pronation. Electrical stimulation, limbering of muscles, and warm packs should precede stretch and spray to relax muscles.
- Exercises and home program: The patient is instructed in exercises for the upper extremities and stretching exercises for the elbow and wrist, as described in Chapter 15. Exercise programs include relaxation, limbering, stretching, and strengthening. When the patient is free of pain and full motion has been achieved, progress to strength and endurance programs.

Injection of Trigger Point

With the patient in the supine position, TrPs are isolated between two fingers or the index finger and thumb. Injection is given directly into the TrP. The entire muscle and neighboring muscles are palpated for possible TrPs. (See Chapter 11 for injection technique.)

Needle size: 1.5, 2.0 in., 21 gauge.

Solution: Any one of the following solutions may be used: 0.5% procaine; 1.0% lidocaine; saline and dry needling in case of allergy. Do not use epinephrine.

Postinjection Follow-up Physical Therapy Program

The patient should receive 3 to 4 consecutive days of treatment. Physical therapy should include electrical stimulation, relaxation, limbering, and stretching of the involved muscle using vaporized coolant spray or ice as needed combined with and followed by an exercise program. Active and active-assisted exercises are an integral part of the physical therapy program. (See Chapter 11 for program details.)

Exercise and Home Program

Exercises should at first be performed under the guidance of a therapist. When the patient is free of pain and full motion has been achieved, progress to strength and endurance programs. Begin and end exercise sessions with stretching and relaxation. (See Chapter 15 for exercise details.)

Corrective and Preventive Measures

- Prescribe a wrist splint to prevent excessive flexion if the patient is symptomatic.
- The patient should avoid activities that promote inflammation and pain (e.g., excessive handshaking).
- Correct faulty tennis stroke technique and inappropriate tennis equipment. The patient should use a proper grip and a lightweight racquet. A stiff racquet should be avoided. The use of a tennis elbow band may relieve symptoms not only during the athletic activity of tennis but also during certain occupational activities that require stress on the extensor forearm muscles.
- Avoid overuse syndromes (prolonged unaccustomed activity in occupational and athletic activities).

Extensor Muscles of the Fingers and Thumb

Extensor Digitorum Communis, Extensor Indicis, Extensor Digiti Minimi, Extensor Pollicis Longus, Extensor Pollicis Brevis, Abductor Pollicis Longus

Symptoms and Pain Pattern

- Local pain limited to the forearm (Fig. 12–56).
- Pain at rest as well as with activity, e.g., handshaking, playing a musical instrument, typing.
- Complaint of grip weakness is usually a result of pain.
- Referred pain to the dorsum of the hand and less frequently to the fingers of individual tendons.[17, 51]
- Pain in the thenar area of the palm and base of the thumb referred from the abductor pollicis longus.[15, 16]

Findings on Examination

- Local or referred pain on palpation of TrPs.
- Limitation in flexion of proximal interphalangeal (PIP) joints due to shortening of the extensors. Pain and limitation are elicited with flexion of the PIP joints while

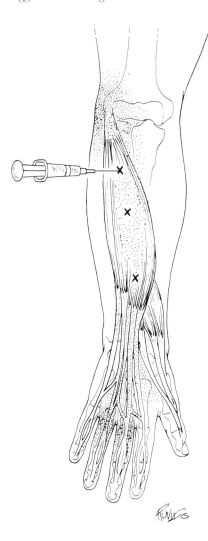

Figure 12–56. Extensor muscles of the fingers and thumb. Injection of trigger points *(X's)* in the extensor digitorum communis. The patient is supine. Neighboring muscles are noted that may also harbor trigger points. Pain pattern is shown by *stippling*.

making a fist as well as with flexion of PIP joints with the metacarpophalangeal joints maintained in extension.
- Weakness of grip.
- Trigger points are most easily detected in the extensor digitorum communis.

Differential Diagnosis

- Tennis elbow.
- Arthritis of wrist or fingers.
- Tenosynovitis of extensor tendons.

Anatomy

Extensor Digitorum Communis

Origin: lateral epicondyle of the humerus.
Insertion: middle base of the second and third phalanges of index, middle, ring, and fifth fingers.
Action: extension of the fingers and wrist.
Nerve supply: deep radial (C6, 7, 8).

Extensor Indicis

Origin: dorsal shaft of the ulna.
Insertion: joins the dorsal extension on the index finger, extends and adducts the index finger.
Nerve supply: deep radial (C6, 7, 8).

Extensor Digiti Minimi

Origin: common extensor tendon.
Insertion: extensor expansion of the little finger.
Action: extends the fifth finger.
Nerve supply: deep radial (C6, 7, 8).

Extensor Pollicis Longus

Origin: lateral side of dorsal surface of the ulna.
Insertion: dorsum of base of the distal phalanx of the thumb.
Action: extends the distal phalanx of the thumb.
Nerve supply: deep radial (C6, 7, 8).

Extensor Pollicis Brevis

Origin: dorsum of the radius and interosseus membrane.
Insertion: base of the proximal phalanx of the thumb.
Action: extends the proximal phalanx, may also act as an abductor of the wrist.
Nerve supply: deep radial (C6, 7).

Abductor Pollicis Longus

Origin: dorsum of the ulna, interosseus membrane of dorsum of the radius.
Insertion: lateral aspect of the base of the first metacarpal of the thumb.
Action: abducts thumb and hand.
Nerve supply: deep radial (C6, 7).

Noninvasive Therapy

The post–trigger point injection follow-up program described in Chapter 11 is recommended as a conservative therapeutic treatment approach. Noninvasive therapy can include:

- Physical therapy modalities (e.g., electrical stimulation and warm packs; see Chapter 19).
- Manual physical therapy techniques (e.g., massage, joint mobilization, and the Trager® Approach [neuromuscular re-education]; see Chapters 16–18 for additional manual techniques).
- Active and passive stretching and limbering of muscles with or without the use of vaporized coolant spray or ice. Active exercise is part of the stretch-and-spray technique. Limbering and relaxation are necessary prior to stretching. Contract-relax techniques may be used.
- Stretch and spray is accomplished by flexing the fingers and hand simultaneously. The elbow is held in extension. The elbow may be flexed when stretching the thumb muscles, stabilizing the wrist. Thumb muscles are stretched in the direction of flexion of the interphalangeal and metacarpophalangeal joints. The thumb is adducted in addition to adduction of the wrist to stretch the abductor pollicis longus. Electrical stimulation, limbering of muscles and warm packs should precede stretch and spray to relax muscles.
- Exercises and a home program for the elbow, wrist, and fingers are described in Chapter 15. The exercise program includes relaxation, limbering, stretching, and strengthening. When the patient is free of pain and full motion has been achieved, progress to strength and endurance programs.

- Prevention and correction of contributing factors.

Injection of Trigger Point

With the patient supine, TrPs are identified. Trigger points may be isolated between two fingers when possible. Injection is given directly into the TrP in addition to needling of the *immediate surrounding area* (see Chapter 11 for injection technique). Palpate the entire muscle and neighboring muscles for additional TrPs (see Fig. 12–56 for injection of TrPs in the extensor digitorum communis). Look for TrPs in neighboring muscles. Trigger points in the extensor forearm muscles are usually treated as a group when involving the finger extensors together with the extensor carpi radialis longus and brevis. This is often seen in symptoms related to tennis elbow.

Needle size: 1.5, 2.0 in., 21 gauge.
Solution: Any one of the following solutions may be used: 0.5% procaine; 1.0% lidocaine; saline and dry needling in case of allergy. Do not use epinephrine.

Precautions

- When injecting the extensor forearm muscles, avoid the superficial and deep branch of the radial nerve.

Postinjection Follow-up Physical Therapy Program

The patient should receive 3 to 4 consecutive days of treatment. Physical therapy should include electrical stimulation, relaxation, limbering, and stretching of the involved muscle using vaporized coolant spray or ice as needed combined with and followed by an exercise program. Active and active-assisted exercises are an integral part of the physical therapy program (see Chapter 11 for details).

Exercise and Home Program

Exercises should at first be performed under the guidance of a therapist. When the patient is free of pain and full motion has been achieved, progress to strength and endurance programs. Begin and end exercise sessions with stretching and relaxation (see Chapter 15 for exercise details.)

Corrective and Preventive Measures

- Avoid overuse syndromes (e.g., excessive writing, typing). Musicians may require limitation in practice sessions and correction in fingering technique as well as instrumental mechanical adjustments that can be made to decrease the demands on the wrist and fingers.
- Perform stretching and relaxation exercises for upper extremities, including hands and fingers.
- Both in occupational and athletic activities tools and athletic equipment should be of the appropriate size to avoid stress on the fingers and wrist, e.g., a hammer handle or tennis racquet that is too large or too small may cause tension in the forearm and hand muscles.

Adductor Pollicis and Opponens Pollicis

Symptoms and Pain Pattern

- Pain over the palmar aspect of the thumb (Fig. 12–57).
- Pain is aggravated with motions of the thumb.
- Pain over the volar aspect of the wrist.
- Shortening of the muscles together with pain may decrease dexterity.[50]

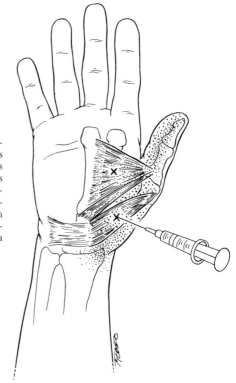

Figure 12–57. Adductor pollicis and opponens pollicis. Injection of trigger points in the adductor pollicis and adductor opponens pollicis (*X's*). The hand is supinated. The needle is inserted into the opponens pollicis trigger point. Trigger points may be approached from the palmar surface. The adductor muscle may be approached from the palm or dorsum between the first and second metacarpal bones. Anatomic landmarks are noted. Pain pattern is shown by *stippling*.

Findings on Examination

- Tenderness over the adductor pollicis noted on palpation of the web space.
- Tenderness over the thenar eminence (opponens pollicis).
- Trigger points may cause restriction of full motion due to pain and muscle shortening.

Differential Diagnosis

- Carpal tunnel syndrome.
- Osteoarthritis of the thumb (e.g., carpometacarpal joint).

Anatomy

Adductor Pollicis

Origin: the oblique head from the front of the base of the second and third metacarpals, capitate, and trapezoid; the transverse head from the distal two thirds of the front of the third metacarpal.

Insertion: both oblique and transverse heads join to insert into the medial aspect base of the proximal phalanx of the thumb.

Action: adduction of the thumb.

Nerve supply:
  a. Oblique head: ulnar (deep palmar branch C8, T1).
  b. Transverse head: ulnar (deep palmar branch C8, T1).

Opponens Pollicis

Origin: trapezium.

Insertion: lateral side of the length of the first metacarpal.

Action: brings the tip of the thumb to the tip of the fifth finger.
Nerve supply: median (C6, 7).

Noninvasive Therapy

The post–trigger point injection follow-up program described in Chapter 11 is recommended as a conservative therapeutic treatment approach. Noninvasive therapy can include:

- Physical therapy modalities (e.g., electrical stimulation and warm packs; see Chapter 19).
- Manual physical therapy techniques (e.g., massage, joint mobilization, and the Trager® Approach [neuromuscular re-education]; see Chapters 16–18 for additional manual techniques).
- Active and passive stretching and limbering of muscles with or without the use of vaporized coolant spray or ice. Active exercise is part of the stretch-and-spray technique. Limbering and relaxation are necessary prior to stretching. Contract-relax techniques may be used.
- Stretch and spray (see Chapter 11): Stretching is performed in the opposite direction of muscle shortening by stretching the web space. Abduction and extension of the thumb are performed passively and actively with the help of vaporized coolant spray or ice. Electrical stimulation, limbering of muscles, and warm packs may precede stretch and spray to relax the muscles. Stretching of muscle is also accomplished actively as well as with assistance during the exercise program. Active exercise is part of the stretch-and-spray technique. Contract-relax techniques may be used.
- Exercises and a home program for the adductor and opponens pollicis are prescribed (see Chapter 15). The exercise program includes relaxation, limbering, stretching, and strengthening. When the patient is free of pain and full motion has been achieved, progress to a strengthening program.

Injection of Trigger Points

Trigger points are identified. Injection is performed directly into the TrP area in the opponens pollicis (see Chapter 11 for technique). The adductor pollicis may be approached from the palm or dorsum of the hand in the web space between the first and second metacarpals (see Fig. 12–57).

Needle size: 1.5, 1.0 in., 22 or 25 gauge.
Solution: Any one of the following solutions may be used: 0.5% procaine; 1.0% lidocaine; saline and dry needling in the case of allergy. Do not use epinephrine.

Postinjection Follow-up Physical Therapy Program

The patient should receive 3 to 4 consecutive days of treatment. Physical therapy should include electrical stimulation, relaxation, limbering, and stretching of the involved muscle using vaporized coolant spray or ice as needed combined with and followed by an exercise program. (See Chapter 11 for details.)

Exercise and Home Program

Exercises should at first be performed under the guidance of a therapist. Begin and end exercise sessions with relaxation and stretching. (See Chapter 15 for exercise details.)

Corrective and Preventive Measures

- Prevent repetitive adduction, opposition, and pinch movements.
- Avoid specific occupational stress, which may occur with constant use of the thumb and fingers. Interrupt work routine for relaxation and stretching of muscles.

Interossei and Lumbrical Muscles

Dorsal Interossei, Volar Interossei, Lumbrical Muscles

Symptoms and Pain Pattern

- Pain in the palm with radiation to the fingers[22] (Fig. 12–58).
- Pain may occur on the dorsum or palmar aspect accompanied by stiffness.
- Pain may occur at rest as well as with finger motion.
- Heberden's nodes have been associated with interosseous TrPs.[51]

Findings on Examination

- Local tenderness on palpation of interossei.
- Local tenderness may cause referred pain to the fingers.
- Trigger points may cause hypoesthesia involving one side of the finger.

Differential Diagnosis

- Carpal tunnel syndrome.
- Digital neuroma.

Anatomy

Dorsal Interossei

Origin: each arises from the adjacent sides of two metacarpals.
Insertion: the first, into the radial side of the proximal phalanx of the second digit; the

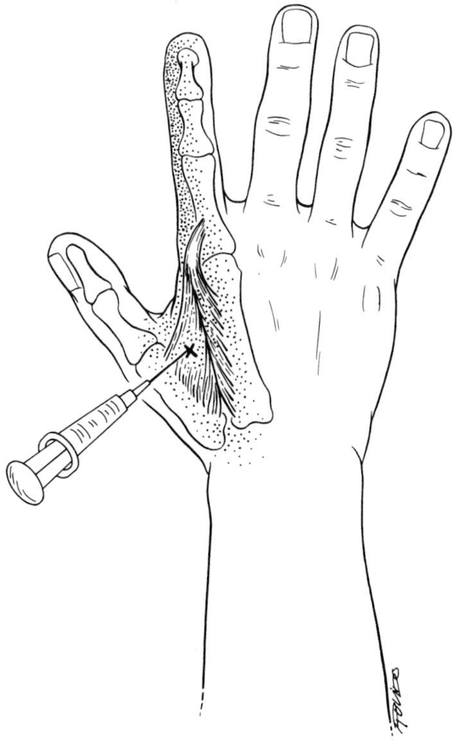

Figure 12–58. Interossei. Injection of trigger point (*X*) in the first interosseous muscle of the right hand. The injection approach for the first dorsal interosseous is from the dorsum of the hand. Trigger point pain pattern of the first dorsal interosseous is shown by *stippling.*

second, into the radial side of the proximal phalanx of the third digit (middle finger); the third, into the ulnar side of the proximal phalanx of the middle finger; the fourth, into the ulnar side of the proximal phalanx of the ring finger.

Action: abduction of the index, middle, and ring fingers from the midline.

Nerve supply: ulnar (deep palmar branch C8, T1).

Volar Interossei

Origin: the first, from the ulnar side of the second metacarpal; the second, from the radial side of the fourth metacarpal; the third, from the radial side of the fifth metacarpal.

Insertion: the first, into the ulnar side of the proximal phalanx of the second digit; the second, into the radial side of the proximal phalanx of the fourth digit; the third, into the radial side of the proximal phalanx of the fifth digit.

Action: each muscle adducts the fingers to the midline.

Nerve supply: ulnar (deep palmar branch C8, T1).

Lumbrical Muscles

Origin: the four lumbricals arise from tendons of the flexor digitor profundus, the first and second from the radial sides of the first and second tendons, and the third and fourth from the adjacent sides of the second, third, and fourth tendons.

Insertion: each inserts into the dorsal expansion on the middle phalanx together with tendons of the extensor digitorum and interossei into bases of terminal phalanges of the middle four fingers.

Action: flexes the metacarpophalangeal joint and extends the interphalangeal joint.

Nerve supply:
   a. First and second lumbricals: median (C6, 7).
   b. Third and fourth lumbricals: ulnar (deep palmar branch C8, T1).

Noninvasive Therapy

The post–trigger point injection follow-up program described in Chapter 11 is recommended as a conservative therapeutic treatment approach. Noninvasive therapy can include:

- Physical therapy modalities (e.g., electrical stimulation and warm packs; see Chapter 19).
- Manual physical therapy techniques (e.g., massage, joint mobilization, and the Trager® Approach [neuromuscular re-education]; see Chapters 16–18 for additional manual techniques).
- Active and passive stretching and limbering of muscles with or without the use of vaporized coolant spray or ice. Active exercise is part of the stretch-and-spray technique. Limbering and relaxation are necessary prior to stretching. Use contract-relax technique.
- Stretch and spray for the interossei and lumbricals is performed. Both abduction and adduction may be required depending on the muscles involved and the restrictions and symptoms noted. Perform extension of the metacarpal joints and flexion of the interphalangeal joints for the lumbricals. Use vaporized coolant spray or ice as necessary. Electrical stimulation, limbering of muscles, and warm packs may precede stretch and spray to relax the muscles. Stretching of muscle is also accomplished actively as well as with assistance during the exercise program. Active exercise is part of the stretch-and-spray technique. Contract-relax techniques may be used.
- Hand exercises should include range-of-motion exercises involving all the muscles of the hand. Add exercises for the wrist. Prescribe the use of clay or putty to strengthen the fingers. Exercise programs include relaxation, limbering, stretching, and strengthening.

Injection of Trigger Point

Identify the TrP by palpation. Inject directly into the TrP area (see Chapter 11 for technique). Needling of the lumbrical muscles is performed on the palmar side of the hand. Figure 12–58 demonstrates injection of the first dorsal interosseous TrP and pain pattern.

Needle size: 1.0, 1.5 in., 25 gauge.
Solution: Any one of the following solutions may be used: 0.5% procaine; 1.0% lidocaine; saline and dry needling in case of allergy. Do not use epinephrine.

Postinjection Follow-up Physical Therapy Program

The patient should receive 3 to 4 consecutive days of treatment. Physical therapy should include electrical stimulation, relaxation, limbering, and stretching of the involved muscle using vaporized coolant spray or ice as needed combined with and followed by an exercise program. Active and active-assisted exercises are an integral part of the physical therapy program.

Exercise and Home Program

Exercises for the hand and wrist are prescribed. Clay or putty is used to improve finger strength. Exercises should at first be performed under the guidance of a therapist. The exercise program includes relaxation, limbering, stretching, and strengthening. Begin and end exercise sessions with stretching and relaxation. (See Chapter 15 for exercise details.)

Corrective and Preventive Measures

- Avoid activities that require a prolonged pinching action of the fingers.
- Patients in occupations requiring repetitive use of the fingers must learn to relax the hand to avoid constant tension. Provide for periods of relaxation and stretching of muscles.

References

1. Barton PM, Grainger RW, Nicholson RL, et al: Toward a rational management of piriformis syndrome [abstract]. Arch Phys Med Rehabil 69:784, 1988.
2. Carlson CR, Okenson JP, Falace DA, et al: Reduction of pain and EMG activity in the masseter region by trapezius trigger point injection. Pain 55(3):397–340, 1993.
3. Daniels L, Worthingham C: Muscle Testing Techniques of Manual Examination, 4th ed. Philadelphia, WB Saunders, 1980.
4. DeJung B: Manual trigger point treatment in chronic lumbosacral pain. Schweiz Med Wochenschr Suppl 62:82–87, 1994.
5. Epstein SE, Gerber LH, Borer JS: Chest wall syndrome: A common cause of unexplained cardiac pain. JAMA 241:2793–2797, 1979.
6. Fricton JR, Auvinen MD, Dykstra D, et al: Myofascial pain syndrome: Electromyographic changes associated with local twitch response. Arch Phys Med Rehabil 66:314–317, 1985.
7. Good MG: Rheumatic myalgias. Practitioner 146:167–174, 1941.
8. Good MG: Diagnosis and treatment of sciatic pain. Lancet 21:597–598, 1942.
9. Good MG: What is "fibrositis"? Rheumatism 5:117–123, 1949.
10. Gutstein M: Diagnosis and treatment of muscular rheumatism. Br J Phys Med 1:302–321, 1938.
11. Hallin RP: Sciatic pain and the piriformis muscle. Postgrad Med 74:69–72, 1983.
12. Hinks AH: Further aid for piriformis muscle syndrome. J Am Osteopath Assoc 74:93, 1974.
13. Hoppenfeld S: Physical examination of the spine and extremities. New York, Appleton-Century-Crofts, 1976.
14. Imamura M, Fischer AA, Iamura ST, et al: Treatment of myofascial pain components in plantar fasciitis speeds up recovery. In Fischer AA (ed): Muscle pain syndrome and fibromyalgia. New York, Haworth Medical, 1998.
15. Kellgren JH: A preliminary account of referred pains arising from muscle. BMJ 2:325–327, 1938.
16. Kellgren JH: Observations on referred pain arising from muscle. Clin Sci 3:175–190, 1938.
17. Kelly M: The relief of facial pain by procaine (Novocain) injections. J Am Geriatr Soc 11:586–596, 1963.

18. Kendall FP, McCreary EK: Muscle testing and function, 3rd ed. Baltimore, Williams & Wilkins, 1983.
19. Kopell W, Thompson AL: Peripheral entrapment neuropathies. Baltimore, Williams & Wilkins, 1963.
20. Kraus H: Prevention of low back pain. J Am Podiatr Med Assoc 6:12–15, 1952.
21. Kraus H: "Pseudo-disc." South Med J 60:416–418, 1967.
22. Kraus H: Clinical Treatment of Back and Neck Pain. New York, McGraw-Hill, 1970.
23. Kraus H (ed): Diagnosis and Treatment of Muscle Pain. Chicago, Quintessence, 1988.
24. Lang M: Die Muskelhädarten (Myogelosen). Munich, JF Lehmann, 1931.
25. Ling FW, Slocumb JC: Use of trigger point injections in chronic pelvic pain. Obstet Gynecol Clin North Am 20(4):809–815, 1993.
26. Lutz EG: Credit card-wallet sciatica [letter to the editor]. JAMA 240:738, 1978.
27. Macdonald AJR: Abnormally tender muscle regions and associated painful movements. Pain 8:197–205, 1980.
28. Melnick J: Treatment of trigger point mechanisms in gastrointestinal disease. NY State J Med 54:1324–1330, 1954.
29. Melnick J: Trigger areas and refractory pain in duodenal ulcer. NY State J Med 57:1073–1076, 1957.
30. Pace JB: Commonly overlooked pain syndromes responsive to simple therapy. Postgrad Med 58:107–113, 1975.
31. Pace JB, Nagle D: Piriform syndrome. West J Med 124:435–439, 1976.
32. Puranen J, Orava S: The hamstring syndrome. A new diagnosis of gluteal sciatic pain. Am J Sports Med 16:517–521, 1988.
33. Rachlin ES: Musculofascial pain syndromes. Medical Times, January 1984:34–47.
34. Rachlin ES: Musculofascial pain syndromes. In Kraus H (ed): Diagnosis and Treatment of Muscle Pain. Chicago, Quintessence, 1988, p 8.
35. Reynolds MD: Myofascial trigger points in persistent posttraumatic shoulder pain. South Med J 77:1277–1280, 1984.
36. Simons DG, Travell TG, Simons LS: Myofascial pain and dysfunction. The Trigger Point Manual, vol 1, 2nd ed. Baltimore, Williams & Wilkins, 1999.
37. Simons DG: Myofascial pain syndrome. In Basmajian JV, Kirby RL (eds): Medical Rehabilitation. Baltimore, Williams & Wilkins, 1984.
38. Simons DG: Myofascial pain syndrome due to trigger points. In Goodgold J (ed): Rehabilitation Medicine. St Louis, Mosby–Year Book, 1988, pp 686–723.
39. Slocumb JC: Neurological factors in chronic pelvic pain: Trigger points and the abdominal pelvic pain syndrome. Am J Obstet Gynecol 149:536–543, 1984.
40. Sola AE: Treatment of myofascial pain syndromes. In Benedetti C, Chapman R, Moriocca G (eds): Advances in Pain Research and Therapy, vol 7. New York, Raven, 1984, pp 467–485.
41. Sola AE: Trigger point therapy. In Robers JR, Hooges JR (eds): Clinical Procedures in Emergency Medicine. Philadelphia, WB Saunders, 1985.
42. Sola AE, Kuitert JH: Quadratus lumborum myofasciitis. Northwest Med 53:1003–1005, 1954.
43. Sola AE, Kuitert JH: Myofascial trigger point pain in the neck and shoulder girdle. Northwest Med 54:980–984, 1955.
44. Sola AE, Rodenberger MS, Gettys BB: Incidence of hypersensitive areas in posterior shoulder muscles: A survey of two hundred young adults. Am J Phys Med 34:585–590, 1955.
45. Sola AE, Williams RL: Myofascial pain syndromes. Neurology 6:91–95, 1956.
46. Steiner C, Staubs C, Ganon M, et al: Piriformis syndrome: Pathogenesis, diagnosis, and treatment. J Am Osteopath Assoc 87:318–323, 1987.
47. Synek VM: The piriformis syndrome: Review and case presentation. Clin Exp Neurol 23:31–37, 1987.
48. TePoorten BA: The piriformis muscle. J Am Osteopath Assoc 69:150–160, 1969.
49. Tortora GJ, Grabowski SR: Principles of Anatomy and Physiology, 8th ed. New York, Harper Collins, 1996.
50. Travell J, Rinzler SH: The myofascial genesis of pain. Postgrad Med 11:425–434, 1952.
51. Travell JG, Simons DG: Myofascial Pain and Dysfunction: The Trigger Point Manual, vol 1. Baltimore, Williams & Wilkins, 1983.
52. Travell JG, Simons DG: Myofascial Pain and Dysfunction: The Trigger Point Manual, vol 2. The Lower Extremities. Baltimore, Williams & Wilkins, 1992.
53. Williams PL, Warwick R: Gray's Anatomy, 36th British ed. Philadelphia, WB Saunders, 1980.

Chapter 13

New Injection Techniques for Treatment of Musculoskeletal Pain

Andrew A. Fischer, MD, PhD

This chapter deals with new treatment techniques based on the concept that spinal segmental sensitization (SSS) is the pathophysiologic basis in the vast majority of musculoskeletal pain (MSP), particularly myofascial pain syndrome (MPS) and other trigger points (TrPs).[9, 10, 14, 16, 17] The clinical significance of SSS is that its presence allows us to understand many conditions that escaped explanation prior to the introduction of this concept.[45] SSS has also led to successful treatment of several conditions in which conventional therapies failed to produce improvement.[14, 17] Treatment of SSS as a component of radiculopathies, myofascial pain, injuries, overuse, and several other conditions substantially speeds up recovery induced by conventional therapy.[14, 17]

This chapter is an update on the new therapeutic procedures that have been described recently.[14, 17] Unpublished observations and more technical details are also provided. The essential conclusions of previous publications[14, 17] regarding treatment can be summarized as follows:

1. Two new trigger point injection techniques were described. They improve substantially the success rate of treatment: Pre-injection block (PIB) anesthetizes the sensitive, painful area, which is supposed to be injected. Needling and infiltration of taut band, particularly if performed after the PIB, provide long-term relief. Such results were documented with pressure algometry in double-blind follow-up studies extending to an average of up to 5 years and by a randomized controlled study.[14, 17, 27–32]

2. *The pain caused by radiculopathy was alleviated and functional limitations improved in 87% of treatments by paraspinous block.* This new injection technique blocks the nociceptive impulses from the sprained supraspinous and interspinous ligaments.[12, 14]

3. It was concluded that new injection techniques can relieve pain and signs caused by radicular compression. Paraspinous block (PSB) frequently produces such improvement instantaneously by relieving paraspinal muscle spasm, which causes the root compression.[6, 9, 10, 13–17] The new injection techniques improved success rates and produced long-term relief of pain caused by TrPs and tender spots.[12, 14, 17, 27–32]

Table 13–1 presents an algorithm for differential diagnosis and treatment of musculoskeletal pain that consists of four phases.[14, 17] Each phase is made up of three steps. In phase I the immediate cause of pain is identified, which is the prerequisite of effective treatment. Phase II involves diagnosis of the SSS corresponding to the tender spots (TSs) and/or TrPs that cause the symptoms. Phase III is the treatment, which consists of injections, physical therapy emphasizing relaxation exercises, and correction of postural deficiencies. Phase IV consists of removal of etiologic factors responsible for the TSs/TrPs. This simple step-by-step approach makes treatment of musculoskeletal pain more effective.[7, 9, 10, 12, 13, 14, 17]

Table 13–2 is a review of components that are part of our treatment regimen for musculoskeletal pain. The reader is referred to previous publications for more details.[6–15] A new exercise regimen, isometric contraction reciprocal inhibition and stretch, has also been described.[7, 9] Our experience indicates that the most effective

Table 13–1.
Algorithm for Management of Musculoskeletal Pain

Goals

Short-term Goals

To alleviate pain before patient leaves the office.
This is achieved by treating the immediate cause(s) of pain, which most frequently consist of tender spots (TSs), trigger points (TrPs), muscle spasm (MSp), or inflammation.

Long-term Goals

To remove perpetuating and etiologic factors responsible for the immediate cause(s) of pain, in order to prevent recurrence of the condition.

Phase I—Identify the immediate cause of pain: TrPs/TSs, MSp, inflammation

1. Ask patient to point with one finger to where the most intensive pain is.
2. Find the point of maximum tenderness of TrP/TSs. Quantify the tenderness (degree of sensitization) by algometer.
3. Reproduction (recognition) of pain. Press over the maximum tender point and ask: Is this the pain you are complaining about?

Phase II—Diagnose the spinal segmental sensitization (SSS) and specify the segment corresponding to the trigger point/tender spot. Dx of SSS:

1. Sensory—Diagnose the hyperalgesic dermatomes by:
   a. *Scratching* along the sensory diagnostic tracks
   b. *Electric skin conductance,* which objectively documents nerve fiber dysfunction
   c. *Pinch & roll (P&R):* tests sensitization of subcutaneous tissue. Can be quantified by Pressure Algometer.
2. Motor—Diagnose the affected myotome:
   a. *TrPs/TSs by palpation and algometry*
   b. *Taut bands by palpation and tissue compliance meter*
   c. *Muscle spasm by palpation and tissue compliance meter*
3. Sclerotome
   a. Enthesopathy
   b. Bursitis, tendinitis
   c. Epicondylitis

Phase III—Treatment: Concentrate on the sensitized spinal segment corresponding to the immediate cause of pain (TrPs/TSs, MSp, neurogenic inflammation), the associated supraspinous ligament sprain, and pentad.

1. Injections for immediate and long-term relief of pain
   a. Paraspinous block to desensitize the SSS.
   b. Pre-injection block to anesthetize the painful sensitive area to be infiltrated.
   c. Needling & infiltration of the taut band (TB), to break up the entire underlying pathology around the TrPs/TSs.
2. Physical therapy—to promote healing after injections, restore function, and prevent recurrence
   a. Modalities—heat or cold; electric stimulation (sinusoid surging and tetanizing currents)
   b. Exercises—*relaxation exercises* and stretching: general and *specific* for the involved myotome, in which the pain-generating TrPs/TSs and MSp are located; relaxation by activation of antagonist muscle(s)
3. Postural correction
   a. *Kraus-Weber* test to specifically diagnose dysfunction (weakness or loss of flexibility) in key postural muscles
   b. *Robin McKenzie: Flexion deficiency of the lumbosacral spine* is indicated by knees-chest—5-cm. *Extension deficiency* is considered if on push-up, pelvis floor distance is over 2.5 cm. On *lateral bending* shoulder should pass midline.
      Induce *corresponding correction* by specific postural exercises[7, 9, 35] (Robin McKenzie, Hans Kraus).

Phase IV—Diagnosis and Removal of Perpetuating and Etiologic Factors

1. *Mechanical:* Overuse, sport injuries, cumulative trauma disorder
2. *Postural deficiencies,* muscle deficiencies (loss of strength or flexibility)
3. *Lab results:* Endocrine, metabolic, electrolyte, vitamin disorders

Table 13–2.
Basic Treatment Components of Trigger Points, Tender Spots, and Segmental (Radicular)
Sensitization

	Specific Injection Techniques	
Procedure	*Conditions in Which Applicable*	*Purpose*
Needling and infiltration of tender area	Local pathology: Tender, inflamed areas, tender spots (TSs), trigger points (TrPs)	Disrupts edema or fibrotic tissue causing pain
Preinjection blocks	Prior to every needling and injection	Prevents pain and sensitization caused by needling and injection
Paraspinous block	Pentad of discopathy, radiculopathy and paraspinal spasm Spinal segmental sensitization	Desensitizes spinal segmental (radicular) sensitization by blocking the irritative focus in supraspinous/interspinous ligament
Diffuse infiltration of spasm	Muscle spasm	To relieve pain and muscle spasm
	Special Physical Therapy Procedures	
Hot packs	Musculoskeletal pain	
	1. Independently	Alleviate pain Promote healing following injection
	2. Postinjection physical therapy	Restore function
Electrical stimulation		Relaxes muscles Increases circulation Squeezes out edema after injection Promotes healing
	Individualized Exercise Regimen Based on Tests of Functional Deficit	
Exercises	1. Muscle spasms, TSs, TrPs, taut band	Relaxation by activation of antagonist relieves spasm and taut band Prevents recurrence
	2. Weakness	Strengthening
	3. Loss of flexibility	Relax and stretch
	4. Tension	Relaxation—general

relaxation of muscle tone, tension, or spasm is the activation of antagonist muscle with minimal intensity. The relaxation is instantaneous.[7, 9] Double-blind studies have proved the efficacy of relaxation exercises.[1, 4] Physical therapy consisting of heat, electrical stimulation, and active relaxation exercises is also a proven concept.[8, 9, 14, 17, 35] Three therapy sessions per week on the days following the injections are recommended. The electrical stimulation is particularly helpful in controlling edema and inflammation caused by needling.[14, 17, 26]

The Pentad of Discopathy-Radiculopathy-Paraspinal Spasm and Supraspinous/Interspinous Ligament Sprain—Treatment by Paraspinous Block

A pentad of signs has been described that is frequently the cause of musculoskeletal pain. *The pentad of discopathy-radiculopathy* consists of (1) narrowed disc space and neural foramen on imaging; this is manifested clinically by (2) narrowed space between spinous processes and (3) a sprained (tender) supraspinous ligament,[19] identifiable also by microedema.[16] (4) There is palpable paraspinal muscle spasm, which causes (5) radicular compression and dysfunction manifested by SSS. It has been established that the interspinous ligament sprain is the irritative focus that causes or maintains the SSS. This conclusion was reached because PSB, which cuts off sensory impulses from the interspinous ligament, reverses the SSS to normal status. Figure 13–1A shows a schematic of the pentad, and Figure 13–1B demonstrates the effect of paraspinous block. The pentad was identified as the cause of symptoms in 82% of patients with MSP.[17]

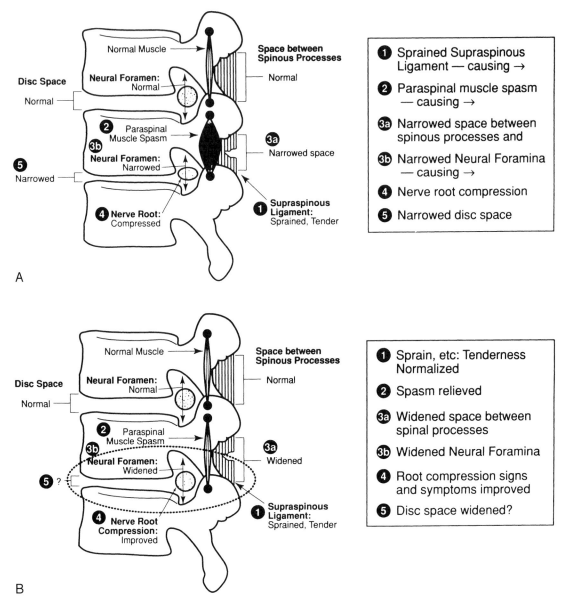

Figure 13–1. *A, The pentad* of discopathy, radiculopathy, paraspinal spinal spasm, and supraspinous ligament sprain. *B,* Changes after paraspinous block.

Paraspinous Block for Alleviation of Pain and Desensitization of Spinal Segment

Paraspinous block consists of spreading the local anesthetic (1% of lidocaine) along the spinous processes and their connection in the form of the supraspinous/interspinous ligaments. These blocks are effective in specifically desensitizing the sensitized segment.[12, 14, 17] The procedure is very simple to perform and no complications were encountered.

A 25-gauge needle, sufficiently long to reach the deep layers up to the vertebral lamina, is employed. At the cervical and thoracic level, a 1.5-in., 25-gauge needle is usually sufficient for PSB, except for very large persons, in whom a 2-in., 25- or 21-gauge needle may be necessary. Similarly, in the lumbosacral area, only in small persons is a 1.5-in. needle sufficient. In larger persons, paraspinous block is performed with a 2-in. needle. Such a needle is also suitable for needling and infiltration of the supraspinous and interspinous ligaments, paraspinal spasm, and bands of fibrotic core following PSB.

Penetration is in the sagittal and going somewhat proximal direction, starting exactly between the spinous processes of the involved segment. The depth of penetration is maximal and usually stops before the vertebral lamina is reached. After careful aspiration in order to avoid blood vessels, one slowly infiltrates a very small amount of anesthetic (less than 0.1 mL). Then the needle is withdrawn to a subcutaneous level and redirected in the proximal direction, ending about 3 mm from the previous deposit. The procedure is then repeated, going as far as the needle reaches. The same procedures are then performed in the distal direction. It is important to penetrate just next to the spinous processes and medially from the spinal muscle, which should be avoided. In case the needle encounters elastic resistance of the muscle, or the fibrotic resistance of a taut band, it is withdrawn to subcutaneous level and reinserted more medially. *The goal is to spread the anesthetic in the loose connecting tissue between the spinalis muscle and the spinous processes.* Here, the anesthetic spreads to the primary dorsal rami or the muscular branches as well as the supraspinous/interspinous ligaments.

Needling and Infiltration of the Sprained Supraspinous/Interspinous Ligaments Combined with Paraspinous Block

After the spreading of anesthetic proximally and distally has been accomplished, the needle is turned medially and the sprained parts of the supraspinous/interspinous ligaments that allow easy penetration are thoroughly needled and infiltrated with very small amounts of lidocaine (Fig. 13–2).[14, 17] If bilateral sensitization at the same levels is present, and the patient tolerates the procedure well, then paraspinous block can be performed on the opposite side prior to the needling and infiltration of the ligament. If needling and infiltration of supraspinous/interspinous ligaments is performed following unilateral paraspinous block, there is some pain, particularly on needling of the deep parts. After bilateral block, needling of the ligaments becomes pain-free.

The effect of paraspinous blocks in reversing the sensitization is very specific: the procedure desensitizes only the segment at which the interspinous ligament has been blocked.[17] Immediately after the block, within approximately 2 minutes, the SSS is reversed to normal. This is manifested by normalization of the hyperalgesic dermatome on scratch, electric skin conductance (ESC), and pinch and roll[16]; on the motor end the TSs/TrPs become less tender and the spasm within the corresponding myotome is relieved. If the patient tolerates the procedure well, follow-up physical therapy is available and the patient can rest after the procedure for 2 to 3 days, then two or three levels can be desensitized by paraspinous block in one session. In the case of severe pain, such as in herpes zoster, four to six levels have been desensitized with a physical therapy session and breaks between the procedures.

Because paraspinous block is very specific, with effects limited to the injected segment, it is crucial to treat the spinal level that is responsible for the patient's symptoms. For example, a patient had demonstrated segmental sensitization of L5–S1–S2. The most sensitive segment was L5, including the dermatome and myotome, with pain present in the lower back, the lateral thigh, and lateral leg. In this case, the choice for first PSB was the L5 level.

Territory of each dermatome is quite consistent, demonstrating very little individual variation in size and location.[16, 17] For example, the L4 dermatome usually includes the lateral thigh, medial leg, and medial malleolus. However, sometimes the TrP within the muscle that is usually supplied by L4 can be partially supplied by the adjacent L5 or L3 segments. Therefore, *it is important to trace back the hyperalgesic dermatomes and myotomes exactly to their origin over the spine.* This is achieved by scratching across the dermatomes from the periphery progressing proximally over the thigh, buttock,

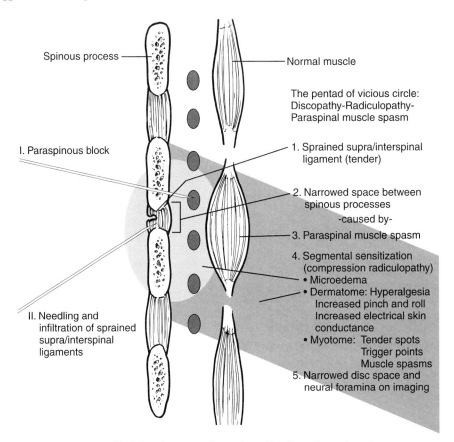

Figure 13–2. *Paraspinous block (PSB)* consists of spreading of local anesthetic along the spinous processes in the space between them and the adjacent spinalis muscle. The block is administered at the level of the spinal segmental sensitization, supraspinous/interspinous (SS/IS) ligament sprain, and microedema. The effect is the immediate relief of pain in the spinal segment and normalization of signs and symptoms of spinal segmental sensitization. Following the paraspinous block, the needle is turned medially and *needling and infiltration (N&I) of SS/IS ligament* is performed.

and paraspinal area. At the involved spinal level, microedema is consistently diagnosable and the pentad is usually also present. At the level where the distance between the spinous processes is narrowed, paraspinal spasm is also palpable. *PSB should be performed at the level where the pentad corresponds to the hyperalgesic dermatome and myotome that harbors the TSs/TrPs causing symptoms.* Following needling and infiltration of the supraspinous ligament, the paraspinal muscles next to the needle are palpated. If fibrotic bands are detected in the paraspinal muscles, they are needled and infiltrated from the same needle penetration by which the paraspinous block had been performed.

PSB is also effective in preventing or reducing pain when *sprained peripheral ligaments* are injected or needling and infiltration of them is performed. Needling and infiltration of the sprained ligaments of the sacroiliac joint is greatly facilitated, and pain is reduced by an S1–S2 PSB administered prior to the needling.

Special paraspinous block techniques are required at the S1 to S3 levels because no spinous processes are present. It has been observed that block at the S1 to S3 levels was effective in desensitization of involved segments similarly to the effect achieved at the L5 level. The probable explanation is that a rudimentary supraspinous/interspinous ligament is present over the sacrum, which can cause the reflex sensitization of the corresponding segments, similarly to the true supraspinous/interspinous ligaments located proximally to the L5 segment. Paraspinous block over the sacrum is performed at the sensitized level, laterally from the midline. The anesthetic is spread deeply to the sacrum. Following the block procedure, needling and infiltration are performed at the same level but over the midline, where the irritative focus that induces segmental sensitization is located. A 2-in., 21-gauge needle is most effective because considerable needling and destruction of the midline structure that corresponds to the interspinous ligaments produces the best results.

Mechanisms of Desensitization and Pain Relief by Paraspinous Block

The correct location of the level where the pentad and supraspinous/interspinous ligament sprain causes the spinal segmental sensitization, or contributes to it, is confirmed by the effect of paraspinous block. Within 1 or 2 minutes following a correctly performed and localized paraspinous block, the treated segment reverts from hypersensitive state to normal sensitivity. This important result is evidently *not* caused by the effect of the local anesthetic on the sensitized structures, which may be the roots or dorsal horn of the spinal segments. The procedure blocks the nociceptive impulses from the sprained interspinous ligament, which is the irritative focus causing the SSS.[14, 17] The mechanism consists of nociceptive impulses bombarding the involved spinal segment through the dorsal primary rami.[43] All peripheral sensitized nociceptors, such as supraspinous/interspinous (SS/IS) ligaments, facet joints, or capsules, internal disruption of discs, trigger points in muscles and other ligaments, sprained ligaments, or pericapsulitis can potentiate the sensitization of the central nervous system through the dorsal horn and thereby aggravate or maintain the SSS.[2, 38, 39, 43, 45]

If eradication of ligamentous and myofascial TrPs fails to eliminate SSS, other possible pain generators or nociceptive foci should be considered, i.e., articular (facet) or discogenic. On the other hand, even when there are imaging studies showing degenerative changes or other pathology in facet joints or discs, *treating the SSS by paraspinous block, needling and infiltration of SS/IS ligaments combined with PIB and needling and infiltration of TrPs can lead to substantial or complete pain relief of long-term duration.* The pain relief in this condition with documented pathology is also associated with elimination of clinical evidence of SSS. The lack of correlation between imaging of disc herniation[9, 17] and pain can be explained best by the concept of SSS and desensitization.[14, 17, 45] It is often possible to perform needling and infiltration of the sprained parts of the SS/IS ligaments from the needle penetration that was performed for paraspinous block. This additional procedure usually provides long-term relief and reduces the risk of recurrence. The possible mechanism involved is the destruction of the inflammation and possibly fibrotic pockets entrapping inflammatory substances along with nerve endings, thereby eradicating the irritative focus.

The effect of paraspinous block in desensitizing the sensitized spinal segment can be explained by Kellgren's studies.[34] He showed that injection of hypertonic saline into the interspinous ligaments induces specific segmental pain patterns. The pain originating from individual interspinous ligaments exactly matches the corresponding dermatomes described by Keegan later.[33] In view of hyperalgesia connected with SSS at all spinal levels, it is obvious that the pain pattern described by Kellgren[34] is a manifestation of SSS caused by irritation of the corresponding interspinous ligament.

Hackett using prolotherapy (sclerotherapy) has provided further evidence of the role of interspinous ligaments as an irritative focus causing segmental pain.[23] He described relief of segmental pain by anesthetic infiltration of the sprained SS/IS ligaments at the corresponding level.(See Chapter 7 in this book.)

Effects of Paraspinous Block

After the PSB, there is usually complete or very substantial relief of the pain located in the periphery within the desensitized spinal segment. Within a few minutes, local tenderness in TSs/TrPs improves (inactivation) very substantially and the increased muscle tone within the myotome (spasm) is also alleviated. The taut band associated with TSs/TrPs shrinks and becomes less tender. These changes make it easier to perform the preinjection block with the goal of anesthetizing the taut band and to follow with needling and infiltration.

The fact that immediately after PSB its effect on sensitization of the spinal segment can be established is of great value. If relief of the sensitization fails to occur, probably the injected SS/IS ligament was not the cause of symptoms and the correct level should be injected.

If multiple levels of SSS are present, the goal is to desensitize several segments. Needling and infiltration of the SS/IS ligaments are limited to one or two levels where the sensitization is most intensive. The number of levels treated during the procedure is limited by a patient's tolerance and by the sensitivity of the individual segments. Only one or a maximum of two hypersensitive segments are injected per session. However, if multiple-level sensitizations are present causing severe pain, several (four to five) levels can be injected in one session. Injection of several levels may cause excessive irritation and pain with exhaustion on the following days.

The percentage of pain alleviation achieved by PSB reflects quantitatively the *component of central sensitization.* After needling and infiltration of the SS/IS ligaments, the peripheral component of sensitization is manifested by the residual pain and related pressure sensitivity caused by TSs/TrPs or muscle spasm in the affected myotome. Needling and infiltration of the TS/TrP reverses also the peripheral component of the sensitization to normal. This is indicated by normalization of pressure pain sensitivity and of palpatory findings, confirming that the taut band in the treated TrPs has been eradicated.

Injection Techniques for Treatment of Local Musculoskeletal Pain

Preinjection Blocks

Preinjection Blocks for Myofascial Trigger Points

The idea of preinjection blocks (PIBs) is to spread the anesthetic along the taut band to be needled and infiltrated. The diffuse infiltration starts next to the TrP or TS, which are the most sensitive parts of the taut band.[17, 41] Consequently, needling and infiltration begins in the region of TrPs/TS and concentrates on it. Following preinjection block, needling and infiltration of the TrPs/TS and taut band can be carried out without causing much pain, employing the technique described later and in previous publications.[9, 13–15, 17] Other advantages of preinjection block include prevention of central sensitization caused by needling or injecting a sensitized area such as TrP/TS. The importance of such preemption is emphasized by modern concepts of pain management.[45] In addition, preinjection block relieves the neurogenic component of the taut band, uncovering the remaining "fibrotic core" that is the sole target for needling and infiltration of the taut band (see Fig. 13–3A and B). Shrinking of the taut band facilitates needling and infiltration, producing better results.[14, 17]

Needle penetration on PIB should be limited to nontender, normal tissue surrounding the taut band in order to prevent pain and further sensitization. This goal cannot always be achieved because the bands may be wide and the anesthesia is ineffective if the procedure is performed too far from the sensitized tissue.

The next important technical feature of the PIB is that the spreading of anesthetic along the taut band should be *on the side where the nerve supply enters the taut band, TrP, or TS.* If spreading the anesthetic along one side of the taut band has not been successful, then the other side can also be blocked in a similar manner.

An important point in technique is that the *main nerve should never be blocked,* only the branches supplying the taut band to be needled and infiltrated. This rule is important for prevention of nerve damage, which can be inflicted if the main nerve is penetrated, and also to prevent paralysis of the entire muscle.

Technique of Preinjection Blocks

Preinjection blocks are performed with a thin needle, usually 25 gauge and 1.5 in. (3.9 cm). Longer needles, if available (2 in., 5 cm), are usually necessary for deeper trigger points in large muscles.

The needles to be used depend on the size of the muscles, as well as how deep the taut band is located. In small muscles of the neck, hands, feet, and forearms, needles of 25 gauge, 1.5 in. (3.9 cm) are used for both PIBs and the following needling and infiltration. Larger muscles, such as the lumbar paraspinals, thigh, arm, and shoulder muscles, require a larger needle of about 2 in. (5 cm), 25 or 21 gauge. For both types of block, a 25-gauge thin needle is ideal. For large and deep muscles, such as the glutei, quadratus lumborum, and piriformis, a 3 to 3.5-in., 25-gauge needle is required for PIB and the same length, but 22 gauge, for needling and infiltration.

The taut bands and TSs/TrPs that are the cause of pain are identified by asking the patient to point with one finger to the site of most intensive pain (see Table 13–1). Reproduction of symptoms by compression of the maximum tender point confirms that this is the cause of pain. TrPs/TSs and the entire taut band, including its attachment to bone, are marked on the skin. The marker avoids the points to be injected later, so cleaning of the skin does not remove the marks. The marks are made along the taut band but not over it; a line is made perpendicular to band length and intersecting it at the spot of maximum tenderness but not reaching it indicates the most sensitive point. The degree of tenderness is then assessed, ideally by using a pressure algometer, or at least by digital compression. The degree of tenderness of the taut band, as well as its size on palpation, is also noted.

The purpose of the procedure is explained to the patient. The area of PIB penetration is cleansed with an alcohol swab. The patient is warned, "I am going to tap your skin so you won't feel the needle penetration through the skin. You may feel some minimal pain, but usually there is no considerable pain on injection." While the patient's skin is being tapped, the needle is pushed into the muscle tissue by a sudden movement. It is best to hold the syringe as a pen, *between the thumb and the index and middle fingers,* which provides the best feedback for resistance. Elastic resistance of normal muscle tissue is easily distinguished from the harder resistance of a contracted taut band. Penetration of the fascia is clearly felt and is an important indicator that the muscle is being entered or, even more important, that it is being exited, with penetration of its fascia on the opposite, deep side. This indicates that the target TrP has been missed; therefore, the needle is withdrawn.

When the tip of the needle reaches the desired depth, aspiration is first performed in order to avoid injection into an artery or vein. Injection into the artery may spread the anesthetic in the muscle or into the nerve supply, temporarily paralyzing the injected muscle or even other muscles. In that case, the patient should not leave the office until the anesthesia and weakness resolve completely. Recovery may take as long as 1 or 2 hours or in exceptional cases even longer.

Depending on the size of the muscle, 0.1 to 0.5 mL of local anesthetic is slowly infiltrated at each stop. Another technique is to slowly inject during needle penetration and/or during withdrawal of the needle in order to spread the anesthetic to different depths of the muscle. Infiltration during movement of the needle carries a minimally increased risk of injection into a vessel.

After the injection is finished to one stop, the needle is carefully withdrawn to subcutaneous level and redirected first proximally because most of the nerves run in a proximal to distal direction. Depending on the size of the muscle injected, the distance between points where the tip of the needle ends can be from a few millimeters in small muscles of the neck, hand, and feet to 2 to 3 cm in large muscles, such as the thigh muscles, gastrocnemius, back, or arm and forearm muscles. *The amount of infiltrated fluid per stop* is also dependent on the size of the muscle and can be 0.1 up to 0.5 mL. The *total number of stops* and, consequently, the length along the taut band that the preinjection block reaches, will depend on the length of the employed needle. The longer the block reaches, of course, the better, because it allows needling and infiltration of a longer section of the taut band.

In very long muscles, if it is necessary to perform the injection in one session, several entries are required in order to spread the anesthetic along an extended section or possibly over the entire taut band. If the attachment to the bones (enthesopathy) will be needled and infiltrated, the preinjection block should reach up to the bone, but again avoiding the attachment of the taut band, which is very painful. From one needle entry, four to six stops can usually be reached proximally, as well as the same number distally. If it is not possible to reach so many stops, the length of the needle is insufficient.

Preinjection block (Fig. 13–3) is also very effective in reducing or preventing pain from injections of sprained ligaments, painful tendons, or other soft tissue irritation. For example, an inverted "V" shaped infiltration, going from a proximal to distal

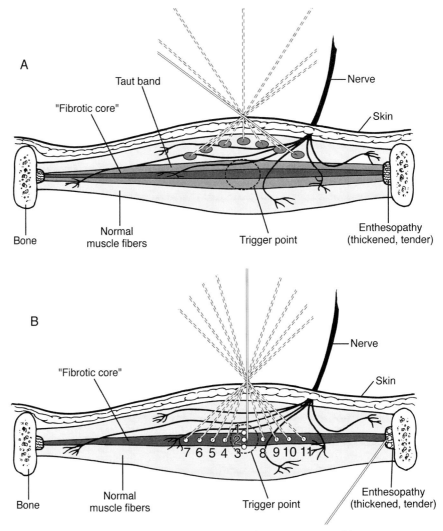

Figure 13–3. *A, Pre-injection block (PIB)* prevents pain and sensitization caused by injection or N&I of a painful, sensitive area. The needle penetrates next to the point of maximum tenderness (tender spot [TS] or trigger point [TrP]) into normal tissue. The anesthetic is spread by infiltration along the taut band [TB], which will be needled and infiltrated following the PIB. *B, The effect of pre-injection block and technique of needling and infiltration of the TB is shown:* Relief of neurogenic muscle fiber contractions shrinks the TB to about 20% of its original thickness (width). The remaining fibers demonstrate very hard fibrotic-like resistance on palpation and needle penetration and are referred to as the *fibrotic core. Needling and infiltration of the TB* are aimed primarily at breaking up the fibrotic core, which cannot be dissolved by any other means. This task is substantially facilitated by PIB, which prevents pain caused by needling and in addition also unveils the fibrotic core of the TB. The N&I is extended over the entire length of the TB.

direction above the biceps tendon, prevents pain and sensitization from injection or needling and infiltration of tendinitis. Needling and infiltration of the tenosynovitis is performed along the length of the tendon, penetrating only the synovial sheath and avoiding the tendon itself. Similarly, preinjection block prior to needling and infiltration of subacromial bursitis is very useful.

Evaluation of Preinjection Block Results

At the end of the procedure, or immediately after it, the patient is asked if there has been any change in the pain. The preinjection block itself induces complete relief of pain and restoration of function if the treated TrPs/TSs had been the cause of the patient's symptoms.

After the preinjection block on the nerve supply side is completed, even before removing the needle, the point of maximum tenderness is compressed digitally or by an algometer in order to assess the results of the block. The pressure pain threshold is increased relative to the preinjection measurement. Following effective PIB, pressure threshold usually increases on the average of 250 to 300%.[11, 13, 17]

Figure 13–4 illustrates changes in pressure threshold over a trigger point caused by lateral epicondylitis in a professional tennis coach. Initial reading was 2.2 kg, which more then doubled to 5.7 kg after the preinjection block, and pain was alleviated completely. Needling and infiltration was performed without pain and further increased the pressure threshold to 9.8 kg. The pain relief and restoration of function lasted a long period.

If the block fails to raise the pressure threshold adequately, the cause is frequently that the depth of the needle penetration was insufficient. Continuing the spreading of the anesthetic into the deeper layers can immediately rectify this. Another possible cause for failure of the block is that it was not performed on the side where the nerve supply enters the taut band. In such cases block on the opposite side of the taut band is performed.

Objective findings of changes induced by preinjection block include shrinkage of the taut band, usually to about 15 to 25% of its original width (see Fig. 13–3B). Relief of neurogenic contraction contributing to the taut band causes this change in size. The remaining part, within the taut band, demonstrates hard fibrotic resistance on palpation. Penetration of the needle also encounters a hard, nonelastic resistance that is typical for fibrotic scar tissue. Therefore, the hard fibrotic resistance remaining after the preinjection block is referred to as the *fibrotic core*. Failure to react to local anesthetic by relaxation is also most compatible with fibrotic tissue.

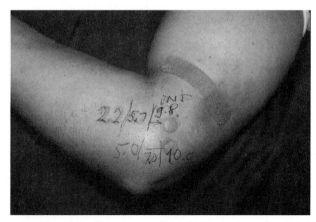

Figure 13–4. *Preinjection block increases pressure threshold over trigger points* (TrPs) *from 2.2 kg to 5.7 kg, more than double value. Following N&I, the TrP was pain-free and further increased the threshold to 9.8 kg. Pain was caused by lateral epicondylitis in a professional tennis coach.*

Technique of Needling and Infiltration of Taut Bands

Following the preinjection block, the taut band, as indicated above, shrinks to about 15 to 20% of its original thickness due to relief of neurogenic contraction of the muscle fibers (see Fig. 13–3B). This facilitates substantially the needling and infiltration that can be concentrated upon the remaining fibrotic core, which is the only goal of the mechanical breakup by this procedure.

Crucial for results is the selection of the *proper length and thickness of the needle.* In small muscles of the neck, the hands, feet, and forearm, a 1.5-in., 25-gauge needle is sufficient. However, in larger muscles, a thicker needle of adequate length is more effective. The point of maximum tenderness is penetrated and after careful aspiration in order to avoid injection into a blood vessel, a very small amount (approximately .1 mL) of lidocaine is deposited at each step. The needle is then withdrawn to the subcutaneous level, where its direction is changed, aiming about 3 to 4 mm proximally. Again, after aspiration, a deposit of .1 mL is made. If the needle is not withdrawn sufficiently from the muscle, and this applies to both preinjection block and needling and infiltration, changing of the direction may cut the muscle fibers. In addition, the needle may be bent, which is dangerous. If the needle is not withdrawn completely from the muscle, the second penetration will repeat the course of the previous one because the direction of the needle cannot be changed. The procedure is repeated step by step, going along the taut band as far as the needle allows. The direction of the needle is changed toward the distal portion of the taut band, and the needling and infiltration are performed again as far as the needle reaches.

Penetration of the needle is aimed at the point of maximum tenderness within the fibrotic core that has remained after the procedure. Sometimes, if the band of the fibrotic core is thick, several parallel needlings and infiltrations are necessary along the abnormal structure. If the taut band is longer than the reach of the needle, another preinjection block is necessary, proximal and distal to the first procedure, followed by corresponding needling and infiltration.

The number of injected sites depends on the patient's tolerance and on other factors. One is whether follow-up physical therapy, particularly *electric stimulation*, is available for the following 2 to 3 days, which assures fast recovery and substantial reduction of postinjection soreness and pain. The electric stimulation also controls edema and allows active relaxation exercises, which again reduce sensitization, pain, and edema. The needling will also be limited in case the patient cannot rest the muscle and avoid strenuous or long-lasting activities for approximately 3 to 4 days.

The amount of lidocaine required for needling and infiltration depends on the size of the muscle and the taut band. In the neck muscles, usually 1.5 mL is the maximum and, together with the preinjection block, it is preferable to limit the amount of anesthetic to less than 3 mL. In larger muscles of the arm, forearm, or leg, 4 to 6 mL are used for preinjection block and a similar amount for needling and infiltration. In large muscles, such as the glutei, quadratus lumborum, piriformis, and large thigh muscles, 8 to 12 mL is required for each of the procedures. The total amount of 1% lidocaine used can be about 50 mL, but more than 15 to 18 mL is rarely exceeded in one session. If acute, widespread pain requires multiple levels of infiltration, one or two levels are started. The patient then receives physical therapy or takes a break to exercise. After approximately 45 minutes, the rest of the areas are injected.

Treatment Results

Dry needling alone is effective in pain relief.[18, 20–22, 24, 36] Adding local anesthetic, however, reduces postinjection soreness.[24] Most experienced clinicians use local anesthetics for TrP injections.[25, 35, 40–42, 44] Because preinjection block has so many advantages, there is no reason for not employing it routinely. In view of the SSS concept, the combination of paraspinous block, followed by preinjection block and ending with needling and infiltration of the most tender residual part of the taut band and TSs/

TrPs, is the best course of treatment. This approach is being employed routinely and renders the best results.

It is important that this approach has been successful also for long-term pain alleviation in patients with *fibromyalgia*. The *immediate cause of pain* in fibromyalgia patients consists of SSS affecting multiple levels characteristically extending to both sides of the involved segment. Best results were achieved by paraspinous block applied *bilaterally* at several levels where pain and sensitization are most severe.

Physicians trained in the injection techniques described earlier reported to the author good results with paraspinous block in patients with *complex regional pain syndrome (reflex sympathetic dystrophy)* and *phantom pain.*

Figure 13–5 shows the excellent correlation between reduction in pain rating by the visual analog scale (VAS) and increase in pressure pain threshold in a group of seven patients with hip pathology scheduled for hip replacement.[29, 32] The pain rating on VAS, shown as full circles, decreased from an average of 5.6 on initial evaluation to 2.1 on discharge and remained practically at the identical level of 1.9 at the 5.1-year follow-up. The pressure threshold over the TrPs that were causing the symptoms, represented by the triangles, increased in a mirror image to VAS reduction from 2.2 kg/cm² on initial evaluation to 4.6 on discharge, ending at 5.6 kg/cm² at the 5.1-year follow-up.[29] Such ideal correlation between changes of pain threshold and pain reduction can be achieved only if the measurement of pressure sensitivity is performed over the TSs/TrPs that are the immediate cause of pain. If the pressure algometry is not performed over the site causing the pain, evidently no correlation between relief of pain and improvement of pressure sensitivity can be expected.[7, 12, 15]

Studies showing that needling and infiltration of the taut band is effective in relieving the pain of different etiology are reviewed next. Long-lasting pain relief, as well as improvement of algometric results, was documented.

Figure 13–6 shows the percentage of patients in whom myofascial TrPs were the immediate cause of pain and the percentage of patients improved after needling and infiltration.[27–32, 37] The table summarizes the published results in conditions with different etiologies. The follow-ups of the studies were double-blind, and their values

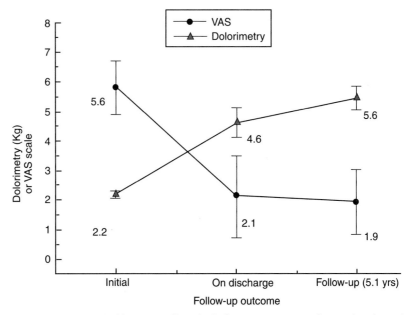

Figure 13–5. Documentation of *long-term effect of N&I* by pain rating using the visual analog scale (VAS) and pressure algometry. The mirror image of the two parameters indicates that the treated trigger points have been the cause of pain. N&I of trigger points was the treatment of patients on a waiting list for total hip replacement. At 5.1-year follow-up, pain control was still effective (VAS = 1.9) and pressure pain threshold was maintained at a high level—5.6 kg/cm².

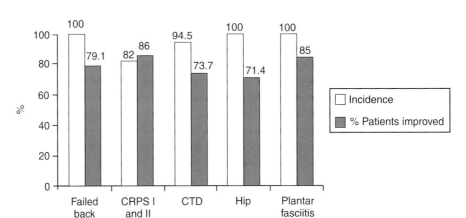

Figure 13–6. *Incidence of myofascial pain syndrome* as cause of pain in different conditions (first column) and *long-term relief of pain by N&I* (second column).

were enhanced by several conditions: First, the studies are crossover; all patients had conventional treatment that failed prior to introduction of needling and infiltration. Previous treatments included physical therapy, in many cases acupuncture, and some patients even received injections using different techniques than those described herein. The percentage of such patients in whom other therapies failed, but who were improved by needling and infiltration, is impressive, ranging from 71.4% to 86% of patients. Second the value of most studies[27, 29–32] was enhanced as the pain relief has been confirmed by corresponding improvement in pressure threshold measurements. This improvement of algometric results serves as evidence that the peripheral sensitization was eliminated and TSs/TrPs have been eradicated.

In patients with *failed back surgery* (n = 24), the myofascial component was cause of pain in 100% of cases. With needling and infiltration 79.1% of patients showed improvement still present at 150 days of follow-up.[30] Of 84 patients suffering from *complex regional pain syndrome*[31] *(reflex sympathetic dystrophy)*, myofascial pain was causing the symptoms in 82% and pain was improved by TrP injections in 86% (n = 84, average follow-up 25.4 months).[31]

From a total of 109 patients with diagnosis of *cumulative traumatic disorders*,[37] the symptoms were caused by myofascial pain in 94.5%, and needling and infiltration achieved improvement in 73.7% of patients.

All 21 patients who were *on a waiting list for total hip replacement*[32] had myofascial pain as a component of their hip pain. Treatment of these patients led to significant improvement in 71.4% (13 month average follow-up). With no additional treatments, at 2-year follow-up, 9 patients out of the initial group of 21 treated by needling and infiltration did not require total hip replacement.[17] The initial VAS of the injected group was 5.72 ± 2.05 (mean ± standard deviation), which at follow-up evaluation was reduced to 2.39 ± 2.85 (P = 0.0023). The 10 patients who underwent total hip replacement had an initial VAS of 6.71 ± 2.86. At 2-year follow-up their VAS decreased to 1 ± 1.41 (P = 0.003). The patients who underwent surgery and the ones who were treated only with needling and infiltration were matched in initial VAS values. There was no statistically significant difference between the two groups on follow-up VAS values (P = 1.000).

At mean follow-up of 5.1 years (range, 49–68 months), from the original group 3 patients had died and 3 could not be found. Of the group, 8 patients had total hip replacement and 7 did not. Initial and 5-year follow-up VAS scores were not significantly different between the remaining groups of patients according to Mann-Whitney-U test (P = 0.87, initial; P = 0.96, follow-up). The Harris functional hip performance scale also failed to show statistically significant differences (79.03 ± 11.71 in the nonoperated group and 78.49 ± 16.61 in the operated group) according to unpaired T test. In addition, the quality of life SF-36 scales showed no statistically significant differences between the two groups according to the unpaired T test. The nonoperated group presented a 113.7 ± 14.09 score vs. 108.9 ± 25.10 in the operated group.

All 29 patients suffering from disabling *plantar fasciitis*[27] had symptoms caused by myofascial TrPs in leg muscles and improved with needling and infiltration in 85%. Nine control patients and 20 injected patients were followed for mean period of 2 years. The control group was treated intensively, three times per week, by conventional physical therapy, including heat, ultrasound, stretching, and special exercises. The experimental group, in addition, received needling and infiltration in the TSs/TrPs of the calf muscles. The results show that the degree of functional improvement, as well as the reduction in pain and increase in pressure pain threshold of the trigger points and TSs, were identical in both groups at the end of the evaluation period of 2 years. However, the statistically significant difference between the groups was in the time to achieve identical functional improvement, alleviation of pain, and normalization of pressure threshold. The control group, with intensive physical therapy, took 21.11 ± 19.5 weeks, while the patients who had needling and infiltration of the TSs/TrPs responsible for pain returned to work in 13.4 ± 2.2 weeks. The shortening of time required to return to work is statistically and clinically highly significant, indicating the efficacy of needling and infiltration concentrated on the etiologic factors.

Figure 13–7 shows results in patients suffering a disabling degree of *plantar fasciitis* in a randomized, controlled study by M. Imamura.[17] This study included 20 control subjects and 13 injected patients. The diagnosis consisted of plantar fasciitis with TrPs in calf muscles. These TrPs were injected. There was no statistically significant difference between both groups in terms of duration of pain complaint, initial VAS, and functional level on a test of the American Orthopedic Foot and Ankle Society (AOFAS). Upon discharge the injected group showed more improvement than the control group, but the difference was not significant. VAS in the injected group dropped from 8.21 ± 1.20 to the final level of 2.92 ± 1.98. The conventionally treated group decreased VAS from 8.46 ± 1.39 to the final 3.73 ± 3.42. Functional improvement on the AOFAS test was significant in both groups, but no significant difference was found between them. The identical level of pain relief and functional improvement allowing return to work has been achieved in the injected group in a

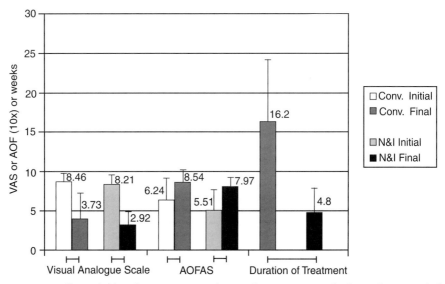

Figure 13–7. Effects of *N&I of trigger points in leg muscles in patients with plantar fasciitis:* Relief of pain, improvement of function, and reduction of time required before returning to work (from 16.2 weeks to 4.8 weeks). Equal reduction in pain and improvement of function have been achieved in the injected group in a statistically highly significantly shorter period of time in the injected group as compared to a control group, which received identical intensive physical therapy.

substantially shorter time: 4.83 ± 3.04 weeks vs. 16.23 ± 7.92 ($P = 0.0002$) in the control group (Mann-Whitney-U test with significant level 5%).

It is important to realize that needling and infiltration of TSs/TrPs alone obtained these results, since preinjection block and particularly paraspinous block were introduced later. When these procedures were added to needling and infiltration, physicians employing the procedures reported to the author substantially improved results. Statistical evaluation of the additional benefits of PIB and PSB is not available; however, instantaneous and impressive improvement has been observed.

Above results and the role of SSS offer an explanation for lack of correlation between pain and disc herniation as documented by imaging.[5]

SUMMARY

A new injection technique, the *paraspinous block (PSB)* alleviates pain associated with SSS by specifically reversing the SSS to normal sensitivity and function. Further, a *pre-injection block (PIB)* prevents pain and sensitization caused by needle penetration into a painful tender area such as a TrP. Finally, the technique of *needling and infiltration of the entire taut band* associated with myofascial TrPs is presented, along with evidence of its long-term efficacy in relieving pain and inducing healing.[6–8, 13, 15, 27–32]

Acknowledgment

The assistance of Hy Dubo, M.D. and Marta Imamura, M.D., Ph.D, in preparation of this manuscript is appreciated.

References

1. Aleksiev A: Longitudinal comparative study on the outcome of inpatient treatment of low back pain with manual therapy vs. physical therapy. J Orthop Med 17:10–14, 1995.
2. Bonica JJ: The Management of Pain. Philadelphia, Lea & Febiger, 1990.
3. Chusid JG, McDonald JJ: Correlative Neuroanatomy & Functional Neurology, 13th ed. Los Altos, Lange Medical Publications, 1967.
4. Deyo RA, Walsh NE, Martin DC, et al: A controlled trial of transcutaneous electrical stimulation (TENS) and exercise for chronic low back pain. N Engl J Med 322:1627–1634, 1990.
5. Ellenberg MR, Ross ML, Honet JC, et al: Prospective evaluation of the course of disk herniation in patients with proven radiculopathy. Arch Phys Med Rehabil 74:3–8, 1993.
6. Fischer AA: Relief of nerve root compression by trigger point injection into the quadratus lumborum muscle. Arch Phys Med Rehabil 74:1263, 1993.
7. Fischer AA: Local injections in pain management. Trigger point needling with infiltration and somatic blocks. Phys Med Rehab Clin North Am 6:851–870, 1995.
8. Fischer AA: Injection techniques in the management of local pain. Journal of Back and Musculoskeletal Rehabilitation 7:107–117, 1996.
9. Fischer AA: New approaches in treatment of myofascial pain. In Fischer AA (ed): Myofascial Pain—Update in Diagnosis and Treatment. Philadelphia, WB Saunders, 1997, pp 153–169.
10. Fischer AA: New developments in diagnosis of myofascial pain and fibromyalgia. Phys Med Rehab Clin North Am 8:1–21, 1997.
11. Fischer AA. Algometry in diagnosis of musculoskeletal pain and evaluation of treatment outcome: An update. In Fischer AA (ed): Muscle Pain Syndromes and Fibromyalgia. New York, Haworth, 1998; pp 5–32.
12. Fischer AA, Imamura ST, Kazyana HS, Imamura M: Trigger point injections and "paraspinous blocs" which relieve segmental spinal sensitization are effective treatment for chronic pain. J Musculoskeletal Pain 6(Suppl 2):52, 1998.
13. Fischer AA: Myofascial pain. In Windsor RE, Lox DM (eds): Soft Tissue Injuries: Diagnosis and Treatment. Philadelphia, Hanley & Belfus, 1998; pp 85–100.
14. Fischer AA: Treatment of Myofascial Pain. J Musculoskeletal Pain 7:131–142, 1999.
15. Fischer AA: Trigger point injections. In Lennard TA (ed): Pain Procedures in Clinical Practice, 2nd ed. Philadelphia, Hanley & Belfus, 2000; pp 153–161.
16. Fischer AA: Functional diagnosis of musculoskeletal pain and evaluation of treatment results by quantitative and objective methods. In Rachlin ES (ed): Myofascial Pain and Fibromyalgia: Trigger Point Management, 2nd ed. Philadelphia, WB Saunders, 2002, pp 145–173.

17. Fischer AA, Imamura M: New concepts in the diagnosis and management of musculoskeletal pain: In Lennard TA (ed): Pain Procedures in Clinical Practice, 2nd ed. Philadelphia, Hanley & Belfus, 2000; pp 213–229.
18. Frost FA, Jessen B, Siggaard-Andersen J: A control, double-blind comparison of mepivacaine injection versus saline injection for myofascial pain. Lancet 8:499–500, 1980.
19. Fujiwara A, Tamai K, An HS, et al: The interspinous ligament of the lumbar spine. Spine 25:358–363, 2000.
20. Garvey TA, Marks MR, Wiesel SW: A prospective, randomized, double blind evaluation of trigger-point injection therapy for low-back pain. Spine 14:962–964, 1989.
21. Gunn CC, Milbrandt WE, Little AS, Mason KE: Dry needling of muscle motor points for chronic low-back pain. A randomized clinical trial with long-term follow-up. Spine 5:279–291, 1980.
22. Gunn CC: The Gunn Approach to the Treatment of Chronic Pain. New York, Churchill Livingstone, 1996.
23. Hackett GS: Ligament and Tendon Relaxation Treated by Prolotherapy, 3rd ed. Springfield, Ill, Thomas, 1958, pp 27–36.
24. Hong C-Z: Lidocaine injection versus dry needling to myofascial trigger point: The importance of the local twitch response. Am J Phys Med Rehabil 73:256–263, 1994.
25. Hong C-Z: Considerations and recommendations regarding myofascial trigger point injection. J Musculoskeletal Pain 2:29–59, 1994.
26. Hseuh T-C, Yu S, Kuan T-S, Hong C-Z: The immediate effectiveness of electrical nerve stimulation and electrical muscle stimulation on myofascial trigger points. Am J Phys Med Rehabil 76:471–476, 1997.
27. Imamura M: Personal communications.
28. Imamura M, Fischer A, Imamura ST, et al: Treatment of myofascial pain components in plantar fasciitis speeds up recovery. In Fischer AA (ed): Muscle Pain Syndromes and Fibromyalgia. New York, Haworth, 1998; pp 91–110.
29. Imamura ST: Personal communications.
30. Imamura ST, Fischer AA, Imamura M, et al: Pain management using myofascial approach when other treatment failed. Phys Med Rehab Clin North Am 8:179–196, 1997.
31. Imamura ST, Lin TY, Texeira MJ, et al: The importance of myofascial pain syndrome in reflex sympathetic dystrophy (or complex regional pain syndrome). Phys Med Rehab Clin North Am 8:207–211, 1997.
32. Imamura ST, Riberto M, Fischer AA, et al: Successful pain relief by treatment of myofascial components in patients with hip pathology scheduled for total hip replacement. In Fischer AA (ed): Muscle Pain Syndromes and Fibromyalgia. New York, Haworth, 1998; pp 73–89.
33. Keegan JJ, Garrett FD. The segmental distribution of the cutaneous nerves in the limbs of man. Anat Rec 102–409, 1948.
34. Kellgren JH: On the distribution of pain arising from deep somatic structures with charts of segmental pain areas. Clin Sci 4:35–46, 1939–1942.
35. Kraus H, Fischer AA: Diagnosis and treatment of myofascial pain. Mt Sinai J Med 58:235–239, 1991.
36. Lewit K: The needle effect in the relief of myofascial pain. Pain 6:83–90, 1979.
37. Lin TY, Teixeira MJ, Fischer AA, et al: Work-related musculoskeletal disorders. Phys Med Rehab Clin North Am 8:113–117, 1997.
38. Mense S, Simons DG: Muscle Pain. Philadelphia, Lippincott Williams & Wilkins, 2000; pp 92–95.
39. Nachemson A, Jonsson E (eds): Neck and Back Pain. Philadelphia, Lippincott Williams & Willkins, 2000, pp 149–163.
40. Rachlin ES: Trigger points. In Rachlin ES (ed): Myofascial Pain and Fibromyalgia. St Louis, Mosby, 1994.
41. Simons DG, Fischer AA: Myofascial pain. In Fields HL (ed): Core Curriculum for Professional Education in Pain, 2nd ed. Seattle, IASP Press, 1995; pp 79–81.
42. Simons DG, Travell JG, Simons LS: Myofascial Pain and Dysfunction. The Trigger Point Manual Vol. 1. Upper Half of Body, 2nd ed. Baltimore, Williams & Wilkins, 1999.
43. Sorkin L, Yaksh TL: Mechanisms of pain processing. In Abram SE (vol ed): Vol VI. Pain Management. In Miller RD (ed): Atlas of Anesthesia. Philadelphia, Churchill Livingstone, 1998; pp 2.1–2.13.
44. Travell JG, Simons DG: Myofascial Pain Dysfunction: The Trigger Point Manual: The Lower Extremities, vol 1. Baltimore, Williams & Wilkins, 1983.
45. Woolf CJ: A new strategy for the treatment of inflammatory pain. Prevention or elimination of central sensitization. Drugs 47(Suppl. 5):1–9, 1994.

Chapter 14

Nerve Block Therapy for Myofascial Pain Management

Winston C. V. Parris, MD

Myofascial pain syndrome may be defined as chronic pain affecting the superficial regions of the musculoskeletal system, though not exclusively. It may be localized and associated with focal pain, affecting a single muscle, or it may affect an entire regional muscle group within the musculoskeletal system. In some cases, the pain may be referred to distant locations.

The presence of multiple trigger points is usually associated with myofascial pain syndromes. Although the trigger points are generally located within the regional part of the body affected, it is not unusual to find trigger points referred to other areas besides the affected area. This situation may lead to errors in diagnosis and management. Myofascial pain syndrome may also be associated with chronic debility, severe stiffness, and generalized fatigue. It is not unusual to have various psychological, emotional, or behavioral comorbidities that may be associated with myofascial pain syndrome.

The etiological factors usually associated with myofascial pain syndrome include residual musculoskeletal pain following major trauma and also lesions associated with extremes of hot and cold temperatures. In the absence of tissue injury, various physical stresses may produce myofascial pain syndrome. These stresses include repetitive microtraumatic events that may be related to occupational or recreational activities, i.e., typing, guitar playing, or assembly-line work. Chronic and extreme fatigue may produce myofascial pain syndrome, and different disease states connected with muscular trauma may also result in myofascial pain syndrome.

The basic treatment of myofascial pain syndromes includes trigger point injections, antidepressant drugs, stretch and spray, physical therapy, and massage and myofascial releases. Heat modalities, ice massage, electrical stimulation, transcutaneous electrical nerve stimulation (TENS), and, more recently, the injection of botulinum toxin type A have been recommended as adjunct therapeutic modalities for the management of myofascial pain. In resistant cases or in patients who do not respond to the aforementioned conservative therapeutic modalities, the use of nerve block therapy may have a prominent place in the management of myofascial pain syndrome. In this chapter, the rationale, prerequisites, classification, indications, contraindications, complications, and description of selected nerve blocks used for myofascial pain syndrome are discussed.

The Role of Nerve Blocks in Pain Management

The late John J. Bonica[1] proposed that chronic pain, including that of myofascial pain syndrome, should be managed whenever possible or practicable under the auspices of an interdisciplinary, multispecialty, and multimodal team. Clearly, not all patients with myofascial pain syndrome fit that model. Nevertheless, it is important to bear in mind that when pain is chronic and when unresponsiveness to treatment exists, it is best to initiate this model so as to avoid duplication of services, misdiagnoses, and unhappiness of patients. Although this therapeutic model is generally considered to be ideal, its absence does not imply that unidisciplinary or unimodal pain management for chronic pain is always unacceptable. Thus, after thorough patient evaluation and assessment, it may be quite effective and satisfactory to use a unidisciplinary or unimodal approach to myofascial pain management. In doing so, it is important to avoid the principle that "one size fits all."

Nerve blocks may have diagnostic, prognostic, and therapeutic uses in the treatment of chronic pain syndromes. In a very few cases, there may be a basis for the use of neurolytic blocks for resistant and localized severe chronic pain.[10] Nerve blocks may also play a useful role in patients who are unable or unwilling to use the recommended pharmacologic agents for managing chronic myofascial pain syndrome. Further, nerve block therapy may be administered as a supplement to other modalities that may be used to manage myofascial pain syndrome. Thus, nerve block therapy may be very effective in the management of chronic pain associated with myofascial pain syndrome when used either alone or in combination with other modalities including physical therapy, physical principles, pharmacologic agents, stretch and spray, TENS unit, and other alternative therapies.

Prerequisites for Nerve Blocks

Nerve blocks by virtue of their actions may produce significant systemic side effects as a consequence of the direct and indirect actions of the nerve blocks. These actions may include respiratory, cardiovascular, and neurologic effects of the nerve blocks or the hemodynamic consequences of the drug effect. Informed consent should also be obtained prior to performing nerve blocks; patients should be evaluated following the block for those side effects and their appropriate management undertaken. The severe complications of nerve blocks should be rare in the management of myofascial pain syndromes because of the volume of medication used and the relatively infrequent involvement of the neuraxial structures that may otherwise produce severe circulatory, cardiorespiratory, and central nervous system effects. Preoperative, intraoperative, and post-block monitoring are always necessary to enhance patient safety and to limit complications that may result from these nerve blocks.

The following precautions are recommended prior to implementing nerve block therapy for the management of myofascial pain[2]:

1. Adequate knowledge of the pathology and the syndrome being treated.
2. Full knowledge of the anatomy of the region to be blocked.
3. Adequate understanding of the risks and benefits of the nerve block and its administration.
4. Familiarity with the equipment, including needles, syringes, nerve block trays being used.
5. Use of appropriate assistance, including a registered nurse or appropriate health care professional to facilitate in monitoring, assessment, and resuscitation should it become necessary.
6. Understanding of the pharmacology of the agents to be used.
7. Availability of a mobile cart stocked not only with the appropriate supplies but also with the equipment and drugs necessary to manage the complications of nerve blocks including cardiorespiratory arrest.[20]
8. Informed consent from the patient and accompanying others prior to performing the block.
9. Personnel adequately trained and appropriately certified in advanced cardiac life support (ACLS) enhance the clinical competency and medicolegal conformity of the team.
10. Adequate pre- and post-block monitoring of essential vital signs including pulse, respiration, blood pressure, pulse oximetry, and pain assessment.

Further, because most patients with chronic myofascial pain syndrome may have associated behavioral, emotional, and psychological comorbidities, it is important to emphasize the promotion of self-reliance, the teaching of coping mechanisms, and the utilization of both physical and psychological rehabilitation in addition to nerve block therapy for the comprehensive management of chronic myofascial pain.

Mechanism of Action

The basic principle underlying the action of nerve block therapy in patients with myofascial pain syndrome is the interruption of sensory and nociceptive pathways in various tissues and muscle groups affected by the disease. Although nerve blocks are not always predictably successful, some reasons for failure include poor technique, inadequate drug and inappropriate dosage, and inappropriate selection of nerve block for treating the specific pain syndrome. Anatomic variation of the myogenic and neural tissue and pathophysiologic dysfunction may be present as a result of either overproduction or underproduction of various vasoactive neuropeptides.

The mechanism of action of local anesthetics in producing effective nerve blockade is thought to be the result of alteration of the resting potential within the nerve and initiation of an action potential that travels orthodromically along the external fiber of the sensory nerve. The consequences include neurotransmitter release inhibiting the generation of an action potential and thus producing conduction blockade. This conduction blockade affects not only sensory fibers but also sympathetic and motor fibers. The sensory and sympathetic fibers are the primary targets for blockade and in the case of myofascial pain syndrome, their resulting motor blockade may produce some rest of the fatigued muscle group, which may ultimately produce pain relief at the expiration of the effects of nerve blockade.

Covino[6] proposed a schema representing a systematic approach to the sequence of events involved in local anesthetic–induced conduction blockade. These events include the binding of local anesthetic molecules to receptor sites in the nerve membrane producing a reduction in sodium permeability. As a consequence, there is a decrease in the rate of depolarization resulting in a failure to achieve threshold potential level producing a lack of development of a propagated action potential. These events cumulatively produce conduction blockade. It is clear that depolarization and repolarization are the key factors in the propagation of an action potential.

The local anesthetics used for nerve block function by blocking the transmission of nociceptive stimuli depending on the individual characteristics of the local anesthetics. Some of the more important pharmacologic characteristics that may influence their activity[19] include (1) molecular weight, (2) structure activity relationships, (3) lipid solubility, (4) PKA or dissociation constant, (5) protein binding, (6) equipotent concentration percent, (7) partition coefficient, (8) intrinsic vasodilator activity, (9) tissue diffusibility, and (10) the rate of local anesthetic biodegradation.

Although supplemental techniques are not usually used for the management of chronic pain secondary to myofascial pain syndrome, they are available to enhance the accuracy of the nerve block. These include radiologic localization of the needle prior to injection of the drug and peripheral nerve stimulation when appropriate as a means of identifying proximity with the nerve structure; in addition, the elicitation of paresthesias may also help to confirm correct needle placement.

Agents Commonly Used for Nerve Blocks

Local anesthetics are by far the most common agents used. The choice of local anesthetic used depends on the pre-block objective and also on the pharmacologic characteristics of the individual local anesthetics. The author's personal preference for typical nerve blocks is bupivacaine (0.25% or 0.5%).

Long-acting steroids including methylprednisolone (Depo-Medrol) and triamcinolone acetonide (Aristocort) also are useful in cases in which an inflammatory component is present. Steroids may be mixed with the local anesthetic and administered, particularly when an inflammatory lesion is either suspected or confirmed.[8] The mechanism of action of long-acting steroids includes (1) anti-inflammatory effect, (2) increased phospholipase A-2 activity, and (3) a hypothesis suggesting the presence of perispinal and intraspinal steroid receptors. Recently, botulinum toxin type A has been advocated as being very effective for severe myofascial pain syndrome.

Complications of Nerve Block

Nerve blocks are incredibly safe when properly administered and appropriately managed. When safety parameters are ignored, severe complications and incapacitating side effects may occur. It is important to stress that many of those complications may not be common in nerve block therapy management of myofascial pain syndrome because neuraxial nerve blocks are rarely performed for the management of pain associated with myofascial pain syndromes. The more common complications that may occur include:

1. Cardiovascular effects including hypotension, bradycardia, peripheral vascular collapse, and cardiac arrest[18]
2. Central nervous system effects including coma, convulsions, and loss of consciousness
3. Respiratory system effects including pneumothorax and respiratory insufficiency
4. Local tissue effects including muscle atrophy[14]
5. Allergic reactions[4]
6. Anaphylactic reactions
7. Hypersensitivity reactions
8. Vasovagal reactions

It is important to emphasize that nerve blocks should be administered using the general principles of multidisciplinary and multimodal applications after a comprehensive physical evaluation preceded by meticulous history taking. These general principles would tend to avoid duplication of services and make the individual therapies more effective and useful. Thus, while a particular nerve block is being administered, it may be appropriate to simultaneously administer biofeedback, physical therapy, and specific pharmacologic agents.

Specific Nerve Blocks for Myofascial Pain

The following is not an exclusive list of nerve blocks used for myofascial pain but is intended to represent some of the nerve blocks that may have some application in the treatment of myofascial pain syndromes. Furthermore, there are specific nerve blocks that may be used for specific myofascial pain syndromes. These would be highlighted when applicable.

Nerve blocks may be conceptually divided into central or neuraxial nerve blocks and peripheral nerve blocks. Peripheral nerve blocks are usually used in the management of myofascial pain syndrome, whereas, although infrequently and for specific indications, neuraxial nerve blocks may have a place in the management of pain associated with myofascial pain syndromes.[3] For purposes of this chapter, neuraxial nerve blocks will not be described; nevertheless, it is quite reasonable in selected cases to use continuous intrathecal or epidural opioid administration for intractable pain associated with myofascial pain syndromes that have been unresponsive to conventional therapies.

The peripheral nerve blocks used for myofascial pain syndrome would be described using a regional format. These include:

1. Nerve Blocks for Myofascial Pain Syndrome Affecting the Head and Neck
   A. Occipital Nerve Block

   Unilateral or bilateral occipital nerve blocks may be used to manage occipital pain emanating from the neuromyogenic structures in the occipital area. The greater occipital nerve block is blocked by using a 3-in., 22-gauge needle that is inserted along the nuchal line just medial to the palpated occipital artery at that level. Aspirations should be performed prior to injection of local anesthetic to avoid intravascular injections or injection through cavernous sinuses in the skull and subsequent intracerebral injection. The lesser occipital nerve is blocked by directing the needle laterally and inferiorly and using the same precautions. More common complications consist of intravascular injections and syncope.

B. Supraorbital Nerve Block

Supraorbital nerve blocks are performed for pain of myofascial origin located in the forehead. This block is performed by inserting a 3-in., 22-gauge needle into the supraorbital fossa, which is located in the supraorbital ridge at a point just lateral to the pupil. Paresthesias are usually sought and elicited as an end point to ideal needle placement. Aspirations are performed prior to injection and pressure should be applied to the supraorbtial ridge (not over the globe of the eye) to minimize hematoma and subsequent swelling over the eye.

C. Supratrochlear Nerve Block

Supratrochlear nerve block is used to supplement supraorbital nerve block and this nerve is accessed a few millimeters lateral to the supraorbital nerve along the supraorbital ridge.

D. Auriculotemporal Nerve Block

The patient is placed in the supine position, and with the head turned away from the site to be blocked. A 3-in., 22-gauge needle is inserted at a point just above the origin of the zygoma and at which the temporal artery is palpated. The needle is advanced perpendicularly until it approaches the periosteum of the temporalis bone. The needle is usually inserted just lateral to the temporal artery and is advanced in a cephalad direction after careful aspiration to avoid intravascular injection.

Auriculotemporal nerve block is useful in the management of atypical facial pain syndrome involving the temporomandibular joint and is also useful in the management of acute herpes zoster involving the external auditory meatus and the management of pain associated with Ramsay Hunt syndrome. Methylprednisolone is usually added to the local anesthetic being injected because the pain may also be associated with an inflammatory component.

E. Greater Auricular Nerve Block

This nerve is blocked with the patient in the sitting position and the cervical spine flexed. This block is performed for the management of painful conditions involving the greater auricular nerve. The nerve is usually accessed as it emerges superficially around the proximal aspect of the sternocleidomastoid muscle at a point approximately 2 to 3 centimeters inferior to the mastoid. Careful aspiration prior to injection is mandatory.

F. Spinal Accessory Nerve Block

Spinal accessory nerve blocks are useful for the diagnosis and occasionally the treatment of spasm associated with the trapezius muscle and/or the sternocleidomastoid muscle. This procedure also has prognostic value when considering the neurolysis of the spinal accessory nerve as a palliative measure of spasm of either the trapezius or sternocleidomastoid muscle.

This nerve is blocked with the patient in the supine position and with the head turned away from the side to be blocked. A 3-in., 22-gauge needle is inserted at a point along the posterior border of the sternocleidomastoid muscle where the proximal one third and the distal two thirds meet. The needle is advanced in a slightly anterior direction and advanced for a depth of approximately 1.5 to 2.5 cm. Careful aspiration is performed to avoid intravascular or cerebrospinal fluid injection. The injection is performed in a fan-like manner so that most branches of the spinal accessory nerve may be blocked. Infrequently, branches of the brachial plexus may be inadvertently blocked.

G. Phrenic Nerve Block

This procedure is frequently used for the management of intractable hiccups associated with diaphragmatic irritation. The phrenic nerve originates from the anterior primary rami of the third, fourth, and fifth cervical nerves with the major contribution coming from the fourth cervical nerve. The phrenic nerve is usually blocked by inserting a 3-in., 22-gauge needle at a point approximately 1 inch above the clavicle in a groove between the posterior border of the sternocleidomastoid muscle and the insertion of the anterior scalene muscle. The needle is inserted in that groove and with a slight anteromedial direction. Careful aspiration is mandatory to avoid intravascular injection and the relationship between the tip of the needle and the apex of the lung should always be borne in mind in an attempt to minimize pneumothorax. If that approach does not give adequate block of the phrenic nerve, the needle may be removed and reintroduced a little more medially behind the posterior border of the sternocleidomastoid muscle. Bilateral phrenic nerve blocks should never be performed for obvious reasons (i.e., bilateral pneumothorax).

H. Facial Nerve Block

Facial nerve blocks may be useful for the management of painful conditions and facial spasms including atypical facial neuralgia and the pain associated with Bell's palsy and herpes zoster involving the geniculate ganglion (Ramsay Hunt syndrome) and also for hemifacial spasms.

The facial nerve is blocked by inserting a 3-in., 22-gauge needle at the level of the anterior border of the mastoid process and immediately below the external auditory meatus. The needle entry should be at the level of the middle section of the ramus of the mandible. The needle should be directed towards the anterior border of the mastoid process while it is advanced in a perpendicular direction to the skin. As the needle makes contact with the mastoid process, it is withdrawn slightly and redirected past the anterior border of the mastoid for approximately 1 to 1.5 cm. This places the needle in close proximity to the stylomastoid foramen and to the point at which the facial nerve exits the skull. Meticulous aspiration should be performed at that point to rule out blood and/or cerebrospinal fluid. An optimum volume of 3.0 to 4.0 mL of local anesthetic with or without steroids is injected with multiple sequential aspirations to ensure that intravascular and subarachnoid injections do not occur.

I. Superficial Cervical Plexus Block

Superficial cervical plexus block is performed by injecting a 3-in., 22-gauge needle at the midpoint along the posterior border of the sternocleidomastoid muscle. The needle is then advanced just past the sternocleidomastoid muscle and is directed along a line that would direct it to a point just behind the lobe of the ear. Local anesthetic injection is carried out in a fan-like direction prior to meticulous aspiration to rule out intravascular injection. Potential complications include intravascular injection of the external jugular vein and other contiguous large vessels as well as hematoma formation, particularly in patients receiving anticoagulants. Inadvertent epidural, subdural, and subarachnoid injection are also possible along with phrenic nerve blockade. Careful monitoring following superficial cervical plexus block is an important part of the post-block monitoring.

J. Deep Cervical Plexus Block

This block is performed with the patient placed in the supine position and with the head turned away from the side to be blocked.[13] It is used for treating painful conditions associated with pain of the strap muscles and contiguous structures in the neck. A marking pencil is used to mark a point approximately 2 inches below the mastoid process on a line drawn between the mastoid process and the posterior aspect of the insertion of the sternocleidomastoid muscle at the clavicle. A 3-in., 22-gauge needle is inserted approximately 2.0 to 2.5 cm anterior to the previously identified point on the line. This places the needle at the C3 or C4 level and allows a single needle to be used to block the deep cervical plexus. The needle is then advanced to a depth of about 2.0 cm in a slightly anterior and a slightly caudad direction to avoid entering the neural foramen or slipping in between the transverse processes and entering the vertebral artery. Paresthesias are usually sought and elicited and are used as the optimal end point of the needle probing. If a paresthesia is not elicited, the needle should be withdrawn and redirected in a slightly anterior direction. Meticulous aspiration is important here. In this situation not only are local anesthetics used but also botulinum toxin may be used to treat a variety of myofascial pain syndromes including cervical dystonias, spasmodic torticollis, and other myofascial pain syndromes of the neck.

K. Stellate Ganglion Block

Stellate ganglion block is useful for most sympathetically mediated pain involving the head, neck, upper extremities, and upper chest down to the T4 level at the nipple. It is useful in myofascial pain syndromes of the face, neck, upper extremity, and upper thorax when a sympathetic component is usually involved in the pathogenesis of that pain.[5]

Stellate ganglion block is usually performed by inserting a 3-in., 22-gauge needle at the level of the anterior tubercle of the transverse process of the sixth cervical vertebra while the carotid artery on the ipsilateral is retracted laterally. The needle is advanced perpendicularly to the skin and when contact with the transverse process is made, the needle is withdrawn for 1 or 2 mm and meticulous aspiration is performed to avoid inadvertent injection of the contiguous vertebral artery. The volume of local anesthetic usually injected is approximately 10 mL and meticulous aspiration should be carried out after every 1 to 2 cc injection to minimize intravascular injection.

A successful end point to this procedure is usually the occurrence of Horner's syndrome, consisting of miosis, enophthalmos, and ptosis. Other side effects associated with a successful stellate ganglion block include inadvertent block of the recurrent laryngeal nerve causing hoarseness and dysphagia and, in a few cases, an exacerbation of the pre-block pain.

L. Cervical Facet Block

Cervical facet blocks are used for the management of painful conditions associated with inflammatory changes of the cervical facet joints, osteoarthritis, and trauma associated with the neck. It is not unusual to have occipital pain, shoulder pain, and suprascapular pain associated with the neck pain.[17]

Before performing a cervical facet block, it is important to consider that each facet is innervated from two separate spinal levels. Each individual facet joint receives fibers from the dorsal ramus at the same level of the individual vertebra and, in addition, another source of innervation comes from the dorsal ramus of the vertebra immediately above the individual facet. Thus, for complete control of pain associated with a disease process from an individual facet joint, it is necessary to block the facet at the level of the lesion and also at the level immediately above the lesion. At each level, the dorsal ramus of the spinal nerve provides a medial branch that surrounds the convexity of the articular pillar of the respective vertebrae. Cervical facet blocks may be performed by using a blind technique or fluoroscopic guidance. Notwithstanding the technique used, a 22-gauge needle is inserted at a point slightly inferior and at a point approximately 2.5 cm lateral to the spinous process and directed in a slightly superior and medial direction toward the articular pillar of the facet to be blocked. After making contact with the transverse process, the needle is withdrawn slightly and then reintroduced toward the lateralmost aspect of the articular pillar. Ideally, fluoroscopic guidance is the technique of choice whenever possible. Careful aspiration should always be performed before injecting local anesthetic and/or steroids into the facet joint. This block is performed with the patient in the prone position and with some moderate flexion of the neck by placing a pillow under the chest.

2. Nerve Blocks of the Upper Extremity
   A. Brachial Plexus Block

   Typically, pain in the upper extremity may be controlled by blocking the brachial plexus.[9] The brachial plexus may be blocked using one of four different approaches. These include (a) the supraclavicular approach, (b) the infraclavicular approach,[15] (c) the interscalene approach,[21] and (d) the axillary approach.[7] There are individual merits and potential complications of each approach. The supraclavicular approach may be associated with pneumothorax whereas the interscalene approach may be associated with epidural and intrathecal injection. The infraclavicular approach is usually used when a continuous infusion is required, and the axillary approach, while being the least invasive of the four approaches, may be usually associated with incomplete pain relief in the entire upper extremity. This may be due to the unpredictable distribution of the local anesthetic as a result of tissue compartmentalization. Prior to blocking the brachial plexus, it is important to review the relevant anatomy and to have a clear appreciation of the roots, trunks, divisions, and cords associated with the brachial plexus.

   B. Suprascapular Nerve Blocks

   Suprascapular nerve blocks are reserved for pain of the shoulder, especially in adhesive capsulitis (frozen shoulder syndrome). This nerve is usually blocked with the patient in the sitting position. A 3-in., 22-gauge needle is inserted one fingerbreadth above the midline of the spine of the scapula and is directed inferiorly and slightly medially toward the suprascapular notch. A paresthesia is usually sought for the performance of this nerve block and, if it is not obtained, the needle is walked off the supraspinous area superiorly and medially while seeking a paresthesia. It is seldom necessary to insert the needle at a depth greater than 1 inch; this measure safeguards against the inadvertent puncture of the pleura, producing pneumothorax.

   Another technique that is used to prevent the onset of pneumothorax in the performance of the suprascapular nerve block is the injection of the patient using the landmarks described above, but doing so with the patient's hand on the side to be blocked being placed over the shoulder of the other side while the paresthesia is sought.[12] This movement serves to rotate the scapula anterolaterally, thus increasing the distance of the scapula from the chest wall and significantly reducing the risk of inadvertent pneumothorax.

   C. Radial Nerve Block at the Elbow

   The radial nerve can be blocked at the elbow by inserting a needle lateral to the insertion of the biceps tendon in the crease of the elbow and advancing the needle in a slightly medial and cephalad direction with the end point being the elicitation of a paresthesia down the lateral aspect of the forearm. Careful aspiration is performed prior to injection and, as a rule of thumb for this block and any other nerve block where paresthesia is sought, opioids should not be used during the performance of these nerve blocks so as to avoid obliterating the sensation of paresthesia.

D. Median Nerve Block at the Elbow

The median nerve may be blocked by inserting a 3-in., 22-gauge needle at a point in the crease of the elbow just medial to the brachial artery in the elbow. The artery is usually immediately medial to the biceps tendon. As the needle is inserted, paresthesias are usually elicited down the anterior aspect of the forearm.

In addition to blocking these nerves at the elbow, the median, ulnar, and radial nerves may be blocked at the wrist. These approaches are relatively straightforward and may be used to manage myofascial pain of the wrist and hand.

E. Intravenous Regional Block

Intravenous regional block with sympatholytic agents may be used for resistant myofascial pain syndromes of the upper extremity. This block is performed by obtaining intravenous access in the dorsum of the affected hand. The limb is then elevated for exsanguination purposes. Then an Esmarch bandage is applied from distal to proximal to the upper extremity and, by careful wrapping of the hand, further exsanguination can be obtained. A blood pressure cuff is applied over the proximal aspect of the Esmarch bandage and the distal cuff (if a two-cuff blood pressure cuff is used) is inflated to a pressure of approximately 100 mm Hg above the patient's systolic blood pressure. This prevents the inflow of blood into the exsanguinated upper extremity. Then the previously obtained intravenous access in the dorsum of the hand of the affected upper extremity is injected with a mixture of local anesthetic, a sympatholytic agent (e.g., guanethidine, labetalol, reserpine), heparin, and a corticosteroid. This solution is kept in the exsanguinated extremity for approximately 15 to 20 minutes and afterward the distal tourniquet is deflated and rapidly reinflated a few times. This process minimizes the release of toxic substances and drug mass into the general circulation.

3. Nerve Blocks Affecting the Chest

Chest wall myofascial pain may be controlled using a variety of nerve blocks. These include the following:

A. Intercostal Nerve Blocks

Intercostal nerve block may be administered by blocking the nerve at its inferior relationship with the continuous rib, and this is performed by using a short-bevel, 22-gauge, 1.5-in. needle that is aimed at the middle of the rib. While the left hand depresses the tissue over the rib, the right hand uses the needle to withdraw the needle over the retracted skin and subcutaneous tissue and walks it off the inferior margin of the rib. As soon as bony contact is lost, the needle is advanced approximately 2 mm deeper, placing it in proximity with the costal groove of the rib, where the intercostal nerve is located. After careful aspiration, approximately 3 to 5 mL of local anesthetic is injected. It is important to recognize that if the lesion causing the pain is at T5, then it is necessary to block the rib above and the rib below in order to optimize adequate analgesia.[11] Further, bilateral intercostal nerve blocks should never be performed, and it is important to recognize that, of all nerve blocks, intercostal nerve block possesses the greatest risk for producing the highest blood level concentration of local anesthetic, thus predisposing to intravascular complications.

B. Interpleural Nerve Block

This technique is usually done via a percutaneous technique and involves the placement of a catheter at a location between the visceral and parietal pleura superior to the rib. The advantage of this technique is that intermittent injections of local anesthetic may be performed to optimize analgesia. The risk of pneumothorax and possible intravascular toxicity is possible with this technique as indeed it is with intercostal nerve blocks.

C. Muscle Infiltration

In myofascial pain syndromes affecting the chest wall, there are a number of muscles that may be affected and may be the major source of pain in these syndromes. When these muscles are identified, they may be infiltrated with a combination of local anesthetics and methylprednisolone or related steroids with satisfactory analgesic results. Commonly affected muscles include:

1. rhomboid
2. pectoralis minor
3. pectoralis major
4. trapezius
5. sternocleidomastoid
6. deltoid

The general principles of nerve block therapy should be observed including meticulous aspiration to avoid intravascular injections and, in the chest wall, precautions against inadvertent pneumothorax.

D. Perichondrial Infiltration

In many patients with myofascial pain syndrome secondary to costochondritis, following median sternotomy for coronary bypass graft, and following chest wall injury, the cartilaginous attachments of the ribs and/or the sternum may be the source of pain. In these two situations, it may be useful to perform perichondrial infiltrations with local anesthetics and methylprednisolone for pain control, especially if the lesions are relatively acute in nature. Perichondrial infiltrations are not very effective if the lesion has been of long-standing duration.

E. Thoracic Field Block

Thoracic field block is usually reserved for patients with resistant chest pain with either a residual myofascial or neuropathic pain component. These are typically seen in patients with postherpetic neuralgia. In these situations, the area of pain is carefully demarcated and after appropriate prepping, a 6-in., 22-gauge needle is inserted subcutaneously in the appropriate tissue plane and is advanced subcutaneously along the borders of the demarcated painful area. It is important to avoid having the needle go internally, in which case pneumothorax may be a high possibility. Thus, the distal end of the needle should always be identified either visually or through palpation. As the needle is withdrawn, a mixture of local anesthetics and methylprednisolone is injected along the demarcated border, and this technique is performed along the area demarcated for the myofascial pain. Careful attention to the total mass of drug injected should always be observed so as to minimize seizure activity secondary to elevated serum levels of local anesthetic.

4. Nerve Blocks to the Abdomen
   A. Ilioinguinal Nerve Block

      Ilioinguinal nerve block is usually performed for myofascial pain present in the affected groin. This technique involves inserting a 1.5-in. needle at a point 2 inches medial and 2 inches inferior to the anterior superior iliac spine. The needle is usually inserted at an oblique angle and aimed towards the pubic symphysis. Paresthesias are usually elicited.

   B. Iliohypogastric Nerve Blocks

      Iliohypogastric nerve block is performed for painful conditions of the groin with a more lateral position in the groin and not involving the scrotal sac or vulval area. In this block, a 1.5-in., 22-gauge needle is inserted at a point 1 inch medial to and 1 inch inferior to the anterior superior iliac spine and is advanced in an oblique direction towards the pubic symphysis. The injections are usually carried out in a fan-like manner as the needle pierces the fascia of the external oblique muscle. Care must be taken not to advance too far internally because perforation of the abdominal cavity and its viscera is possible.

   C. Genitofemoral Nerve

      This nerve originates from the anterior primary rami of L1–2 and has a genital branch and a femoral branch. The genital branch innervates the perineal area and may be blocked by inserting a needle at a point just lateral to the pubic tubercle and injecting approximately 3.0 to 5.0 mL of a local anesthetic at that level. The femoral branch is blocked by identifying the middle third of the inguinal ligament and infiltrating a point just below the middle portion of the inguinal ligament with approximately 3.0 to 5.0 mL of local anesthetic.

   D. Injection of Hasselbach's Triangle

      Hasselbach's triangle is formed by lines connecting the following points: umbilicus, anterior superior iliac spine, and pubic symphysis. Pain in that lower quadrant of the abdomen usually follows groin injuries and postoperative inguinal hernia repair. Infiltration of that area may be used in critically ill patients who are not good candidates for general anesthesia or spinal anesthesia. Also, it may be used as a form of preemptive analgesia for patients undergoing inguinal hernia repair.

5. Nerve Blocks for the Back Area

   Trigger point injections are frequently performed in the back area because most of the muscles of the back including the longus colli and the paravertebral muscles are subject to trauma and inflammatory lesions causing pain. Trigger point injections of those areas are frequently performed for myofascial pain syndromes.

   An assortment of neuraxial nerve blocks including paravertebral nerve blocks and facet blocks may be performed using local anesthetics and, more recently, radiofrequency lesioning to manage persistent myofascial pain.

   Sacroiliac nerve blocks are very useful when sacroiliac arthropathy is present.

6. Pelvis and Perineal Nerve Blocks

   Myofascial pain of the pelvis and perineal areas is usually a part of a larger syndrome that generally responds to more invasive nerve blocks. These nerve blocks include caudal epidural nerve blocks, subarachnoid saddle blocks, ganglion impar blocks (Walther ganglion blocks), and superior hypogastric nerve blocks.

7. Nerve Blocks of the Lower Extremity

The lower extremity is typically innervated by four major nerves. The anterior thigh is innervated by the femoral nerve, the posterior thigh by the sciatic nerve, the medial thigh by the obturator nerve, and the lateral thigh by the femoral cutaneous nerve. In myofascial pain syndromes referable to the specific anatomic locations, those nerve blocks may be performed with good effects.[16]

A. Sciatic Nerve Block

The sciatic nerve block is usually blocked by inserting a 6-in., 22-gauge needle at a point midway between a line connecting the greater trochanter and the ischial tuberosity. The needle is advanced until a paresthesia is elicited down the posterior aspect of the leg.

B. Femoral Nerve Block

The femoral nerve is usually blocked by inserting a needle immediately lateral to the palpated femoral artery in the groin and advancing perpendicularly seeking paresthesias. In this situation, meticulous aspiration should be carried out prior to and during the injection to avoid intravascular injection.

C. Obturator Nerve Block

The obturator nerve block is performed by inserting a needle 1 inch laterally and 1 inch inferior to the pubic tubercle and injecting in a fan-like direction because the obturator nerve usually begins dividing at a very proximal level in the groin.

D. Lateral Femoral Cutaneous Nerve Block

The lateral femoral cutaneous nerve is very useful for treating pain along the anterolateral aspect of the thigh. This condition is usually called neuralgia hyperesthetica and may be associated with various inflammatory lesions or trauma in the region of the anterior superior iliac spine. This pain may also follow radiotherapy to the pelvis as a result of trauma to the lateral femoral cutaneous nerve of thigh. This nerve is usually blocked by inserting a 1.5-in., 22-gauge needle at a point 1 inch medial to the anterior superior iliac spine and just inferior to the inguinal ligament. Occasionally, the nerve may be just inferior to the ligamentous structure—the tensor fascia lata—and this is usually identified by feeling a popping sensation as the needle goes through this ligament. Fan-like injection is recommended so that all the divided branches of this nerve may be effectively blocked.

E. Modified Sciatic Nerve Block

The sciatic nerve block may be blocked at the posterior knee level in a modified sciatic nerve block technique. This is useful for children and is a good measure of preemptive analgesia for foot surgery. In this situation, the needle is inserted in the apex of the popliteal fossa in the posterior aspect of the knee and paresthesias are sought.

F. Ankle Blocks

Ankle blocks are usually effective in dealing with ankle and foot pain. The nerves to be blocked for comprehensive analgesia of the ankle area include:

1. Sural nerve
2. Posterior tibial nerve
3. Deep peroneal nerve
4. Superficial peroneal nerve
5. Saphenous nerve

Singly or collectively, these nerves when effectively blocked would provide effective analgesia of the affected foot.

Conclusion

Myofascial pain syndrome may be effectively treated if all the appropriate therapeutic modalities are applied. Nerve block therapy represents an added therapeutic advantage in the management of persistent and/or unresponsive cases of myofascial pain syndromes. Meticulous history taking and physical examination with appropriate diagnosis are important prior to the application of appropriate therapeutic modalities. Thus, the various nerve blocks described in this chapter may play a significant role in the management of myofascial pain syndromes.

References

1. Bonica JJ: The Management of Pain. Philadelphia, Lea & Febiger, 1953.
2. Bonica JJ: Clinical Applications of Diagnostic and Therapeutic Nerve Blocks. Springfield, Ill, Thomas, 1959.
3. Bridenbaugh PO, Cousins MJ: Neural Blockade in Clinical Anesthesia and Management of Pain. Philadelphia, Lippincott, 1988.
4. Brown DT, Beamish D, Wildsmith JAW: Allergic reaction to an amide local anesthetic. Br J Anaesth 53:435, 1981.
5. Carron H, Litwiller R: Stellate ganglion block. Anesth Analg 54:567, 1975.
6. Covino BG: Pharmacology of local anesthetic agents. Br J Anaesth 5:701, 1986.
7. deJong RH: Axillary block of the brachial plexus. Anesthesiology 22:215, 1961.
8. Delaney TJ, Rowlingson JC, Carron H, et al: The effects of steroids on nerves and meninges. Anesth Analg 59:610, 1980.
9. Kulenkampff D: Anesthesia of the brachial plexus (German). Zentralbl Chir 38:1337, 1911.
10. Moore DC: Regional Block, 4th ed. Springfield, Ill, Thomas, 1975.
11. Parris WCV: Nerve block therapy. Clin Anesthesiol 3:93, 1985.
12. Parris WCV: Suprascapular nerve block: A safer technique. Anesthesiology 72:580, 1990.
13. Parris WCV: Nerve block therapy. In Contemporary Issues in Chronic Pain Management. Boston, Kluwer, 1991, p 171.
14. Parris WCV, Dettbarn WD: Muscle atrophy following bupivacaine trigger point injection. Anesthesiol Rev 16:50, 1988.
15. Raj PP, Montgomery SJ, Nettles D, et al: Infraclavicular brachial plexus block: A new approach. Anesth Analg 52:987, 1973.
16. Raj PP, Pai U: Upper and Lower Extremity Blocks. In PP Raj (ed): Practical Management of Pain, 2nd ed. St Louis, Mo, Mosby, 1992, p 743.
17. Raj PP, Pai U, Rawal N: Techniques of regional anesthesia in adults. In PP Raj (ed): Clinical Practice of Regional Anesthesia. New York, Churchill Livingstone, 1991.
18. Reiz S, Nath S: Cardiotoxicity of local anaesthetic agents. Br J Anaesth 58:736, 1986.
19. Ritchie JM, Ritchie B, Greengard P: The active structure of local anesthetics. J Pharmacol Exp Ther 150:152, 1965.
20. Standards for cardiopulmonary resuscitation (CPR) and emergency cardiac care (ECC). JAMA 227(Suppl.):883, 1992.
21. Winnie AP: Interscalene brachial plexus block. Anesth Analg 49;455, 1970.

Part III

Physical Therapy and Rehabilitation

Chapter 15

Muscle Deficiency

Hans Kraus, MD†

Myofascial Pain

Myofascial pain can be categorized into four types: (1) muscle spasm, (2) muscle tension, (3) muscle deficiency, and (4) trigger points.

Medical literature tends to concentrate on trigger points and injection therapy to the exclusion of the other types of myofascial pain. The clinical facts contradict such emphasis. I can find no better way to clarify this than to describe my own experience with the history of myofascial pain.

When I was a resident in 1931 at the fracture service of Wienna University's Department of Surgery, it was the custom to treat acute muscle spasm—following sprain, strain, or fracture—with either immobilization or traction. My coach, Heinz Kowalski, taught me differently. The way he treated an injured extremity was to wrap it in towels soaked with alcohol, expose it to live steam, and follow up with gentle limbering movements. This method produced much more rapid and satisfactory results than our usual immobilization.

Taking a cue from Kowalski, I used the same treatment on two skiers with sprained ankles and was surprised to find how quickly their pain was relieved and full function restored. Later, in an attempt to improve on this cumbersome method involving alcohol and live steam, I experimented with various fluids. Eventually, I hit on ethyl chloride as the most effective means of relieving discomfort and facilitating movement.[7, 8] Ethyl chloride is superior to procaine (Novocain) injections because it does not mask pathologic conditions; the hypoesthesia it produces is only temporary and does not affect major injuries. With ethyl chloride I began to obtain consistently favorable results in treating sprains, muscle strains, partial ligament tears, back pain, and certain types of impacted fractures.[16]

I followed this treatment with exercises to strengthen, limber, and stretch the affected muscles. Not only was the period of disability shortened considerably, but improvement was usually permanent. I became so involved in therapeutic exercise that I established an exercise department: adjacent to the fracture service. However, although exercise helped increase function, I discovered this same treatment frequently to be ineffective in alleviating chronic pain.

Fortunately, I came across a book written in 1931 by Max Lange,[19] with a lengthy description of "myogelosis" or muscle hardening, which he treated with deep point massage on or glucose injections. Lange's coworkers, Glogowsky and Wallraff,[4] performed biopsies on these tender spots and found them to be degenerated areas of muscle tissue. In 1959, Steindler[25] described these tender nodules as trigger points. Lange discussed not only all the most common trigger points but also indicated their locations at the myofascial or myotendinous junction. After studying his book, I added trigger point injections and needling to my treatment of chronic muscle pain. Later, I discovered that gentle relaxing and limbering exercises, in combination with ethyl chloride spray and 15 minutes of sinusoidal current, were an important follow-up to injection and notably improved the chances of success.

---

†Deceased. Revisions to this chapter by Isabel Rachlin, P.T.

I was now aware of three types of muscle pain: muscle deficiency (weakness and stiffness), muscle spasm, and trigger points.

Between 1940 and 1946, at the Posture Clinic at Columbia Presbyterian Hospital in New York, Dr. Sonya Weber and I developed a test chart to appraise faulty posture and scoliosis.[13] This chart included six tests for strength and flexibility of key posture muscles. In 1946, we used these so-called Kraus-Weber tests to evaluate patients in a multidisciplinary back clinic organized by Dr. Barbara Stimson at the same hospital. Eighty-two percent of the 3000 back patients we saw in the clinic had no pathologic condition[3]; their back pain was of postural or muscular origin. These patients often turned out to be deficient in one or more of the six key posture muscles. An exercise program aimed at correcting these deficiencies obtained satisfactory results.[8] I was now even more convinced of the value of properly prescribed therapeutic exercise.

Because back pain was endemic in the United States, we wondered how children would fare on the Kraus-Weber tests. Although children rarely suffer from backache, the unfitness of their trunk muscles seemed to prognosticate future problems. Accordingly, we examined 5000 youngsters between 5 and 16 years of age. Almost 60% failed one or more of the tests.[15] This result seemed to explain the frequency of back pain among adults.

To verify these facts, we traveled to Europe in 1951 to test 1000 children each in Switzerland, Austria, and Italy. We selected these countries because at that time they had a much smaller incidence of back pain than the United States. Fewer than 10% failed the tests.[15] In fact, none failed more than one of the six components of the test, whereas our children frequently failed two or three components. Our children were better nourished but sat much more than their European counterparts, who had to walk everywhere. The U.S. children spent more time watching television than engaging in active play. Schools concentrated their physical education efforts on sports and games that involved the fittest children while neglecting the others.

When President Eisenhower was informed of the unfit condition of children, he established the President's Council on Youth Fitness, since renamed the President's Council on Physical Fitness and Sports.

We found the same kind of sedentary lifestyle in our adult back pain population, who were also exposed to tension-creating stress. Suppression of the normal biologic fight-or-flight response[1] meant that people had no physical release for stress. Tension thus appeared to form another link in the pathogenesis of myofascial pain. We recognized tension as the fourth important cause of muscle pain. The absence of a normal response to stress and the role of underexercise in the development of balanced physiology became important aspects of our approach to treating myofascial pain.

Myofascial back and neck pain may frequently be one indication of hypokinetic disease (disease produced by stress and lack of exercise).[18] It has been shown that duodenal ulcers, coronary heart disease, overweight, diabetes, and emotional problems may be due, at least in part, to the imbalance between stress and physical release.[18]

It is obvious that injections alone will not help a person who has no physical outlet, exhibits weakness and stiffness of key postural muscles, and leads a tension-filled life. A concerted effort is required to manage muscle deficiency with exercise and to manage tension in various ways: with relaxation exercise, medication, biofeedback, and psychiatry, when needed. A patient's lifestyle, working posture, and physical activities may require modification.

Injecting trigger points is important in chronic cases. The use of surface anesthesia (cold) and gentle motion is essential for breaking spasm in the acute phase. In chronic cases, all four types of myofascial pain may be present. The patient may present with acute muscle spasm. When spasm is relieved, we may find trigger points, muscle deficiency, tension, or any combination of these. We then proceed with trigger point injections, exercises directed at muscle deficiency, and relaxation. Merely relieving pain is simplistic. Any treatment that does not include specific exercises and relaxation training and fails to modify pathogenic activities and lifestyle will yield only temporary results.

Treatment

The best way of treating muscle deficiency, which is the diminution of strength or flexibility, or both, is with exercise. Exercise is also an essential element in treating tension, muscle spasm, and the aftereffects of trigger point injection.

Exercise is the most effective and frequently needed modality in managing myofascial pain. Unfortunately, it is prescribed cavalierly. Few physicians know the basic principles of exercise. Even fewer are familiar with the details.

When properly prescribed and executed, exercise can be a very important therapeutic agent. It deserves the same careful attention as prescribing medication. This includes the correct indication, type, and quality of exercise. No physician would consider prescribing "heart medicine" as such, and yet therapeutic exercise is often prescribed as "back exercise" and its execution left haphazardly to a therapist. Therapists are frequently trained to give a standard set of exercises to all comers, regardless of the complaint.

In order to prescribe exercise properly, one has to evaluate the patient's individual needs. This is achieved by testing strength and flexibility.[10] The basic qualities of muscle function are contraction, strength, and flexibility. Flexibility consists of two parts: (1) physiologic elasticity, i.e., the ability to relax, give up tension, and decontract; and (2) mechanical elasticity, i.e., yielding to active or passive stretch.

How can muscle strength be gauged? For the extremities we advocate the old Lovett[21] approach, which is still useful and does not require any machines. The Lovett scale tests 0, if the muscle cannot contract at all; 1, if it can contract but cannot produce movement; 2, if it can contract and move with assistance; 3, if it can move against gravity and minimal resistance; 4, if it can overcome gravity and increased resistance to 70% of normal function; and 5, if it has full strength in comparison with the contralateral side or the patient's previous ability.

To assess strength and flexibility of key posture muscles, we use the Kraus-Weber tests[13, 14] (Fig. 15–1A–F). The most common findings in back problems are stiffness of back and hamstring muscles and weakness of abdominal muscles.

To test total flexibility of a joint, we first appraise the patient's ability to relax. When the patient has relaxed as much as possible, we ask him or her to extend the joint to full range. We measure the excursion with a goniometer. In the Kraus-Weber tests, we gauge flexibility by noting the difference between the spontaneous floor reach and the floor reach after the patient is told not to try hard but to let go. The increased reach correlates with tension.

There are two types of strengthening exercises: anisometric and isometric.[6, 20] In anisometric exercise, the patient goes through the full range of motion. This means contracting or gradually lengthening against weight or resistance. Anisometric exercises are the most frequently used exercises, especially gradual shortening against resistance (concentric contraction). In isometric exercise, the muscle is tightened against resis-

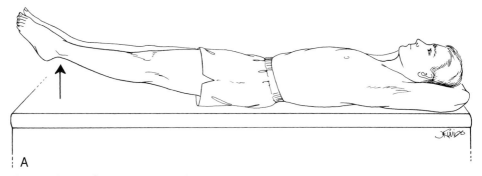

Figure 15–1. A, the patient is supine, hands behind the neck, and legs extended with the knees straight. The patient is asked to lift both feet 10 in. off the table, holding that position for 10 seconds. This is a test for hip flexor muscles.

Illustration continued on following page

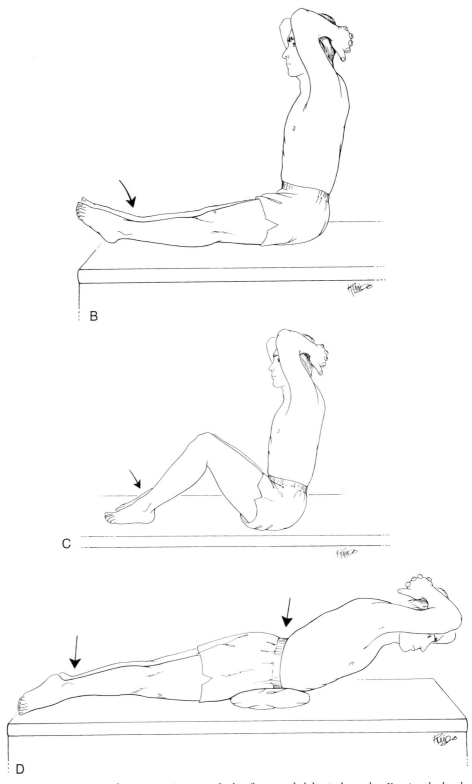

Figure 15–1. *Continuued. B*, test no. 2 is a test for hip flexors and abdominal muscles. Keeping the hands behind the neck, the patient is asked to roll up to a sitting position, with the legs straight, and the ankles held down. The arrow indicates the point at which the patient's body is stabilized by another person. *C*, this is a test for the abdominal muscles. With the patient in the supine position, hands behind the neck, with knees flexed, the examiner holds the patient's feet down on the table (indicated by arrow). The patient is asked to "roll up to a sitting position." *D*, test for upper back muscles. Lying prone with a pillow under the hips, the hands behind the neck and the feet and hips held down, the patient is asked to raise the trunk and hold for 10 seconds. Arrows indicate point at which the patient's body is stabilized by another person.

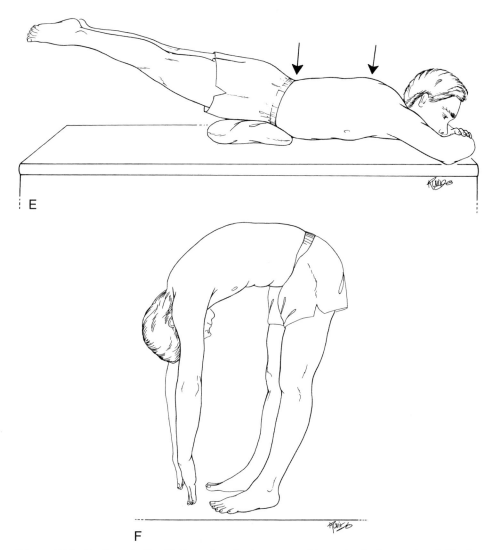

Figure 15–1. *Continuued. E,* with the patient in the same position as in *D,* the examiner holds the shoulders and hips down (indicated by arrows). The patient is asked to raise both legs and hold for 10 seconds. This tests the muscles of the lower back. *F,* this is a test for muscle flexibility and muscle tension. With the patient standing erect with the feet together, the knees extended, and his hands at his sides, he is asked to try to touch the floor with the fingertips. If the patient cannot touch the floor he is asked to try again, this time being asked to relax, drop the head forward, and try to let the torso "hang" from the hips. The patient is told not to try hard but to let go. The increased reach on the second attempt correlates with the presence of muscle tension.

tance but without movement. Isometric exercises can be useful as part of a program, but should never be attempted without warm-up, relaxation, and stretching before and after.

We always give the muscle sufficient rest between movements. In the case of the extremities, we first have the patient warm up with general exercises for the whole extremity, then concentrate on the muscle group that needs strengthening. We never give multirepetitions but have the patient perform various movements in turn. If the extremity is weak, we work each muscle group three or four times, then proceed to the next group, and the next, before returning to the first. When we notice that the patient is beginning to tire, we stop. Gradually we add more demanding exercises.

In our back program,[11] we try to alternate prone and supine exercises in which, by working the antagonists, we give the muscles alternate chances to rest. Here again, patients are limited to three repetitions at a time.

The successful possibilities of such a program are evidenced by the "Y's Way to a Healthy Back"[22] program, which we devised in 1972 and which operated until December 1986. These exercises were intended to address the main deficiencies seen in our population at the Columbia Presbyterian Hospital's back clinic.[9] The program included strengthening abdominal muscles and limbering, relaxing, and stretching back muscles and hamstrings. In a one-on-one situation in private practice, we add further exercises, if needed. For example, we may work at strengthening upper or lower back muscles, although these muscles are seldom weak enough to require such exercises.

Thanks to the work of its organizer, Mr. Alexander Melleby, the "Y's Way to a Healthy Back" was eventually offered in a thousand YMCAs and YWCAs throughout the country. Six thousand physical educators were trained in a program that developed trainers as well as exercise instructors. All were taught to give the same exercises in a standardized way. At its height, the program functioned in the United States, Canada, Japan, Taiwan, and Australia.

The results of these original exercises were reviewed in a study of 11,809 participants,[17] who were tested with the Kraus-Weber tests before and after taking part. Of these, 80.7% said they felt better after completing the exercise series, which consisted of two sessions a week for 6 weeks.

Unfortunately, when Mr. Melleby retired, his successors found it necessary to alter the exercises and to leave out some essential movements and alternating positions. The program was gradually used less and less. In my opinion it cannot be as effective as the original program.

When administering strengthening exercises, we must be aware of just how much the patient can tolerate. While it is necessary to give an "overload,"[5] i.e., somewhat more than the patient can accomplish easily, working to fatigue is contraindicated.

Peder Palmen[23] showed that fatigue exercises for healthy young athletes result in declining performance. Improvement takes place only after 4 days of exercise during which performance decreases. If you put a patient's weak muscles onto a similar regimen, he or she will not be able to perform at all and will require a few days of rest, after which you will have to start all over again. If the same process is repeated, the same result will occur. In other words, in order to strengthen a weak muscle, we have to increase our demands gradually instead of working to maximum capacity. This precept is often overlooked.

In the case of patients who have had a leg encased in plaster following surgery or injury to knee or ankle, the muscles tend to be quite weak. Nonetheless, patients are often instructed to walk as much as possible. The result is stiffness, pain, and the frequent development of trigger points.

Before addressing flexibility, we must first treat the tension that is inherent to some degree in almost everyone. For this reason, we begin all flexibility exercises with relaxation. Next, we treat mechanical flexibility by stretching the muscle, first actively, by using the antagonists to gain full range, and then passively, by stretching the muscle gently. Before giving passive stretch, we often use "reflex relaxation,"[24] giving resistance to the antagonist of the tight muscle. For example, we give resistance to extensors, which causes the flexors to relax, or vice versa. Reflex relaxation increases muscle range. When the patient cannot go beyond that range, the therapist helps with passive stretching.

Passive stretching or violent active stretching without prior relaxation and warm-up can lead to muscle strain and diminished range. Just as we do not work to full capacity in our strengthening exercises, we do not attempt to obtain maximum range in our flexibility treatment. Maximum stretch will cause discomfort and result in limited rather than increased range. The basic rule is never to exceed existing pain limits. In stretching, however, we sometimes have to raise the pain threshold by using cold (ethyl chloride spray or ice).

After the patient has been fully rehabilitated, he or she should continue therapeutic exercises, to which can be added more strenuous physical activities such as swimming, fast walking, bicycling, or jogging. Demanding exercises have a relaxing effect that can be measured by electromyogram. DeVries and Adams[2] have shown that exercises which raise the heartbeat to 100 or 120 beats/min produce greater relaxation than 500 mg of meprobamate.

The most common mistakes incurred in prescribing therapeutic exercises are the following[11, 12]:

1. Prescribing a program without previous muscle testing.
2. Omitting warm-up and cool-down exercises, which should include relaxing and limbering.
3. Handing out an exercise sheet, thereby leaving the entire treatment to the patient.
4. Giving multirepetition exercises.
5. Prescribing isometric exercises as the main part of the program, without stressing relaxation and stretching of the same muscle groups.
6. Giving too many or too strenuous exercises instead of gradually adding more demanding ones.
7. Doing the exercises in rapid succession without relaxing between movements.
8. Omitting the home program, which the patient should perform daily.
9. Discharging the patient too soon, i.e., before he or she is fully capable of resuming all normal activities. This means strengthening the muscles far above their minimal ability.

One back patient whom we saw had a job which required him to lift 200-lb weights. After treatment, his lifting ability was only 100 lbs. His insurance carrier insisted against our advice that he return to work and that he perform weightlifting exercises until he regained his former strength. After a few weeks, the patient returned with the same injury.

In treating acute muscle spasm, we give the first three or four exercises of the respective program (back, shoulder, neck), while relieving pain with electrotherapy and ethyl chloride spray. We have the patient perform these exercises frequently at home, using ice. We avoid bed rest and immobilization whenever possible.

The following is a list of exercises we have used for many years, first in rehabilitation fracture patients at the Vienna University Medical School, later in treating posture and back patients at Columbia Presbyterian Hospital with Dr. Barbara Stimson, and in over 50 years of private practice.

Exercise for the Extremities

In the acute phase: Perform only the first two or three exercises, using ice or ethyl chloride spray. Gradually increase the number and intensity of exercises.

In the chronic phase: Always relax between movements. Provide resistance to antagonists in order to achieve reflex relaxation. Stretch gently, always within pain limits.

Begin all exercises with relaxation. Have the patient lie on his or her back with a pillow under the knees (Fig. 15–2). Tell the patient to close the eyes, take a deep breath, exhale slowly, drop the head to the left, then to the right, pull up the shoulders,

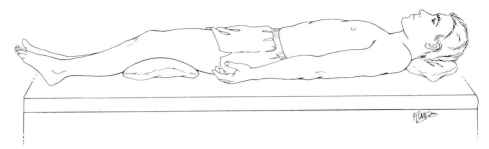

Figure 15–2.

and let go. Continue until the patient is relaxed. Perform the first four relaxation exercises of the neck program (exercises 50–53).

Exercises should be performed no more than three times in succession, with rest between each movement. Perform each series in sequence, forward and backward, several times. *The most frequent mistakes are:*

- Starting antigravity exercises before the patient is adequately strengthened.
- Giving too strenuous resistance or stretching.
- Using wall climbing or pendulum exercises (the latter are insufficient to increase range or strength).
- Omitting relaxation.
- Giving isometric exercises alone, without the full program.

Exercises for the Upper Extremities

Shoulder. The first five exercises should first be performed lying down, then sitting up.

1. Close the fist, touch the shoulder, and extend and unclench the fist (Fig. 15–3).
2. With hands on chest, abduct, sliding the elbows upward, and then bring them back to the original position (Fig. 15–4).
3. Extend arm straight up, bring it down, and relax (Fig. 15–5).
4. Bring the arm across the chest and return to the standing position (Fig. 15–6).
5. Join hands, bring them down in front of the legs, then raise the arms above the head (Fig. 15–7).

The following exercises should be performed sitting up or standing:

6. Touch the back of the neck reaching down as far as possible (Fig. 15–8).
7. Touch the lower back and slide the hand up as far as possible (Fig. 15–9).
8. Continue the previous exercise by pulling the hand up with the help of the injured arm or by pulling the end of a towel (Fig. 15–10).
9. Fold the arms behind the neck and bring the elbows back. Bring elbows forward, then relax (Fig. 15–11).

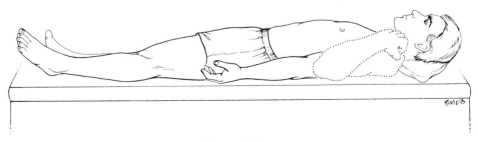

Figure 15–3.

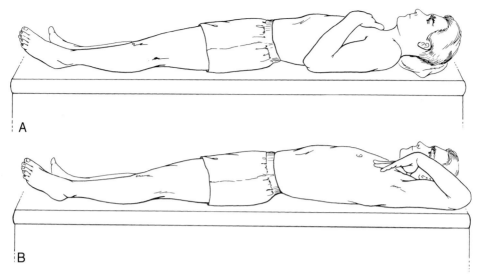

A

B

Figure 15–4.

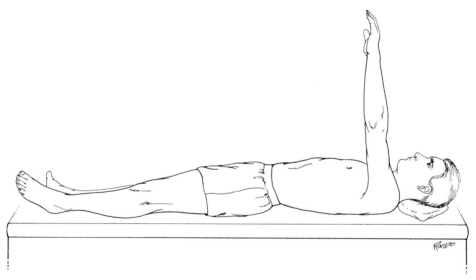

Figure 15–5.

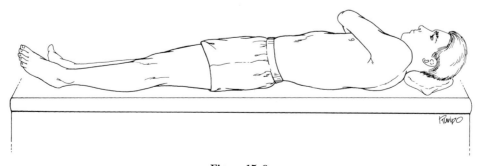

Figure 15–6.

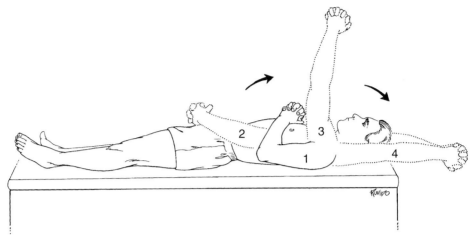

Figure 15–7.

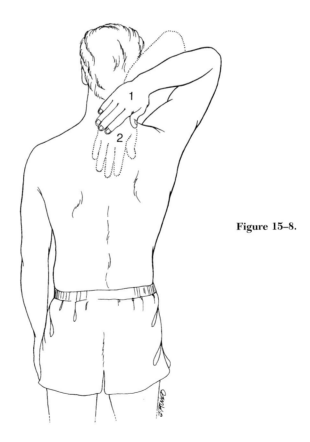

Figure 15–8.

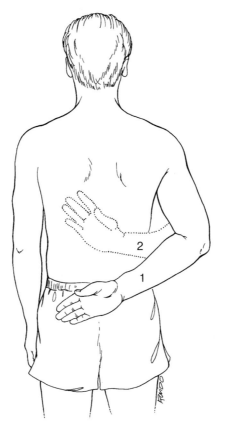

Figure 15–9.

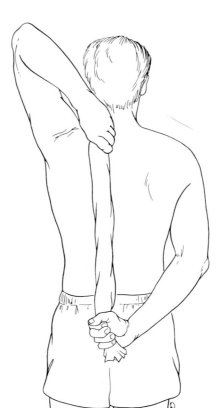

Figure 15–10.

447

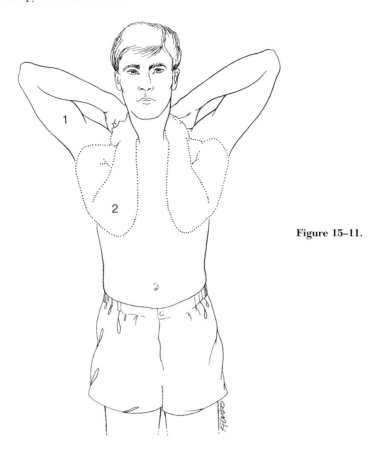

Figure 15–11.

Elbow. Use shoulder exercises as warm-up. All exercises are first performed lying down, then sitting or standing:

10. Bend and extend the elbow with the palm facing up and then with the palm facing down (Fig. 15–12).
11. Bring the hand across the chest to the opposite shoulder, turn out, turn in (Fig. 15–13).
12. To stretch elbow flexors, join hands, raise to shoulder height, pronate, and extend as far as possible, using the good hand to increase range (Fig. 15–14).

Wrist and Hand. Use shoulder and elbow exercises as warm-up. The following exercises may be performed sitting.

13. Flex and extend the wrist over the edge of a table or pillow.
14. Use exercise 11 for supination and pronation.
15. Close and open the fist, first with the thumb inside the fingers, then with the thumb outside.
16. Spread and close the fingers.
17. Knead clay or putty to increase the strength of the flexors.

Exercises for the Lower Extremities

Begin with relaxation exercises (exercises 50–53), as earlier. Perform each exercise in a sequence of three. At first, while there is discomfort and the leg is weak, all lower extremity exercises should be done lying down. Slide the leg along the surface in the beginning. Later, lift against gravity. As the patient gets stronger, use the entire exercise program as a warm-up and follow with specific exercises and gradually increasing resistance. Lastly, use weights for work at home.

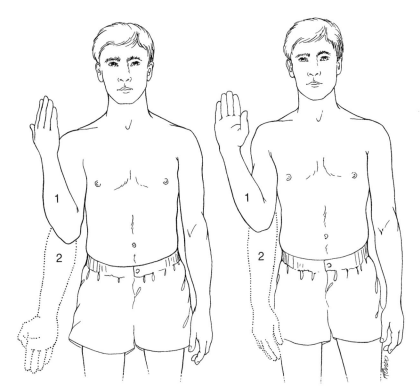

Figure 15–12.

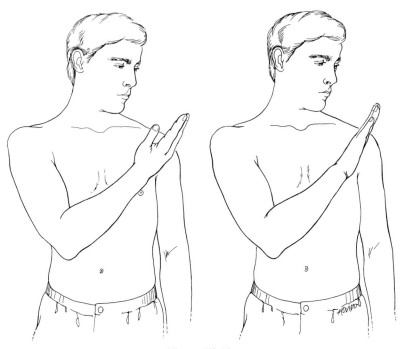

Figure 15–13.

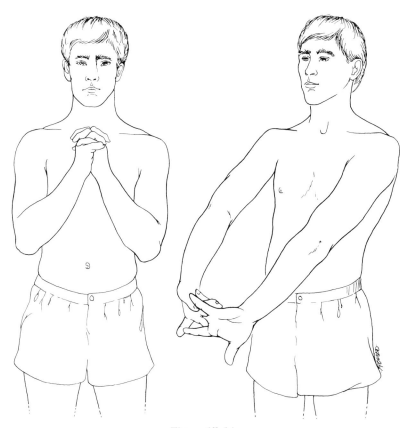

Figure 15–14.

Hip

18. Lying on the back, bring the knee to the chest, then straighten out. Relax (Fig. 15–15A).

19. Lying on the back with the knees flexed, bring the knee to the chest, slide to full extension, and return to the flexed position. Alternate with the other knee (Fig. 15–15B).

20. Perform the same movement while lying on the side. Alternate legs (Fig. 15–16).

21. Prone, tighten buttocks, and relax (Fig. 15–17).

22. Again supine, abduct and adduct extending the legs (Fig. 15–18).

23. Supine, with knee flexed, abduct and adduct (Fig. 15–19).

24. Lying on the side, abduct with a straight leg, lower it, and relax (Fig. 15–20).

25. Lying on the side, abduct with flexed knee.

The last two exercises should be performed with a therapist's assistance. The patient should not attempt them at home until he or she can do so without strain or discomfort. The following four exercises are all performed prone.

26. Flex and extend the knee (Fig. 15–21).

27. Flex knees and rotate hips out and in (Fig. 15–22).

28. Flex the knee and lift the leg (Fig. 15–23).

29. Repeat exercise 28, with the knee extended.

30. Sitting with the legs hanging over the edge of the table, with the good leg resting on the floor or a stool, bring the affected knee to the chest, bring the leg down, and relax (Fig. 15–24).

31. Sitting in the same position, extend the knee fully. Keep foot outwardly rotated in order to strengthen the vastus medialis (Fig. 15–25).

Text continued on page 455

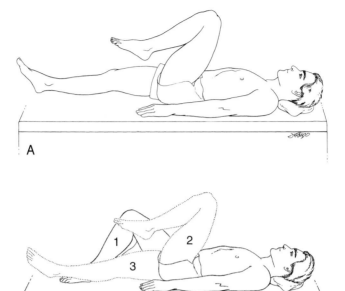

A

B

Figure 15–15.

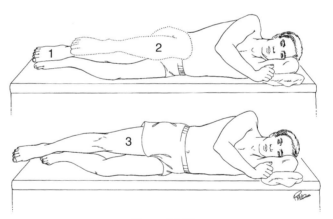

Figure 15–16.

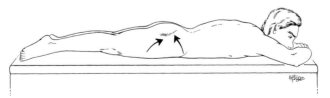

Figure 15–17.

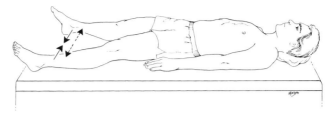

Figure 15–18.

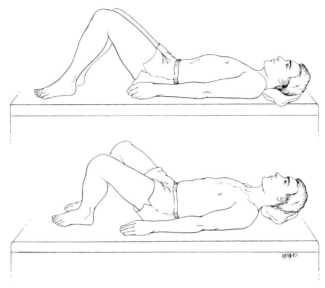

Figure 15–19.

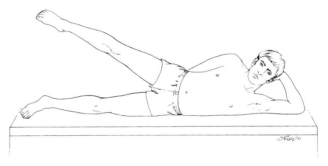

Figure 15–20.

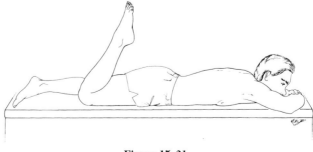

Figure 15–21.

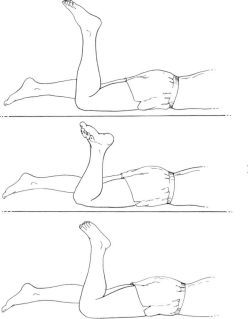

Figure 15–22.

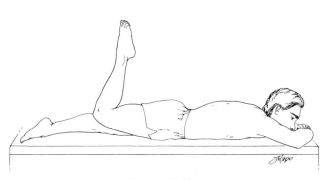

Figure 15–23.

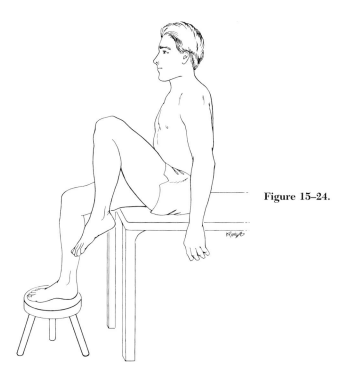

Figure 15–24.

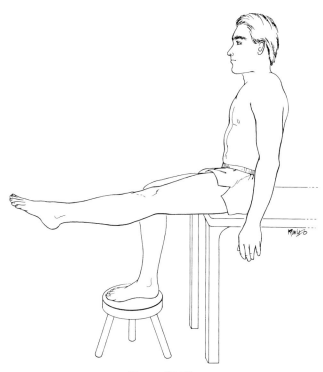

Figure 15–25.

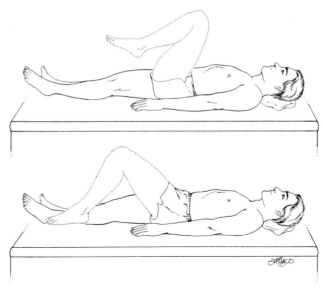

Figure 15–26.

Knee

32a. Supine, gently bend and extend the injured knee (Fig. 15–26).

32b. Supine with the knees flexed, extend the knee, and flex back to the starting position (Fig. 15–27).

32c. Supine, with the knees flexed, bring the knee to the chest, extend, and return to flexed position.

33. With a pillow under the knee, extend the leg (Fig. 15–28).

34. Tighten quadriceps and let go.

35. Prone, flex and extend the knee (see Fig. 15–21).

36. Supine, do bicycle stretch. Bring knee to chest, extend toward ceiling, stretch out, and slowly return to the flexed position. Do this first with the toes pointed, then with the heel first (Fig. 15–29).

37. Sitting with the legs hanging over the edge of the table, with the good leg supported, extend the knee. Hold foot in outward rotation. The patient may add weights when flexibility is achieved and the pain is gone (see Fig. 15–25).

Isometric Exercises

38. Supine, with the leg straight and outwardly rotated (held down by the therapist or by a heavy piece of furniture), tighten the quadriceps and attempt to raise the leg against resistance. Hold for 10 seconds and release.

39. Repeat exercise 38, holding the leg extended for 10 seconds against resistance.

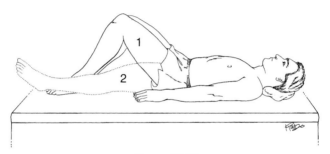

Figure 15–27.

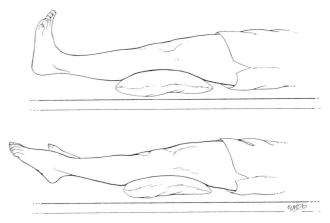

Figure 15–28.

Ankle

40. Supine, with the knees straight, dorsiflex and plantarflex ankle.
41. Repeat, with the knees flexed.
42. With the knees straight, pronate and supinate (Fig. 15–30*A*).
43. Sitting with the legs hanging over the edge of the table, dorsiflex and plantarflex.
44. Repeat, with pronation and supination.
45. Flex and extend the toes (Fig. 15–30*B*).

The following four exercises are performed standing:

46. Holding onto the table, stand on toes and increase lifting body weight as tolerated (Fig. 15–31).
47. Holding onto the table, bend the knees, keeping the heels on the floor.
48. Holding onto a table or leaning against a wall, with heels on floor, lean forward from the hips (Fig. 15–32).
49. Stand on the outside, then on the inside, of the foot, holding onto a table if necessary.

The most common mistakes in lower extremity exercises are:

- Permitting walking and weight-bearing when these cause pain or limping.
- Administering antigravity exercises too soon.

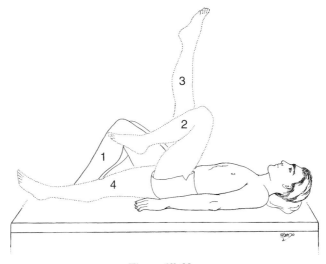

Figure 15–29.

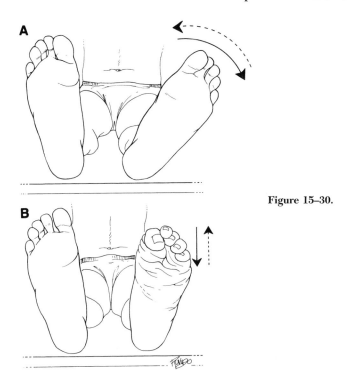

Figure 15–30.

• Performing multirepetition straight leg raises, which can produce backache and tight quadriceps.

Neck Exercises

The basic position is supine with the knees flexed. Exercises should always be done slowly, with rest between movement. No exercise is performed more than three times in succession. The exercise order is reversed as a cool-down.

50. The patient, positioned comfortably in the supine position with the knees flexed, takes a deep breath and exhales slowly with the eyes closed. Slide one leg out and slide it back, alternating legs. Tighten both fists, then let go and take another deep breath. Bring up the shoulders and let go. Breathe in when shrugging up, exhale when letting go of the shrug. Drop the head to the left, return to the normal position, then permit the head to drop to the right. Repeat until completely relaxed (Fig. 15–33).
51. Turn the head to the left, return to a normal position in front followed by rotation to the right, returning to the normal front and center position (Fig. 15–34).
52. Tilt the head to the left, then to the right.
53. Pull the shoulder blades together; relax.

Repeat the above movements sitting up. In addition, flex and extend the neck. Add gentle passive and active stretching, first supine, then sitting.

Back Exercises*

54. Perform the first four relaxation exercises (50–53) of the neck program.
55. Supine, with the knees flexed, bring the knee to the chest, extend, and return to the flexed position. When extending the leg the foot is returned to the floor permitting the leg to slide out and slide back (see Fig. 15–15B).

---

*A videotape, *Say Goodbye to Back Pain,* including neck exercises, is available by calling 1-800-383-8811.

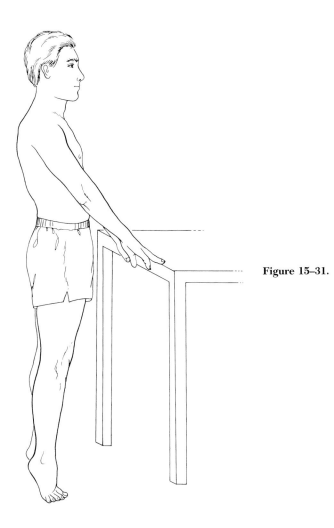

Figure 15–31.

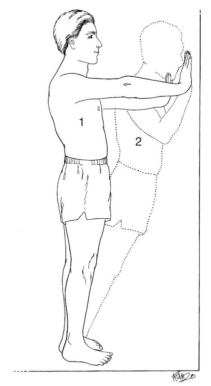

Figure 15–32.

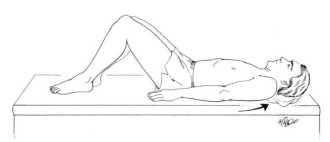

Figure 15–33.

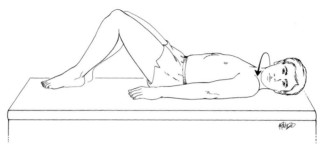

Figure 15–34.

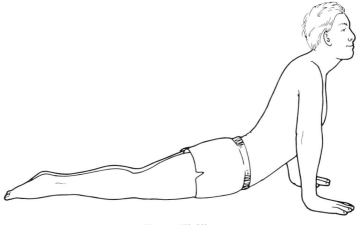

Figure 15–35.

56. Repeat, alternately lying on either side. Remember to slide the leg when it is extended. Do not tense the top leg. The leg should be "dead weight" (see Fig. 15–16).

57. Prone, tighten buttocks and relax (see Fig. 15–17).

58. Prone, hands under shoulders, straighten the arms while keeping the hips on the floor (Fig. 15–35).

59. In the basic position, bring both knees to the chest, then return to the basic position. Do not raise the hips off the floor (Fig. 15–36).

60. On hands and knees, arch back, then collapse to swayback position ("cat back") (Fig. 15–37).

61. In the basic position, raise the head and shoulders reaching toward the knees. Perform the exercise slowly. Relax (Fig. 15–38).

62. Kneeling with the forearms resting on a plinth, slowly slide hands forward, stretching the pectoral muscles. Maintain the thighs perpendicular to the floor (Fig. 15–39).

63. From hands and knee position, bring the hips back (buttocks resting on heels), relaxing the torso, neck, and face (Fig. 15–40).

64. Sitting on the edge of a table or chair with the feet on the floor or a stool, slowly drop the head and arms between the legs. Return to the upright position and relax (Fig. 15–41).

65. In the basic position, with the feet held down, slowly curl up to a sitting position. If the patient has weak abdominal muscles, begin with the hands along the sides. Later, the hands can be crossed over the stomach, then over the chest, and lastly behind the neck (Fig. 15–42).

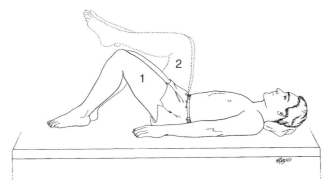

Figure 15–36.

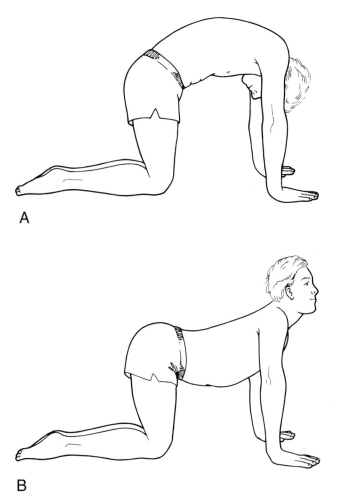

A

B

Figure 15–37.

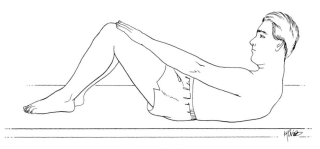

Figure 15–38.

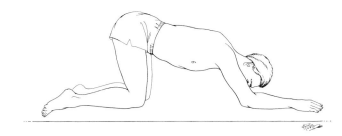

Figure 15–39.

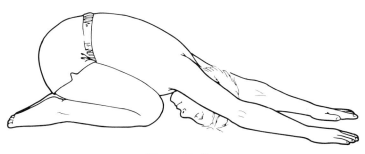

Figure 15–40.

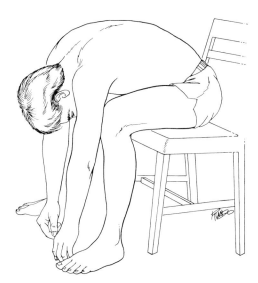

Figure 15–41.

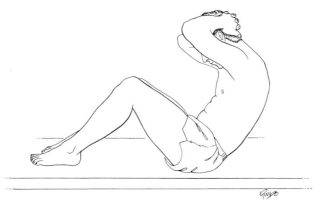

Figure 15–42.

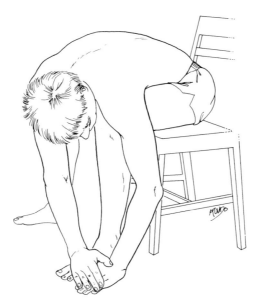

Figure 15–43.

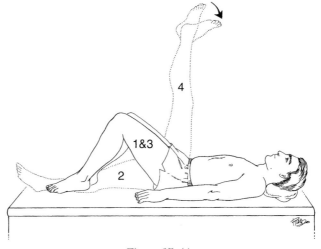

Figure 15–44.

66. Sitting as in exercise 62, twist the trunk to the left, dropping the head and arms, and then straighten up and repeat to the right (Fig. 15–43).

67. Bicycle stretch: Bring the knee to the chest, extend toward the ceiling, stretch out, and return to the flexed position, first with the toes pointed, then with the heel first (see Fig. 15–29).

68. Straight leg stretch: From the basic position, straighten the leg, raise as high as possible, lower, and return to the basic position. Do this first with pointed toes, then with the ankle in dorsiflexion (Fig. 15–44).

69. Standing with the hands joined behind the back and the arms straight, slowly bend forward as far as possible from the waist until you feel stretching in the back of the legs. Keep your back and neck straight when bending forward from the hips (Fig. 15–45).

70. Calf muscle stretch: Holding on to a table or leaning against a wall, with the heels on the floor, lean forward from the hips (see Fig 15–32).

71. Standing with the feet together and the knees straight, slowly reach toward the floor (see Fig. 15–1F).

Lower Back Weakness

72. Lying prone with a pillow under the hips, raise and lower each leg in turn, relaxing between movements.

73. When stronger, in the same position as exercise 72, raise both legs simultaneously, lower them and relax (see Fig. 15–1E).

Upper Back Weakness

74. Prone with a pillow under the hips, raise the arms and shoulders; lower them and relax. Repeat with the other arm (Fig. 15–1D).

75. In the same position as exercise 74, with the legs stabilized, raise the head, shoulders, and upper back while the arms are held alongside the body. Relax. When stronger, perform the same movement with the hands clasped behind the neck.

In acute cases of back pain, begin with exercises 54 through 57, gradually adding others as tolerated. Always keep within pain limits. The *most frequent mistakes are:*

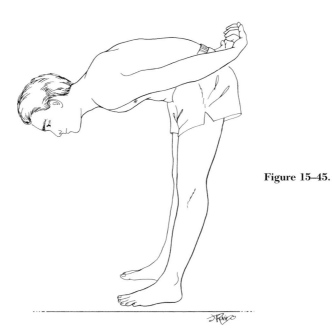

Figure 15–45.

- Neglecting relaxation.
- Omitting warm-up and cool-down.
- Giving multirepetition exercises.
- Giving too many exercises too soon, or giving exercises that are too demanding.
- Handing out written exercise sheets instead of teaching and monitoring the patient.
- Forgetting to use ice or ethyl chloride to relieve discomfort.

References

1. Cannon WB: Bodily Changes in Pain, Hunger, Fear and Rage, 2nd ed. New York, Appleton-Century-Crofts, 1929.
2. DeVries HA, Adams GM: Electromyographic comparison of single doses of exercise and meprobamate as to effect of muscular relaxation. Am J Phys Med 51(3):130–141, 1972.
3. Gaston S: Personal communication, 1946.
4. Glogowsky G, Wallraff J: Ein Beltrag zur Klinik und Histologie dier Muskelhärten (Myogelosen). Z Orthop 80:237–268, 1951.
5. Hellbrandt FA: Application of the overload principle to muscle training in man. Am J Phys Med 35:278–283, 1958.
6. Hettinger T, Muler EA: Muskelleistung and Muskeltraining. Arbeltsphysiologie 15:111–126, 1953.
7. Kraus H: New treatment for injured joints [abstract]. JAMA 104:1261, 1935.
8. Kraus H: Use of surface anesthesia in the treatment of painful motion. JAMA 116:2582–2583, 1941.
9. Kraus H: Diagnosis and treatment of low back pain. Gen Pract 5:55–60, 1952.
10. Kraus H: Therapeutic Exercise. Springfield, Ill, Charles C Thomas, 1963.
11. Kraus H: Clinical Treatment of Back and Neck Pain. New York, McGraw-Hill, 1970.
12. Kraus H (ed): Diagnosis and Treatment of Muscle Pain. Chicago, Quintessence, 1988.
13. Kraus H, Eisenmenger-Weber S: Quantitative tabulation of postural evaluation [report]. Physiother Rev 26:235–242, 1946.
14. Kraus H, Eisenmenger-Weber S: Fundamental considerations of postural exercises. Physiother Rev 27:361–368, 1947.
15. Kraus H, Hirschland RP: Minimum muscular fitness tests in school children. Res Q 25:178–188, 1954.
16. Kraus H, Mahoney JW: Fracture rehabilitation. In Covalt DA (ed): Rehabilitation in Industry, New York, Grune & Stratton, 1958.
17. Kraus H, Nagler W, Melleby A: Evaluation of an exercise program for back pain. Fam Physician 28:153–158, 1983.
18. Kraus H, Raab W: Hypokinetic Disease—Diseases Produced by Lack of Exercise. Springfield, Ill, Charles C Thomas, 1961.
19. Lange M: Die Muskelhärten (Myogelosen). Munich, Lehmann, 1931.
20. Liberson WT: Brief isometric exercises. In Basmajian JV (ed): Therapeutic Exercise, 4th ed. Baltimore, Williams & Wilkins, 1984.
21. Lovett RW: The Treatment of Infantile Paralysis. Philadelphia, Lea & Febiger, 1916.
22. Melleby A: The Y's way to a healthy back, Piscataway, NJ, 1982, New Century.
23. Palmen P: Über die Bedeutung der Nährung für die Erholung der Leistungsfähigkeit der Muskeln. Scand Arch Physiol 24:174, 1911.
24. Sherrington CS: Reciprocal innervation of antagonist muscles: 14th note on double reciprocal innervation. Proc R Soc Lond [Biol] 81:249–268, 1909.
25. Steindler A: Lectures on the Interpretation of Pain in Orthopedic Practice. Springfield, Ill, Charles C Thomas, 1959.

Chapter 16

Physical Therapy Treatment Approaches for Myofascial Pain Syndromes and Fibromyalgia

Isabel Rachlin, PT

This chapter examines a number of subjects important in the treatment of patients with myofascial pain syndromes, fibromyalgia, and other chronic pain conditions. The topics covered include the use of massage, with an emphasis on practitioner care, neuromuscular re-education, significant contributing and perpetuating factors, and patient education. The modality of massage is given extra attention due to its relevance in the treatment of myofascial pain syndromes.

Therapeutic Massage in the Treatment of Myofascial Pain Syndromes and Fibromyalgia

Massage is an excellent tool in the treatment of myofascial pain syndromes and at times the sole treatment necessary. A reasonable course of therapeutic massage along with other modalities may be tried before an invasive procedure such as injection is pronounced necessary. Two attributes not present in mechanical modalities are:

1. The ability of the practitioner to feel the exact tissue quality and the degree to which it responds during every moment of the treatment.
2. The well-known therapeutic effect of touch, whether for medical conditions or relaxation purposes.

Physiologic Effects of Massage

The scientific community has documented the physiologic effects of massage, providing understanding of the mechanisms by which massage causes therapeutic results.[4] Deep or kneading massage strokes, like muscle contraction, have been found to mechanically aid blood and lymph movement, thereby increasing blood supply and nutrients in an area and speeding up the removal of metabolic waste products.[25, 26, 61] The stretching force of massage on muscle fibers or across muscle fibers (as in deep friction massage) can mechanically break down adhesions and increase normal movement and flexibility of the tissues.[46, 55]

Pain relief as a result of massage has a number of physiologic explanations. Massage aids the body's removal of metabolic waste products, which can be responsible for cramping and soreness in muscles. The pressure and movement of the massage stimulates the non-nociceptive nerve endings, thus reducing pain. Massage can also contribute to the release of endorphins, a neurotransmitter that acts as a "central pain suppressant,"[63] and to increasing serotonin levels, which inhibit transmission of pain signals to the brain.[11] Reflex responses of massage can also include the reduction of blood pressure and general relaxation.[26]

Massage Techniques

The massage techniques discussed in this chapter are some that specifically address the following myofascial pain conditions: trigger points, muscle spasms, and fibromyalgia.

Dozens of massage strokes from around the world have been defined. The massage techniques described in Table 16–1 are intended to expose the reader to some possibilities for therapeutic soft tissue mobilization. As is true with any hands-on modality, massage cannot be fully learned from a book. It is recommended that the practitioner seek hands-on guidance and practice in massage techniques. (Also see Chapters 17 and 18.)

Applications of Massage

Therapeutic Massage for Trigger Points

Trigger points (TrPs), palpated as tender "knots" or "taut bands" in muscles or ligaments, may cause local as well as referred pain in a predictable and reproducible pain pattern.[23, 52] Trigger points develop when muscles are overstressed or fatigued. Acute injury, insufficient sleep, and chilling of muscles may be precipitating factors. Most often TrPs are the result of accumulated tension and muscle shortening due to poor postural and ergonomic factors and emotional stress. Some TrPs may cause symptoms only when excessive physical or emotional stress is present; other TrPs may create symptoms while the patient is at rest.

A combination of massage techniques can be used when treating TrPs. As with any condition, the practitioner must be attentive to the needs of the particular patient and how those needs change during the course of treatment. The practitioner cannot mindlessly rub a patient's muscle and consider this to be treatment. The quality, texture, and temperature of the tissues will change in response to massage and the practitioner should use this feedback (as well as verbal feedback from the patient) to guide him or her in the technique appropriate at each moment.

The area to be treated should be warmed up with gentle stroking and kneading. Do not begin the treatment by working too deeply. As the tissues become warmer and more elastic, the practitioner is able to sink more deeply into the muscles without hurting the patient and may then employ deeper strokes such as compression. A TrP is often palpable with superficial pressure at the onset of treatment; at other times it is not until the superficial layers have been relaxed with stroking, kneading, or stripping that a TrP is revealed in the deeper layers of tissue. The patient's reported site of pain may be referred from the TrP. Massaging the area of reported pain without treating the active TrP will not provide the patient with lasting relief. Fibrositis (a diffuse hardening of muscles) may obscure TrPs. A "pinching" and "rolling" massage of the tissues can be used in conjunction with kneading massage to soften these areas.[12, 23] The deep massage techniques such as compression, used to try to break down TrPs and adhesions in muscle or ligament fibers, may be painful to the patient. Kneading strokes, which gently "milk the muscle," may be used periodically to soothe the area, facilitate circulatory exchange to speed up evacuation of metabolic waste products, and to rest the practitioner's hands. Gentler, lighter strokes should also be used to conclude the treatment for similar reasons: to encourage increased blood exchange to prevent soreness and to promote relaxation. Stripping massage can also be used with the aforementioned techniques. Overall, a combination of deep concentrated attention to the TrP and general kneading or broader strokes is recommended. The practitioner will, with practice, find a rhythm of making transitions smoothly from one technique to another.

Beth Paris, a physical therapist with over 20 years of experience treating patients with TrPs and teaching courses on the subject, advocates a specific manual approach (see also Chapter 18).[44] Paris teaches the therapist to put the treated muscle on gentle stretch, and to find the taut bands and TrPs by using finger pressure *perpendicular* to the direction of the muscle fibers (Fig. 16–6). Fingertips are used to "sift" through the muscle, feeling for "ropey" tissue, taut bands of dense tissue, and TrPs (small dense nodules), which elicit patient symptoms and referred pain patterns. Feedback from patients is essential to let therapists know when they have located the most reactive TrP (which is the goal) and to inform therapists how sensation changes during the treatment.

Table 16–1.
Massage Techniques

Stroking

Stroking employs gentle strokes gliding over and into the tissue. This superficial massage technique is utilized to warm up an area for deeper strokes, to use as periodic rests during deeper work, and for calming and relaxation at the end of the treatment[12, 55, 63] (Fig. 16–1A–C).

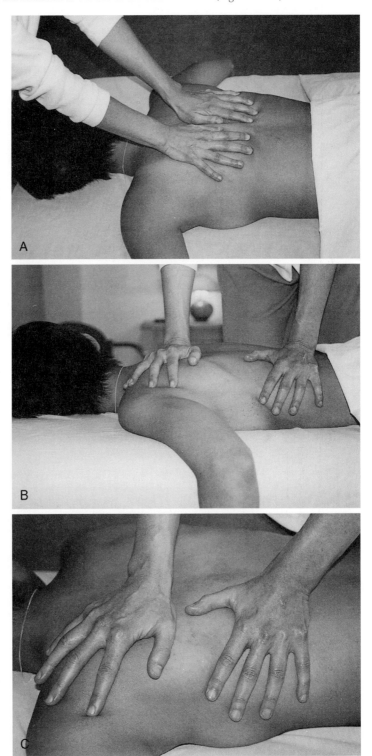

Figure 16–1. *A–C*, Stroking technique—gentle strokes gliding over and superficially into the tissue.

Kneading

Kneading can be a moderately deep massage technique. This technique is performed by contouring or "sinking" the hands into the underlying tissues, then lifting and gently squeezing the tissues as they roll out of the hand, creating a "milking" of the muscles[12, 17, 55] (Figs. 16–2 and 16–3). Kneading may be used to warm up muscles for deeper massage work, decrease soreness in an area (due to the increased blood flow and removal of metabolic waste), increase muscle flexibility, decrease muscle spasm, and facilitate relaxation. Stroking and kneading are both applied with slow rhythmic strokes.

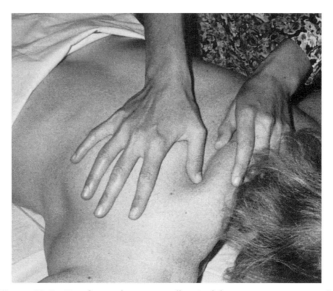

Figure 16–2. Kneading technique—"milking" of the upper trapezius muscle.

Compression

A number of practitioners advocate applying sustained compression in an effort to "inactivate" a trigger point.[6, 46, 59] The practitioner administers deep pressure directed on a trigger point using thumb, finger, knuckles, or elbow depending on the area addressed (Figs. 16–4 and 16–5). The initial pressure should be enough to cause tolerable discomfort and then pressure is gradually increased as the pain lessens. The pressure can be held for 5 to 25 seconds and repeated after a brief rest until the pain or referred symptoms of the trigger point cannot be reproduced.

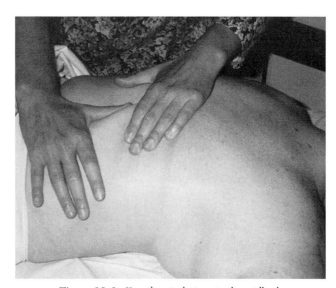

Figure 16–3. Kneading technique in the midback.

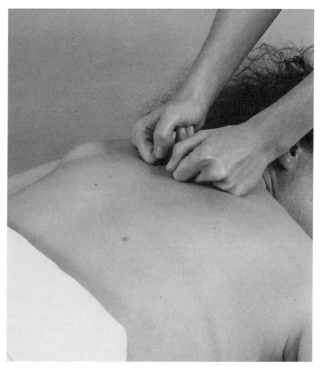

Figure 16–4. The use of the knuckles to apply compression or deep massage.

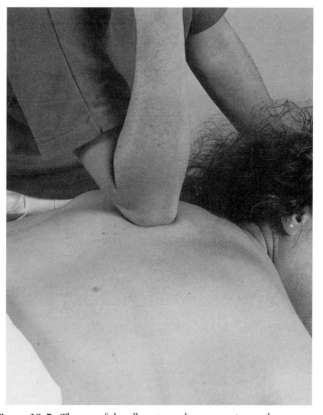

Figure 16–5. The use of the elbow to apply compression or deep massage.

Stripping Massage

Stripping massage is used in the treatment of trigger points. This technique, as described by Travell and Simons,[52, 59] employs slow, progressively deeper strokes using full hand contact beginning at the distal end of the muscle, sliding up toward the trigger point and beyond it. The practitioner is able to feel the area of the trigger point as a "nodular obstruction"[59] and repeats the strokes until the lump decreases and the patient no longer experiences referred pain or tenderness when pressure is applied.

Shiatsu and Acupressure

Shiatsu and acupressure are two types of massage that utilize pressure to specific points on the body.[55] These techniques are based on the ancient Oriental view of the body as being comprised of meridians (energy pathways). Because one must have a knowledge of these theories to understand why and how these techniques are applied, I will not give instruction in, but rather acknowledge, these techniques and propose further study and practice of them.

Ice Massage

Ice massage, a technique of ice application, is useful in the treatment of muscle spasms.[24] Many physical therapy departments keep paper cups of ice in their freezers so that the cup can be held upside down by the practitioner and peeled away as the ice melts. The practitioner should *keep the ice moving* over the affected area so no one spot becomes too cold. When the muscle is numbed and cold to the touch, enough ice has been applied for therapeutic effect. This may take approximately 5 minutes depending on the size and depth of the area as well as the patient's individual tolerance and response to cold. Cold therapy relieves pain "by elevating the pain threshold as a direct effect of temperature reduction on nerve fibers and receptors."[27] Other beneficial physiologic effects of cold treatment include local hyperemia due to reflex vasodilation of the vascular system following an initial constriction of the vessels, and lowered tone in muscles as a result of its effect on the autonomic nervous system.[41] Contraindications to the use of ice massage include poor circulation, allergy to cold, and extreme discomfort or aversion to cold.

When a TrP has been located, it is crucial to sustain pressure (compression) on the smallest and most irritable point. Force is delivered through the fingertips with the fingers and wrist straight (neutral), approaching the muscle at a steep angle. The least pressure necessary to induce sensation should be used. Excessive force may cause unnecessary pain and will not be productive. The patient must continue to give feedback, informing the therapist of pain level, referral patterns, and changes in symptoms. As the compression is sustained, approximately 10 to 20 seconds, symptoms may begin to diminish (the TrP has become less irritable) and increased pressure is tolerated.

Paris suggests that compression be held still on the TrP without moving back and forth over it, because the movement can cause increased patient discomfort. "Micromovements" on the spot can be used, as can passive motion of the patient

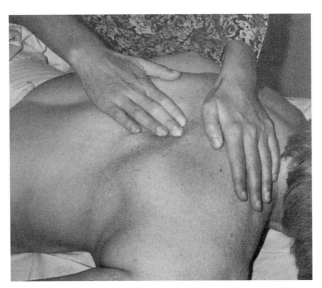

Figure 16–6. Finger pressure is applied perpendicular to the direction of the muscle fibers.

while the pressure continues to be held still on the TrP. How much pressure should be used? This will be determined by many factors including the sensitivity of the patient, the reactivity of the TrP, and the density of the tissues. "Listening" to the tissues, patient feedback, and experience become the guides. The same variables apply to duration of sustained compression. In the treatment of TrPs, accurate point location is crucial. If the therapist is not directly treating the TrP, therapeutic results will not be achieved.

Patients will commonly experience some level of discomfort during this treatment but often describe it as a "good hurt," a characteristic of accurate point location. Gentle massage strokes may be used periodically and at the end of the session to soothe the patient and to give a feeling of integration.

When treating the patient with multiple TrPs, the most irritable TrP should be treated first. If another area is dense and ropey but pain-free, it is not the priority. In Chapter 18 Paris details how to perform an in-depth soft tissue examination. She describes the need to treat bilaterally and elaborates on commonly found patterns of TrPs. Knowledge of these patterns can aid the therapist in recognizing involved muscles and the typical sequence for treatment of TrPs in frequently seen pain complaints.

Trigger points in the midscapulae, and upper trapezius and levator scapulae muscles, are probably the most frequently treated TrPs by physical therapists. The treatment usually needs to address multiple areas along with the area harboring the primary pain or primary TrP (see Chapter 9 for classification of TrPs). It is common that once the primary TrP has been treated, TrPs in neighboring muscles or antagonistic muscles will become more obviously symptomatic. Often patients with pain and TrPs in the mid and upper back or neck area have a forward-head and rounded-shoulder posture. The anterior muscles (i.e., pectoralis and sternocleidomastoid muscles) should be treated to achieve normal muscle length and long-lasting results. Many practitioners, myself included, find that the more holistically the patient is treated, that is, integrating the whole body rather than treating an isolated symptomatic area, the greater the ultimate results and prevention of recurrence. This is especially true for stretching and exercise as discussed later in this chapter and is also true for massage and other modalities.[64] One can understand that restoring full length and relaxation to lower back musculature allows upper back muscles to maintain balance and relaxation. Tight hamstrings, for instance, can "pull" the lower back into an inefficient shortened position; the need for attention to multiple muscle groups is apparent.

The type of massage treatment described may take 30 to 60 minutes depending on the endurance of the practitioner and the patient's needs. Some TrPs may become deactivated after only a few minutes of treatment whereas others may take multiple treatments of 30 to 60 minutes. Regardless of the time spent, postmassage passive and active stretching of the involved muscle groups is ideal to further increase the elasticity and normal length of the muscle fibers. Shaw emphasizes the need to retrain shortened muscles (especially those harboring TrPs) in order to maintain results achieved with hands-on treatment.[51] Along with postural and ergonomic corrections, Shaw advises stretching bilaterally in a pain-free range of motion every one to one-and-a-half hours. The frequency of performance facilitates re-education of the muscles.[51]

Patients should schedule one to three appointments per week so that there is time for the tissues to respond to the last treatment before the next is administered. The practitioner should tell the patient that soreness may occur 24 to 48 hours following treatment owing to direct stimulation of the TrP area, but that this soreness should subside without ill effects. (If the soreness does last longer, the practitioner may have overworked the area and should move more slowly with this particular patient.)

Massage for Patients with Fibromyalgia

Fibromyalgia is a chronic pain syndrome characterized by a history of widespread pain for a minimum of 3 months. It usually includes low back pain as well as palpable pain in 11 of 18 defined bilateral tender points (see Chapters 1 and 2). Many people who have fibromyalgia find exercising or even activities of daily living too uncomfortable and strenuous and have difficulty finding pain relief.[3, 35] Massage may provide some welcome relief from that chronic pain and has been shown to help decrease stiffness and fatigue, and to improve sleep.[11] The massage should be gentle and general, focusing on relaxation; it should not create pain. Patients with fibromyalgia may not be able to tolerate deep pressure on specific areas owing to the tender points that characterize the illness. Stroking and kneading are usually appropriate, always applying pressure within the patient's pain tolerance. Because many people with fibromyalgia have difficulty exercising and moving in general, the increased circulation to muscles provided by massage will help maintain healthy tissues as well as increase comfort.[61]

Special attention to positioning is often warranted for these sensitive patients; be flexible about treating patients in their position of maximum comfort. For some this position may be side-lying with a pillow between the knees for comfort (Fig. 16–7). For others it may mean an extra pillow under the stomach, chest, or ankle in the prone position. If a patient cannot tolerate the head turned to one side while lying prone, try placing a folded towel or very small pillow under the side of the head pressing on the table; this bolstering will decrease torque on the neck. For some elderly or differently abled patients, climbing on and off the treatment table may be too difficult. Massage, therefore, can be performed with the patient sitting in a chair with attention to proper lumbar support. From this position the therapist may still reach the patient's face, neck, upper back, arms, hands, legs, and feet.

Another consideration in the case of sensitive patients is the advantage of working on areas distant from reported sites of pain. For example, if the patient complains of pain in the upper trapezius but can tolerate little touching of this area, massaging the face, pectoralis muscles, neck, and midback helps to relax the patient and often helps to decrease pain in the shoulder or problem area. Similarly, if a patient complaining of low back pain cannot comfortably attain or maintain a prone or side-lying position, massage of the feet, belly (the "front of the back"), legs, psoas muscles, and neck in the supine position (with a pillow placed under the knees) may still address the back musculature and provide pain relief.[63] Massage chairs, designed to allow back massage with the patient seated, are available from many massage table manufacturers.

When treating chronic pain patients with syndromes such as fibromyalgia, the practitioner must sometimes be satisfied with achieving a lower level of the patient's

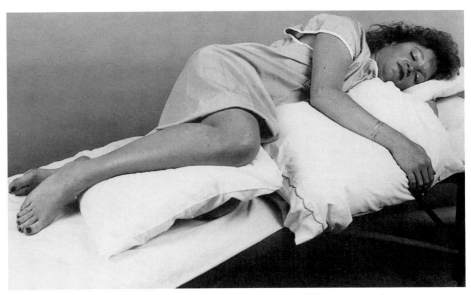

Figure 16–7. Side-lying position with pillows placed for patient comfort.

pain; the goal of abolishing the patient's pain may still be reasonable but the practitioner should not blame himself or herself (or the patient) if this goal is not reached, even after many sessions. Remember, frustration can lead to burnout, and most chronic pain patients are grateful for *any increased comfort gained.* Many people with chronic pain have lost sight of ever attaining a pain-free state. Until the patient is able to believe that he or she *can* live without pain, it is unlikely that such an outcome will be reached. As the course of treatment progresses and the patient is experiencing greater pain relief, the ultimate goal of "zero pain" becomes more possible. Massage, even after the first treatment or two, may create enough pain relief needed for the patient to do some active exercises or activities of daily living that he or she was otherwise unable to perform. Stretching exercises, and active range of motion, and in particular cardiovascular exercises as tolerated should be included in the physical therapy programs of these patients (as with other physical therapy patients).[34, 35] (See Chapter 2 for further discussion of exercise in the treatment of fibromyalgia.)

Fibromyalgia: Clinical Observations

Over the past decade health care providers have become increasingly aware of fibromyalgia as a diagnosis and are using it much more frequently. It is positive that providers are utilizing new ideas in addressing patient complaints; however, many are using this diagnosis for almost any complaint of lasting muscle pain and may not be aware of the actual diagnostic criteria (see Chapter 1 for diagnostic criteria of fibromyalgia). I have treated patients with numerous conditions ranging from symptomatic disc bulges, back pain due to poor posture and tension, somaticized psycho/emotional issues, undiagnosed pancreatic cancer, to undiagnosed food sensitivities and allergies, all coming in with the diagnosis of fibromyalgia. Often patients were told by their physicians that fibromyalgia is a lifelong condition. It is of great concern that these patients are being told, and believing, that they have a "lifelong" condition when there are many precipitating causes and perpetuating factors that have not been explored or treated.

Musculoskeletal issues including poor posture and ergonomics, muscle weakness, imbalance and inflexibility, and TrPs must be addressed as possible contributors to the patient's condition. Food sensitivities or allergies (e.g., to wheat, dairy, chocolate, and refined sugars) and environmental allergies (e.g., to dust, mold, pollen) can cause migraine, fatigue, muscle aches, morning stiffness, and gastrointestinal symptoms.[5, 13, 20, 30, 33, 42] These factors may also have to be ruled out as responsible for the patient's discomfort before arriving at a fibromyalgia diagnosis. Refined sugar and processed foods may also contribute to fatigue and muscle and joint stiffness.[5, 13, 40] To determine if particular foods are contributing factors, a patient can simply omit suspected foods from the diet for one or more weeks to check for a change in symptoms, and then add them back into the diet one at a time to observe the effects. A specialist in environmental testing may also be consulted to test for food and environmental hypersensitivities.

Psychological and emotional issues may be the root of physical complaints for some patients, and no course of physically based treatment alone will ultimately alleviate their symptoms (see Chapter 5).

Now that the diagnosis of fibromyalgia has become more widely accepted, the next step is for practitioners to make sure they are using it accurately and not overlooking other treatable causes of symptoms.

Massage for Muscle Spasms

The cause of a muscle spasm should be assessed before massage is considered as treatment. If the cause of a muscle spasm is, for example, a dislocated joint, massage will not usually suffice as treatment of the underlying problem. In many cases, though, the muscle spasm masks the underlying problem and until the muscles are relaxed, the causative problem is not apparent. Ice massage is known to help decrease pain and can be used to help "break a vicious cycle of secondary muscle spasm with ischemia and pain and more muscle spasms."[27] Stroking and kneading techniques are also used to increase blood flow to an area and aid in relaxation. In the case of muscle spasm, the practitioner should proceed slowly and gently, progressively deepening the strokes as the muscle spasm decreases. Often other modalities such as ice, tetanizing electrical stimulation, hot packs, contract-relax, and postisometric relaxation exercises may be used instead of or prior to massage.[28, 60]

Contraindications to Massage

There are many conditions that necessitate precautions when performing massage. The context, condition of the patient, and knowledge and skill level of the practitioner must be taken into consideration. The patient's physician should be consulted if the patient has a questionable health issue or risk. Precaution should also be taken when massaging someone who, for any reason, cannot provide adequate feedback during the treatment session.

The following conditions are regarded as contraindications to massage treatment:

- Systemic viral or bacterial infections.
- Inflammation secondary to bacterial infection.
- Calcification of soft structures when myositis ossificans may be a consideration.
- Hemophilia.[12] (Consult the patient's physician.)
- Hematoma.
- Deep venous thrombosis.
- Inflamed rheumatoid and gouty arthritis.
- Bursitis. (Do not massage the bursa itself. Massage of muscles thought to be contributing to the bursitis may be indicated, such as massage of the gluteal and lateral thigh muscles in cases of greater trochanteric bursitis.)
- Pain due to nerve entrapment, e.g., with carpal tunnel syndrome. (Do not massage over area of nerve entrapment. Suspected involved muscles may be treated.)
- Phlebitis and cellulitis.
- Pitting edema.
- The presence of metastatic cancer. (Consult the patient's physician. Light massage may be permissible.)[31]
- Presence of a tumor or "local" malignancy. (Do not massage over or around a tumor. Consult the patient's physician prior to massage for a patient with a "local" cancer lesion.)
- Infectious skin diseases.[22, 61]

Lubrication

Use of lubrication for massage purposes will be determined by the technique used, the practitioner's preference, and the sensitivity or preference of the patient. Lubrication is used to decrease friction between the practitioner's hands and the patient's skin, thereby decreasing uncomfortable pulling of skin or body hair and allowing the practitioner's hands to stay relaxed.

Many brands of oils and lotions are marketed specifically for massage use and can be found in drugstores, health food stores, and medical supply stores and catalogues. Popular oils are almond oil, coconut oil, arnica oil, mineral oil, and combinations of these and other oils. Commonly used solid lubricants include cocoa butter, Abolene cream, and non–oil based creams. A variety of lotions exist and offer a consistency between an oil and a solid lubricant. A lotion manufactured for the purposes of dry skin may be absorbed too quickly for therapeutic massage treatment. I have found that ultrasound media such as ultrasound gel and lotion are frequently used as massage lubricants in physical therapy departments. It is my experience that these are inferior lubricants *for the purpose of massage;* they are too slippery or sticky for good hand-tissue contact and therefore cause decreased sensitivity and increased tension in the practitioner's hands.

Generally, some type of lubricant is used with stroking and kneading techniques because of its ability to reduce surface friction. Friction massage and compression are often performed without lubrication because nonslippery skin contact is desired. Powder or corn starch may also be used as a medium for massage. It can actually decrease slipping on skin when that is desirable as in the case of sweaty hands on a hot day.

Nonscented lubricants should be used in the clinical setting. Many people have sensitivities or allergies to perfumes and scents. Similarly, there are people who have sensitivities or allergies to oils and lotions in general and this must be assessed before a lubricant is applied.

The practitioner should try a variety of media to find which ones work best for him or her. I prefer using small amounts of a combined almond/olive oil or arnica oil—just enough to decrease surface friction but still allow firm nonslippery hand contact. I have found that this type of lubrication is suitable for TrP treatment that includes stroking, kneading, stripping, or compression techniques. The practitioner's hands must not be sliding over the muscles to the extent that the tissue quality cannot be sensitively assessed throughout the treatment; too much oil or lotion or the use of ultrasound media will not allow this level of sensitivity.

The medium to be used should be applied onto the practitioner's hands rather than poured directly onto the patient. This enables the practitioner to better control the amount applied and to warm up the medium before it touches the patient's skin.

Adjuncts to Massage

Adjunctive modalities are often used to enhance the therapeutic effects of massage. Hot packs when used for 15 to 20 minutes prior to treatment warm up the area to be treated, inducing pliability in the tissues and allowing the practitioner to use deep pressure earlier in the treatment. Hot packs or ultrasound treatment may be helpful after the massage to prevent or decrease possible postmassage soreness and to further relaxation and increased blood flow to the area. The use of vaporized (vapocoolant) spray or ice with stretch can be an important adjunct in the treatment of TrPs, muscle spasm, or shortened muscles in general. The use of the quick cold stimulus applied by a stroke of ice or vapocoolant spray (fluorimethane or ethyl chloride) causes an anesthetizing effect allowing increased stretching of a muscle.[56] Low-level laser therapy appears to be useful in treating many musculoskeletal conditions including myofascial pain syndromes.[53] This modality, though widely utilized elsewhere, has not yet gained approval for widespread use in the United States. Electrical stimulation is used to induce muscle relaxation and pain relief and is often used in combination with ultrasound in the treatment of TrPs and muscle spasm. (See Chapter 19 on physical therapy modalities.) Acupuncture has been used for treatment of muscle pain and musculoskeletal disorders for thousands of years and can be extremely effective when provided by an experienced well-trained practitioner.[2, 7, 21, 45]

Numerous manual techniques involving muscle contraction and reflex relaxation are used in conjunction with massage. Contract-relax, postisometric relaxation, proprioceptive neuromuscular facilitation, and muscle energy technique are some of these methods.[28, 59, 60]

There are a number of products that allow patients to perform self-massage for TrPs and muscle pain. Theracane and Backbuddy are examples of tools that use leverage to apply deep pressure to hard-to-reach areas (Fig. 16–8). Taping two squash balls together and lying down on the floor with them under the desired back muscles delivers deep pressure to these areas. Electric-powered vibrators, such as the Magic Wand by Hitachi, can be used at home by the patient. Sustained pressure of the vibrator on TrPs and tight muscles can help decrease or alleviate pain.

Positioning the Patient

Patient comfort is essential during massage therapy. The patient's body or body part must be fully supported so that the patient is able to completely relax. Tension

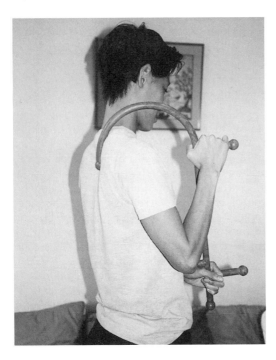

Figure 16–8. The use of a Theracane for self-massage to the upper back.

in the muscles is counterproductive. Proper bolstering can aid in positioning, so it is wise to have pillows, bolsters, and towel rolls available for this purpose (see also discussion of massage for fibromyalgia). In the supine position, a pillow under the knees removes stress on the low back and a towel roll under the neck may be helpful to remove stress from the neck. The prone position can be made more comfortable by placing a pillow or low bolster under the ankles and a pillow under the stomach or chest when necessary. As mentioned earlier, if a patient in the prone position cannot tolerate lying with the head turned to one side, try placing a folded towel or a very small pillow under the side of the head touching the table; this will decrease torque on the neck (Fig. 16–9). (Some treatment tables have face cradles that allow the neck to stay straight instead of turned to the side.)

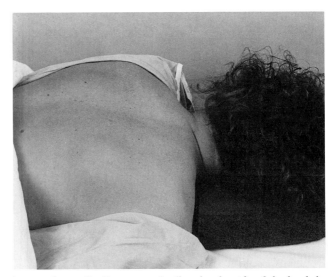

Figure 16–9. The use of a small pillow or towel roll under the side of the head decreases torque on the neck.

If the patient is receiving massage seated in a chair, be attentive to the posture and support of the entire patient, not only the part being treated. One or two pillows on the patient's lap can act as an arm support and take stress off the neck, shoulders, and arms. A lumbar support will decrease stress on the neck and back. Proper draping will also facilitate comfort and relaxation. Only those areas being worked on should be exposed; clothing or a sheet can cover the rest of the body to prevent unnecessary embarrassment or chill. Extra lightweight blankets should be on hand; cold will cause muscles to tighten.

Positioning and Self-Care for the Practitioner

Practitioner comfort is equally as important as patient comfort. The practitioner who is a martyr and strains all day will suffer injury and have nothing to give the next day. The table height should be low enough so that the practitioner can use his or her body weight to lean into the massage; if the table is not adjustable in height, some low platforms or step stools may be necessary. Standing with the feet shoulder width apart will enable the practitioner to shift weight easily with the direction of the massage. Proper posture must also be maintained to avoid back and neck strain; do not hunch over the patient. Keep knees, shoulders, and back relaxed. Comfortable supportive shoes should be worn. Many practitioners prefer to sit when performing massage on small areas such as a limb or TrP in the upper back. If choosing to sit, one must still be aware of keeping the body weight over the area being treated so as not to overstress the hands. The main concerns for practitioner comfort are keeping the back relatively straight and making sure that body weight, not hand or arm strength, is the force behind the massage.

Practitioners who do massage must be careful to prevent hand and wrist injuries due to improper use and overuse. Many physical therapists and massage therapists develop thumb and wrist strains, tendinitis or tenosynovitis, as well as carpal tunnel syndrome. Correct practice includes keeping the hands, wrists, and shoulders relaxed while working. If the hands become tense or cramped, gently shake them out and come back to the patient with relaxed hands. *Relaxed hands will also allow the practitioner heightened sensitivity in assessing the quality of the underlying tissues.* The wrists should remain relatively straight to prevent wrist strain and carpal tunnel syndrome. Do not overuse the thumbs! An invitation to strain and eventual arthritis is to continually use the thumbs as the main tools of massage treatment. Instead of using the thumbs, allow the force of the movement to come through the entire arm (not the finger or wrist joints) and lean body weight into the movement. Substitute the thenar eminence, the flat back of the fingers and hands, knuckles, elbow, or other fingers if a lot of force is required on an area.

Another way to prevent overuse injury is to avoid scheduling two or more patients consecutively who require deep massage work; have rest time between these patients.

Neuromuscular Re-education

Patients often suffer pain long after the original injury or precipitating cause is gone and the injured tissues have healed. In many of these cases, the nervous system and unconscious are still guarding the area and associating it with pain, maintaining a pain and tension cycle. Crowley and Kendal[8] described this process in their article on developing a questionnaire for measuring fear-avoidance:

> An individual suffers an initial injury causing tissue damage and pain. In this acute stage the pain may be aggravated by certain movements and activities and, as a result, these are reduced in an attempt to control pain levels. In time the individual starts to avoid these movements and activities in anticipation of increased pain and/or increased damage. Once the injury heals, the person may continue this avoidance through fear of experiencing increased pain. Current theory suggests the avoidance of movements and activities leads to muscle weakness, muscle tension and joint disuse as well as sensitization

of central pain transmission pathways which in turn may maintain pain levels and disability.

The nervous system may learn so successfully to identify the "injured" area with pain, and be so hypersensitized that just *thinking* about an activity that the patient perceives as painful will create the pain, without even performing the activity! Bringing this phenomenon to the patient's conscious attention is the first step in the re-education process. Informing patients that they can have some control over their pain is very empowering. In fact, a patient's condition may begin to shift immediately, without any other intervention when the unconscious perpetuating factor is brought to his or her conscious attention.

There are numerous techniques of neuromuscular re-education (see Chapter 17). Two excellent approaches are the Trager Approach of Psychophysical Integration and Mentastics Movement Re-education and the Feldenkrais Method of Functional Integration and Awareness through Movement.[10, 39, 50, 57, 62] Both of these approaches are composed of two components. One is a hands-on component that utilizes gentle pain-free movement to re-educate the body and mind (the central nervous system). This manual communication provides the patient with an experience of pain-free movement, relaxed muscles, improved firing of motor units, and integration, thus "reprogramming" and "overriding" the dysfunctional patterns. The second component is teaching the patient self-care "exercises" that promote increased body awareness, improved posture, and increased pain-free, efficient movement. These approaches may be extremely beneficial to patients with myofascial pain, chronic pain, and fibromyalgia, as well as numerous other conditions.

Patient Education and Pertinent Topics

Massage treatment or treatment by any modality is almost worthless in the long run if causative factors and follow-up care are not addressed. Instruction in proper posture is essential in the case of any neck, shoulder, or back problem. It is pointless to give a 45-minute TrP treatment to someone who then drives home with a slumped, forward-head posture. Patients must be instructed in the use of lumbar supports, wedges, and sitting options, i.e., therapeutic balls or "kneeling chairs," and the like (Fig. 16–10A–C). Flexibility and strengthening exercises must be performed by the patient when shortened or weak muscles are contributing factors. Full body stretching and exercise is often more beneficial than locally targeted exercises. For instance, upper back and neck tension is addressed far more effectively with yogic "sun salutations" (which stretches multiple muscle groups) or aerobic exercise than with local neck or upper back stretches alone. Also, core conditioning exercises (i.e., Pilates) that emphasize strength and balance of the core muscle groups of the body (abdominals, back and pelvic musculature) help support tissues throughout the body. When possible, patients should be encouraged to do aerobic exercise. Aerobic exercise promotes general health and well-being, increases circulatory flow promoting healthy tissues, and helps reduce muscular and emotional tension.[34] McCain has studied and observed the effects of aerobic exercise on people with fibromyalgia. He writes, "Exercise, therefore, may lead directly to observable improvements in mastery over pain, enhanced self-esteem, and to better social support behaviors by significant others."[34]

Exercise and Movement

In my practice I draw on many types of strengthening, stretching, and limbering exercises including yoga, core-conditioning, tai chi, qi gong, the McKenzie Approach, Mentastics® Movement Re-education, and more traditional physical therapy exercises. However, encouraging patients to "feel into themselves" and take time to move and stretch in ways that feel good and necessary to them in the present moment is of even greater importance. Taking some time each day (i.e., 5 to 60 minutes) to move in

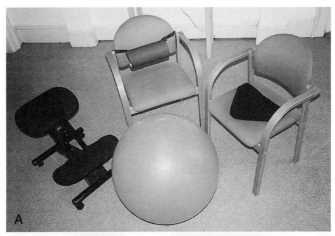

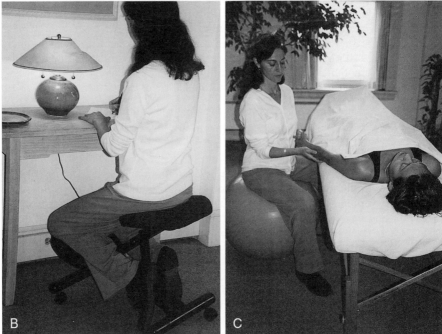

Figure 16–10. *A,* Seating options. *B,* Use of "kneeling chair." *C,* Use of therapeutic ball for seated activities.

uncontrived, pleasurable ways can be beneficial for recovering from and preventing injury and painful conditions. I call this "giving oneself a massage from the inside out."

This experience differs from "exercises" in that patients "listen" to what their bodies "tell" them to do rather than performing a preconceived movement prescribed by someone else. This type of activity can take many forms, such as dancing to music or simply lying on the floor and breathing. Prescribed exercises often take place in limited planes of motion (e.g., flexion/extension, sidebending, rotations). Moving and stretching in the infinite angles that muscles and joints can move in allows for greater release of tension, more complete stretching, and better flow of information to the central nervous system, fostering increased body awareness. As mentioned earlier, incorporating multiple muscle groups and full-body stretching and movement instead of isolating body parts (i.e., cervical stretches for neck pain) promotes greater pain relief.

Patients should be advised to incorporate more free and spontaneous movement and self-care (i.e., correct posture, full breathing, stretching) into their everyday activities. Despite our cultural inhibitions and protocols of "proper" public physical behavior, we are still biologic organisms who need to move and stretch our bodies throughout the day, not just when "it's time to do my exercises." Many pain complaints, such as neck and back pain, are often simply due to lack of movement. The Trager Approach of Psychophysical Integration and Mentastics Movement Re-education,[39, 58, 63] and Emily Conrad's Continuum Movement are useful training for practitioners who want to explore these ideas and gain structure and language with which to teach them to clients.

The Effect of Emotional Tension on Myofascial Problems and Chronic Pain

The effect of emotional tension on myofascial problems and chronic pain cannot be overemphasized. Just as in the case of poor posture, a TrP, e.g., can be treated for 45 minutes, but if the patient has problems which cause him or her to be tense or angry, the physical therapy will probably have little long-term effect (see Chapter 5). We only do patients a disservice by making this topic taboo or pretending it does not exist as a contributing factor. Psycho/emotional issues are equally as significant as postural and ergonomic factors. Numerous studies show the effects of mental or emotional stress and tension on the musculoskeletal system.[14, 18, 37, 49] Skubick[54] postulates two mechanisms that account for this relationship:

1. Inappropriate and excessive extrafusal muscle fiber contraction, i.e., muscle tension as defined by Kraus[23, 24]—prolonged contraction beyond postural functional need. And
2. Activation of myofascial trigger points via sympathetic innervation as proposed by Hubbard.[19]

Of course for many patients psycho/emotional factors will not necessarily play any role in their condition. For others, these issues may be either at the root of their symptoms or are significant perpetuating factors. The symptoms and stressors may be of "temporary" nature such as a job the patient does not like or anger at a supervisor or spouse. In the case of some patients, particularly those with chronic pain, the stressor may be older and more chronic (i.e., anger at a parent or a childhood history of emotional or physical maltreatment). I have treated many patients whose (unconscious) coping strategy for the stresses of life appears to be continual physical symptoms for which they seek medical attention, and which impair their ability to function fully in social or work situations. Most of these patients have seen numerous practitioners and show a similar course in therapy: some initial improvement the first two to four treatments followed by reports of increased symptoms, then plateauing at their original status. They report that treatment is helpful but never seem to improve. This pattern is repeated with every type of intervention tried.

Naturally, a physical therapist should not attempt to be a psychotherapist. However, as mentioned earlier in this chapter, sometimes simply bringing unconscious behaviors to the conscious attention of the patient results in an almost immediate positive shift in the patient's condition, without any further intervention.[48] Other patients may benefit from counseling with an appropriate provider or behavior modification and physical therapy (see Chapter 5). This combination can sometimes help patients with chronic pain become progressively less fearful of activity and increasingly strong, flexible, and empowered in their bodies and lives.[1, 8, 15, 29, 36] Often family members (i.e., spouses, children, parents) have been unconsciously enabling the patient to stay ill or impaired. Family therapy should be used in these situations.

It is difficult to address these issues without a team approach. How do we discuss these issues with referring physicians who have treated the patient as though their condition is due solely to physical origins? This will be an ongoing question and dialogue into the next decade and highlights the importance of an integrated or multidisciplinary approach.

McClaflin[36] advises practitioners (and primary care physicians in particular) to

Table 16–2.
Active and Passive Therapy

Passive Therapy	Active Therapy
Administered to patient by provider	Requires patient involvement
• Medication	• Sense of control and shared responsibility
• Trigger point injections	• Exercise
• Injections used in pain clinics	• Postural/movement re-education
• Massage/modalities	• Relaxation/meditation/biofeedback
	• Psychotherapy/behavior modification techniques
	• Support groups
↓ Often leads to	↓ Often leads to
• Temporary pain relief	• Feeling of improved self-esteem
• Longer expected course of treatment	• Coping strategies
• Lower chance of permanent success	• Sense of control over pain
	• Better chance of Rx success

Data from references 34 and 36.

intervene early with "at risk to chronic pain" patients. He advises communicating a plan of care, emphasizing "the patient's active role in the success or failure of the plan." He prescribes active therapies (Table 16–2) and referral to medical, physical, occupational, psychological, and family therapy practitioners when needed. Ozer[43] describes a similar approach. He emphasizes goal setting with the active participation of the patient. Ozer finds that goal setting and successful treatment planning helps patients to gain clarity regarding their concerns about their condition and its impact on their lives.

As the patient develops functional goals, it may facilitate a positive and hopeful view of the future. People who live with chronic pain often feel a lack of power and control over their pain, their bodies, and their lives. Any type of treatment that results in providing the patient with a greater sense of control over these matters is constructive.

Important Contributing Factors

Other factors that undermine treatment if neglected include insufficient sleep, poor diet, and food and environmental sensitivities (Table 16–3). The necessity for arch supports or corrective footwear should also be assessed, particularly when lower extremity complaints are present. Ergonomic considerations in the car, home, and workplace should be addressed (see Chapter 20).

Women's pocketbooks are a common contributing factor to neck and shoulder pain. Women can be encouraged to avoid carrying a pocketbook on one shoulder, causing asymmetry and tension in the shoulder and neck muscles. The pocketbook may be worn across the body for better weight distribution and to decrease muscle tension (Figs. 16–11A and B). A wide shoulder strap is also helpful. Lightening the load is of equal importance. Only essential items should be carried, ideally keys and wallet; other items may be left in the car or at home or workplace. A hip sack (fanny pack)

Table 16–3.
Commonly Overlooked Contributing Factors to Neck, Back, and General Muscle Pain

• Shallow breathing	• High heels or uncomfortable shoes
• Clenched jaw	• Heavy coat/leather jacket
• Rushing throughout the day	• Insufficient sleep
• Lack of full, free movement	• Poor diet (refined sugar, food sensitivities)
• Women's pocketbooks	• Overeating (past the point of "feeling full")
• Long, heavy hair	• Ill-fitting furniture and exercise equipment
• Tight pants, waistband, or bra	

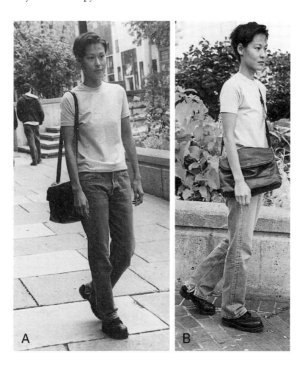

Figure 16–11. *A,* Wearing a pocket-book on one shoulder can contribute to neck, shoulder, and upper back injury. *B,* Wearing a pocketbook across the body distributes the weight more safely.

is an excellent alternative (Fig. 16–12). A knapsack worn correctly is also a better option for carrying moderately heavy loads.

Uncomfortable clothing is a little-discussed contributor to muscle tension. Tight clothing, such as tight waistbands, bras (including "jog bras"), and pantyhose can contribute to back pain. Heavy coats and leather jackets may cause neck, levator scapulae, rhomboid, and upper trapezius muscle strain and pain (Fig. 16–13). High heels may be responsible for neck, back, and knee pain. It seems obvious, but dressing warmly in cold weather can help keep muscles relaxed. When we are dressed inappropriately for cold temperatures, muscles tense, tighten, and shorten. I advise all of my patients to wear a scarf and extra sweater, and often a hat, when they come for

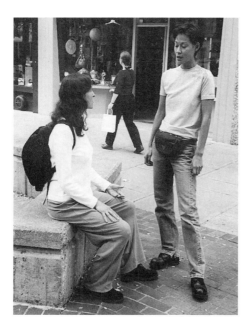

Figure 16–12. Wearing a knapsack or fanny pack instead of a pocketbook can help prevent shoulder and neck injuries due to carrying weight on one shoulder.

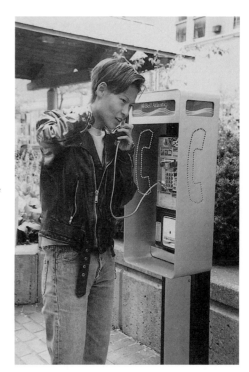

Figure 16–13. Heavy jackets and coats can cause neck, shoulder, and upper back pain.

their physical therapy appointment so that they do not go out in the cold and tighten up again following treatment.

"Breathe, Slow Down, Let Your Jaw Relax."

I often tell my patients, "If you don't remember anything else you learned in physical therapy, remember to BREATHE!" I have observed that most people do not breathe fully, depriving themselves of the thousands of micromovements and stretches breathing provides to the rib cage, torso, and back muscles throughout the day. When these structures are not taken through their full (functional) range of motion, they become tight and the muscles develop tension.

Many people unconsciously hold their breath intermittently throughout the day and most exhibit shallow breathing in general. I teach patients to relax their jaw and to do a couple of minutes of full expansive breathing (rib cage, back, chest, and abdomen) a few times daily to stimulate the diaphragm and the nervous system to breathe more fully in general. Deep breathing can help release mental and muscular tension. Fritz writes, "Breathing patterns are a direct link to altering autonomic nervous system patterns, which in turn affect mood, feelings, and behavior."[12] Simply lying down on the floor, or sitting comfortably and breathing fully from the diaphragm for 5 or more minutes can facilitate profound relaxation and significant pain relief. Most good yoga teachers emphasize breathing instruction as an integral part of their classes. Yoga incorporates breathing, strengthening, and stretching, and may be helpful to many patients.

Conclusion

A practitioner rarely "cures" a myofascial pain syndrome. Successful results are gained only when therapy by a health professional is one tool in the patient's active attempt to take care of himself or herself. It is a disservice to massage patients and create a situation where patients are merely passive recipients of treatment and feel they must rely on someone else to "fix" them. As a physical therapist, it is my practice to try to empower all patients by first teaching them what they can do for themselves; secondly, to encourage and guide patients in carrying out their home program; thirdly, applying hands-on treatment and modalities when self-care treatment is not enough; and finally, referring them to other health professionals when necessary.

References

1. Arnoff GM: Myofascial syndrome and fibromyalgia: A critical assessment and alternative view. Clinical J Pain 14:74–85, 1998.
2. Arnold MD, Thornbrough LM: Treatment of musculoskeletal pain with traditional Chinese herbal medicine. Phys Med Rehab Clin North Am 10(3):663–672, 1999.
3. Backstrom G: When Muscle Pain Won't Go Away. Dallas, Taylor, 1992.
4. Braverman DL, Schulman RA: Massage techniques in rehabilitation medicine. Phys Med Rehab Clin North Am 10(3):631–649, 1999.
5. Brosroff J, Callacombe SJ (eds): Food Allergy and Intolerance. Philadelphia, WB Saunders, 1987.
6. Chaitow L: Osteopathic Self-treatment. Wellingborough, UK, Thorsons, 1990, p 43.
7. Coan R, Wong G, Coan PL: The acupuncture treatment of neck pain: A randomized controlled study. Am J Chin Med 9:326–332, 1982.
8. Crowley D, Kendall N: Development and initial validation of a questionnaire for measuring fear-avoidance associated with pain: The fear-avoidance of pain scale. J Musculoskeletal Pain 1(3):3–20, 1999.
9. Cyriax J: Textbook of Orthopaedic Medicine, vol 2, 8th ed. Baltimore, Williams & Wilkins, 1971.
10. Feldenkrais M: Awareness through Movement. New York, Harper & Row, 1977.
11. Field T. Massage therapy effects. American Psychologist 53(12):1270–1281, 1998.
12. Fritz S: Mosby's Fundamentals of Therapeutic Massage. St. Louis, Mosby, 2000.
13. Golan R: Optimal Wellness. New York, Ballantine Books, 1995.
14. Grzesiak RC: Psychological aspects of chronic orofacial pain: Theory, assessment and management. Pain Digest 1:100–119, 1991.
15. Grzesiak RC: Psychological considerations in myofascial pain, fibromyalgia, and related musculoskeletal pain. In Rachlin ES (ed): Myofascial Pain Syndromes and Fibromyalgia. St. Louis, Mosby, 1994.
16. Guadagno-Hammond C: Trager Mentastics: Movement as a Way to Agelessness. New York, Stanton Hill Press, 1987.
17. Hofkosh JM: Classical massage. In Basmajian JV (ed): Manipulation, Traction and Massage, 3rd ed. Baltimore, Williams & Wilkins, 1985.
18. Holmes TH, Wolff HG: Life situations, emotions, and backache. Psychosom Med 14:18–33, 1952.
19. Hubbard DR, Berkoff GM: Myofascial trigger points show spontaneous needle EMG activity. Spine 18(13):1803–1807, 1993.
20. Hughes EC, Gott PS, Weinstein RC, Binggeli R: Migraine: A diagnosis test for etiology of food sensitivity by nutritionally supported fast and confirmed by long-term report. Ann Allergy 55:23–32, 1985.
21. Kho HG, Robertson EN: The mechanisms of acupuncture analgesia: Review and update. American Journal of Acupuncture 25(4):261–281, 1997.
22. Knapp ME: Massage. In Keottke FT, Stillwell GK, Lehman JF (eds): Krusen's Handbook of Physical Medicine and Rehabilitation. Philadelphia, WB Saunders, 1982.
23. Kraus H (ed): Diagnosis and Treatment of Muscle Pain, Chicago, Quintessence Books, 1988.
24. Kraus H: Clinical Treatment of Back and Neck Pain. New York, McGraw-Hill, 1970.
25. Kuprian W (ed): Physical Therapy for Sports. Philadelphia, WB Saunders, 1982.
26. Le Postollec M: Massage therapy: History, physiology and research. Advance for Physical Therapists and PT Assistants, Oct 30, 2000:6–7.
27. Lehmann JF, DeLateur BJ: Cryotherapy. In Lehman JF (ed): Therapeutic Heat and Cold. Baltimore, Williams & Wilkins 1982.
28. Lewit K: Manipulative Therapy in Rehabilitation of the Motor System. London, Butterworths, 1985.
29. Lipowski ZJ: Somatization and depression. Psychosomatics 31:13–21, 1990.
30. Little CH, Stewart AG, Fennessy MR: Platelet serotonin release in rheumatoid arthritis as studied in food intolerant patients. Lancet ii:297–299, 1983.
31. MacDonald G: Medicine Hands: Massage for People with Cancer. Tallahassee, Fla, Findhorn Press, 1999.
32. Maisel E (ed): The Resurrection of the Body; The Essential Writings of F. Matthias Alexander. New York, Delta Books, 1980.
33. Mansfield LE, Vaughan ST, Waller SF, et al: Food allergy and adult migraine: Double-blind and mediator confirmation of an allergic etiology. Ann Allergy 55:126–129, 1985.
34. McCain G: Treatment of fibromyalgia and myofascial pain syndromes. In Rachlin ES (ed): Myofascial Pain and Fibromyalgia. St. Louis, Mosby, 1994.
35. McCain GA: Management of fibromyalgia syndrome. In Fricton JF, Awas EA (eds): Advances in Pain Research and Therapy. New York, Raven Press, 1990, p 297.
36. McClaflin R: Myofascial pain syndrome: Primary care strategies for early intervention. Postgraduate Med 96(2):56–71, 1994.

37. McNulty WH, Gevirtz RN, Hubbard DR, Berkoff GM: Needle electromyographic evaluation of trigger point response to a psychological stressor. Psychophysiology 31(3):313–316, 1994.
38. Miller B: Alternative somatic therapies. In White A, Anderson R (eds): Conservative Care of Low Back Pain. Baltimore, Williams & Wilkins, 1991.
39. Murphy J: Trager. Advance for Physical Therapists, July 11, 1994:4.
40. Murray M, Pizzorno J: Encyclopedia of Natural Medicine, 2nd ed. Rocklin, Prima Publishing, 1998.
41. Ork H: Uses of cold. In Kuprian W (ed): Physical Therapy for Sports. Philadelphia, WB Saunders, 1982.
42. Ortolani C: Atlas on mechanisms in adverse reaction to foods. Allergy 50(Suppl. 20):5–81, 1995.
43. Ozer MN: Patient as partner: Patient involvement in rehabilitation. Presented at Focus on Pain '98, March 15, 1998, San Antonio, Texas.
44. Paris B: Myofascial Pain/Dysfunction: Level II Trigger Point: Head, Neck, and Jaw; Level II Trigger Point: Back Pain. Ithaca, New York, April 10–11, 1999.
45. Pomeranz B: Scientific basis of acupuncture: In Stux G, Pomeranz B (eds): Acupuncture Textbook and Atlas. Berlin, Springer-Verlag, 1987.
46. Prudden B: Pain Erasure: The Bonnie Prudden Way. New York, Ballantine Books, 1980.
47. Rickover R: Fitness without Stress: A Guide to the Alexander Technique. Portland, Ore, Metamorphous Press, 1988.
48. Sarno J: The Mind Body Prescription: Healing the Body, Healing the Pain. New York, Warner Books, 1998.
49. Sella GE: Surface EMG in the investigation and treatment of myofascitis. Presentation at the Janet G. Travell Seminar Series-Focus on Pain '98, March 12–15, 1998, San Antonio, Texas.
50. Shaeferman S: Awareness Heals: The Feldenkrais Method for Dynamic Health. Reading, Mass, Perseus Books, 1997.
51. Shaw N: On the trigger. Advance for Physical Therapists and PT Assistants, December 11, 2000:35–36.
52. Simons DG, Travell TG, Simons LS: Myofascial Pain and Dysfunction. The Trigger Point Manual, vol 1, 2nd ed. Baltimore: Williams & Wilkins, 1999.
53. Simunovic Z: Low-level laser therapy with trigger point technique, a clinical study on 243 patients. J Clin Laser Med Surg 14(4):163–167, 1996.
54. Skubick D: The upper quadrant myofascial syndrome from a biomechanical, ergonomic, and psychophysical perspective. Paper presented at Focus on Pain '98 Conference, March 12–15, 1998, San Antonio, Texas.
55. Tappan F: Healing massage techniques. A study of Eastern and Western methods. Reston, Va, Reston Publishing, 1978.
56. Torg J, Vegso J, Torg E: Rehabilitation of Athletic Injuries. An Atlas of Therapeutic Exercises. St. Louis, Mosby-Year, 1987, p 6.
57. Trager M: Trager mentastics: Movement as a Way to Agelessness. Tarrytown, NY, Station Hill Press, 1989.
58. Travell JG, Simons DG: Myofascial Pain and Dysfunction. The Trigger Point Manual, vol 1. Baltimore, Williams & Wilkins, 1983.
59. Travell JG, Simons DG: Myofascial Pain and Dysfunction. The Trigger Point Manual, vol 2. Baltimore, Williams & Wilkins, 1992.
60. Voss DE, Ionta MK, Myers BJ: Proprioceptive neuromuscular facilitation, 3rd ed. Philadelphia, Harper & Row, 1985.
61. Wakim K: Physiologic effects of massage. In Basmajian JV (ed): Manipulation, Traction and Massage, 3rd ed. Baltimore, Williams & Wilkins, 1985.
62. Watrous IS: The Trager approach: An effective tool for physical therapy. Physical Therapy Forum, April 10, 1992:22–25.
63. Wook EC, Becker PD: Beard's Massage, 3rd ed. Philadelphia, WB Saunders, 1981.
64. Yue SK: Compartment approach to the shoulder and pelvic girdles related pain syndrome. Presentation at the Janet G. Travell Seminar Series-Focus on Pain '98, March 12–15, 1998, San Antonio, Texas.

Chapter 17

Manual Therapy for Myofascial Pain and Dysfunction

Brian Miller, PT, OCS

According to Lewit, "The structure in the motor system that reacts most to stimuli and is the effector of the nervous system is the muscle. As a result, it is also the structure that most regularly and intensively expresses pain."[42] In other words, myofascial tissue, owing partly to its dynamic and mutable nature, is highly susceptible to dysfunction and pain. This, fortunately, also makes it highly amenable to positive change via physical means of treatment, specifically orthopedic manual therapy. The exact nature of the pathologic changes in myofascial tissues has not been elucidated. There appears to be no simple answer, and possibly a complex combination of factors is involved. This area is in urgent need of further research. We can, however, speculate about various hypothetical mechanisms of myofascial pain and dysfunction (MPD) and how they may relate to management of the problem.

These mechanisms can be categorized in various ways, but I have found three main classifications helpful. This chapter is in no way offered as a comprehensive or scientifically exacting investigation of this area but provides a modicum of organization for directing future study.

The first category includes biomechanical influences. These range from simple mechanical inefficiency to actual muscle and connective tissue changes. Mechanical inefficiency can result from intratissue as well as intertissue and extratissue sources. Intratissue sources include increased muscle tension levels, which can include increases from passive sources such as muscle edema[62] and also from active sources such as excessive muscle tonus (as indicated by elevated electromyographic activity)[25] associated with dysponesis.[65] Intertissue sources involve increased friction or drag between adjacent structures (or even actual adherences), which are manifested in decreased layer mobility or decreased muscle play as defined by Johnson.[29] Myofascial tissue changes can include tissue dehydration (as occurs in many aging connective tissues), tissue or collagen creep (as occurs with diminished or absent movement), sources of tethering ranging from the microlevel (e.g., collagen cross-linking) to the macrolevel (e.g., post-traumatic scarring), and other changes (e.g., alterations in the extracellular matrix, ground substance, and so on). These changes range from microscopic ultrastructural to macroscopic. Extratissue sources are discussed later.

The second category includes neurophysiologic influences. This category can include reflex action, cyclic stereotypical action, and habitual conditioned action.[16] At the reflex level, such reflexes as the stretch reflex or the Golgi tendon organ (GTO) reflex may be involved. Also, more obscure "reflexes" may be involved (which may possibly be classified as cyclic stereotypical action) such as the protective arthrokinematic reflex[3, 68] and the startle pattern.[56] Overlapping with this area are both conscious and unconscious aspects of instinctive and learned behavior. Because the musculature of the body is a primary means of emotional expression, emotional and cognitive states can have a profound influence on neuromuscular behavior and can contribute to MPD.

The third category involves fluidochemical influences. This category includes micro- and macrocirculatory changes affecting fluidochemical transport and exchange (such as altered chemical exchange on the cellular level, impaired lymphatic flow, and vascular stasis or ischemia). Rolf[50] discussed changes in the chemical state of the muscle from a gel to a solid state, a hypothesis that has been shown to be invalid yet that may offer insights into the nature of change in myofascial tissues. Various chemical substances may influence myofascial tissue, such as metabolites (both substrates and byproducts), electrolytes, hormones, neurotransmitters, and neurogenic and non-neurogenic pain mediators). One or more of these chemicals may be lacking, overabundant, or present in balanced qualities. Tsujii[62] has shown the relationship of mechanical stimulation of polymodal receptors to neurogenically based inflammatory and immunologic activity.

Electrochemical influences may also be involved because most essential biologic functions are composed of biochemical and bioelectric phenomena such as membrane depolarization and repolarization, with the accompanying production of weak electromagnetic fields. The interactive nature of biologic tissues and electromagnetic fields is a fascinating area that is just beginning to be studied and could yield valuable information related to MPD as well as many other areas in medicine. In addition, such phenomena as the piezoelectric effect are well known in the physical sciences; there may be a parallel phenomenon in biologic tissues. A mechanism similar to this phenomenon could explain why practitioners can touch tissues in different ways utilizing differing therapeutic forces but still produce similar beneficial effects when the touching is performed with a clear intention and purpose. Certainly this is an area worthy of investigation.

Obviously, these categories and the proposed hypothetical mechanisms are not mutually exclusive but involve significant interaction and overlap. Both the mechanically based intention of orthopedic manual therapies and the re-educational emphasis of neurologic manual therapies can operate through any number of the mechanisms proposed earlier.

The lack of precise knowledge regarding pathologic changes in myofascial tissues does not preclude effective treatment, however. Maitland discusses "not allowing theoretical knowledge (which in fact may be quite false), or lack of it, to obstruct seeing and finding clinical facts."[44] A balance of both the science and the art of myofascially directed manual therapy is needed. Although laboratory and clinical science provides the framework and guidelines for treatment, historically many scientific discoveries have been made in accordance with the adage that "empiricism adjusts the path of science behind it."[26] Maitland states that "there is much in medicine that is still unknown, and although precise diagnosis is not always possible, this need be no bar to precise, effective, and informative manipulative treatment. . . ."[44] Herein enters the art of treatment, which ultimately determines how successfully this information is utilized.

The approach discussed in this chapter is eclectic but is based heavily on the functional orthopedic perspective developed by Johnson[29] and is also influenced by the more recent research of Tsujii.[62]

Evaluation

Although MPD is wide-reaching in its scope and influence and can involve virtually any body area, I have chosen to present illustrative examples from the cervical region—the upper cervical region in particular. This choice was made to adapt this information to a single chapter. The reader should keep in mind that in no way does this selective presentation indicate that I advocate a reductionist approach whereby a region of the body is evaluated and treated in isolation. On the contrary, unless the therapist adopts a systems-based approach and looks at whole body functioning in relation to the symptomatic or dysfunctional area, it is likely that the patient's full rehabilitation potential will not be attained and therapeutic benefits will be both incomplete and temporary.

Subjective

Subjective evaluation has been thoroughly presented by others and extensive discussion here would be redundant. Nevertheless, a methodical and meticulous subjective examination will provide the clinician with most information necessary to obtain an accurate clinical impression. One point that deserves special mention is the importance of tracing the patient's actions as thoroughly as possible through the entire course of a typical day and night. This process is indispensable in uncovering the habitual positions, postures, activities, or movements that contributed to the patient's problem. An outline of key points in taking a history follows:

I. Type of onset
   A. Sudden
      1. Nontraumatic
      2. Traumatic
         a. Microtraumatic
         b. Macrotraumatic
   B. Gradual or insidious
      1. When was it first noticeable? Problematic?
      2. What was the time frame of its development?
II. Occurrence
   A. First time
   B. Occurred previously (episodic)
      1. Sporadically
      2. Predictably
   C. Past occurrence
      1. Course of the problem
      2. Response to treatment
      3. Recovery time
III. Symptom location
   A. Pain
      1. Body chart
      2. Quality of location
         a. Localized or diffuse
         b. Superficial or deep
      3. Does it change distribution (size, depth, etc.)?
         a. Location at its worst
         b. Location at its best
   B. Dysesthesias
   C. Other symptoms
      1. Stiffness or immobility
      2. Weakness
      3. Swelling
      4. Instability, giving way
      5. Locking
      6. Other
IV. Nature of pain
   A. Pain quality—MMPI
V. Presence
   A. Constant
      1. Fixed intensity
      2. Variable intensity
   B. Intermittent
      1. Duration when present
      2. Frequency of appearance
VI. Quantitative ranking of intensity (on an analogue scale)
   A. In the last 24 hours
   B. Since problem began
      1. At its best
      2. At its worst
VII. Influence of motion and position
   A. Aggravating factors

    B. Easing factors
        1. Activity level
            a. Rest
            b. Prolonged postures
            c. Activity
                (1) Prescription—how much?
        2. Posture
            a. Recumbent
                (1) Supine
                (2) Side-lying
                (3) Prone
                (4) Other
            b. Sitting
                (1) Unsupported or supported
                (2) Slouched or upright
            c. Standing
        3. Movements
            a. Transfers
                (1) Rolling
                (2) Lying-to-sitting
                (3) Sitting-to-standing
            b. Walking
            c. Squatting
            d. Stairs
            e. Bending
            f. Lifting
            g. Carrying
            h. Twisting
            i. Reaching
        4. Valsalva maneuver
        5. Sensitivities[68]
            a. Weight-bearing sensitivity
            b. Stasis sensitivity
            c. Pressure sensitivity
            d. Positional sensitivity
VIII. Rest factors
    A. Sleeping position
    B. Movements related to bed
        1. How they roll over
        2. How they arise from bed
    C. Bed
        1. Type and condition of bed
        2. Side slept on
        3. Position relative to bed partner
    C. Pillow
        1. Composition of pillow
        2. Number and thickness of pillows
        3. Positioning of pillows
    D. Sleep quality
        1. How much sleep
        2. Quality of sleep
        3. How easy to fall asleep and wake up
    E. Pre- and post-sleep activities
        1. Activities just prior to sleeping
        2. How patient wakes up first thing in morning
        3. Activities just after waking

IX. State of health
    A. General appraisal of health
    B. Recent weight change
        1. Explained (dieting, stress, etc.)
        2. Unexplained
    C. Medications
        1. Possible contraindications to manual therapy
           a. Steroids
           b. Anticoagulants
    D. Nutrition
        1. Hydration levels and factors affecting hydration such as alcohol and methylxanthine (especially caffeine) intake
        2. Overall food quality and health
        3. Macronutrient profile and composition
        4. Vitamin and mineral intake
        5. Phytochemical intake
        6. Bacterial flora in gastrointestinal tract
        7. Consumption of nonessential substances
    D. Night pain
        1. None noticed
        2. Pain provoked with position change but then allows patient to fall asleep again
        3. Pain keeps patient awake but patient can stay in bed
        4. Pain keeps patient awake and requires that patient periodically get out of bed to obtain relief
X. Personal information
    A. Age and weight
    B. Family and other psychoemotional, psychosocial, and socioeconomic factors
XI. Personal habits
    A. Bowel and bladder function
    B. Menstruation
    C. Sex
    D. Diet
XII. Lifestyle
    A. Occupation
        1. Physical demands
        2. Workplace design
        3. Psychological demands
    B. Recreation
        1. Leisure activities
        2. Sports, performing arts, etc
XIII. Test results
    A. Imaging tests—x-rays, computed tomography, magnetic resonance imaging, bone scan, etc.
    B. Blood tests
    C. Electrodiagnostic tests
    D. Others
XIV. General leading questions
    A. "Are you under any unusual stresses?"[47]
    B. "Is there anything else I should know about?"

Some excellent references in this area include the works of Maitland[44] and McKenzie.[47] Although these monographs are intended for joint-oriented therapies, their principles apply to myofascially directed therapies as well. Maitland's discussion of communication is particularly noteworthy. Refined communication skills are fundamental in the management of any neuromusculoskeletal condition, including MPD. One of the best known and respected clinicians in this area of patient-clinician communication was Milton Erickson. Although he practiced psychiatry, the principles that he developed and expounded upon are highly applicable to myofascial and other musculoskeletal problems.[16] It would behoove both the novice and the experienced practitioner to study works written by and about this consummately skilled physician.

Information more specifically related to myofascial disorders is provided by the classic works of Travell and Simons.[60, 61] In particular, the stereotypical patterns of local and referred pain from myofascial tissues that these authors documented should be noted during the subjective aspect of the evaluation. For example, myofascial dysfunction in the suboccipital muscles such as the rectus capitus posterior major may cause local pain in the posterior suboccipital region as well as pain referred from the occiput to the orbital region.

Objective

Objective findings are obtained through both visual and tactile/kinesthetic means. The therapist observes the patient's static structure and observes as well as feels the quantity and particularly the quality of his or her movements.

Observation

The therapist observes both the patient's skeletal and soft tissue structure. In observing skeletal structure, the therapist uses "x-ray eyes," noting the skeletal orientation, alignment, and position from an impression of the underlying skeletal configuration and visible bony landmarks. The skeleton should optimally be aligned such that a vertical plumb line would symmetrically bisect the skeleton when viewed in the frontal plane. Left and right symmetry relative to this central bisecting line should also be noted. Although lack of symmetry does not necessarily indicate myofascial dysfunction (because asymmetry tends to be the norm in the human body), myofascial dysfunction is often reflected in structural asymmetry.[23]

Laterally, the alignment of bony parts and joints should match up with those parameters that have been well established for so-called "good" posture.[25] This alignment involves the center of gravity of each body part being aligned vertically above the one below it. In addition to optimal vertical alignment of the axial skeleton (cranium, spine, and pelvis) and the limbs with the vertical line of gravity, the appendicular skeleton (shoulder and pelvic girdles) should be level horizontally as well. The ideal skeletal alignment is that assumed by a freely articulated skeleton if it were suspended from the cranium with its component parts hanging downward. Although alignment is typically determined via front, rear, and side views, standing on a chair or stool and looking down on the patient from above provides an additional valuable visual perspective and enables one to see patterns that are not often seen with the more standard views.

The three-dimensional position in space of each skeletal part should also be noted. Deviations from normal can be expressed in biomechanical terms as rotations (flexion and extension, left and right rotation, left and right side-bending) and translations (anterior-posterior positioning, left-right or medial-lateral positioning, and compressed-distracted positioning).[66] For example, common deviations noted in the position of the cranium are anterior translation (i.e., forward head), extension (usually in the upper and midcervical joints), and lateral translation (lateral shift).

In addition to the relationship of each skeletal part with the whole body base of support (the feet in standing and primarily the pelvis and thighs in sitting), each inferior part provides an individual base of support for the superior part. For example, the rib cage provides the base of support for the shoulder girdle. A forward shoulder position results in inadequate inferior support for the shoulder, so that a large portion of the support comes through suspensory muscles such as the upper trapezius and the levator scapulae hanging from the cervical spine. The result is that not only are these muscles overstressed but also other synergistic supporting muscles in the kinetic chain, such as the posterior cervical muscles, are overloaded.

Another way of viewing the body has its origins in spatial aesthetic considerations as opposed to traditional orthopedic considerations. With this spatial perspective in mind, the therapist notes the dimensions of a specific region of the body, i.e., length, depth, and width. Because muscle overactivity involves a process of shortening, the resulting decrease in span can be readily detected by noting comparative differences in dimensions. For example, cervical muscles that are in a chronic state of co-contraction will often pull the neck into a shortened configuration, roughly akin to a turtle withdrawing its head into a shell. Thus, the dimension that is diminished is length. Tight pectoral muscles will pull the shoulder girdles anteriorly and medially, causing an anterior narrowing. In this instance, the decreased dimension is width. Noting these alterations in body dimensions can be a useful guide in identifying myofascial restriction and subsequently directing treatment.[29]

In addition to noting posture, the configuration and distribution of the myofascial tissue mass are observed. A two-dimensional perspective can be gained via an outline or "silhouette" view. This view is obtained from looking at a body part profile or, conversely, by observing the negative space around a body part. When artists draw the human body, they composes it as an amalgam of ellipses. The curves in this profile view should present with that same characteristic elliptical quality. Overly flat curves suggest muscle underdevelopment or underutilization, whereas excessively rounded or bulging curves suggest muscle overdevelopment or overuse. Because these patterns of myofascial development accurately reflect the patterns of use in the body, they enable the therapist to identify sites of stress and potential dysfunction. This myofascial development can also be assessed three dimensionally as a contour rather than simply a profile.[17]

One also needs to consider the proportions of muscle development, i.e., is a particular region of the body under-, over-, or appropriately developed relative to adjacent areas of the body? The junctions between disproportionately developed areas are prime sites for tissue overload and potential sites for future degenerative changes. An example of this is the individual with overdeveloped extensor muscles in the cervical spine and underdeveloped deep flexors. This person will probably develop an excessively lordotic cervical curve and eventually demonstrate degenerative changes in the posterior articular structures as well as other related problems.

Although these observation schemes show how the appearance of the body may deviate from the ideal, appearances can be deceptive. The patient can often be using excessive effort to maintain what appears to be an ideal orthostatic position but is, in fact, inefficient and stressful. Although the experienced eye can appreciate the degree of ease or effort in posture and movement, there is a subtleness to this quality that is difficult to express. It is more concretely detected by the feel of resistance with the induction of small early-range passive motions (i.e., initiation feel) as described in the next section. An even more objective and quantifiable means of measuring this inappropriate muscle effort would be the use of surface electromyography (EMG).

Motion Testing

The therapist assesses active motion from the micro- to the macrolevel, noting (1) both spinal segmental motion and regional motion in the symptomatic region, (2) how that region participates in whole body motion, and (3) how motion in other parts of the body relates to and affects the symptomatic region. Turning the head, for example, should involve not only cervical spine segmental rotation but, for optimal efficiency, should also involve participatory action of the upper thoracic spine and rib cage, slight motion in the shoulder girdle (particularly the clavicle and the scapula), avoidance of any respiratory holding pattern in the rib cage, a very subtle torsioning down through the torso, and a slight lateral weight shift in the base of support (Fig. 17–1A and *B*). If any one of these components has disturbed motion, the resulting inefficient motion contributes, either directly or indirectly, to overload of the myofascial tissues (as well as other structures such as the joints).

Both passive and active motions are examined. Active-assistive motions with the

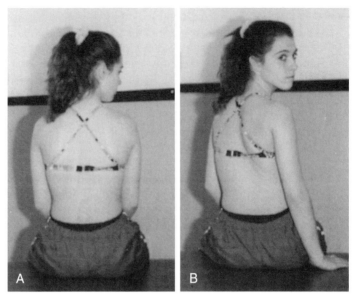

Figure 17–1. A, Rotation of cervical spine performed in isolated fashion with lack of participation of inferior segments. **B**, Rotation of cervical spine performed with integrated participation of pelvis, rib cage, and shoulder girdle, and utilization of weight-shifting.

patient in a functional weight-bearing position are of particular value. The therapist gently moves the body part a few degrees in each direction with light, gentle, slow movements, noting the patient's responsiveness to the movement, i.e., how readily, easily, and willingly the patient moves (Fig. 17–2A). This induced motion not only has the quality of passive motion because it is manually initiated by the therapist but also has the quality of active motion because the patient actively participates and does not remain totally passive. The feel of resistance to this movement is noted and can be described as an initiation feel[20, 48] (early-range). If the amplitude of motion is pro-

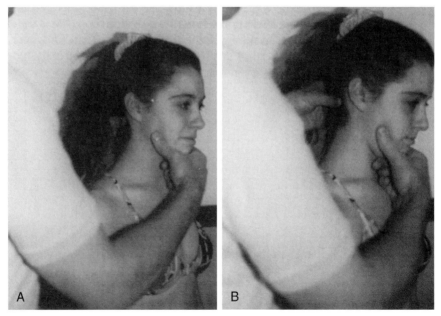

Figure 17–2. A, Assessing initiation feel of head movements. **B**, Assessing through-range feel of head movements.

gressed further (into the midrange), a through-range feel[48, 52] is assessed (Fig. 17–2*B*). Both of these forms of motion resistance assessment offer information that differs somewhat from the more commonly assessed end feel (end-range). In general, active motions are assessed more easily in a functional weight-bearing position whereas passive motions can be often be assessed more accurately in a relaxed, non–weight-bearing position.

One can also observe the length of individual muscles via well-documented muscle length tests,[12, 17, 60, 61] involving combinations of various physiologic movements. One common error made by the novice is to assume that a muscle is normal simply because it can be stretched in one direction to its full range. A large percentage of muscles have a complex muscle fiber arrangement or unusual muscle belly morphology. Multi-angular (as opposed to pure parallel) fiber direction may be present, such as in the twisted fibers in the levator scapulae muscle. The levator scapulae muscle has long, more vertically oriented, and more superficial fibers as well as shorter, more horizontally oriented, and deeper diagonal fibers.[60] In other muscles, there are also pennate and bipennate muscle fiber arrangements to consider. Therefore stretches—both for evaluation and treatment—will usually involve motion in an arcuate pathway that contains more than one plane of movement.

The therapist can also assess the accessory lengthening ability (or extensibility) of soft tissues (including muscle, fascia, and neuromeningeal elements) by applying a light tensile load, sustaining it, and noting the resulting distribution of tensile deformation.[17, 64] One common way of assessing this is with the arm pull technique (Fig. 17–3). Restrictions will be perceived as a remote "tethering"—i.e., the tissue fails to elongate in proportion to adjacent tissues. The restriction can be perceived along the linear extent of the upper quarter (in the neck region, shoulder, upper arm, and so on) as well as in the cross section of the upper limb and forequarter (anterior or posterior, superficial or deep, and so on). Although this is a highly subjective method of assessment, it can often provide information unobtainable by other means. Also, correlating the therapist's findings with results of other motion tests and findings on direct palpation as well as with the patient's subjective experience can add to the validity and reliability of the information.

Observation and motion testing are useful for determining the structural and/or functional dysfunction that is causing the problem. In terms of localizing the source of the problem, however, they are rarely as specific as palpation. Although these assessment tools may have the sensitivity to determine which motion or muscle is affected and possibly why, only palpation is discriminating enough to determine exactly which part of the muscle is affected and to direct treatment accordingly.

Note that it is of vital importance to recognize that the cause of the problem may be distinctly different from the source of the problem. Although a myofascial pain

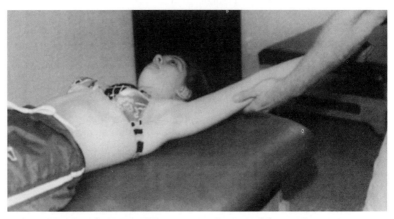

Figure 17–3. Assessing and treating deficits in muscle extensibility in forequarter region with arm pull technique.

arising from a previous traumatic injury may respond beautifully to locally directed treatment of the source (i.e., the lesioned tissue), a long-standing chronic problem, particularly one of apparently insidious but usually repetitive microtraumatic onset, usually requires treatment by a systems approach. Therefore, for successful treatment of MPD, the thinking therapist always considers both the cause and the source in developing a treatment plan.

Palpation

The high degree of sensitivity and precision possible with palpation allows one to accurately locate a lesioned area. Palpation can often detect subtle changes that would go undetected with observation alone. The therapist first notes the subjective response to palpation. Is an area tender to palpation and, if so, how easily is that area provoked? Is the area very sensitive and will light, superficial palpation provoke pain or is firmer, deeper palpation necessary to provoke pain? How irritable is the area to palpation? Does the pain subside rapidly once pressure is withdrawn or does it linger for a considerable period? With sustained pressure to the area (5–15 seconds), does the pain begin to spread and refer to another area or does it remain local or even begin to abate?

Next, more objective findings are noted with palpation. Does the condition of the area suggest a more acute lesion (i.e., is it warmer with a sense of bogginess, congestion, swelling, or inflammation) or does it appear to be more chronic (i.e., is it cooler with a sense of "dryness," stringiness, ropiness, or hardness)? Does it have qualities of both (i.e., is there a harder, denser core surrounded by an outer "sheath" layer of apparent edema)? Is the location of the sensitive indurated area very focal (i.e., does it resemble a discrete nodule), is it more linear (i.e., does it resemble a band or fibril), or does it involve a more general area (i.e., an entire region of a muscle belly)? Does the sense of tenseness and fullness involve the entire muscle or just discrete areas and does it resemble that of turgor (such as would occur with intramuscular edema) or does it have a more elastic, "twangy" property (such as would occur with muscle spasm and hypertonicity)? Does palpating the sensitive area provoke a local twitch response or a jump sign,[60] suggesting high reactivity? To develop an overall view of patterns of increased muscle tension and/or hardening, palpatory findings can be plotted on an actual body chart.

In assessing tenderness of an area, some additional points need to be clarified. While tenderness of a particular structure may be present in the majority of individuals, tenderness should not be present in a healthy, optimally functioning structure. Consequently, while tenderness may be "the norm" for that individual, it is not truly normal nor an ideal state and indicates a subclinical dysfunction. However, in detecting dysfunction beyond the baseline level, one should check if this same level of tenderness is present on the contralateral side. Virtually every myofascial structure is represented bilaterally in the human body; therefore, we have this basis of comparison. To determine if a patient is unusually sensitive to palpation in general, we may also consider palpating a healthy muscle belly in an unrelated area and noting his or her reaction to it.

Other tissue characteristics are examined with palpation that have been well described by Johnson.[29] These are (1) the intrinsic mobility of the skin as detected by sliding one's finger through the tissue and noting its inherent extensibility (finger sliding) or stretching the skin apart between two points (dual contact extensibility), (2) the sliding mobility of the skin in relation to the underlying tissue (skin sliding to assess superficial fascial mobility), (3) the side-to-side (i.e., lateral) mobility of a muscle and its freedom from adjacent structures (muscle play), and (4) the texture and consistency of the muscle itself in response to focal, linear, and general pressures and frictioning (the latter indicating both muscle tonus and muscle condition). The distinct separation of these factors for didactic purposes should not be construed as being entirely accurate in the clinical presentation. In fact, there is a considerable degree of mutual interdependency and fusion of characteristics.

Assessment

When the examination is completed, the findings are sorted and correlated and a hypothesis formed regarding the tissue(s) at fault and the possible causes of that dysfunction. For example, if the posterior suboccipital muscles are found to be dysfunctional, several hypotheses may be considered. Some possibilities might include a somatic manifestation of systemic stress, abnormal use patterns related to improper head positioning, and disturbed neuromuscular or biomechanical relationships with other areas. Discussion of some of these possibilities follows as an illustration of the complexity involved in determining etiology.

Systemic stress can be manifested somatically in the form of the startle reflex as described by Tengwall[56] (Fig. 17–4A and B), sympatheticotonia as described by Korr,[39] Selye's general and local adaptation syndromes,[54] and so forth. Each of these physiologic occurrences is an explanation for increased local and general hypertonicity that could overstress the suboccipital region.

One set of abnormal use patterns in the cervical spine is related to how the head can be postured in various ways to accommodate vision. Prolonged work on a computer monitor with a fixed visual focus involves static contraction of the suboccipital muscles. The suboccipital muscles have approximately the same motor unit to nerve fiber ratio (5:1) as the ocular muscles, suggesting a strong functional connection as aptly demonstrated with normal eye-head coordination. Any time we turn to look at something, the eye and neck movements are well synchronized. This static positioning at the monitor, the protracted position often adopted with strained vision, the forward tilt position that is necessary with using bifocals, and the backward tilt position that is often employed in using glasses that slide down the nose are but a few of the aberrant use patterns that can contribute to pain and dysfunction in the cervical musculature, especially the suboccipital area.

The suboccipital region is related to other areas of the body both neuromuscularly and biomechanically. Besides its direct relation to the eyes as discussed, the suboccipi-

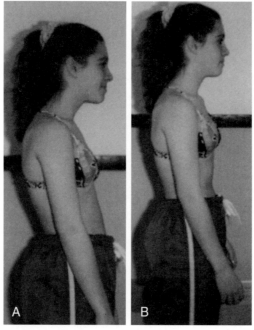

Figure 17–4. A, "Startle" response or somatic retraction posture. Note the posterior inclination of the thorax and the withdrawn position of the sternum, which dictate the dysfunctional shoulder girdle, neck, and head position. **B**, Less overt, more subtle "startle" response posture.

tal region is also related to the temporomandibular joint, because an increase in tone in the masticatory muscles sets off a kinetic chain reaction involving other muscles such as the hyoidal muscles. This in turn requires a proportional increase in the suboccipital muscle tone to maintain a balanced, level position of the cranium in the sagittal plane. The sacroiliac joint is also related to the suboccipital region, especially the occipito-atlantal joint. The exact nature of this relationship is unclear—perhaps it has to do with horizontal balance in the axial skeleton. Nevertheless, many astute clinicians including Grieve[22] and Lewit[43] as well as by the chiropractic profession—the Lovett "brother" relationship. Numerous other clinical situations contribute to dysfunction in the suboccipital region.

In summary, both in evaluation and treatment, a systems type of approach needs to be taken in addressing MPD. Otherwise, the practitioner is in danger of perpetually chasing symptoms but constantly overlooking the source of the problem. The postural, movement, functional, and behavioral patterns of the entire system must be considered in determining causation. It will often be discovered that what first appears to be a local myofascial problem is one involving the overall organization and use pattern of the entire organism.

Treatment

I have found that a three-pronged approach to managing MPD is effective. This approach involves manual ("hands on") therapy, movement and exercise therapy, and education (Fig. 17–5). Manual therapy includes a host of techniques with primary emphasis on soft tissue mobilization, neurosensorimotor re-education, and to a lesser extent joint mobilization. Movement and exercise therapy can include such activities as somatic education procedures[15, 32] and loosening exercises,[1, 11, 58] as well as more traditional stretching, strengthening, and conditioning exercises. Education involves both cognitive and behavioral techniques and can range from teaching improved rest and work positions to offering somatically based stress management strategies.

The goal of treatment is to restore normal intra- and intertissue mobility in the myofascial tissues. These forms of mobility are influenced by such factors as muscle

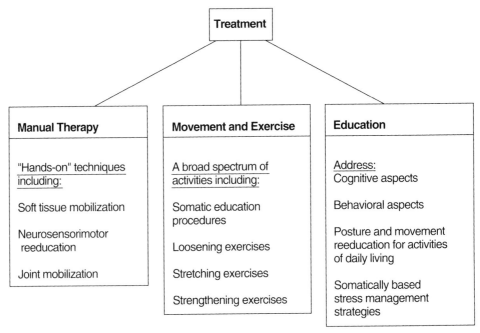

Figure 17–5. A three-pronged approach to managing myofascial pain.

play, condition, tone, length, control, and "strength" (meaning aspects of strength, power, endurance, and conditioning). Most of these factors are interrelated and to some extent inextricably intertwined. Separation is largely artificial and more for didactic purposes. From the standpoint of pure mechanics, the therapeutic goal is to improve biomechanical efficiency in the system, thereby reducing "wear and tear" on the tissues and the pain that accompanies it.

This treatment philosophy addresses both pain and dysfunction. To treat pain exclusively leads the practitioner down a deceptive path, chasing pain here and there in the body, occasionally winning "battles" but ultimately always losing the "war." Failure results because symptoms of the problem are addressed rather than the problem itself and its cause. Conversely, treating dysfunction to the exclusion of pain can lead to an approach that is overly mechanistic and frequently interpreted by the patient as cold and insensitive. The latter situation may lead to a loss of rapport with the patient and a disappointing therapeutic outcome. Rather, a balance between the two is sought, addressing both cause and symptoms, and addressing not only the problem but also the whole patient. The practitioner must be open-minded and flexible in his or her approach and have a wide variety of treatment options available. Particularly in dealing with chronic myofascial pain, a broad armamentarium of treatment principles and procedures can be invaluable because individual patient sensitivities and preferences often preclude "cookbook" or overly orthodox approaches.

Indications and Contraindications

The lack of normal soft tissue condition and mobility is the prime indication for treatment. Although pain is what brings the patient to us and it certainly guides the course of treatment, accurate and fruitful assessment requires that we have more objectively verifiable findings to base our treatment on. These findings consist of the structural (i.e., biomechanical) and functional (i.e., neuromuscular and behavioral) restrictions that make up soft tissue dysfunction. Patients' problems can be categorized according to a number of emerging classification schemes. One particular scheme that I have found especially useful in selecting treatment is that of the McKenzie[47] paradigm. The postural (or positional, or both) syndrome is well suited to a neurosensorimotor re-education approach, whereas the dysfunction syndrome lends itself well to a soft tissue mobilization approach. Although the derangement syndrome can be addressed with either of these two manual approaches, it lends itself to more direct and rapid improvement with joint-oriented techniques involving repeated or sustained end-range positioning or joint mobilization and manipulation, individually or in combination. Although such cookbook generalizations can sometimes be inaccurate, they do provide a useful starting point for less experienced clinicians.

Contraindications are similar to those well documented with joint-oriented manual therapy,[12] but soft tissue–oriented techniques are much safer. Conditions involving active infection, inflammation, neoplasia, or other dangerous disease processes; severe neurologic changes; instability; fresh tissue injury; and similar circumstances should be avoided. However, the actual extent of these conditions, the specific way in which manual therapy is administered, and the practitioner's skills make many contraindications relative rather than absolute. Travell and Simons[60] mention the danger involved with pressure over the posterior triangle of the neck, but I have never personally encountered a difficulty with this procedure, and in informal surveys of fellow clinicians performing similar work, no difficulties of that specific type have been encountered. On three occasions, I have had patients experience mild autonomic reactions involving sweating, lightheadedness, and diffuse uneasiness, similar to an acute stress reaction, but these were transient reactions only. The patient was allowed to rest quietly in a recumbent position and was given a small amount of drink or food if requested. The problem passed within 30 minutes and the patient experienced no ill effects the following day.

Manual Therapy Options

The therapist is presented with various therapeutic dichotomies when selecting from among the different manual therapy options. For example, either a hypo- or a hyperstimulation approach may be used. A hypostimulation approach (light force and strong avoidance of any discomfort) has many applications but can be particularly useful for the anxious, sensitive, or more acute patient. A hyperstimulation approach[30, 62] (heavier force and some tolerance for producing moderate discomfort) is used less often but can be of value for an athletic or heavily muscled patient with tight or thick connective tissue or for a chronically involved patient with lower levels of irritability (Fig. 17–6).

One can also choose between sustained and rhythmic techniques. Sustained techniques can be useful if repetitive motion is irritating, whereas rhythmic techniques have a neuromodulatory influence and are useful for tonus and nonirritable pain reduction. Monophasic techniques are normally used, but polyphasic techniques (involving several simultaneous directions or rhythms of motion) can be employed when needed to disrupt dysponetic[65] patterns of muscle activity. Likewise, one can select between non–weight-bearing and weight-bearing treatment. Treatment in a non–weight-bearing position facilitates overall relaxation, whereas treatment in weight-bearing position simulates a more functional position.

Surprisingly, under certain circumstances, as when the neck is treated, patients may actually feel more secure in a weight-bearing position as opposed to a non–weight-bearing one. This situation occurs because in the supine position, patients are obliged to surrender much of their muscular control in the neck to allow passive movement. If they fail to do so, they may experience even more pain with manual therapy than without. Similar dichotomies are specific vs. generalized treatment and an isolated vs. an integrated approach.

Of a more specific and practical nature, numerous mechanical options in technique application exist. Therapeutic force can be applied tangentially to more superficial tissues or perpendicularly to deeper tissues; the contact area can be focal or broad; pressures can be lighter or firm, involve a moving contact and a stationary muscle or a stationary contact and a moving muscle; the contact site can be fixed or variable; and movement rhythm can be sustained or intermittent. In addition, intermittent rhythms can range from slow repetitive (approximately 0.5 Hz), to medium rhythmic (approximately 0.5–2.0 Hz), to fast oscillatory (approximately 2–4 Hz) rhythms.

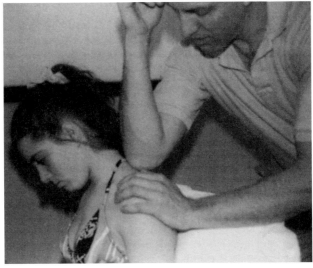

Figure 17–6. A hyperstimulation technique utilizing deep focal pressure technique in the left superomedial interscapular region with patient's upper quarter slumped into flexion, the cervical spine rotated mildly to the right, and the left arm hanging relaxed.

One may need to consider the patient's belief system in selecting the type of intervention that would be of most benefit to them. If the patient has a particular bias in preference for a treatment approach, it would behoove the wise practitioner to work with the patient in accordance with that person's wishes.

Soft Tissue Treatment Options

The number of techniques that can be applied is almost infinite, with each individual technique being a composite of a number of variables depending upon the desired therapeutic effect. The following are some of the variables that can constitute the characteristics of specific techniques:

1. The particular soft tissue characteristic to be addressed
   a. Layer mobility
   b. Muscle play
   c. Muscle tonus
   d. Muscle condition
   e. Myofascial length and extensibility (including muscular, fascial, neuromeningeal, and other components)
2. The position of the patient
   a. Supine, prone, side-lying, sitting, and other traditional positions
   b. Nontraditional static positions such as those adopted from Rolfing, Feldenkrais, yoga, qi gong, martial arts, dance, and other nontraditional sources
   c. Dynamic movements involving active motion adopted from Rolfing as well as newer bodywork approaches
3. The anatomic region addressed
   a. Specific
   b. General
4. The manual "tools" (and hence the contact area and pressure)
   a. Combinations of fingers and thumbs
   b. Knuckles
   c. Hands
   d. Elbows and forearms
   e. Feet and other body parts
5. The intensity of the technique
   a. Hypostimulatory
   b. Neutral
   c. Hyperstimulatory
6. The temporal nature of techniques
   a. Sustained
   b. Rhythmic and the variation of the rate
   c. Monophasic or polyphasic activities
7. The dynamics of the technique
   a. Body part relatively stationary and manual contact moving
   b. Manual contact relatively stationary and body part moving
8. The topographic distribution of manual therapy attention
   a. Isolated
   b. Integrated and balanced

The mechanical actions performed with soft tissue mobilization have been described as pressure, pressing, compressing, frictioning, cross-fiber stroking, snapping, strumming, rubbing, pumping, bending or breaking, stripping massage, light or firm stroking, jostling, shaking, kneading, ironing, effleurage, petrissage, and the like. The specific type of action depends on the desired effect, the patient's response to the variety of tissue deformation being performed, the morphology of the muscle being treated, and so forth.

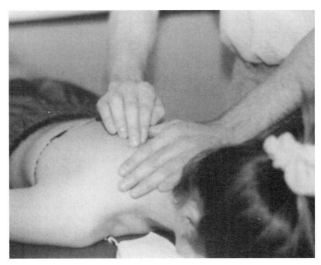

Figure 17–7. Treating focal deficit in superficial fascia layer mobility.

Layer Mobility

Techniques can be specific to tissue characteristics. In addressing layer mobility, one can treat restrictions both focally and generally. A focal technique, described by Johnson[29] as a superficial fascia technique, involves (1) locating a specific point and direction of maximum sliding restriction in the superficial plane of tissue, (2) applying a light sustained force with the fingertip(s) to that specific point in the specific planar direction of restriction, and (3) allowing soft tissue deformation to occur with the sustained application of this load (Fig. 17–7). A general technique involves a broader contact such as with the entire palmar surface of the hand and fingers and again uses sustained application of a low-level force in the superficial plane (Fig. 17–8) with the addition of spiral twisting as an option. The spiral twist can be performed in the direction of maximum ease (for the indirect technique) or the direction of maximum bind (for direct technique).

When the intrinsic mobility of the superficial fascia is restricted (i.e., restricted

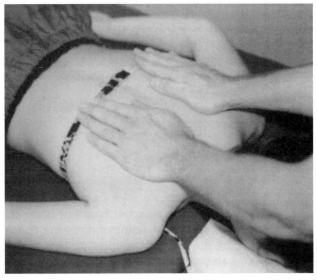

Figure 17–8. Treating generalized deficit in layer mobility of superficial fascia in the inferior direction.

extensibility of the superficial layer itself as noted between two specific points) as opposed to a restriction in the extrinsic mobility of the superficial fascia (i.e., restricted mobility of the superficial fascial layer relative to the underlying tissues), a dual contact type of technique can be utilized. With this technique, a restricted area is bracketed by finger contact at specific points on either side of the restricted area and the two contact points are slowly stretched apart. To enhance this type of treatment even further, the direction of distraction can be rhythmically rotated on a central axis (first clockwise, then counterclockwise, then clockwise again, and so on) in synchrony with any one of several inherent bodily rhythms until the restriction releases.

A common error made when addressing superficial fascial mobility is to note the amplitude of mobility rather than the quality of end feel. Just as amplitude of mobility can vary from joint to joint, so will the mobility of superficial fascia vary throughout the body, depending on whether it is on a softer ventral surface or a tougher dorsal surface, whether it is in close proximity to or distant from a bony attachment, and so forth. Johnson[29] makes the important distinction of noting that the crucial factor is an abrupt, harder end feel that exists with a restriction as opposed to a softer, more resilient end feel that is present in the absence of a restriction.

Muscle Play

In addressing muscle play, therapeutic force can be applied (1) transversely to the muscle fiber direction obtaining a perpendicular deformation of the muscle or (2) longitudinally alongside the muscle obtaining a parallel separation of the muscle from adjacent tissues. The transverse technique can be sustained or repetitive with either a slow rhythmic stretch or a more rapid oscillatory stretch. The contacts can be focal, allowing greater specificity (Fig. 17–9), or broad, allowing more comfort and dispersal of possibly irritating forces (Fig. 17–10). The longitudinal technique may consist of long continuous strokes, optimally suited for promoting fluid (i.e., lymphatic) flow or it may consist of short interrupted strokes designed to prevent the accumulation of annoying tissue tension (Fig. 17–11). This longitudinal technique can be performed along the muscle belly or similarly along the bony attachments of the muscles,

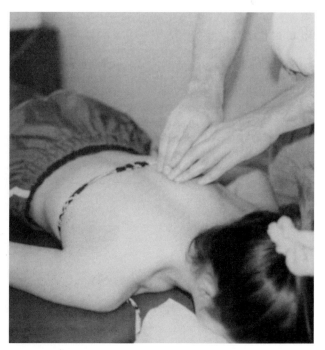

Figure 17–9. Soft tissue mobilization using focal contact in a transverse direction to improve the muscle play of the thoracic paraspinal muscles.

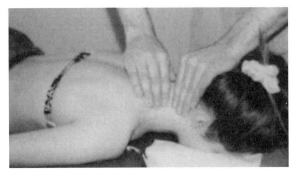

Figure 17–10. Using broad contact to effect gross muscle play in a posterior direction of the cervical extensors.

described by Johnson as a "bony contours" technique[29] (Fig. 17–12). It can function to separate muscles from other adjoining muscles or other noncontractile soft tissues, or from adjacent bones or bony attachments. Johnson[29] emphasizes the specific location, depth, and direction of the muscle play restriction. This is turn requires that the therapist position and angle the therapeutic pressures accordingly.

The sternocleidomastoid (SCM) muscle is an example of one in which play can be easily examined (Fig. 17–13). The therapist must examine this muscle along its entire course, from its attachment to the mastoid process down to its attachments into the sternum and clavicle. The muscle must have free play along its entire length from the underlying structures, just as its constituent muscle bellies must be free to move relative to one another. The SCM is generally thought of as having both a sternal and a clavicular head, but often more than two muscle bellies are apparent. In fact, Kapandji[34] states that this muscle has four distinct bands. The mobility of a muscle relative to its bony attachment is also important. An example is mobility of the upper trapezius muscle along its attachment at the superior nuchal line. These bony contours[29] must be addressed along with play movements along the belly of the muscle to ensure normal muscle play in its entirety.

Muscle Condition

Of particular importance is muscle condition. A variety of techniques can be used here, most of which fall into the category of pressures applied directly into the substance of the muscle. Rather than the emphasis on intertissue mobility as with

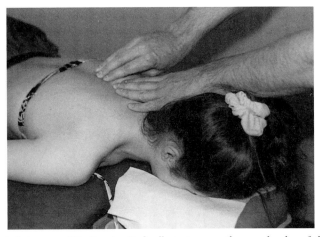

Figure 17–11. Soft tissue mobilization longitudinally to improve the muscle play of the thoracic paraspinal muscles.

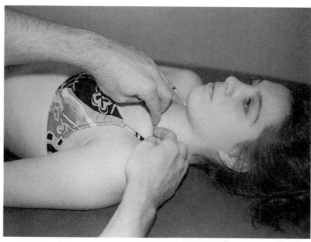

Figure 17–12. Soft tissue mobilization along the "bony contours" of the posterior border of the clavicle.

muscle play techniques, with muscle condition techniques the emphasis is on intra-tissue mobility and condition. The goal of these pressures is to break up hardened, indurated, and edematous areas of the muscle interstitia and restore the muscle to its normal resilient, supple, and homogeneous condition. Travell and Simon's[60] trigger points fall into the category of abnormal muscle condition; therefore, some of these techniques are similar if not identical to the "ischaemic compression" and "stripping massage" mentioned by these authors.[60] The pressures can be applied in a variety of forms including stationary sustained pressures and circular pressures, but most commonly, the pressures will again be applied either longitudinally in the direction of the muscle fibers or perpendicularly at right angles to the muscle fibers.

Longitudinally applied techniques can involve either focal or generalized pressures (Fig. 17–14). Focal pressures can be applied as short repeated longitudinal strokes that resemble Travell and Simon's stripping massage.[60] The emphasis with these techniques is on a circumscribed area within the muscle. Larger areas of the muscle

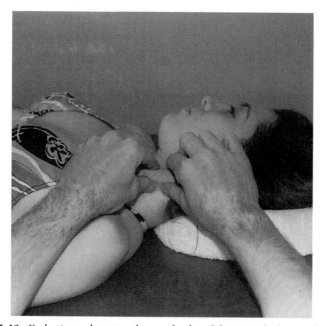

Figure 17–13. Evaluating and treating the muscle play of the sternocleidomastoid as a whole.

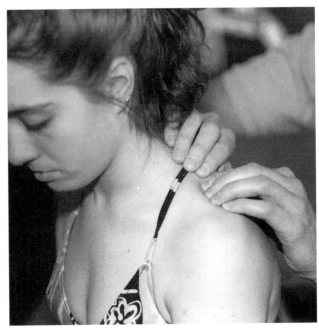

Figure 17–14. Focal longitudinally directed soft tissue mobilization improving the muscle condition of the upper trapezius.

can be addressed with generalized techniques that employ broader contact areas and long continuous, longitudinal strokes. These techniques are more dynamic and can be performed in several ways. In one way, the patient is passive and the therapist applies "ironing" pressures to the muscle (Fig. 17–15). Alternatively, the patient performs active physiologic movement while the therapist applies more or less stationary pressure against the muscle, guiding it in the proper direction and improving the "tracking" of the movement (Fig. 17–16). This latter technique is derived from Rolfing.[50]

Perpendicular pressures can also be applied in a variety of forms. One form is known as strumming.[29] It is performed by sliding the fingers against the muscle and then slipping on top of and over the muscle belly rhythmically, perpendicular to the direction of its fibers (Fig. 17–17). The site within the muscle that is addressed by this technique can be relatively constant and yet not quite fixed. This sounds paradoxical but involves the therapist constantly maneuvering the placement and angle of contact to give maximal access to the restrictions in muscle tone, play, and condition

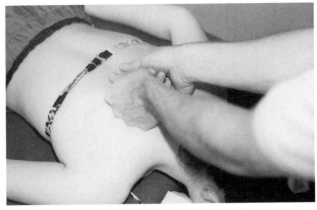

Figure 17–15. Inferiorly directed pressures to improve paraspinal muscle condition bilaterally.

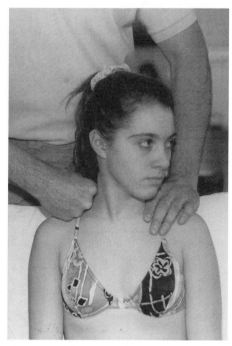

Figure 17–16. Dynamic soft tissue mobilization involving posteriorly directed sustained pressure against the shawl muscles while the patient actively rotates to the left (pressure stationary but muscle moving).

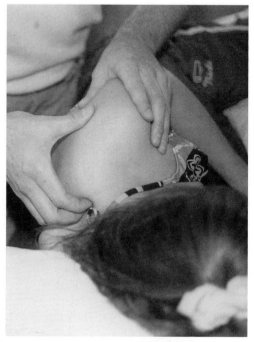

Figure 17–17. "Strumming" on the levator scapulae near its insertion in the superomedial angle of the scapula.

that can be addressed with this technique. While strumming can be used to treat muscle condition, play, and tone simultaneously, subtle variations in how it is performed usually shift the emphasis more from one to another. Strumming can be performed softly as a hypostimulation technique to mainly reduce tone or it can be performed more vigorously as a hyperstimulation technique to produce an irritating response accompanied by a reactive production of neuroanalgesic substances.[62] When the technique is performed in this more aggressive manner, both muscle condition and muscle play are affected more. Perpendicular pressures can also be performed in a firm manner on a fixed site on the muscle or tendon to facilitate tissue analgesia and healing (Cyriax's transverse friction massage[9]).

Muscle Tonus

Muscle tonus can be addressed with a wide array of techniques designed to reduce hypertonicity. *Hold* or *contract-relax techniques* at minimal levels of activation can be used to eliminate excessive muscle tonus that the patient was often unaware of using (owing to the sensorimotor amnesia phenomena described by Hanna[24]). In addition to addressing tonus at the whole muscle level, sustained focal pressure can be used to direct the individual's awareness to specific points of elevated tonus within a particular muscle in a manner similar to tactilely directed biofeedback[29] (Fig. 17–18). This useful procedure allows the patient to achieve improved muscle control and relaxation at a specific focal point within a muscle. Various adjunctive learning strategies involving visualization, imagery, breathing, and so forth can be used to assist in the development of this control.[29] Variations on this method can involve applying sustained pressure to a threshold of either pain or resistance and maintaining that pressure until the threshold changes, as demonstrated by a lessening of pain or a lessening of resistance.[10]

The *Feldenkrais method*™ uses a variety of procedures to eliminate extraneous tone.[11] One is performing passive movements slowly, smoothly, and gently, with frequent pauses and then repetition of the motion, so that the patient can become aware of and "turn off" any parasitic muscle activity. Another is to carefully shorten a muscle a very small amount through a variety of means (e.g., joint compression, support of a bony part against gravity). With this technique, the patient's central nervous system recognizes that the muscle effort previously required is no longer necessary for support and, therefore, reduces the muscle effort to the lowest essential level. This latter method is described by Rywerant[52] as an effort substitution technique.

The *Trager® approach* uses gentle, flowing rhythmic oscillations of not only local and regional structures but also the whole body to achieve a lessening of both local

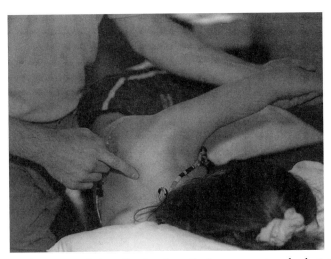

Figure 17–18. Focal pressure technique directing the patient's awareness to redundant muscle activity in simulation of forward-reaching movement.

and systemic tonus.[58] The way this effect is achieved is unclear but it may be either through peripheral mechanisms such as stimulation of skin, joint, or muscle receptors or through a central mechanism such as stimulation of the vestibular apparatus. The latter mechanism functions in much the same way that rocking soothes and calms a baby.

An additional approach is *Aston's functional massage*.[2] This unique technique involves the use of flowing massage strokes that are applied in an alternately counter-directional manner and are shaped to the contours of the patient's body.[2]

In addressing restrictions in muscle play, condition, and tone, there is considerable overlap in these factors, and accordingly their respective techniques, because one tissue mobility factor is often closely linked to another. They are presented as totally distinct entities for teaching purposes only. Often one technique is combined with another such as using the oscillations from the Trager® approach to enhance muscle play techniques (associated oscillations).[29]

Muscle Length and Extensibility

Muscle length can be restored with stretching techniques. Stretching can be specific for certain muscles or for certain directions and can be facilitated via activation of antagonists followed by activation of the agonists.[38] Considerations with regard to the direction of stretching include (1) the anatomic direction of the preponderance of fibers; (2) the precise three-dimensional direction of maximum perceived restriction; and (3) the fact that most muscles have multiangular fiber architecture (at times even involving a twist in the muscle) and compartmentalized design and function. Therefore, stretching in similar but slightly varied directions is often helpful.

Other aspects to consider with stretching include (1) heating the muscles, either extrinsically or, better yet, intrinsically via exercise; (2) fully and completely relaxing the muscles and related "control" regions of the body such as the gut, the head/neck region, fingers, toes); (3) coordinating stretching with respiration, with stretching performed primarily during the relaxation that occurs during the exhalation phase; (4) utilizing the "five S's:" slow, small, soft, smooth, and sensitive;[48] (see under Sensorimotor Control); (5) engaging the end-range barrier in a gentle, inquisitive, exploratory manner rather than in an abrupt and coercive manner; (6) doing the more restricted side first and last so that it gets proportionally more attention; (7) allowing for a refractory period of at least several seconds for the muscle tonus to subside to baseline levels after activation of the antagonists; and (8) releasing from the stretched position slowly and carefully to avoid rebound tightening.

A whole host of stretching methodologies[43] exists, but the details of these go beyond the scope of this discussion. Such types include static passive (relaxed), static active, (including so-called active isolated), isometric, and dynamic. Besides the traditional physiologic stretching, stretching can also be performed euthytatically with application of sustained, low-level, tensile forces (Fig. 17–19). Variations include adding a spiral twist to the linear forces and using hold and contract-relax variations[30] as well as including positional variations that facilitate stretching neuromeningeal elements. The myofascial release techniques described by Ward[64] fall into this category.

Neurosensorimotor Treatment Options

Any one of the methods of this category encompasses a wealth of detail that goes beyond the scope of this chapter and therefore is mentioned here only in terms of general principles. Both traditional methods such as neurodevelopment treatment (NDT) and proprioceptive neuromuscular facilitation (PNF) as well as alternative methods such as those of Alexander,[32] Feldenkrais,[17] and Trager®[58, 59] may be utilized.

A particular program that I have found useful in dealing with many cases of MPD consists of elements of the previously mentioned disciplines and includes the following strategies: (1) inhibiting redundant, dysponetic, or otherwise inappropriate muscle activity that would interfere with the desired movement; (2) selectively recruiting

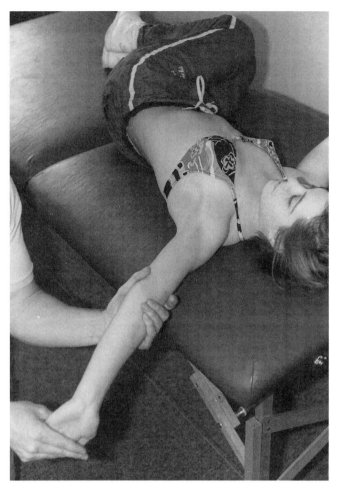

Figure 17–19. Stretching technique combining trunk rotation, shoulder external rotation and abduction, and wrist extension to achieve functional stretching of the pectoral muscles, upper extremity and forequarter fasciae, and neuromeningeal elements.

minimal muscle effort in a controlled manner to achieve the desired movement with less effort and more efficiency; and (3) adding progressively graded resistance to smoothly amplify these minimal efforts into stronger ones, thereby facilitating the power and functionality of these desired movements. Depending on the clinical situation, one or more of these strategies can be used, either alone or in combination.

Inhibitory strategies can include (1) rhythmic oscillatory movement; (2) light sustained touch and handling having a directional intent and employing extremely low-load compressive or tensile forces; (3) light exploratory touch that cultivates kinesthetic awareness; (4) very slow, smooth, gentle, guided, and supported movements; and (5) sustained and supported positions and postures.

The selective recruitment strategy uses many of the same techniques in a process of taking an unskilled habitual movement, differentiating it into its component deliberate movements, and then reorganizing and integrating these deliberate movements back into a more efficient, skilled, and integrated movement.[5] This process can be achieved with gentle, slow, and precise "communicative" handling and use of a variety of nonhabitual movement patterns.

The resistance strategy involves taking the new, more efficient movement and progressively applying resistance incrementally, maintaining the quality of movement yet improving its power and quickness. With this strategy, it is desirable to develop muscle control through the full spectrum of facilitation, from minimal to maximal levels of muscle activation.

Although the word *movement* has been used earlier, a more appropriate term may be the *neuromuscular organization* of the body. This latter term reflects both the more static aspects of posture and dynamic aspects of movement and avoids the tendency to view posture and movement as separate rather than interrelated entities. Certainly, all of these strategies are applicable to both posture and movement.

An extremely common example of an aberrant neuromuscular pattern that can lead to MPD is the stiffening of the muscles of the neck that accompanies the initiation of movement. In time, this neuromuscular habit often progresses to a maintained co-contraction of the muscles of the neck that, in fact, is entirely unnecessary. This phenomenon is discussed in depth with regard to the Alexander technique under Sensorimotor Control. Considerable overlap exists between manual therapy and movement therapy because manual therapy is often needed to create the desired neuromuscular state, whereas movement therapy is required to train the patient to develop and maintain this state through regular practice with ongoing awareness.

Joint Mobilization Options

The role of joints in myofascial dysfunction must also be considered. Korr[39] has described the presence of somatosomatic and viscerosomatic reflexes in which both joint dysfunction and visceral dysfunction result in referred pain or even referred tenderness in the myofascial tissues.[8] Although treating the myofascia can often produce relief of pain, ultimately the source of the problem must be addressed to avoid relapse. Thus apparent myofascial pain can arise from structures other than the myofascia, and in instances when joint dysfunction is causing this pain, it is most effectively treated with joint mobilization or manipulation.[24]

Distinction between the different causes of apparent MPD is not easy and requires thorough evaluation and treatment of all problems affecting the associated structures with the potential for contributing to the pain, particularly joints but also including such structures as the neuromeningeal elements.[4] These structures can be those located in the area of pain, those capable of referring pain into the area, and those in other locations that can produce adverse effects. Assessment of the treatment response will further corroborate the source of the dysfunction and whether that source is in the condition of a structure itself or in the nature of its function(s).

Assistive Methods and Devices

While the therapist is working on soft tissues, various methods can be used to facilitate normalization. One such active-assisted method is the "sustained pressure" technique of Johnson,[29] which is actually the use of the therapist's finger to direct the patient's conscious awareness to focal areas of increased tone within a muscle. The area of increased tone is palpated and pressure is applied up to a certain critical amount and no more. This amount of pressure is determined by the patient's motor reflex threshold,[41] with the therapist applying enough pressure so that his or her finger sinks down into the muscle without resistance but not so much pressure that a protective response is evoked whereby the muscle tightens against the pressure. At this point, various visualization and imagery strategies as well as directed breathing or focal muscle contraction and relaxation strategies can be used to bring about a local reduction of tonus.

More dynamic active-assisted methods can also be used. The patient can perform active physiologic movements of a body part while soft tissue mobilization is applied to the muscles involved in the movement. Other nonlocal isotonic movements such as eye or respiratory movements can be used to direct movement while simultaneous soft tissue mobilization is being applied to the involved muscles. Eye movements are useful in directing movements of the spine (most notably, the upper cervical spine),

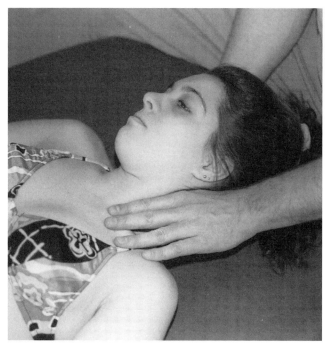

Figure 17–20. Repeated oscillatory mobilization into cervical rotation with the therapist's right hand while the left hand encourages inhibition of the sternocleidomastoid by the supportive quality of contact.

whereas respiratory movements are useful for directing movements of the trunk (particularly, the thoracic cage).

A valuable passive-assisted method is the use of associated oscillations.[29] These are rhythmic, oscillatory, wavelike movements developed from the Trager Approach of Psychophysical Integration[59] that the therapist applies to a local region or to the entire body. They can be used alone or in combination with soft tissue mobilization (Fig. 17–20) for inducing both local muscular and systemic relaxation (via neural and possibly circulatory mechanisms), for using the momentum of the body to loosen restrictions, and for providing movement education by creating a sensory experience of effortless movement.

Assistive devices such as specialized taping[45] can be used to apply external tension (Fig. 17–21). This tension can be corrective in nature—the soft tissues are guided into a new position, thereby relieving stress on overloaded or overstretched tissues or providing a low-level stretch to overshortened and overtightened tissues or both. This tension can also serve as a simple behavioral reminder, regularly cuing the patient to assume a more optimal position. Both nonelastic and elastic (i.e., kinesiotaping)[36] forms of taping can be used, the latter being a more recent development and having the advantage of more closely approximating the actual action of muscle.

Various types of therapeutic devices ranging from rubber balls to more specialized tools such as the J-bar[53] can be used to apply therapeutic pressure to dysfunctional areas. Also, foam rolls can also be used in many ways, including longitudinally along the spine in the supine position to teach more vertical alignment and horizontally across the spine to facilitate posterior segmental pressure over soft tissues and stretching of opposing anterior soft tissues (Fig. 17–22).

Movement Therapy Options
Sensorimotor Control

A common error with application of movement therapy is to begin working on stretching and particularly strengthening before the patient develops fine motor con-

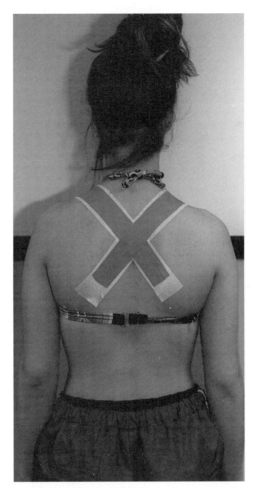

Figure 17–21. Taping for postural correction and reeducation.

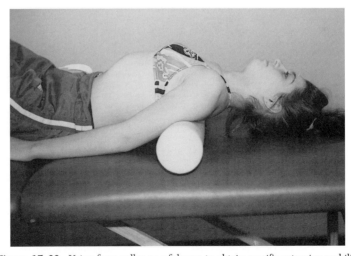

Figure 17–22. Using foam roller as a fulcrum to obtain specific extension mobility.

trol. The principles described by Miller[48] adapted from the Feldenkrais approach are instructing patients to perform mobility exercises with emphasis on the five S's: slow, small, soft, smooth, and sensitive. Moving as slowly and to the smallest degree possible, at least initially, allows the patient to perceive every part of the movement, to receive feedback as the movement is being done, and to do the movement with the lowest effort possible and thereby have the greatest awareness of what is occurring, as is physiologically dictated by the Weber-Fechner law.[13] Performing the movement softly means with as little effort as possible, with maximum awareness of all components of the movement, and performing it smoothly means an absence of unnecessary acceleration or deceleration, again resulting in lower forces and higher sensitivity. Performing movements this way creates a highly favorable environment for motor learning. As an example, the head retraction exercise, which is often performed for reducing forward head position, is typically performed in an overly abrupt manner with redundant co-contraction and associated motions and some degree of flexion or extension rather than a more pure translatory motion (Fig. 17–23A and B). Applying the five S's to the performance of this movement allows the person to refine that movement into a more fluid, beneficial one.

Loosening exercises[1, 11, 58] allow elimination of extraneous levels of muscle tonus, thereby furthering improved movement efficiency. An example of a loosening exercise for the neck is slow, relaxed, rolling rotation of the head from side to side in non–weight-bearing position (to facilitate relaxation of the extrinsic cervical muscles) or soft left-and-right bouncing of the shoulder girdles alternately into elevation and depression to relax and release tension in the shawl muscles. These rhythmic oscillatory exercises can be particularly useful for patients experiencing MPD largely from chronic muscle hypertonicity (Fig. 17–24). If a patient with irritable myofascial tissues does not relax his or her muscles to the baseline level of optimal tone prior to stretching, stretching can become an exercise in futility and result in minimal or no gains in range of motion and/or provocation of unnecessary soreness. As such, loosening exercises can be a useful preliminary measure.

Feldenkrais[14] developed hundreds of Awareness Through Movement lessons designed to reprogram habitually performed, inefficient movement patterns into more

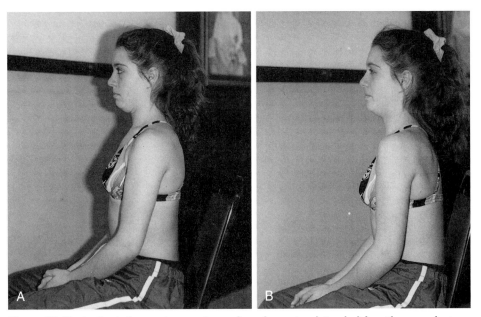

Figure 17–23. **A,** Cervical retraction exercise performed as a translational glide with an emphasis on lengthening and utilizing minimal effort. **B,** Cervical retraction exercise performed in a faulty manner with head extension, excessive effort, and undesired associated motions.

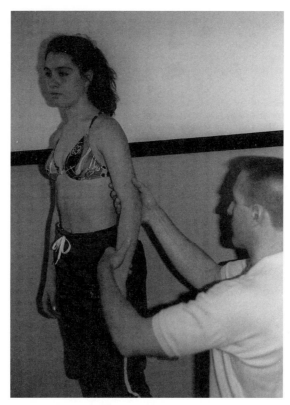

Figure 17–24. Loosening mobilization to the arm to begin training in active inhibition of muscle hypertonus.

intelligent, skilled, and efficient movement. Although many aspects of function are addressed in these lessons, a particularly important aspect is the correlation of movement in any one part of the body with movements in other parts. Thus, in performing a motion such as cervical rotation, a sample lesson might introduce how movement from the pelvis, the rib cage, the shoulder girdle, the eyes, and even the tongue will enhance the comfort and ease of another movement, improving both its quantity and quality. For example, in rotating to look behind the body, the patient will find this motion easier if there is a lateral weight shift in the pelvis in sitting whereby the base of support shifts from being equally distributed on both ischial tuberosities more toward one tuberosity.

Among other things, the Alexander technique[32] teaches the patient how to dissociate the cervical muscles from the initiation and implementation of motor tasks involving other parts of the body. An example would be training the patient to inhibit the stiffening of the neck that commonly occurs upon raising the arm. This inhibitory type of training can be applied to teaching someone to perform numerous functional tasks more efficiently, from light tasks such as writing and working at a keyboard to heavy tasks such as lifting and carrying. A light, guiding, directional touch with a "suggestive" quality can impart the necessary kinesthetic sensations to achieve this inhibitory effect. One can supplement the Alexander technique with generic postural re-education employing various forms of auditory, visual, and kinesthetic cuing. Patients who habitually hold their head in a slightly extended position can be told to imagine that they have eyes on the back of the head and to align them with an imaginary horizon. Patients who are tightly bracing with the neck muscles can be taught to visualize the head being like a gently floating balloon or a golf ball balanced on a golf tee. Obviously, a multitude of ideokinetic strategies can be employed.[34]

Stretching and Strengthening

Active stretching should follow the same general guidelines described under the passive technique. Again the point should be emphasized that stretching should be preceded by or accompanied with tonus reduction methodologies to derive maximum benefit.

Strengthening is another area that is vast in its scope. One point that should be kept in mind is designing the exercise to match the functional demand placed on a muscle. The best exercise for improved posture occurs via tonic activation as opposed to performing a few phasic exercises periodically throughout the day and then relapsing into previous poor postural patterns. However, the way in which the patient attempts to do this is crucial. Typically, patients try to hold a new posture until they tire or until it becomes so uncomfortable that they will not attempt it in the future. Rather, the patient should realize that much repetition is required, and the patient should phase in and out of the "old" and the "new" postures until the distinction between them blurs and either one, or any posture in between, can be assumed with equal ease.

Another important point is that posture should be improved through increasing efficiency via selective muscle inhibition rather than gross muscle facilitation. That means that using more muscle effort to overcome a poor posture is doomed to failure because it requires too much effort. Superimposing more tension upon pre-existing tension only increases the total muscle effort and the resulting compressive and shearing forces imposed upon the osseoarticular system. In comparison, releasing or inhibiting the unnecessary and inappropriate muscle tone that pulls the body out of an ideal position allows the automatic postural mechanisms of the nervous system to maintain an effortless upright stance with minimal opposition, thereby reducing stress on the system and greatly increasing patient compliance because of its more natural feel and effortless quality.

I believe that both in the health care community and among the public there is still too much emphasis on improving "strength." Although strength development is certainly important, improving neuromuscular control is even more vital and will translate back into more efficiently increasing strength. A specific strengthening exercise in the neck involves activation of the deep flexors such as the longus colli and capitis and the rectus capitis anterior. These muscles are often inhibited by the overactivity of the posterior extensor muscles, and the overaccentuated lordotic curve in the cervical spine is frequently a reflection of this.[17] To strengthen these muscles, a slow sequential "curl-up" of the cervical spine (similar to that in the lumbar spine) should be performed with emphasis on maintaining the length of the cervical spine and avoiding shortening motions as would occur with protraction of the neck by excessive use of the sternocleidomastoid muscles (Fig. 17–25A–C). An additional point in this exercise is to encourage the upper thoracic spine and rib cage to participate in the segmental motion.

In summary, technically precise movement and exercise performance as well as intelligent exercise prescription are key factors in addressing MPD.

Behavioral and Cognitive Re-education

Behavioral and cognitive re-education is a valuable complement to kinesthetically implemented movement re-education, although the two often merge in practical application. The patient needs to be taught and then demonstrate back to the therapist various options for rest and work positions, especially prolonged positions such as those used when sleeping, reading, and performing stationary occupational tasks. The patient must also be taught problem-solving skills for optimizing functional posture and movements, both in the workplace and at home.

A particularly common fault is confusing organizational intent with movement intent. For any extended positioning or movement task, from working at a desk to walking, the body should be organized so that it assumes its maximum length (the "up" direction of the Alexander technique) and to a lesser extent its maximum width. This neuromuscular configuration constitutes the organizational intent of the body.

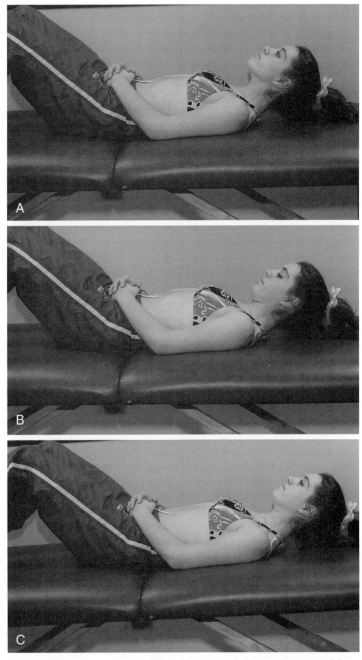

Figure 17–25. A, Faulty attempt to strengthen deep cervical flexors characterized by protraction or shortening of the cervical spine. **B,** Faulty strengthening of deep cervical flexors characterized by excessive flexion of the lower cervical and cervicothoracic segments. **C,** Correct strengthening of deep cervical flexors characterized by flexion distributed down into the upper thoracic spine with participatory action of the rib cage and abdominal muscles. Note that attempting to maintain the horizontal length of the cervical spine helps to minimize undesired sternocleidomastoid activity.

The movement intent has to do with a desired direction of travel such as the forward direction when reaching or moving from one place to another. A person can maintain an upward organizational intent of the body (an optimally aligned vertical posture) while still having a forward movement intent. However, the two are commonly confused during function. Hence, the person reaching forward to grasp an object frequently flexes in the lumbar spine, collapses through the thorax, excessively protracts the shoulder girdle, and compensatorily extends the neck to maintain level eye position. The result is that the person achieves forward movement but the body shortens (Fig. 17–26A). The more optimal version of the movement would involve maintaining the head, neck, torso, and shoulders in near-neutral yet relaxed posture, achieving the forward movement with a simple hip flexion "hinging" at the hips (Fig. 17–26B).

Dysfunctional breathing is an very common but rarely recognized source of myofascial pain. For example, inappropriate and excessive use of accessory muscles of respiration can overload both those muscles and the joints in the region. While a person's unconscious breathing pattern is a deeply ingrained motor pattern and difficult to change, more superficial interferences to free, unconstrained breathing can be removed or inhibited, thereby alleviating these subtle chronic myofascial stresses.

In addition, the therapist needs to educate the patient as to how chronic negative emotional states (anxiety, fear, anger, sadness, depression, bitterness, resentment) can have an adverse influence on the neuromuscular configuration of the body, particularly the axial musculature. This circumstance is a commonly overlooked but widely pervasive perpetuating factor in MPD. It is one that may require psychotherapeutic consultation and major lifestyle change to rectify, and obviously the patient's improvement rests heavily on an acknowledgment of the problem and a desire to resolve it.

Nonmechanical Treatment Considerations

Although beyond the scope of this chapter, various physical therapy modalities can be utilized for their anti-inflammatory and healing action (see Chapter 19). If the patient is unresponsive to therapy that is normally successful and especially if the therapist notes any unusual quality of the myofascial tissues or atypical behavior, it is important to consult with the referring physician. Then the physician can decide to re-examine the patient or refer him or her to a specialist. Referral to other specialists, either to facilitate ongoing physical therapy or as a precursor to further physical therapy, can often provide the key to a patient's progress.

As an example, psychotherapeutic intervention may be indicated for MPD. A number of my colleagues and I have encountered patients who were marginally responsive to physical therapy. These patients did, however, demonstrate symptoms and objective signs of MPD. Either through rapport with the patient or through some

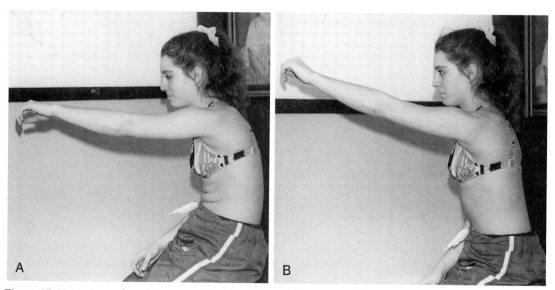

Figure 17–26. A, Forward reaching accomplished by collapse of the spine into flexion. **B**, Forward reaching initiated by hip flexion, maintaining the vertical integrity of the spine.

other means, it was revealed that a large percentage of these patients were childhood or sometimes adult victims of physical, sexual, and/or psychological abuse. The distinction between the somatic and the psychological components of dysfunction in these cases is blurred, and the therapist needs to inform the physician of these findings so that psychotherapeutic help can be arranged. It should be emphasized that although a therapeutic relationship often involves counseling the patient in many aspects of his or her life, the physical therapist should refrain from providing psychotherapeutic counseling per se unless trained and licensed to do so.

Nutritional counseling can also be invaluable, as pointed out by Travell and Simons.[60, 61] I have seen profound alterations in soft tissue quality after only a few weeks of dietary modification. Whereas prior to the dietary changes the patient was refractory to physical therapy, afterward she responded positively.

Possible Treatment Reactions

Soft tissue mobilization is normally a safe procedure. The majority of adverse reactions can be avoided or minimized by refining communication and treatment skills. Soreness following treatment, however, is not uncommon. This soreness is most likely to occur with the initial treatments, especially in a case of long-standing dysfunction. Soreness may be immediate but is more often delayed. Warning of possible exacerbation prepares the patient for this contingency and avoids any possible panic reaction in which the patient's fear of the pain provokes a secondary reaction that is often more intense and long lasting than the initial reaction. Proper patient rapport minimizes the likelihood of this development. An ideal treatment would result in minimal soreness to soreness lasting several hours. Soreness lasting beyond 24 hours usually indicates that the treatment was excessive in terms of its vigor, duration, or amount of work done or that the patient is more sensitive than others and needs to be treated with extra caution.

Patients with congenitally loose or fragile connective tissue might experience bruising if the treatment is vigorous. Relative contraindications that would compromise tissue integrity such as anticoagulant and steroid use should cause the therapist to be especially careful with their manual treatment. The rare occurrence of an autonomic reaction and how to deal with it was mentioned previously. Another unusual reaction is a somatoemotional episode. In cases already mentioned previously in which there was a history of abuse, it is not rare for the patient to experience flashbacks either in a conscious waking state or in dreams of the episode(s) or to experience an emotional release associated with the triggering of this memory. The therapist should be supportive and understanding at this juncture because the patient is often embarrassed by these episodes. Again, directing the patient toward appropriate counseling sources may be indicated in these situations. This situation should, of course, be managed with tact, kindness, and understanding.

Positive reactions to treatment may include sensations of looseness, lightness, and ease of movement, reduction or abolition of pain, and sometimes evidence of reduced sympathetic activity such as a general feeling of well-being or of sleepiness.

Special Considerations

The treatment of MPD should be considered as different from the treatment of fibromyalgia, although many of the same general principles apply. Owing to a lack of understanding as to the exact cause of fibromyalgia, there is no consensus on the best way of managing it. Although exercise can be helpful, the acute pain present during stages of exacerbation often make it intolerable for the patient to perform any but the gentlest of exercises. In these cases, an approach such as that derived from qigong,[7] yoga, and related classic mind-body disciplines that sensitively focuses on alignment, relaxation, breathing, and general enhancement of internal awareness will often be the most fruitful. I can recall one patient who after being taught the yogic "breath of fire"[38] experienced a 60% reduction of pain from that intervention alone. Similarly, manual therapy must be gentle and avoid hyperstimulation modes of treatment.

Inhibitory modes of treatment (such as described under Neurosensorimotor Treatment Options including techniques such as positional release) can often be useful in these situations. Furthermore, strong emphasis should be placed on optimizing postural and movement efficiency so as to minimize the stresses upon the myofascial tissues. At times during stages of exacerbation, manual therapy should be avoided altogether, with treatment shifting away from corrective therapy and toward palliative therapy and medical management. Much research remains to be done in this area.

Reassessment Following Treatment

Following treatment, the therapist should look for a change in subjective findings such as tenderness to palpation, local pain, and referred pain. The therapist should also examine for objective alteration in function. Motion should be re-examined, noting both range of motion and resistance to motion (the latter including end feel and through-range feel). Structural restriction could be differentiated to some degree from functional restriction with hold-relax techniques. Changes in tissue quality would also be noted with palpation. Lastly, one would observe how these changes carry over into changes in postural and movement habits and functional ability.

Conclusion

Treatment of myofascial pain and dysfunction by manual means has been performed as far back as history records. Only in recent decades, as "high-tech" machinery for the application of therapeutic modalities and elaborate but often nonphysiologic exercise regimens came into vogue and as "massage" fell into disfavor, has this therapeutic means been de-emphasized and neglected. Fortunately, there has been a recent resurgence in its popularity owing to its demonstrated effectiveness and an evolution in its sophistication. Various forms of manual therapy have been integrated into and are now being applied in conjunction with movement therapy and more enlightened educational procedures. This integration is vital in making the transition from a passive treatment modality that may be effective but often has limited carryover to a comprehensive treatment program that has as its ultimate goal educating the patient, kinesthetically, behaviorally, and cognitively, so that he or she can progress to self-management and independence.

The drawbacks to this approach are that it requires time—considerable time for effective training of the therapist and much time spent with the patient in a one-on-one relationship. With the increased emphasis on cost-effectiveness, this time spent with the patient is threatened. One should remember, however, not to confuse cost-effectiveness with results-effectiveness. In the long term, only methods that produce results satisfactory to the patient (and not necessarily to third parties) are truly cost-effective.

Acknowledgments

The author expresses his indebtedness and gratitude to Gregory S. Johnson, P.T., who has developed and organized many of the concepts presented here and contributed immeasurably to the advancement of clinical treatment of MPD as well as to musculoskeletal treatment in general.

References

1. Aston J: Overview of Aston patterning, course notes. Omega Institute, Rhinebeck, NY, July 7–11, 1986.
2. Aston J: Aston patterning functional massage, course notes. Mill Valley, Calif, April 16–24, 1987.
3. Boers T: Arthropraxis: Lumbar spine and sacroiliac joint evaluation and specific joint manipulation, course notes. Columbus, Ga, April 5–7, 1990.
4. Butler D: Mobilisation of the Nervous System. New York, Churchill Livingstone, 1991.

6. Chaitow L: Neuromuscular Technique. New York, Thorsons, 1980.
7. Cohen K: The Way of Qigong. New York, Ballantine Books, 1997.
8. Cyriax J: Textbook of Orthopaedic Medicine, 7th ed. London, Baillière Tindall, 1978.
9. Cyriax JH, Cyriax PJ: Illustrated Manual of Orthopaedic Medicine. Boston, Butterworths, 1983.
10. Diehl B: Personal communication, 1990.
11. Eitner D: Physical therapy for sports. In Kuprian W (ed): Physical Therapy for Sports. Philadelphia, WB Saunders, 1981.
12. Evjenth O, Hamberg J: Muscle Stretching in Manual Therapy—A Clinical Manual: The Spinal Column and the TM Joint, vol II. Sweden, Afta Rehab Forlag, 1985.
13. Feldenkrais M: Body & Mature Behavior: A Study of Anxiety, Sex, Gravitation, and Learning. New York, International Universities Press, 1949 (8th printing, 1981).
14. Feldenkrais M: Awareness Through Movement. New York, Harper & Row, 1977.
15. Feldenkrais M: The Elusive Obvious. Cupertino, Calif, Meta, 1981.
16. Feldenkrais M: The Potent Self: A Guide to Spontaneity. San Francisco, Harper & Row, 1985.
17. Feldenkrais method (practitioner training). Presented by Mia Segal, New York, 1986–1988.
18. Fricton JR, Awad EQ: Advances in Pain Research and Therapy. Vol 28: Myofascial Pain and Fibromyalgia. New York, Raven, 1990.
19. Garlick D (ed): Proprioception, Posture, and Emotion. Kensington, NSW, Australia 2063, Committee in Post-Graduate Medical Education, The University of New South Wales, 1982.
20. Greenman PE (ed): Concepts and Mechanisms of Neuromuscular Functions. New York, Springer-Verlag, 1984.
21. Greenman PE: Principles of Manual Medicine. Baltimore, Williams & Wilkins, 1989.
22. Grieve GP: Common Vertebral Joint Problems, 2nd ed. New York, Churchill Livingstone, 1988.
23. Hanlon WH: Taproots: Underlying Principles of Milton Erickson's Therapy and Hypnosis. New York, WW Norton, 1987.
24. Hanna T: Somatics. Reading, Mass, Addison-Wesley, 1988.
25. Headley BJ, North BA: Myofascial Exams & Biofeedback. St. Paul, Minn, Pain Resources, 1990.
26. Herbert F: Dune. Berkeley, Calif, Berkeley Books, 1965.
27. Janda V: Manipulative medicine in the management of soft tissue pain syndromes, North American Academy of Manipulative Medicine, October 19–21, 1983, Alexandria, Va.
28. Janda V: Muscles and cervicogenic pain syndromes. In Grant R: Clinics in Physical Therapy: Physical Therapy of the Cervical and Thoracic Spine. New York, Churchill Livingstone, 1988.
29. Johnson GS: Functional Orthopaedics. Institute for Physical Art, 45 Tappan Road, San Anselmo, Calif, 1985.
30. Johnson GS: Personal communication, 1986.
31. Johnson GS: Lumbar protective mechanism. In White AH, Anderson R (eds): Conservative Care of Low Back Pain. Baltimore, Williams & Wilkins, 1991.
32. Jones FP: Body Awareness in Action: A Study of the Alexander Technique. New York, Schocken Books, 1970.
33. Jahan D: Job's Body—A Handbook for Bodywork. Barrytown Ltd., Barrytown, NY, 1988.
34. Kapandji IA: The Physiology of the Joints. Vol 3, The Trunk and Vertebral Column. New York, Churchill Livingstone, 1974.
35. Kase K: Illustrated Kinesio-taping. Tokyo, Ken'I-Kai Information, 1997.
36. Kendall HO, Kendall FP, Boynton DA: Posture and Pain. Malabar Fla, Robert E. Krieger, 1952 (reprinted 1981).
37. Khalsa DS: Brain Longevity. New York, Warner Books, 1997.
38. Knott M, Voss DE: Proprioceptive Neuromuscular Facilitation: Patterns and Techniques, 2nd ed. New York, Harper & Row, 1968.
39. Korr I: The Collected Papers of Irvin M. Korr. Colorado Springs, Colo, American Academy of Osteopathy, 1979.
40. Kurz T: Stretching Scientifically: A Guide to Flexibility Training. Island Pond, Vt, Stadion, 1994.
41. Lee D: Principles and practice of muscle energy and functional techniques. In Grieve GP: Modern Manual Therapy of the Vertebral Column. New York, Churchill Livingstone, 1986.
42. Lewit K: Management of muscular pain associated with articular dysfunction. In Fricton JR, Awad EA: Advances in Pain Research and Therapy. Vol 28, Myofascial Pain and Fibromyalgia. New York, Raven, 1990.
43. Lewit K: Manipulative Therapy in Rehabilitation of the Locomotor System, 2nd ed. Boston, Butterworths, 1992.
44. Maitland GD: Vertebral Manipulation, 5th ed. Boston, Butterworths, 1986.
45. McConnell J: McConnell patellofemoral treatment plan, course notes. Kailua-Kona, Hawaii, November 30–December 1, 1990.
46. McGeary MP: Personal communication, Richmond, Va, 1992.
47. McKenzie RA: The Cervical and Thoracic Spine: Mechanical Diagnosis and Therapy. Waikanae, New Zealand, Spinal Publications, 1990.
48. Miller B: Somatokinetic approaches, course notes. Somerset, NJ, 1990.
49. Miller B: Alternative somatic therapies. In White AH, Anderson R (eds): Conservative Care of Low Back Pain. Baltimore, Williams & Wilkins, 1991.
50. Rolf IP: Rolfing: The Integration of Human Structures. New York, Harper & Row, 1977.
51. Ruth S, Keggereis S: Facilitating cervical flexion using a Feldenkrais method: Awareness through movement. J Spinal Phys Ther 16:1, 1992.

52. Rywerant Y: The Feldenkrais Method. San Francisco, Harper & Row, 1983.
53. Sellers LS: Personal communication, Columbus, Ga, 1991.
54. Selye H: The Stress of Life. New York, McGraw-Hill, 1978.
55. Sweigard LE: Human Movement Potential: Its Ideokinetic Facilitation. New York, Harper & Row, 1974.
56. Tengwall R: Toward an Etiology of Malposture. Somatics 3(3), Autumn/Winter, 1981–82.
57. Todd ME: The Thinking Body. Brooklyn, NY, Dance Horizons, 1937.
58. Trager M: Trager Mentastics: Movement as a Way to Agelessness. Barrytown, NY, Station Hill, 1987.
59. Trager practitioner training. Betty Fuller, New York, October 30–November 1, 1986.
60. Travell JG, Simons DG: Myofascial Pain and Dysfunction: The Trigger Point Manual. Baltimore, Williams & Wilkins, 1983.
61. Travell JG, Simons DG: Myofascial Pain and Dysfunction: The Trigger Point Manual. Vol 2: The Lower Extremities. Baltimore, Williams & Wilkins, 1992.
62. Tsujii Y: Myotherapy of the upper quarter. LaCrosse, Wis, February 27–29, 1992.
63. Vollowitz E: Furniture prescription for the conservative management of low back pain. Topics in Acute Care and Trauma Rehabilitation, April 1988: 18–37.
64. Ward R: Myofascial release, course notes. East Lansing, Mich, Michigan State University College of Osteopathic Medicine, April 13–15, 1984.
65. Whatmore GB, Kholi DR: The Physiopathology and Treatment of Functional Disorder. New York, Grune & Stratton, 1974.
66. White AA, Panjabi MM: Clinical Biomechanics of the Spine. Philadelphia, JB Lippincott, 1978.
67. Witt PL: Trager Psychophysical Integration: An Additional Tool in the Treatment of Chronic Spinal Pain and Dysfunction. Whirlpool, Summer 1986.
68. Wyke B: Seminar on Articular Neurology. New York, February 1981.

Chapter 18

The Practical Application of Trigger Point Work in Physical Therapy

Beth Paris, PT, LMT

The purpose of this chapter is to demonstrate for the physical therapist how to incorporate the body of knowledge about myofascial pain syndromes into the day-to-day practice of physical therapy (PT). Dr. Travell believed that there would be no area of medicine untouched by her research regarding the nature of the trigger point and its bodily effects.[1] Likewise, there is no area of PT specialization that would not benefit from a thorough understanding of this work. No doubt, the existence of the trigger point (TrP) has already become common knowledge in PT and is incorporated in evaluation and treatment in some settings, but the degree of success experienced by the practitioner is directly proportional to the skill of the examiner, the thoroughness of application of this therapy, and a deep understanding of the behavior of TrPs in the long-term process of recovery or management of bodily dysfunction.

This chapter aims first to underscore the ubiquitous presence of myofascial dysfunction in the PT setting, then to elucidate the evaluation of patients for the presence and relative importance of TrPs, with the focus on streamlining the physical examination, organizing it around the common patterns of muscle involvement seen daily in practice. Developing a plan to successfully treat patients with a myofascial pain component is explored, including a discussion of modifications to our other treatment modalities. The interpersonal relationship between the therapist and the myofascial pain patient is emphasized. It is hoped that the information presented here will provide a level of confidence in the practical application of TrP work in physical therapy practice that will inspire its use in every appropriate situation.

The Clinical Significance of Trigger Points in Physical Therapy Practice

We find only what we are looking for! We need to realize that we should be looking for TrPs in our clinical examination of just about every patient who enters the PT clinic.

The mechanism by which this can be explained is: *TrPs develop in response to "stress" to the muscle.* What is stressful to muscle? The myofascial system itself is sensitive to environmental stressors acting on it, such as temperature and pressure, and internal factors such as position, movement or rest, kind of work performed, or degree of stretch. Additionally, it could be said that our myofascial system sensitively monitors noxious inputs from all body systems; thus, potentially every source of pain or dysfunction may be recognized as a stressor to muscle. This relationship between the TrP and all body systems is demonstrated well in Figure 9–1 (see Chapter 9).

The clinical manifestations of the TrP:

1. TrPs present as *a primary source of pain and dysfunction*. They are the muscular response to specific stresses acting on those muscles, be they tensional holding patterns (tension headache), muscle injury or strain, or postural stresses, to name a few.

2. TrPs are often a *component of any pain or dysfunction* arising from any body system.

Muscles are stressed by noxious inputs from joints, nerves, vascular or visceral structures. Examples include nearly global involvement of shoulder muscles in disorders such as subacromial bursitis or tendinitis of the supraspinatus tendon or bicipital tendon, involvement of gluteal and lateral rotator muscles in sacroiliac dysfunction, and pectoral triggers that develop in response to cardiac dysfunction and pain.[3]

3. TrP symptoms *mimic many diagnoses*, and are often missed in standard medical practice. Again, we find only what we are looking for. Triggers cause pain at a distance (referred pain), tingling and numbness in their referral zone, and limitations of function that may well be attributed to other structures if the trigger is not identified. For example, sciatica, impingement syndromes of the shoulder, thoracic outlet syndrome, cervical radiculopathy, and many others are diagnoses that in some cases would be better described as myofascial pain syndrome if a differential diagnosis were sought.[4]

4. TrPs *persist as residuals of many other disorders*, so that persistent symptoms may continue for weeks, months, and years after the primary disturbance is rectified. This helps to explain diagnoses such as postlaminectomy syndrome, "failed back" syndrome, and poor response to many other surgical procedures and interventions. It also illuminates the long-term sequelae of motor vehicle injury, radiculopathies, and some sports injuries. Dr. Travell first became interested in this work when patients successfully treated for cardiac disease continued having persistent chest or even arm pain that had been attributed only to their cardiac status.[8]

5. TrPs *can cause or contribute to other somatic dysfunction*, by virtue of the secondary effects of the TrP such as loss of range of motion (ROM), loss of strength, altered proprioception, altered biomechanics, and altered blood flow. Travell suggests that tendinitis may be caused by persistent pulls on the tendon from the taut bands created by TrPs.[5] Wear and tear on joints of the spine, shoulder, or patellofemoral joint may arise from the altered biomechanics that stem from those secondary effects as well.

The list of possible permutations in diagnosis, symptomatology, and cause-and-effect reverberations between the myofascial TrP and all other bodily systems is endless, but our response to this seemingly complex problem is simple—view every person who comes through our door as a possible "carrier" of myofascial TrPs. Systematically examine each client, treat the myofascial components along with any other clinical problems that are identified as well, and evaluate the outcome of treatment. Clinical success will be magnified many times over by adding this crucial element to patient care.

Guidelines for the Evaluation of the Patient

The Interview

Evaluation begins with a thorough history-taking session (Table 18–1). This conversation may occupy the entire first visit with the patient, and its importance in the whole course of treatment cannot be underestimated. We are listening for *etiology* (specifically, historical events that implicate the primary structures involved, the progression of symptoms that might suggest secondary involvement of muscle, emotional relationship to the problem, and so on). We are listening for the *behavior of symptoms* (Does this suggest a myofascial component? What else does it sound like?). We want to get an almost exhaustive list of the *subjective limitations* generated by the condition,

Table 18–1.
Components of the Interview

1. Elements of history—identifying etiology, behavior of symptoms, subjective description of limitations (including pain diagram), perpetuating factors
2. Establishing a documented baseline of symptoms, limitations
3. Creating an environment of rapport and trust to build a therapeutic relationship

so that we may evaluate our progress as we enter into treatment, and also very importantly, so that we can develop a set of "outcomes" measurements. We also need to find out about the individuals' *lifestyle*—what are their work and recreational activities, how do they see the stress level in their work and home life, what support systems do they have in family or friends—so that we can identify perpetuating factors that might be central to their care and discharge planning. Brian Miller's chapter in this volume covers many of the questions that should be asked in the interview (see Chapter 17).

Another part of this initial conversation must be the completion of the *pain diagram*, and possible pain-rating scale or clear descriptions of the symptoms described on the diagram. Ideally, patients depict the problem, unless they are unable to translate from their body to the page, in which case they demonstrate the area of pain and the therapist enters it on the picture. This eliminates misunderstanding generated by words—shoulder can mean anything involving the upper quarter, low back may be mid-thoracic to coccygeal regions, so a verbal description of pain zones is nearly useless.

The picture and description are important for many reasons. They provide a visual record of the starting point in the relationship with the patient to this course of therapy. They are a ready reference guide to be consulted at the beginning of every session, they provide documentation to the insurance companies, and they may serve as a comparative record if they are done periodically, demonstrating progress in the difficult subjective realm of pain. Periodic charting of this sort may also demonstrate progress to patients who can no longer remember their condition when they began treatment. In general, it is also useful for the practitioner to see the way patients picture their symptoms, providing clues to their emotional relationship to the pain, and their ability or inability to sense their body and to differentiate between a variety of sensations.

The initial interview is important for fact-finding and documentation, and it contributes to the development of the therapist's plan for effective examination and treatment. This initial session is also extremely important in the establishment of rapport with the patient. Persons with myofascial pain have several barriers to overcome in establishing a truly therapeutic relationship. First, they may have already seen numerous people who have not helped them, or have hurt them or misunderstood them, or, very often, have discounted them. Often no one has taken the time to listen and give the impression that they understand the full impact of the patients' distress. Patients may also have significant apprehension about treatment, inasmuch as they are already in pain and are often mystified by their symptoms. They may have fear about the real nature of their problem because it has often not been definitively diagnosed or explained to them. In addition, they are facing a treatment that involves body contact and exposure, and this may generate anxiety for reasons unknown to the practitioner, including religious or social mores, prior history of abuse, and low self-esteem.

Individuals with myofascial pain will already experience therapeutic effects at the outset if they feel understood, and they will be convinced of the practitioner's professional expertise in the realm of pain management as demonstrated by the nature of the questions asked in the initial interview and subsequent conversation. The next step is an explanation of the physical examination and its purpose, and with this, patients will in most cases be prepared to participate fully in the process in the most positive manner. The initial history taking and conversation would be followed by the physical examination, including a demonstration by the patient of any positions or movements that exacerbate the symptoms, postural evaluation, appropriate strength or ROM measurements, and, importantly, detailed hands-on assessment as described later.

Developing a Hypothesis to Streamline the Physical Examination

Following the interview and review of the prescription, diagnostic studies, and any other materials regarding this person that are available, it is necessary to assess the patient by physical examination. As stated earlier, the examination may include all elements of physical therapy assessment, but this discussion will follow only the assessment of the patient's myofascial involvement—*that is, the presence and extent of irritability of TrPs in the patient's muscular system.* Consideration of even this single aspect of patient involvement might ideally involve a complete top-to-toe assessment, which may in fact be necessary along the way, but it is essential to streamline the initial physical examination to arrive at a plan of care. The therapist must be able to hypothesize about the zone of involvement, thus the zone of priority for TrP examination. The chosen zone must be comprehensive enough to identify all the key muscles involved.

Consideration of the Etiology

Consideration of the precipitating events and subsequent history will provide information about muscles that may have been directly involved in the trauma, and muscles that may be involved due to their relationship to the injured or painful tissues (e.g., joint movers in the case of ligamentous or joint injury, or muscles innervated by compressed nerves).

If a complete history has been taken that identifies the progression or change in symptoms over time, it will be possible to consider the initial and then successive acquisition of triggers through the spread via satellite and secondary mechanisms, and also through coping strategies of the patient, which ultimately engage more and more muscles in aberrant patterns. Satellite TrPs are those that develop by virtue of being in the reference zone of other activated muscles. Due to the proximal to distal nature of pain referral, we can expect a domino pattern of muscle involvement down the limb or up or down the torso. *Secondary trigger points* are those that develop in any muscle of the myotatic unit of the primary affected muscle. It may be necessary to scan an entire quarter of the body to conduct a thorough examination.[5]

Subjective Reporting of Symptoms

The *pain diagram* will be the primary clue to the specific muscular involvement that is directly causing the pain symptoms. Many common muscle patterns will be described so frequently by patients that they become totally familiar, and their names begin to leap off the page, but less common muscles must also be considered. Drs. Travell and Simons delineated two zones within the pain referral pattern, the essential pain zone (that area most frequently encountered as a reactive zone) and the spillover pain zone (the area less frequently reported in relation to that particular muscle).[5] It is important to remember that these patterns are composites—they reflect the whole range of possibilities seen in patients, and any given patient may manifest only a portion of the pattern.[7] It may be that the individual's pain is arising from a muscle that less frequently generates pain in this area (the spillover zone of referral); therefore, all muscles with pain patterns that include the zones described in the diagram must ultimately be considered. For example, the person with active TrPs in the latissimus dorsi may complain only of ulnar forearm pain or tingling throughout the ulnar aspect of the arm, or with longissimus thoracis activation, the chief complaint might be lumbar pain. Priority would be given, however, to muscles with the essential pain zone overlapping the picture (Fig. 18–1).

The demonstrated or described functional loss—movements that cause pain, activities of daily living (ADL) that are impaired, or positions of discomfort—will also clearly implicate particular muscles or groups of muscles. *The triggers will be activated, that is, they will produce referred pain, when they are stretching, contracting, or are compressed by outside forces.* They may also be activated when fatigued, so their pain referral may appear only following a period of activity. Pain that seems to occur at rest may be due to this, or to compression of the trigger by the weight of the body, e.g., resting on one's back compresses the infraspinatus; sitting in a chair compresses the gluteus maximus. *TrP activity is exacerbated by prolonged immobilization,* especially in suboptimal positions. Positions of rest may activate triggers in muscles that

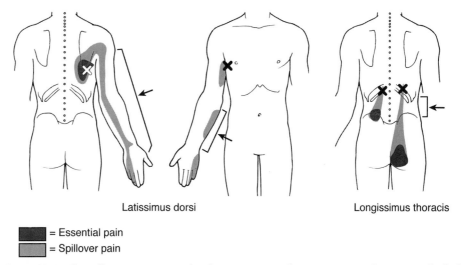

Latissimus dorsi   Longissimus thoracis

■ = Essential pain
■ = Spillover pain

Figure 18–1. The spillover pain zone may be the primary zone of pain or symptoms for a given individual; therefore, all potential muscles must be considered.

are on a prolonged stretch or in a shortened position, as in activation of trapezius or levator scapulae triggers when turning the head to sleep prone, or side-lying activation of quadratus lumborum triggers on the down-side (stretch) or up-side (shortening).

The muscle harboring an active TrP has an altered threshold of excitability. This refers to the broadcasting of symptoms from the affected muscle. The more reactive the TrP, the less stress the muscle can tolerate before symptoms are felt. As we listen to patients' complaints, this will be confirmed by their reports that ordinary activity causes pain. The extent of their limitations is a reflection of the severity of the TrP, i.e., the more reactive the TrP, the lower the threshold of excitability in the muscle and the less stretch, loading, repetition, cooling, immobilization, and so forth tolerated. Treatment will increase this threshold if it is successful, and this concept will guide our evaluation of progress in therapy (Fig. 18–2).

With all of these considerations kept in mind, it should be possible to identify the most likely muscle or group of muscles that produces the symptoms and the related muscles that may be reinforcing or perpetuating the same. In summary, the hypothesis of where to begin and what to include in the muscular examination will be based on the thorough understanding of the behavior of the patient's symptoms, matching the muscles with pain referral patterns that fit. This includes identifying the pain diagram, and muscles that are implicated by the patient's loss of function. In this way the "primary" muscles of involvement are identified, and the muscles related to them by

Figure 18–2. There is an inverse relationship between the reactivity of the trigger point and its threshold of excitability. Point A indicates a highly reactive TrP, with a low threshold of excitability. It takes minimal stimulus to produce symptoms. Point B shows the effects of treatment—as the reactivity of the TrP diminishes, the person can tolerate greater levels of activity.

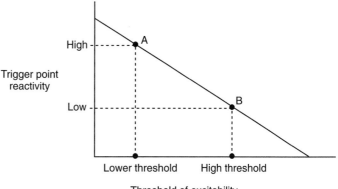

function (secondaries) and central influences (satellites) complete the picture. This is the starting point, but the physical examination provides the only accurate information from which we can develop a treatment plan.

The Mechanics of Physical Examination

General Guidelines for Hands-on Evaluation

1. Patients must be *maximally relaxed*—positioning for comfort, draping, and temperature of the room are important. A conversation describing your intention—what you are going to do, why you are doing it, what the patient's role in the process is—will be helpful toward this end as well.

2. The examination follows from the *general to the specific*—that is, looking at response to touch in general, which zone within the examining area is most prominent—i.e., comparing one side to the other, comparing layers of muscle tension, then zeroing in on a given muscle, comparing sections of the muscle and then individual fibers to each other.

3. We are *comparing the person only with himself or herself*. We may have a sense of what is tight, loose, and so forth, but the ultimate distinction is as mentioned earlier—ultimately, how does one muscle fiber compare to the one next to it?

4. The examination should proceed *proximal to distal*—thinking here of the myotatic unit, the "domino effect" of satellite TrPs, and the progression and perpetuation of the problem over time. *This particular rule should dominate not only examination but also treatment of the patient at every session.* Pressure or manipulation of the TrP may activate its referral zone of influence, and it may activate the satellite TrPs inadvertently. Examination and treatment from proximal to distal, following the general trend of pain referral, will prevent the reactivation of muscles already treated or examined during the session. It is also an extremely common experience that once the proximal triggers have been adequately treated, much of the distal pain and/or other sensory changes disappear, and the distal triggers become latent or inactivated with little or no effort.

Location of Active Trigger Points

The starting point for locating the TrP (Table 18–2) is the identification of the taut band. The only thorough way to locate taut bands in the muscle is to examine the muscle perpendicular to the direction of the muscle fibers. This is true of a flat palpation or pincer palpation technique. The direction of palpation may change in different portions of the muscle, as the fiber direction may be changing in different sections of the muscle. *The examination must always be conducted at right angles to the fibers* (Fig. 18–3).

Once the person is relaxed and comfortable and the individual muscle is also positioned for relaxation, the muscle is placed on a gentle stretch to increase the tension difference between the affected and unaffected fiber groups, and the cross-fiber examination can begin. Once the taut band is located, location of the actual point is required. The standard pain diagrams provide the guidelines for streamlining the examination process. The X marks indicate the most likely sites of TrPs if the muscle is involved, so this is the first place to attempt cross-fiber palpation. If this zone is

Table 18–2.
Qualities of a Trigger Point

To assist in the location of TrPs, the qualities of the TrP are listed:

- Taut band located within the contractile portion of the myofascial unit
- Spot tenderness within the taut band and/or differences in tissue quality at this site
- Local twitch response when point is palpated or manipulated
- Jump sign—excessive reaction to stimulation of the point
- Production of pain referral pattern with sustained pressure on the point (10 seconds)

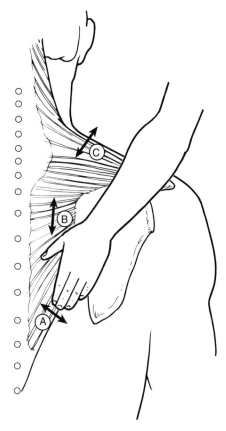

Figure 18–3. Muscles must be examined at right angles to their fiber direction to locate taut bands. Fingers align with fiber direction but palpation is transverse. A, For lower trapezius the fingers are oblique. B, For middle trapezius, fingers are horizontal and palpation is vertical. C, Upper trapezius fibers are oblique at 90-degree angles to lower trapezius.

active, then a thorough palpation of the muscle is necessary to gain full appreciation of its involvement. Numerous triggers may be found within the muscle. If, however, the key zones are not taut or tender, that muscle may be considered less significant and the examination can continue.

How do you know when you are on the TrP? The tissue quality is the objective guide to specific point location. In general, the most reactive section of the taut band will feel more dense and less compressible than the tissue nearby. It may feel wider than the rest of the band. On occasion it will feel gritty, or fibrous, or indurated. Most often, it feels *different*. But our fine-tuning in point location will also depend on the subjective reporting of the patient.

The Role of Patient Feedback

The importance of patient reporting during the examination cannot be overemphasized. Although the TrP's exact location may be identified by careful examination, it is not uncommon for the most irritable site to be unremarkable in texture and its location on the band difficult to ascertain without this feedback. The TrP may be a millimeter in diameter, and a spot may even be insensitive at one angle of palpation and excruciating with a slight alteration in direction of pressure. Examiners should be aware that their expectation that a ropey or tense muscle will be reactive may not always be borne out. The first examination is crucial for assessing how to "read" that individual's tissues—some people are more ropey, without pain; some are just minimally taut and experience a lot of pain; some are so taut that they are virtually numb to pain; and people with fibromyalgia or other disorders that alter pain perception may have a high level of discomfort even in zones with no perceivable taut bands.

It is extremely important to realize that truly accurate assessment depends on patient cooperation. The person who can and will give good feedback during the

Table 18–3.
Guidelines I Use for Patient Feedback

Patients are asked to use specific language to report reactions to pressure, and I explain what my response will be as follows:

1. If they say it *hurts*——I won't stop.
2. If they say it *hurts too much*——I'll lighten up or stop.
3. If *they report any sensation outside the place I am touching*——I will continue.

---

entire examination process is assured a more complete plan of care. Therefore, much attention needs to be paid to this dynamic. As described earlier, the establishment of rapport early in the interview is invaluable for success, and during the physical examination further efforts to aid communication and trust are important. Specifically, patients must be encouraged to give feedback during the examination process—this will happen if they understand the reason for the probing palpation and the importance of reporting strong sensations.

Patient compliance with reporting their experience during the *examination* is often a significant problem. There may be many reasons for this, including fear of judgment about their pain tolerance, or a "no pain no gain" sense that will propel them to tolerate excessive pain, or a fear that the examiner will not treat them adequately if they complain. Some other people will over-report, jumping and reporting each discomfort very dramatically, because they have great fear of the process. They need to be forewarned that the examination may be painful, and there can be agreed-upon guidelines for the examination that will empower them and encourage their feedback. I explain that I would like a specific type of reporting that will guide my examination, as indicated in Table 18–3.

I further clarify that "hurts too much" is the appropriate response when they feel they cannot relax into the sensation. The examiner will be monitoring for muscular response as well, still not relying solely on patient feedback.

These multiple tiers of response eliminate patient concerns that if they report pain they will be judged, or fear that I will stop the pressure, which is often perceived as "a good hurt," or just a sense that pressure is needed there. People will often need frequent reminding to continue to report their subjective experience as the examination progresses. They may need continued encouragement that it is proper to report the pain, or they may start to think you know exactly what is happening to them, or they become absorbed in their experience and forget to report what they are feeling.

The notion of "a good hurt" is the unofficial hallmark for accurate location of a trigger point. The experience can otherwise be sharp, burning, aching, or just intense. A common experience is of deep relief—the sense of discovery of a significant spot that literally aches to be touched. Some patients will not be able to initially distinguish these different qualities of pain; others will be very articulate about the sensations experienced at different spots.

The TrP has been located by palpation and patient feedback. The degree of reactivity of the point has to be assessed. This will be determined on the basis of:

• The tissue quality at the site
• The intensity of pain experienced and reported
• Presence or absence of a local twitch response
• Manifestation of the jump sign (intensity of pain response)
• Referral of pain or other distressing sensations

In particular, in relation to the last item, the assessment of pain referral can only be made if the examination is done properly. The pressure on the point must be sustained for 10 seconds,[5] and patients *must* report their reactions. There is no other way to determine if the person is experiencing referred symptoms. They must also be encouraged to report *any* sensations they have outside the zone of pressure—the referral may be experienced as tingling or numbness or even weakness, a tightening sensation, or other paresthesias, possibly just a feeling that "something" is happening.

Hands-on Evaluation of the Soft Tissues

This discussion of examination has focused on the location and analysis of a single TrP. To provide a sense of the overall process, a step-by-step examination of the interscapular region will be described (Table 18–4). This region is chosen because of its prime importance in many pain syndromes, and the particulars of the region's anatomy that will illustrate significant features of examination.

Patients are positioned prone on the examining surface, with arms at their side up on the table. This is a good anatomic position for muscle location, and it puts the interscapular muscles on a gentle stretch as the shoulder girdle abducts slightly toward the table. The area is stroked with mild pressure to assess response to touch, to make a quick comparison of one side to the other, and to get an immediate sense of the muscular layers on each side—if the rhomboid or erectors are more reactive than the overlying trapezius, they are readily perceived through the superficial tissues. To follow the discussion of step-by-step layer examination of the region, refer to Figure 18–4.

The lower trapezius will be the first muscle examined. TrP3 is located in the lateral border of the muscle, found near the medial border of the scapula, medial to the trapezius point of attachment on the spine of the scapula. The fibers of the lateral border of the trapezius are oblique, and the examiner places fingertips along that edge of muscle. The tips of the fingers are used for palpation, as the smaller the surface area, the clearer the information will be. A gentle small motion across the fibers will identify taut bands in the border, and gliding along the located band, with repeated small cross-fiber motions, will locate the point itself. This will be perceived as textural difference, a local twitch response, jump sign, or the patient reporting of sensation. The lateral border may be very taut and on careful examination often seems to be like a washboard, with multiple fibers palpable. This region may be explored crosswise to locate several reactive points, all possibly painful and radiating. When a key spot is identified, sustained pressure should be maintained over the point for 10 to 15 seconds to see if a referral pattern develops. The muscle should then be further examined, moving medially toward the midline, examining crosswise, and also gliding along the bands superior to inferior, to be sure the most tender point on each band has been identified and fully examined for referral patterns.

At this point, the examination can proceed to deeper levels. The rhomboids are examined nearly perpendicular to the lower trapezius, as the fiber direction shifts 180 degrees and the TrPs in this level generally cluster near the muscular attachment to the scapula. The muscle may be directly palpated at the lower third of the scapular border, where the lower trapezius is absent, although this muscle can be easily examined through the trapezius as well, due to the opposing fiber directions of muscle layers. Proceed proximally along the medial border of the scapula to identify other possible TrPs, and be sure to palpate medially along taut bands as well. The three divisions of the erectors can be examined similarly, with the palpating fingers aligned nearly vertical, and the examination proceeding with gentle cross-fiber motions lateral to medial, scanning the interscapular zone from the medial border of the scapula to the spinous processes. Once the interscapular region is examined thoroughly, the examination can then continue into the referral zones of these muscles, the muscles of the suprascapular region, neck, and head.

At each point, a mental note is made of the extent of involvement—level of reactivity, tissue quality, pain referral. After a region is examined, care should be taken

---

Table 18–4.
Steps in Examination

The flow of the physical examination is as follows:
- Positioning for comfort
- General sensing of tissue layers and comparison of symmetrical zones
- Thorough examination of muscle layers
- Effleurage and stretch to diminish intensity of sensation

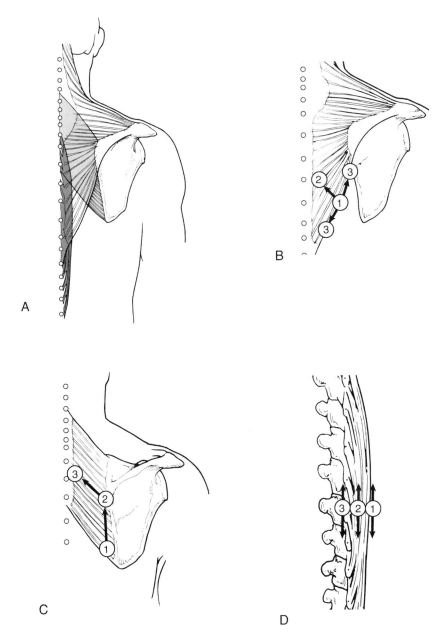

Figure 18–4. The examination of the interscapular region includes the lower and middle trapezius, rhomboids, and thoracic erector spinae. *A,* Three layers of muscles in the interscapular region. *B,* Lower trapezius. *C,* Rhomboid. *D,* Thoracic erector spinae. By following steps 1, 2, and 3, you can be assured of thorough examination of each muscle.

to reduce the sensation of intensity at particular points. An effleurage type stroke is indicated, to "smooth" the skin, eliminating the "polka-dot" sensation that may linger, especially if the points were tender. Gentle stretches to the area may also be beneficial, again to offer a change of stimulus and to provide an integrative sensation for the patient. It is also important to examine both sides, even if the complaint is unilateral. In this region, the spine as connection between the two sides requires a bilateral examination, but in general this is good practice—again it gives the person a sense of integration rather than dissection, and it also puts into perspective the examination that has been done. Ultimately, each person can be compared only to himself or herself as the "normal" toward which we move in treatment. At this point it should be mentioned that it is very common for a person to have "mirror" TrPs on the opposite side from the pain that are less irritable, and, also, that most individuals are harboring many latent TrPs in general, so their relative intensity must be weighed.

Common Patterns of Muscle Involvement—
Streamlining the Examination Based
on Symptom Patterns

The Upper Quarter
General Comments on the Region

First, if we look at the upper extremity patient stripped of specific diagnosis, there are some extremely common complaints that are reported by patients:

1. Pain localized around joints but also diffusely in the limb or part of the limb
2. Limitations of ROM, usually due to pain
3. Sharp pains near a joint with small movements or jarring forces
4. Tingling and numbness
5. Exacerbation of symptoms during the night and an inability to get comfortable in bed, especially in shoulder pain syndromes

The diagnosis will often emphasize the joint included in the pain zone or limitation rather than naming it as an accurate rendering of all the tissues involved. It is up to the physical therapist to identify the offending structures of the muscular system.

The interscapular zone is the prime starting point for examination and a rich source of TrPs in the upper quarter. Following our awareness of proximal to distal relationships, and the kinesiology of movement of the shoulder, the scapular movers are key:

1. *Lower Trapezius, Middle Trapezius, Rhomboid*—Movers and stabilizers of the scapula, they influence and participate in glenohumeral movement. Painful shoulder motion for any reason will activate and exacerbate these TrPs. Their inhibition (due to the presence of TrPs), weakness, and taut bands limiting motion contribute to all upper extremity dysfunction.

2. *Levator Scapulae, Scalenes*—The levator scapulae TrP radiates into the posterior shoulder/scapular zone, and often the scalenes are activated simultaneously, referring into the interscapular zone and, especially, biceps area of the brachium. Their referral patterns instigate the activation of triggers in these referral zones. They are the important link when motions of the neck and head cause arm pain, so often described as "possible cervical radiculopathy."

3. *Serratus Posterior Superior* (SPS)—This is so extremely important and so frequently missed in assessment as to be criminal. The pattern of radiation of pain and other distressing symptoms makes the SPS a prime player for perpetuation of TrPs throughout the limb. It is located deep to the interscapular movers (lower and middle trapezius, rhomboids) and attaches to the ribs, so it does not actually move the scapula at all. It is a respiratory muscle, probably activated by accident—just "being in the wrong place at the wrong time"—that is, in the zone of referral of the more superficial muscles. The SPS may also be activated by paradoxical breathing, a not uncommon problem for people with pain, and by pressure of the scapula against the muscle belly, as with resisted or forceful horizontal abduction. It generates deep subscapular pain and activates the posterior deltoid, triceps, and ulnar flexor patterns characteristic of ulnar nerve syndromes.

4. *Infraspinatus*—Another muscle that must be highlighted in consideration of upper extremity complaints is the "busybody" of the shoulder, the infraspinatus. This muscle is involved in virtually every upper extremity patient this therapist has ever examined. Perhaps the ratio of external to internal rotators of the glenohumeral joint overloads the infraspinatus as it modulates the activities of the larger latissimus dorsi,

pectoralis major, teres major and subscapularis with very little other help, or perhaps it is the muscle's proximity to the joint and therefore its role as joint stabilizer, or the muscle's location in the referral zone of proximal TrPs. Nevertheless, this muscle almost always harbors painful and often radiating triggers, even in asymptomatic persons, and in most symptomatic ones.

Common Upper Extremity Patterns

1. *Infraspinatus, Pectoralis Major and Minor, Coracobrachialis, Biceps Brachii*—"Shoulder Joint Pain" with localized intense sensation around the glenohumeral and biceps tendon area. Symptoms are worse in bed. This group is associated with bicipital tendinitis, supraspinatus tendinitis, and joint pain, as well as radicular pain.

2. *Scalenes, Biceps Brachii, Common Extensors of the Forearm, Adductor Pollicis, and First Dorsal Interosseus*—These are highly suspect in persons with thumb symptoms, which are so often associated with carpal tunnel syndrome. The person usually will report a prior history of neck problems, and symptoms around the shoulder, elbow, or forearm as well; often treatment of the proximal muscles drastically reduces the hand symptoms.

3. *Latissimus Dorsi/Teres Major—Triceps—Supinator/Common Extensors of the Forearm*—Lateral elbow and forearm pain, tingling and numbness in the forearm and hand, diffuse arm aching. Symptoms are worse in bed, especially when the arms are stretched overhead during sleep. These muscles mimic and accompany the inflammatory diagnoses of lateral epicondylitis, tendinitis of the elbow, and olecranon bursitis, and also mimic thoracic outlet syndrome.

4. *Subscapularis—Latissimus Dorsi—Pectoralis Major*—Significant loss of ROM, especially in flexion, abduction, and external rotation. Frozen shoulder due to or exacerbated by muscular limitations always implicates this triad, with the infraspinatus involved as usual in almost all shoulder complaints.

5. *Infraspinatus, Posterior Deltoid, Triceps, Ulnar Flexors and Extensors*—Often instigated by the serratus posterior superior, this group offers an explanation for several particular and less common kinds of complaints—deep subscapular pain, back of the shoulder pain, olecranon pain, and ulnar forearm pain, tingling, or numbness. All of these pains are aggravated by computer or desk work.

Why are these patterns common in practice? The explanation generally is related to the proximal to distal nature of referral and the development of satellite TrPs, and/or the functional patterns of the extremity that activate groups of muscle for coordinated actions of the limb, even those apparently focused in the distal limb. For example, when writing with a pen or pencil causes pain, the latissimus/triceps/supinator combination will kick into action, and treating the forearm alone is a frustrating endeavor. The infraspinatus and serratus posterior superior, both muscles not necessarily central to a particular activity of the extremity, are nevertheless activated by most actions of the limb and act as silent perpetuators all day long. Mabel Todd compared the shoulder to a wheel, with the glenohumeral joint at the hub and with the muscles as spokes radiating out from the center in all directions. This image depicts the extensive myotatic unit of the shoulder and orchestration required for its coordinated action.[6]

Examination of the extremity may be streamlined by following these groupings above as a basic framework for examination, but over time a complete muscular assessment should be done, especially if initial treatment aimed at these key muscles is not completely successful. Any muscle with patterns of referral in the zone of complaints, whether it is the essential pain zone or spillover pain zone, may be a very significant player if not the key muscle in a given individual. The orderly examination and treatment of the limb from proximal to distal, with particular patterns in mind and complete thoroughness at key levels of the examination, will permit much greater success in developing a proper treatment plan that will have long-term benefit to the patient.

Headache

General Comments on the Region

Headache may be simple or complex. The muscle tension headache diagnosis represents the mainstream understanding that pain actually can be referred by muscle and suggests that tension in the individual causes tightness in the muscles of the neck or head that somehow causes a headache. This describes myofascial pain! Migraine headaches may be vascular in origin and are thought to be multifactorial in cause, with muscle reactivity one of the factors, and much of the actual pain in migraine may be myofascial in nature. Another prime source of head pain is actually related to dysfunction of the masticatory apparatus and this too usually has a significant myofascial component. There are other causes of headache, and volumes have been written on the subject.

The headache diagnosis simply implies that the person's head hurts. Once again the therapist must ascertain if there is a muscular component to the person's complaints, then treat this component and observe the effects on symptoms. These effects may be measured by several parameters of change—frequency of headache, intensity of headache, scope of headache zone, duration of headache, and other associated symptoms (nausea, sensitivity to light or noise, loss of ROM). The particular pattern of headache reported will guide the examination, keeping certain patterns of involvement in mind.

Once again the importance of the interscapular zone as the starting point for examination in headache patients cannot be overemphasized. The interscapular muscles are extrinsic movers of the head and neck, so they are functionally linked to the zone of pain, and their patterns of referral are all upward. Their referral patterns will directly produce headache. These muscles also activate triggers in cervical and masticatory muscles that produce headache. If the interscapular muscles are not treated adequately, they will also reactivate the cervical and masticatory muscle triggers after these have been inactivated through direct treatment. They must be considered regardless of etiology and zone of head pain.

The lower trapezius is of prime importance. It produces occipital headaches and activates triggers in the upper trapezius and posterior cervical muscles. The middle trapezius causes pain around the seventh cervical vertebra and may activate the posterior cervicals from this level. The thoracic erector spinae originate here and continue into the cervical range, potentially causing vertebral mechanical difficulties due to their taut bands or inducing transient weakness in the cervical region, which overloads intrinsic cervical muscles. It also directly causes radiating pain into the neck, activating satellite triggers in the splenii and semispinalis muscles. When patients with head and neck pain are examined, cervical stretch into any direction is often felt all the way down into the interscapular zone, activating pain there and upward into the head.

Common Headache Patterns

1. *Lower Trapezius, Upper Trapezius, Levator Scapula, Temporalis*—The individual usually clearly describes the progression of symptoms from a pain in the interscapular region, progressing to tightness moving up the angle of the neck and back of the neck, then developing into a pain in the neck and then temples. They often sense that if they can relax or otherwise treat their pain early on, the headache does not develop. These are often described by persons with multiple types of headache as their "tension headache." These headaches may be unilateral, switch from side to side, or occur on both sides at once, with each felt as a separate pattern.

2. *Sternocleidomastoid (SCM), Suboccipitals, Occipitofrontalis, Temporalis*—This person often describes a "sickening, all-over headache," often accompanied by dizziness or nausea, affected by changes of position of the head. They may be one sided or bilateral, and often the person wants to close his or her eyes and ears, reducing input from the kinesthetic and other senses. This group easily mimics migraine.

3. *SCM, Pectoralis Major, Scalenes, Splenius Capitis*—As above, but especially

linked with poor sitting posture. Stiffness and pain in the neck may accompany the headache.

4. *Migraine Mimickers and Concomitants—SCM, Upper Trapezius, Semispinalis Cervicis, Suboccipitals*—Eye pain, unilateral intense pain, and tenderness of the occiput and scalp characterize these muscular patterns.

Sciatica
General Comments

One of the most common pain complaints involving the lower extremity is the pattern of symptoms that almost invariably lead to the diagnosis, by the physician or by patients themselves, of sciatica. This handy catchword is used very lightly to describe pain that is felt in the buttock primarily, or radiating from the buttock into the back or side of the leg, and in its fullest manifestation, wrapping down the leg to the outer calf and perhaps causing pain in the foot. Tingling and numbness, usually the cardinal signs of neurologic involvement, may also be described in these zones. The implication of the diagnosis is that the sciatic nerve is the source of the problem, and the cause of the pain. However, if we look at the pain referral diagrams of Travell and Simons, we see numerous muscles that generate the same distribution of symptoms, manifesting as pain, numbness and tingling, or both. If we carefully examine our patients, we will almost always find a significant myofascial contribution to the symptoms and perhaps TrPs that exactly mirror their complaints (Fig. 18–5).

Muscular Pattern of Involvement

Quadratus Lumborum, Gluteus Medius and Gluteus Minimus, Peroneus Longus and Brevis—The quadratus lumborum is the most often missed cause of back pain and is a frequent silent culprit in perpetuating the sciatic-like lower extremity syndrome.[9] It radiates into the buttock, activating any and all muscles both superficial and deep in this zone, but most frequently the gluteus medius and mimimus. The medius radiates locally in the buttock and posteriorly into the thigh, suggesting deep nerve pain, and the minimus radiates extensively into the posterior thigh and down the lateral thigh to the ankle. This last most convincingly mimics the dermatomal pattern of pain with sciatic nerve root disturbances. The peroneal muscles of the lateral compartment of the calf may become involved as satellite triggers of the more proximal muscle and convincingly augment the pain felt in the lower leg.

Sciatica—A Case in Five Points

At the start of this chapter, the clinical significance of TrPs was outlined, and five manifestations of the TrP were delineated. To illustrate their importance in the practical setting of the PT clinic, a brief analysis of "sciatica" in relation to these five points is made. It is hoped that this will offer unequivocal proof of the essential role of careful examination and treatment of all our patients who walk in with any label, providing us with rich opportunities to truly understand the nature of their pain.

The person who has a diagnosis of sciatica usually has a history involving intermittent episodes of back pain prior to leg symptoms, perhaps over years, or has had a traumatic injury such as a fall from a height, motor vehicle accident, or heavy lifting event. Pain has usually progressed from back to buttock and eventually into the leg. Sharp electrical pains in the posterior thigh may or may not be present, but often the patient has some tingling or numbness in the extremity. Pain may be linked to movement of the lumbar region, especially turning over in bed, twisting to get in or out of a car, and coughing or sneezing.

TrPs occur as a primary source of pain and dysfunction—Virtually all these symptoms may be generated from the soft tissues. There may be low back pain over years, and eventually the reactive muscles begin to generate symptoms radiating into the buttock, activating satellite triggers there as described earlier.

Triggers are a component of any pain or dysfunction—The wear and tear on the disc that so often eventuates to pressure on nerve roots is not occurring in isolation.

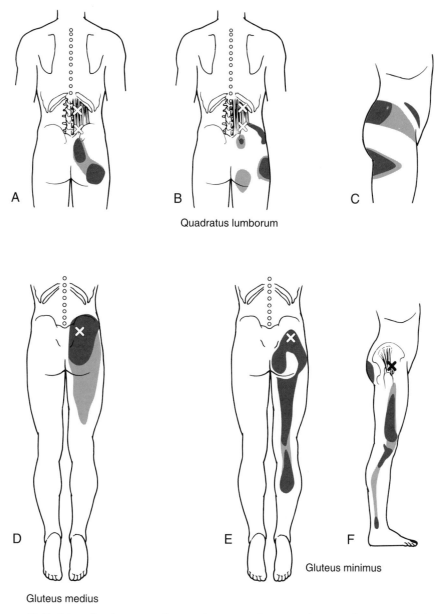

Figure 18–5. Pain referral patterns that together mimic discogenic disease with sciatica include the quadratus lumborum, gluteus medius, and gluteus minimus.

The soft tissues of the back also experience the same stresses, generating TrP activity. The noxious input from the disc pressure against the soft tissues and the nerve root irritability also act as instigators of muscle involvement. The actual symptoms the person experiences may still be due to or exacerbated by the myofascial system, even in the presence of disc disease.

TrP symptoms may mimic many diagnoses—The quadratus lumborum attaches to the 12th rib and will be activated by coughing and sneezing. It links the leg symptoms to movements of the back in general. The gluteus medius and minimus can produce tingling and numbness in radicular patterns in the absence of nerve root irritability.

TrPs persist as residuals of other disorders—As stated earlier, the muscular involvement may accompany organic disease. Repair of the disc may or may not eradicate the TrPs that accompany the disease, which may continue to produce symptoms after surgery. This may be an important feature of the devastating diagnoses "failed back syndrome" and "postlaminectomy syndrome."

TrPs can cause other somatic dysfunctions—The continual pressure exerted on the facet and disc joints of the lumbar spine from the quadratus lumborum, the erectors, and deeper paraspinal muscles, as well as the abnormal biomechanics of these joints due to abnormal muscle patterns generated by taut bands, inhibition, and chronic holding patterns associated with TrPs may all contribute to the degeneration of the joints, or changes in the intervertebral spacing that impinge on the nerve roots. TrPs arising in the gluteals will affect gait, may affect sacroiliac alignment or movement, and ultimately affect the lumbar region from below. The gross patterns of inactivity and diminished blood flow that arise secondarily from chronic muscle pain also have their effect on the vitality of other tissues in the region.

Developing a Treatment Plan

The Components of Each Session

After evaluation, the therapist should have one or more hypotheses about the myofascial health of the person. These hypotheses will be explored, beginning each session with a plan of action that will test a particular idea. The components of each session should include direct manipulation of a particular group of muscles, passive and active stretches of these muscles to increase the length of taut bands and to "reset" proprioceptors, and ideally instruction in exercises that reinforce the learning that occurred in the session. Each session should start with a check-in to assess the effects of the last session and overall progress, and to get an idea of the individual's needs that day. This check-in reinforces the therapeutic relationship—that of give and take between collaborators. By listening to patients and then responding to them, we gain useful information and improve patient compliance and outcomes.

The extent to which hands-on treatment of the TrP will be used in managing patients is based on therapist preferences, clinic policies and priorities, and the knowledge of the practitioner. To some degree, there will be benefits to the patient in proportion to the time spent in this endeavor, but whether it is brief or central, it will improve treatment outcomes.

Even when the hands-on management is the central focus of care, other modalities may be used as well. Heat may precede direct work to increase overall relaxation or follow manipulation of the TrPs as a means of reducing post-treatment soreness and to augment the effects of treatment. Short applications of ice may be used for massage of the TrP directly instead of fingertip pressure. Vapocoolant spray may be used in conjunction with stretch to "reset" the resting length of the muscle. Electrotherapies may be well tolerated for direct stimulation of the TrPs. These modalities are best used to support the hands-on work, not to replace it.

The techniques for direct manual manipulation of the TrP are numerous. Compression of the point is central, with the duration and the extent of pressure varying in relation to several factors, including the thickness and depth of the muscle, the irritability of the point, and the intention of the examiner. Movement of the fingertip and passive or active movement of the muscle may be incorporated with the pressure. Positional release techniques that use only minimal pressure are sometimes the method of choice. The guidelines for these parameters of treatment will essentially be patient tolerance and preference, therapist style and skills, and the goals of the particular session. (See Chapters 16 and 17 for further discussion of this topic.)

Exercise Regimens

Exercise plays an important role in overall physical therapy management. The goals are generally increasing strength, flexibility, and endurance, with functional goals of improved posture, muscle balance, or stability. Toward these ends, progressive resistive protocols are used, often accompanied by specific muscle stretches. This entire approach needs to be re-examined and ultimately modified for the person experiencing myofascial pain. Although poor strength, low endurance, and inflexibility may be perpetuating factors or obvious effects of myofascial pain syndromes, the individual with active TrPs will often not tolerate programs aimed at improving these parameters of function. Repetition and resistance are stressful to muscles with a diminished threshold of excitability, as is prolonged or full–end range stretching, and will often exacerbate the symptoms, activating referral patterns and increasing local stiffness and pain. (See Chapters 15, 16, and 17 for further discussion and recommendations.)

For myofascial pain patients, initial efforts at developing a home program need to focus first on relaxation and awareness. Chronic pain patients may be actively seeking to move as little as possible, either consciously or through splinting and compensatory motor patterns. They may also be actively tuning out sensation, as this has been a coping strategy for living with pain. But the process of recovery involves a reclaiming of awareness of the body, and increasing ease in living and moving in it. Movement is the means by which the person may begin to explore sensation and push the parameters of comfort therein. Small movements at first, such as slow pelvic tilts, isolations of the rib cage, and small oscillations of the head on the neck, will begin to bring movement to frozen areas. Pleasurable movement such as dancing to music, even gentle swaying, will suggest to the nervous system that sometimes the body can be a comfortable place to inhabit. These baseline activities will go a long way toward a positive involvement in rehabilitation. Modifications to activities of daily living and postural re-education can follow and/or be part of this process of increasing awareness.

Exercises to increase ROM or flexibility will also be a part of the program, of course, but should initially be gentle, without overpressure, and preferably take the form of "active stretching" in which the antagonist performs the action, taking advantage of the reciprocal inhibition that develops during muscle contraction, and greatly reducing the risk of overstretch, while also accomplishing some strengthening.[2] An example of active stretch would be supine straight leg raising to stretch the hamstrings, using the quadriceps to perform the act of stretching rather than a gravity assisted long-sitting type of stretch. Postisometric relaxation may be another method for increasing ROM and involves a moderate isometric effort, followed by a relaxation phase, and then a gentle passive stretch of the muscle.[10] This technique (also known as contract-relax-stretch in the proprioceptive neuromuscular facilitation [PNF] language) can be used during sessions as well as be a component of the home program.

Once the threshold of excitability is reduced through direct therapies to the TrP, more extensive stretching and strengthening can be offered, but always with a very cautious attitude—minimal repetitions to start, no resistance, and then very gradual resistance.[5] In this practitioner's experience, the typical sports medicine approach of heavy strengthening and stretching is damaging to the person with severe myofascial pain. Not uncommonly, persons with latent or active TrPs who attempt "self-improvement" through health club fitness programs of their own making, or even programs of running, cycling, or athletics, soon find themselves experiencing acute pain syndromes.

The emphasis in the home program will be on brief but frequent exercise moments throughout the day rather than longer periods of exercise with many repetitions in a session. This will serve to remind the person to pay attention to posture, to relax, and to directly interrupt the tensional holding patterns of the day that generally perpetuate if not cause their TrPs. Other aspects of a home program include the use of heat for pain relief and relaxation and self-massage of TrPs using a Theracane or other device that would minimize the effort and distortion involved in self-treatment. Attention to ergonomics and to causal relationships that exacerbate symptoms are important as well. In fact, paying attention in general is an essential part of the home program.

Frequency of Treatment and Prognosis

The plan for the frequency of visits depends on the severity and scope of the myofascial involvement, as well as other aspects of the disorder. Considering the myofascial elements, it is important to remember that a muscle goes through a process

Table 18–5.
Factors Influencing Prognosis

- Duration of the problem—the longer the pain has been present, the slower to change.
- Progression of symptoms over time—if the problem has been complicated by satellite TrPs and many compensatory patterns, the unraveling will be slower.
- Extent of muscle involvement—sheer numbers of muscles involved influence the rate of response.
- Degree of excitability of TrPs at the outset—sometimes therapy is focused initially at simply desensitizing the person to touch, and effective treatment of triggers cannot even begin for some weeks.
- Patient response to treatment!

of reaction to treatment, which Dr. Travell considered to be a 10-day process. She actually thought that the effect of a treatment could not be fully assessed until this time.[1] There is often a period of post-treatment soreness that may occur immediately, or up to 2 days following treatment, and may continue for one to several days. After this time, the improvement is noted, and there may be a pain-free phase, or significantly diminished symptom phase, and then a slow return of symptoms to a new reduced level. The response to treatment is one of the best tools for truly accurate evaluation and may take several sessions to complete. Only after four to six sessions does this therapist seriously consider prognosis and long-term goals.

The frequency of treatment will take all the factors in Table 18–5 into consideration. To summarize, if the person has very severe or very complex problems, treatment frequency will be twice a week or more, with the idea that each session in a week may address different aspects of the problem, allowing any given muscle to have at least a week or more to react before it is treated again. In the case of extreme sensitivity, the interval between treatments will be short so that gentle desensitization can be repeated often. In general, this therapist aims for once a week treatment, so that the effects of a session can be more accurately assessed and so that post-treatment soreness does not interfere in the next session. As the whole process of working with TrPs is one of re-education and habit breakthrough, the ideal interval between treatments may become the period that includes maximal improvement but does not allow significant backsliding. This interval should increase as the patient recovers.

Reassessment is an ongoing part of therapy and involves some objective parameters such as ROM or strength improvements, improved posture or gait, and reduction in the number and intensity of TrPs, but subjective reporting will continue to remain central in patient care. For this reason, the establishment of desirable functional outcomes should be established early on, generated by the extensive list of symptoms defined in the inteview. The threshold of excitability should increase with successful treatment, and this should be evident in greater tolerance for ordinary activity. Repeating pain diagrams may provide a visual clue to changes in subjective sensation. Depending on the extent of involvement, some measures of improvement should be noted within the first six sessions, although the course of recovery is highly variable, from total recovery within a few sessions to many months of slow and even intermittent or wavering progress. Patients who do not show significant progress should be re-evaluated for "reasons for failure," which will most often be primarily perpetuating factors that have not been or cannot be adequately addressed.

Conclusion

A physical therapy practice that emphasizes manual examination and treatment of TrPs will attract people who want and need touch in their recovery process. The practice will develop a reputation for thorough, personalized care, and will offer people an experience they have been waiting for—someone who will actually listen carefully and ask the right questions, will understand their complaints rather than be stupefied by them, and most importantly, will touch them where they hurt and will seem to be able to zero in as no other practitioner has on the pertinent, pain-causing sites in their bodies. Not everyone who leaves this practice will be cured; some will be frustrating and frustrated by their poor response to the work, but almost all will be much better educated about themselves and have a truly expanded sense of their bodies, with more ability to personally have an impact on their pain. A high percentage will leave the rehabilitative process without the problem they came in with, and for the practitioner, there can be no greater satisfaction than this.

References

1. Bobb AL, personal communication, 1985.
2. Peters JM, Peters HK: The Flexibility Manual. West Grove, Pa, Sports Kinetics, 1995.
3. Rachlin ES: Myofascial Pain and Fibromyalgia: Trigger Point Management. St. Louis, Mosby-Year Book, 1994.
4. Rubin D: Myofascial trigger point syndromes: An approach to management. Arch Phys Med Rehabil 62:107–110, 1981.
5. Simons DG, Travell JE, Simons L: Myofascial Pain and Dysfunction: The Trigger Point Manual. Vol 1, Upper Half of Body. Baltimore, Williams & Wilkins, 1999.
6. Todd ME: The Thinking Body. Princeton, Princeton Book Company, 1937.
7. Travell J, Rinzler S: The myofascial genesis of pain. Postgraduate Medicine 11(5):425–434, 1952.
8. Travell J: Office Hours: Day and Night: The Autobiography of Janet Travell MD. Cleveland, The New American Library, 1968.
9. Travell JG, Simons DG: Myofascial Pain and Dysfunction: The Trigger Point Manual. Vol 2, The Lower Extremities. Baltimore, Williams & Wilkins, 1992.
10. Wells PE, Franpton V, Bowsher D: Pain Management in Physical Therapy. Stamford, CT, Appleton and Lange, 1988.

Chapter 19

Electrical Modalities in the Treatment of Myofascial Conditions

Joseph Kahn, PhD, PT

The administration of electrical modalities to patients with myofascial conditions presents few problems for the physical therapy clinician. Most tissues involved lie within the superficial layers and are especially favorably suited to this approach. Electrical stimulation (impulses) travels along the first moist conductor encountered and so the depth of penetration becomes less of a factor than direction and fiber recruitment. Increased penetration may be obtained with higher frequencies, following the laws of electrophysics that indicate "the higher the frequency (or shorter the wavelength), the deeper the penetration." Increased intensities (voltage, amperage) may also be utilized to increase the depth of penetration, but dermal irritation, burns, and discomfort accompany higher electrical amplitudes. Present equipment employs differential frequency control for increased depth. It should also be noted that not every fiber responds to the same frequency, and that a unit offering variable frequencies is desired in order to provide a wide spectrum of fiber stimulation and maximum recruitment.

Electrode placement is an essential factor in success. Size and conformity of electrodes are also important. With myofascial stimulation, it is recommended that the electrodes parallel the shape of the target tissue as closely as possible. In specific cases, however, a transarthral approach may be preferred to ensure stimulation *around* an entire joint (or target tissue) because, as mentioned previously, the current will follow a good conductor between electrodes rather than *across* a highly resistant region. Stiff, or nonflexible, electrodes do not make good skin contact, leaving air spaces with high resistance, which leads to discomfort and often burns. Well-moistened electrodes are essential for good transmission, comfort, and recruitment. Flexible commercial electrodes, paper towel or aluminum foil electrodes (requiring "alligator clips"), and self-adhering electrodes are recommended.

With two electrodes on the same muscle, maximum recruitment may be obtained. This has traditionally been termed "bipolar" placement, even though it has nothing to do with polarity! With only *one* electrode on the target muscle, i.e., motor point stimulation, the correct term is *unipolar* placement. With *low-volt* procedures two electrodes complete the circuit, or four with dual-channel operations. With *high-volt* apparatus, three electrodes (or more) complete the circuit(s), using a large reference electrode and smaller active pads. This arrangement facilitates reciprocal techniques, possible only with low-volt dual-channel apparatus and special parameter controls. Interferential currents require four electrodes in a crossed pattern over the target area for maximal effectiveness. Microampere stimulation may be administered via pad electrodes, probes, or manually, with the physical therapist in the circuit (explained elsewhere in this chapter). Transcutaneous electrical nerve stimulation (TENS) electrode placements include nerve roots, trigger points, points of pain, and, of course, acupuncture points. With iontophoresis, yet another requirement is recommended and is explained under Iontophoresis.

Although the concepts and rationales for electrical modalities have remained intact since the original edition of this volume, there have been many beneficial additions to the hardware available.

Electrical Stimulation

Electrical stimulation comes in many forms. Each mode and waveform is individualized for specific therapeutic purposes. The three main divisions of electrotherapeutic stimulation are: (1) continuous or tetanizing, (2) surged or ramped, and (3) pulsed or interrupted modes. These forms apply to alternating current (AC), direct current (DC), and, when offered, faradic current. Alternating current consists of a biphasic waveform with variable polarity changes ("frequency") in waveform. Direct current is represented by a monophasic (unipolar) form. Faradic current is a form of AC current with sharply defined phases, not generally offered on American-made equipment.

With the continuous or tetanizing mode, so long as the frequency is greater than 50 Hz, although the range is 30–100 Hz, smooth tetanic contractions will be elicited. This mode is advantageous in inducing relaxation in tense myofascial tissues, as well as enhancing production of β-endorphins for mild analgesia. This optimal frequency may be obtained from AC at 50 Hz, pulsed DC at 50 pulses per second (pps), or other carrier frequencies pulsed at 50 pps. Clinical experience suggests this continuous mode prior to exercising modes, i.e., ramped or pulsed, or both.

The ramped or surged modes reach peak intensity over a short duration, usually in milli- or microseconds, and are primarily used to produce contractions with mainly "slow-twitch" fiber involvement. Pulsed or interrupted modes reach peak intensity instantaneously and are utilized to produce contractions with mainly "fast-twitch" fiber involvement.

With each of these modes, *amperage* will determine the intensity of contractions, whereas the *duty cycle* will establish the on/off relation. Current amplitudes usually run in the low- to mid-amperage range, e.g., 1 to 75 mamp. *Pulse durations* provide relative comfort and are measured in milliseconds in the 1 to 300 ms range. Many clinicians utilize all three modes in a general treatment session: tetanizing for relaxation, followed by the ramped or pulsed mode for exercising.

The advantages of electrical stimulation are relatively weight-free exercise, increased fiber recruitment, enhanced reticuloendothelial waste removal, increased circulation, and endorphin-release analgesia. It should be noted that electrical stimulation is far from "passive" because the target myofascial tissues contract. The work of Dr. Rosemary Jones in England[7] indicates the possibilities of changing slow-twitch fibers to fast-twitch fibers and the reverse, by selected differential frequency stimulation—truly, a form of bioengineering! It is interesting to note that two other British researchers report success with specialized electrical stimulation with specific conditions: Nobuku Shindo[15] reported obtaining active contraction and relaxation with spastic paraplegics using low-volt parameters, and Diane Farragher[5] administered low-volt pulsed DC with physiologically matched parameters for chronic Bell's palsy.

Traditional low-volt stimulation utilizes both AC and DC to produce contractions in normally innervated musculature and the associated myofascial tissues. However, in the presence of nerve damage (reaction of degeneration, or "RD" to physical therapists), the ability to respond to AC and Faradic current is lost, and *only pulsed DC will be effective.* Low-volt procedures usually fall below 100 V and 1 kHz. Current amplitudes lie in the 1- to 75-mamp range (Figs. 19–1 and 19–2).

Clinicians can now utilize a computerized programmed electric stimulation device, the "Neurotech NT 2000" made by Bio-Medical Research, Ltd. in Donegal, Ireland. A small computer module is connected to the device. The clinician then adjusts the parameters desired and programs a complete program into the device. The computer is then disconnected, and the patient takes the unit home for daily applications as programmed. Other than returning for changes in the program, the patient has only to turn the unit on for a treatment exactly as designed by the clinician (Fig. 19–3).

Iontophoresis

Iontophoresis is not a form of electrical stimulation per se, although the current used may offer some stimulatory effects indirectly. The continuous low-volt DC mode

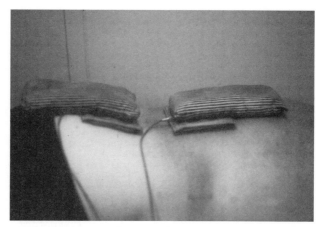

Figure 19–1. Low-volt AC stimulation to the lumbosacral region.

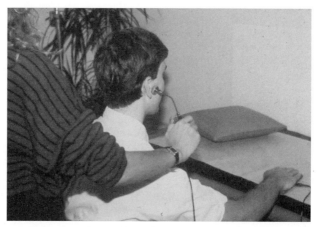

Figure 19–2. Low-volt stimulation for nerve degeneration using pulsed DC.

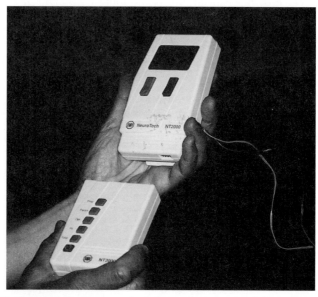

Figure 19–3. The lower portion (computer) of the device is separated from the stimulator after the clinician has programmed the desired treatment parameters.

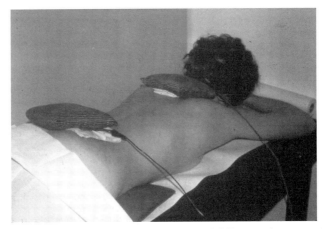

Figure 19–4. Double iontophoresis, administering two ions of different polarities simultaneously with a standard DC generator.

is utilized for ionic transfer, or iontophoresis, and is the *sole* current form for this purpose. Despite the DC characteristics of high-volt pulsed DC, it is not used for iontophoresis owing to the extremely short duration of the pulses (in the microsecond range) and low microamperage involved. The formula for ionic transfer requires amperage over a period of time, negating the effectiveness of any *pulsed* waveforms. The successful introduction of chemical substances into the body is accomplished via the continuous polarity of DC (Fig. 19–4).

Electrode placement with iontophoresis becomes a most important aspect of technique. Since the cathode (−) is considerably more irritating to the skin because of the sodium hydroxide formed at the skin-electrode interface with DC, it is advisable to keep the cathode at least twice the size of the anode (+) at all times, *even if the cathode is the active electrode. This reduces current density on the cathode and lessens the chance of burns.* One commercial source[3] now offers "buffered" electrodes for iontophoresis that are claimed to be effective in reducing the chemical irritation formed at the cathode as well as the weak hydrochloric acid formed at the anode. Consequently, their electrodes are almost of equal size. Whether the buffering substance or mechanism affects the ionic transfer itself remains to be seen (Figs. 19–5 and 19–6).

Iontophoresis is slowly achieving recognition as an ideal method of introducing chemicals into the human body. Several manufacturers have made innovative additions to their existing equipment to facilitate administration. Dexamethasone is being touted

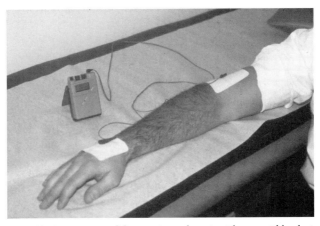

Figure 19–5. Compact unit delivering iontophoresis with compatible electrodes.

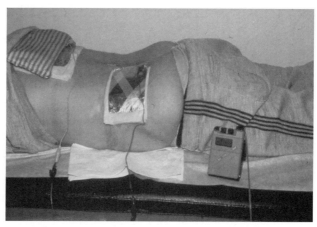

Figure 19–6. Compact unit with traditional electrodes.

by most workers as the preferred chemical (ion). However, there is still much controversy regarding the correct polarity to be used with this substance. Early practitioners obtained fairly good results with anodal applications. Later, recommendations to use the cathode as the active electrode also provided reasonably good results. Dexamethasone is primarily an anti-inflammatory (sodium dexamethasone phosphate, with or without lidocaine). I believe, however, that there is a need for more than just this one ion in practice. There is no single ion that can "do it all." (In baseball, a utility infielder may adequately cover all of the bases and the shortstop positions when needed. However, an experienced professional first, second, or third baseman or a veteran shortstop is much preferred.) There are many ions of proven effectiveness to be used other than dexamethasone for conditions other than inflammation: acetic acid with calcific deposits, mecholyl for ischemia, magnesium for muscle spasm, ibuprofen as a nonsteroid anti-inflammatory, salicylate and iodine as sclerolytic agents, and, of course, traditional low-percentage hydrocortisone. Clinicians are advised to use these specialized physiologic agents when anti-inflammatory effects alone are not primary.[9]

High-Voltage Stimulation

High-volt pulsed DC was originally considered for deeper penetration than obtained with low-volt. The extremely short pulse durations in the microsecond range, as well as the microamperage attained, necessitate increased power up to 500 V in order to obtain muscular contractions. This neatly falls under the aegis of the traditional strength-duration curve phenomenon so familiar to physical therapy students. The relative comfort of this mode is a matter of individual sensitivities. The quality of the contractions, however, remains similar to those with traditional low-volt techniques. The typical waveform is a twin-spiked DC, 7- to 20-µs duration, pulsed at 1 to 100 pps at microamperage levels, with selected active electrode polarity[1] (Fig. 19–7).

Interferential Currents

Interferential currents use the penetrating quality of the medium frequencies, i.e., 4000 Hz, to reach greater depths than with low-volt equipment. Here, two different medium frequencies are "crossed" to produce "beat" frequencies in the optimal range of 50 to 100 Hz *deeper than what is available with low-volt procedures at the same frequencies.* By maintaining one of the two frequencies constant (4000 Hz), and taking the second through a range of frequencies (4001–4100 Hz), a broad spectrum of beat frequencies is obtained, stimulating a wide number of fibers with differential frequency response capabilities. Thus, a greater recruitment possibility is realized, as are diagnos-

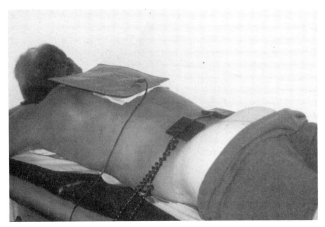

Figure 19–7. Typical high-volt pulsed DC for a low back syndrome (sandbags removed).

tic clues regarding stronger responses to the lower beat frequencies where partial denervation is present. Because the interferential currents are normally biphasic (AC), near-normal innervation is necessary. Power runs in the 1- to 100-V range, with continuous and variable beat frequencies used singularly or in a "sweep" mode, covering many frequencies. "Vectoring" is also available on many models, and is a method of pinpointing the exact location of the crossing point and permitting variation of frequency ranges and targeting (Fig. 19–8).

Russian Stimulation

So-called Russian stimulation is usually 2500 Hz, pulsed at variable rates from 1 to 100 pps, with an asymmetrical biphasic waveform. Here again, patient comfort is determined by individual sensitivities. At the 2500-Hz frequency, higher voltages are again required, i.e., 300 to 500 V (Fig. 19–9).

Microampere Stimulation

The latest entry into the field is the microampere stimulation devices. The mnemonic MENS is incorrect because the N (neural) is out of place. Stimulation here is to the "second circuit" in the body, advocated by Dr. Bjorn Nordenstrom[13] and others.

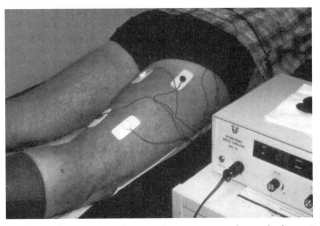

Figure 19–8. Interferential current stimulation with circuits crossed over the hamstring musculature.

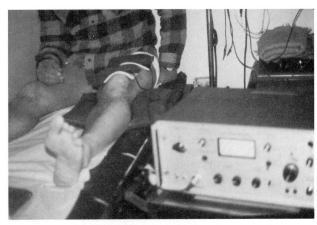

Figure 19–9. Russian stimulation to the quadriceps muscle groups.

The microamperage is hardly sufficient to affect the primary *neural* system. It is designed to reach the circulatory ionic transfer routes within the capillaries rather than the sensory or motor nerve circuitry. Microampere stimulation is programmed to enhance healing of damaged tissues by bringing blood-borne nutrient materials to the target zone. The naturally high resistance of damaged tissues is overcome by the addition of microcurrents to the ion transport system in the capillaries, simulating the intrinsic microcurrents of the body's own system. Polarity is obtained via square wave DC, with alternating polarity capabilities of the symmetrical square waveform. Frequency capabilities range from less than 1 Hz through 100 Hz. Amplitude range is up to 500 μamp. In many instances, microampere stimulation provides a modicum of analgesia. Little or no sensation or contractions are noted by the patient, since neither sensory nor motor points are stimulated with these parameters (Fig. 19–10).

Transcutaneous Electrical Nerve Stimulation

TENS is designed to block the pain sensation's pathway along the ascending neural tracts. Explained in Melzack and Wall's "gate theory"[10] and by the endorphin release phenomenon, this modality has gained in popularity despite unjustified criticism. Most TENS devices today use an asymmetrical biphasic waveform, with frequency ranges from 1 to 150 Hz, pulse widths from 50 to 300 ms, and amplitudes through 75 mcmp. Frequency and pulse width modulation are usually available to minimize

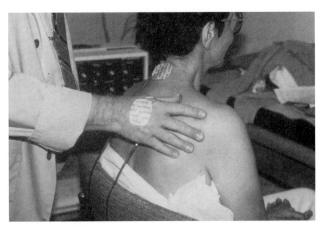

Figure 19–10. Manual technique with microampere stimulation.

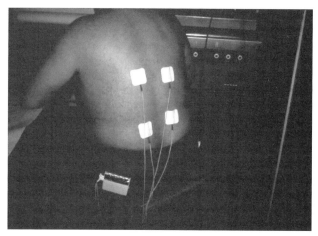

Figure 19–11. TENS administered to the dorsolumbar region.

accommodation. Several models also offer a "burst" mode, with stimulation in a pulselike form, found by some clinicians to be an effective temporary analgesic mode. Very few, if any, TENS models offer the polarity found with square waves. An asymmetrical biphasic waveform will indicate a slight polar phenomenon, but not at clinically significant or detectable levels. This would explain the differential color coding on lead wires, i.e., red (+) and black (−) (Figs. 19–11 and 19–12). TENS has also been found effective in osteogenic enhancement for nonunited fractures (Fig. 19–13).[9]

Ultrasound

Ultrasound, although not electrical in nature, behaves much like electrical phenomena. Household current, 110 V at 60 Hz, is amplified to 500 V at 1 MHz, and is imposed on a piezoelectric crystal (usually PZT: lead zirconate titanate) to produce sound waves at 1 Mc for therapeutic purposes. Currently there are units available that operate at 3 Mc. Unlike electromagnetic phenomena, increased absorption levels are obtained with *lower* frequencies with ultrasound. The 1-Mc units, therefore, are utilized for deeper penetration, whereas the 3-Mc units are suggested for superficial tissues, i.e., myofascial (Fig. 19–14). Subaqueous techniques with ultrasound are recommended for anatomic problem areas (Fig. 19–15).

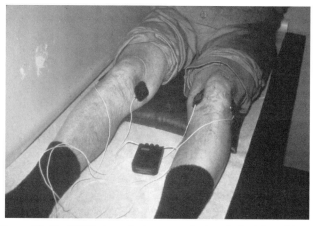

Figure 19–12. TENS shown in the transarthral mode for bilateral knees.

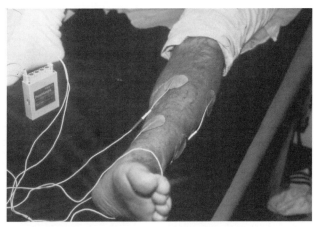

Figure 19–13. TENS administered for osteogenic enhancement with a nonunion fracture.

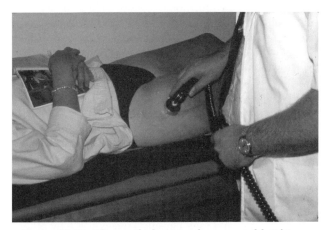

Figure 19–14. Ultrasound administered over a painful, tight scar.

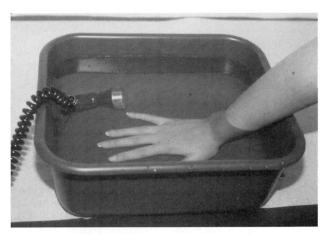

Figure 19–15. Subaqueous ultrasound.

Phonophoresis

The introduction of chemical substances into the body with sound waves, *phonophoresis*, offers clinicians a convenient, noninvasive procedure to obtain the benefits of specific therapeutic chemical agents. Phonophoresis should not be confused with iontophoresis, however; they are two distinctly different concepts. Phonophoresis is the introduction of entire *molecules* into the tissues, which then must be broken down into usable components by the body's systems. Iontophoresis is the introduction of *ions*, which are chemically active and ready for recombination. Ultrasound provides slightly deeper penetration than the 1 mm offered by iontophoresis. At deeper levels, however, the circulating blood washes away the introduced molecules sooner than the ions deposited at a shallower level where there are fewer blood vessels. Many clinicians take advantage of these phenomena by utilizing both procedures whenever possible. (Solutions may be used with iontophoresis, as well as ointments, as ion sources.) Phonophoresis is not recommended with solutions—only with ointments. If an ointment is used as an ion source, the treatment may be followed by application of ultrasound with the usual gel or other transmission medium superimposed over the remaining ointment (Fig. 19–16).

Simultaneous ultrasound with electrical stimulation has been a popular procedure for many years. Unfortunately, there is little in the literature to document the advantages of this technique other than the saving of time. After all, ultrasound is utilized to obtain muscle relaxation, whereas electrical stimulation favors contraction. It is difficult to conceive of maximum benefit of either if administered simultaneously. Ultrasound treatments usually require a much shorter time than effective electrical stimulation procedures. Pulsing the ultrasound in order to use a longer treatment time has satisfied some practitioners, but not the die-hards!

Shortwave Diathermy

Shortwave diathermy remains in our armamentarium as the single modality able to produce heat deep within the tissues without heating the superficial layers. It becomes a very valuable procedure when the target tissues are within the thorax, abdominal cavity, sinuses, and joint capsules, inaccessible by other means. With myofascial targets at *deeper* levels, shortwave diathermy becomes a modality of choice (Fig. 19–17).

Shortwave diathermy in a *pulsed* mode offers the effects of electromagnetic energy without the build-up of undesired heat. This concept is unusual because it is exactly the deep heat that is wanted for therapy.

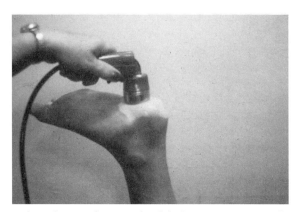

Figure 19–16. Phonophoresis administered with hydrocortisone ointment for a painful heel.

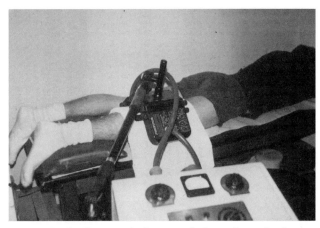

Figure 19–17. Shortwave diathermy applied over the popliteal region.

Cold Laser

The helium-neon cold laser offers the clinician a unique opportunity to penetrate the cell membrane in order to facilitate healing (Fig. 19–18). The selected wavelength of 632.8 nm, obtained from a helium-neon mixture, has been shown to penetrate the cell membrane and effectively stimulate the mitochondria responsible for production of DNA, adenosine triphosphate (ATP), and the like. Operating at only 1 mW, the cold laser also serves as a point stimulator over known Acupuncture points, trigger points, and inflammatory sites. (A familiar analogy often made by practitioners is the laser as "acupuncture with a beam of light instead of a needle.") Developments have led to the addition of units operating at higher milliwatt levels. Canadian and European models utilize milliwattage *considerably higher* than domestic models[2, 8, 10, 12, 16] (Fig. 19–18).

Cold laser therapy is on hold as of this writing. Failure to obtain FDA premarket approval has limited the use of this modality to those willing to operate under the "clinical investigational" status. As of this writing, sales of the cold laser equipment in the United States have been minimal. Reluctance to become involved with an investigational device deters many practitioners, facilities, and institutions from purchasing and/or using this modality. In Canada, Argentina, Israel, Britain, and other countries, cold laser is utilized regularly, and at much higher intensities than the 1 to 5 mW of United States models. (Recently I was privileged to serve as a speaker at a sports

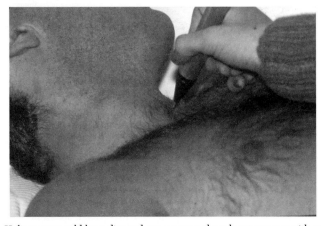

Figure 19–18. Helium-neon cold laser directed at a contracted tracheostomy scar with a postcoma patient.

medicine conference in Buenos Aires, Argentina, where I found that cold lasers were used there as commonly as we use ultrasound here, with many on display in the exhibit hall.) An excellent text on the topic from Britain is listed under Suggested Readings. The value of cold laser in a wide spectrum of pathologies has been underestimated in the United States: some of these are wound healing, dental and associated conditions, trigger point/acupuncture point radiation for pain, and sclerolytic action over scars and fibrotic tissues. It is unfortunate that this modality is not being used to its fullest at this time (Fig. 19–19).

Trigger Points

Special attention to trigger points is warranted here. These mysterious points, when stimulated, elicit reactions at distant points. Generally, these reactions lie within dermatomes, myotomes, or the oriental "meridians" familiar to acupuncturists. The ideal practitioner to treat trigger points is the physical therapist, because much of his or her training is at the "hands-on" level of care. Manual palpation remains the best method of locating trigger points. Once located, however, the method of stimulation becomes a matter of choice, experience, and training for the clinician. There is an extensive menu for the clinician: heat (moxibustion), cold (cryotherapy), digital pressure (shiatsu), ultrasound (sonopuncture), electricity (TENS and microampere stimulation), light (cold laser), and invasive techniques (injections and acupuncture). For the practicing physical therapist, the choices usually are limited to TENS, cold laser, ultrasound, or manual pressure, individually or in varied combinations. With the exception of TENS, the others are clinical or office procedures. TENS, however, is mainly designed for use at home, by the patient, *after* clinically ascertaining efficacy. Manual techniques may be included during massage or mobilization, as well as during the initial evaluation procedures. Ultrasound, because it is a short procedure, may be added to and included in any of the scheduled treatment sessions. Heat has been used to reduce pain for decades in the form of diathermy, microthermy, moist heat, and infrared radiation. Cold has been used in acute conditions but has also been used over trigger points for temporary analgesia. Electric stimulation, in the form of TENS, is widely used for analgesia, with electrode placements including trigger points, nerve roots, and known acupuncture points. Neither the motor nor sensory circuitry in the

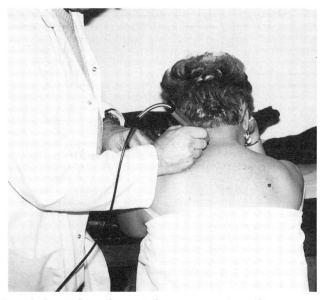

Figure 19–19. Here the laser is directed to cervical acupuncture points and/or nerve roots for analgesic effects.

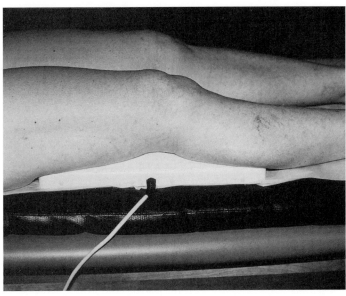

Figure 19–20. The electromagnetic pad is placed under the popliteal regions for the management of knee pain and/or dysfunction, in the office or at home.

body will respond readily to microamperage. The healing characteristics and polar phenomena with microamperage apparently account for its efficacy.

Magnet therapy is the latest in alternative methods. Two basic modes of magnetism are involved: electromagnets and "natural" magnets. Electromagnetic fields are produced electronically and the patient placed within the operational field. Treatments are devoid of sensation, even heat, and are approximately 30 minutes in length. Models for use at home by the patient are also available (Fig. 19–20). The other mode involves "natural" magnets, e.g., magnetite, lodestone, and the like, which are worn by the patient as needed (Fig. 19–21).[5] Sized for various anatomic areas, they are quite effective. Reasonably priced, they are not yet reimbursable, nor is a prescription

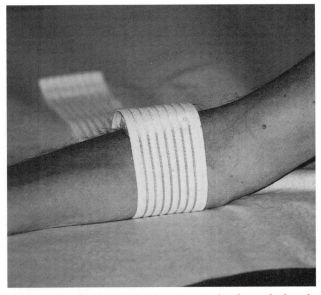

Figure 19–21. A natural magnet to be worn by the patient is placed over the lateral epicondylar region for pain control in the lower forearm, wrist, and hand.

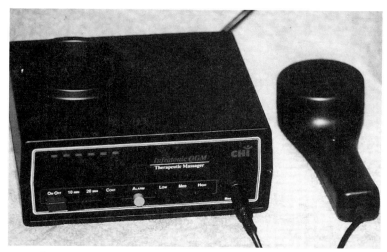

Figure 19–22. The unit ("CHI GONG") is small and portable and provides the desired low-frequency infrasound to affected areas, much like traditional ultrasound.

needed. Before I retired, I found that I was prescribing fewer TENS units and was instead prescribing magnets for analgesia between office visits or at discharge. Several manufacturers and/or dealers[6] offer these magnets, and they even may be found at most local pharmacies. Magnetic therapy is to be considered as an alternative medicine approach.

The latest addition to the modality field is infrasonic deep massage units. This concept, derived from many years of study and practice in China, provides deep massage using the penetrating qualities of very low sound frequencies. Operating at 8 to 14 Hz, this device can administer massage through clothing and will even penetrate a plaster cast. There is no sensation other than a gentle massage, with no accompanying heat produced. Details regarding history, studies, and techniques may be obtained from the manufacturer and/or dealer (Figs. 19–22 and 19–23).[6, 14]

In summary, the physical therapist's noninvasive approach to trigger point treatment

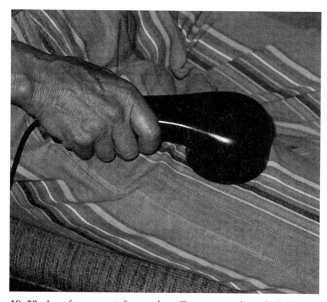

Figure 19–23. Low-frequency infrasound is effective even through clothing, as shown.

is a matter of selective, personal experience, and expertise with each of the listed modalities, leaving invasive methods by physicians as a last resort.

Commentary

I generally favor a mixed-modality approach in designing an appropriate treatment for a patient. Utilizing the benefits of each in a single session, I see the patient less frequently, and usually obtain favorable results more quickly. Then, it is a matter of elimination to determine which of the modalities offers the best results. This also assists with billing and collections from carriers, most of whom limit their reimbursements to a few procedures. Utilizing many modalities, one is reasonably assured of adequate payment even if some of the procedures are denied.

In recent years, emphasis has been placed on manual techniques and exercises, leaving modalities on the "bottom rung" of the rehabilitation ladder. I am pleased to say that many clinicians are returning to more traditional modalities to provide ongoing relief before, during, and after use of other modalities.

The history of electrotherapy is long and complex but follows the same pattern as is exhibited with most other medical concepts: early acceptance followed by skepticism and doubt, and even ridicule. Then, perseverance and continuing good clinical results in the hands of those who understand and master the procedures usually engenders a rebirth and overwhelming acceptance of the earlier concepts . . . however, *now* at a higher level of technical advancement.

References

1. Alon G: High Voltage Stimulation. Chattanooga, Tenn, Chattanooga Corp, 1984.
2. Barnes JF: Electro-acupuncture and cold laser therapy as adjuncts to pain treatment. J Craniomandibular Pract 2:148, 1984.
3. Empi Inc: Dupel System, St Paul, Minn.
4. Enmeweka C: Laser biostimulation of healing wounds: Specific effects and mechanisms of action. J Spinal Phys Ther 9:333–338, 1988.
5. Farragher D: Personal communication, 1985.
6. G.E. Miller Inc., 45 Saw Mill Rd., Yonkers, NY 1070.
7. Jones R: Personal communication, 1985.
8. Kahn J: Open wound management with the HeNe cold laser. J Spinal Phys Ther 6:203, 1984.
9. Kahn J: Principles and Practice of Electrotherapy, 2nd ed. New York, Churchill Livingstone, 1991.
10. Kleinkort J, Foley RA: The cold laser. Clin Manage 2:30, 1982.
11. Melzack R, Wall PD: Pain mechanisms, a new theory. Science 150:971, 1965.
12. Mester E: The effect of laser rays on wound healing. Am J Surg 122:532, 1971.
13. Nordenstrom B: An electrifying possibility, reviewed by Gary Taubes in Discovery, April 1986:22–27.
14. Scientific Investigators into Chinese Qi-Gong. Chiva Healthways Institute, 117 Avenida Granada, San Clemente, CA 92672.
15. Shindo N: Personal communication, 1985.
16. Snyder L, Meckler C, Borc L: The effect of cold laser on musculoskeletal trigger points. Phys Ther May 1984: 745.

Suggested Reading

Baxter GD: Therapeutic Lasers. New York, Churchill Livingstone, 1994.
Gersh MR: Electrotherapy in Rehabilitation. Philadelphia, FA Davis, 1992.
Kaplan PG, Tanner E: Musculoskeletal Pain and Disability. East Norwalk, Conn, Appleton & Lange, 1989, pp 291–303.
Kauffman TL: Geriatric Rehabilitation Manual. Philadelphia, Churchill Livingstone, 1999.
Low J, Reed A: Electrotherapy Explained. London, Butterworth-Heinemann, 1990.
Scully M, Barnes MR: Physical Therapy. Philadelphia, JB Lippincott, 1989.
Washnis GJ, Hricak RZ: Discovery of Magnetic Health. Rockville, Md, Nova Publishing, 1993.
Whitaker J, Adderly B: The Pain Relief Breakthrough. Toronto, Canada, 1998.
Wilder E: Obstetric and Gynecologic Physical Therapy. New York, Churchill Livingstone, 1988, pp 113–129.

Chapter 20

The Role of Ergonomics in the Prevention and Management of Myofascial Pain

Elsayed Abdel-Moty, PhD ▪ Tarek M. Khalil, PhD, PE
Renee Steele-Rosomoff, BSN, MBA
Hubert L. Rosomoff, MD, DMedSci ▪ Shihab S. Asfour, PhD

Musculoskeletal injuries and the resulting pain and soft tissue changes often produce significant changes in the manner by which people perform daily tasks. In order to manage these injuries and prepare the patient to engage in a productive lifestyle, medical professionals have relied on traditional therapeutic interventions and pain management approaches. The application of this "medical model" alone may not be as effective if the casues of pain/injury are not adequately addressed. For this purpose, ergonomic interventions for community re-entry and environmental modification become essential in order to prevent injury and re-injury.

This chapter outlines a selected number of proven ergonomic contributions for the prevention, rehabilitation, and disability management of myofascial pain and fibromyalgia. These interventions were developed and tested by the ergonomics team at the University of Miami Comprehensive Pain and Rehabilitation Center (CPRC) and have proven valuable to postinjury management and return to work.

What Is Ergonomics?

Ergonomics is the scientific study of work and of the relationship between people and their working or living environment. This relationship comprises humans, equipment, tools, tasks, and environmental conditions. On one hand, humans have certain capabilities. These can be described in terms of anatomic (structural), physiologic (functional), and psychological (behavioral) attributes. Humans also have limitations arising from factors such as gender differences, aging, fitness, diet, stress, as well as pain and injury. Our abilities—and limitations—combined with acquired skills determine how well we perform daily tasks. Ergonomics helps people recognize their abilities and limitations for safe and effective performance within the environment.

The term "fitting humans to the job" describes the process of matching people's capabilities with the task demands as well as designing equipment that best meets human expectations. When there is a mismatch between the physical requirements of the job and human capabilities, musculoskeletal disorders can result.

The Premise of the Ergonomic Approach

The basis of the ergonomic approach to the management of musculoskeletal injuries is based on the model of the *human-environment-machine system* (HEMS) (Fig. 20–1). The goal of ergonomics is to establish a HEMS that ensures a match between people and their surroundings while reducing the levels of stresses resulting from our interaction with work, machines, and the environment. In a safe HEMS, ergonomics strives to:

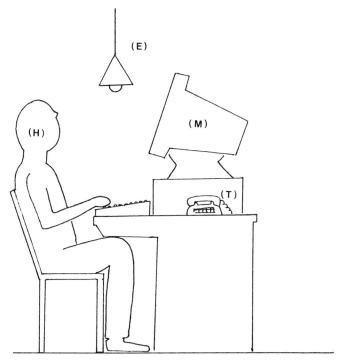

Figure 20–1. The basis of the ergonomic approach to the management of myofascial pain is the study of the "human-machine system." The components of this system are humans (H) having certain capabilities and limitations; machines (M) and tools (T) having specific design and layout characteristics; and environment (E) being physical (light, heat, etc.) as well as social (family, job satisfaction, etc.).

1. Design and/or recommend machines and equipment based on human capabilities.
2. Structure tasks in order to enhance ease, efficiency, and safety.
3. Match job demands and human capabilities.
4. Make people aware of their capabilities, limitations, and the environment within which they perform.

Ergonomic Disorders

Poor ergonomic design of tasks, equipment, or workplaces has resulted in a newly recognized group of injuries referred to as "ergonomic disorders." These are disorders caused by repetitive motions, forceful exertions, and sustained or awkward postures. Among ergonomic disorders are back and neck pain, soft tissue injuries, eye fatigue and strain, numbness of fingertips, headache, skin problems, stress, and cumulative trauma disorders (also known as repetitive motion injuries or overuse syndromes).

Musculoskeletal disorders are common workplace injuries with low back pain (LBP)—accounting for about 20% of all injuries and illnesses in the workplace and costing the nation more than 60 billion dollars anually.[14] Another common problem is cumulative trauma disorders (CTDs), also known as the "disease of the information age." A special case of CTD is carpal tunnel syndrome (CTS). CTDs and CTS are the most frequently reported on-the-job ailments, affecting over one half of the American work force.

Causes of Ergonomic Disorders in the Workplace

Work-related musculoskeletal injuries are equally likely to afflict people who perform sedentary-type jobs and those involved in heavy labor.[12] A common characteristic in this class of injuries is that job tasks require excessive force, repetitive movements, excessive bending, twisting, and reaching, and constant deviation from the body's neutral postures. Soft tissue injury can also result from activities such as lifting, slips and falls, driving, and accidents. They can also develop gradually due to disuse, muscle weakness, and as a result of the cumulative "wear and tear" placed on the body when daily tasks are carried out incorrectly.

Several activities and job tasks are more likely to result in ergonomic disorders. Examples are checkout scanning in a supermarket, keypunching, working at an assembly line, meat processing, sewing and knitting, packing, stapling, polishing and buffing, surface grinding, painting, and sports activities (e.g., golf). In particular, computers have been blamed for causing or contributing to workplace injuries. Prolonged keypunching, constant switching of the eyes between the document and the computer screen, using the telephone while typing or mousing, and inadequate visual attributes of the operator are but some of the conditions that have resulted in disabling disorders in the workplace user.

Ergonomic Contributions

Ergonomic contributions to the management of musculoskeletal injuries and disorders can take place at the various stages of injury occurrence. The first stage represents efforts in the prevention and avoidance of injury *(injury prevention phase)*. Once an injury occurs, the second stage becomes pain management, rehabilitation, and disability prevention *(rehabilitation phase)*. The third stage follows rehabilitation, when efforts aim to ensure safe return to a productive lifestyle while minimizing the chances of reinjury *(post-rehabilitation phase)*.

Ergonomics and Injury Prevention

Ideally, the thrust of the ergonomics approach is to control the risk factors that can contribute to injury rather than take corrective actions after a mishap. In this primary stage of prevention, the implementation of established ergonomics guidelines for safety and accident prevention reduces the exposure to the risk factors. Following the theme of the HEMS, these ergonomic guidelines address humans, equipment, and the environment. Prior to implementation of the guidelines, the risk factors must be identified.

Idenfi cation of the Problem

It is important to pinpoint, as early as possible, the cause of the problem. The majority of workplace disorders may be induced environmentally or occupationally or through a combination of many factors. The scientific ergonomic approach does not subscribe to the notion that people who claim to have injuries or pain are "malingerers." Several factors are linked to the onset or development of soft tissue injuries. These are:

1. Physical factors (e.g., posture, strength, flexibility, body build, reflexes)
2. Individual factors (e.g., age, medical history, education, fitness level)
3. Psychological factors (e.g., depression, family problems, anxiety, job dissatisfaction, personality traits)
4. Task factors (prolonged sitting, high repetitiveness, high force, poor posture, fatiguing tasks, high speed, mechanical vibration, mental stress)

Human Safety

Safety is everyone's responsibility (Fig. 20–2). People should be trained to recognize their abilities and limitations. They should also be trained to identify the stresses resulting from work, home, sports, or leisure activities. Safety awareness should be individualized for the person and for the job with a sufficient degree of generalization

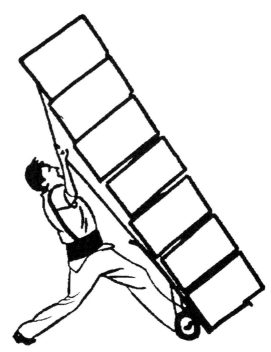

Figure 20–2. Safety is everyone's responsibility. Careless acts, whether resulting from poor safety aware-ness, human error, or problems in the engineering design of tools and equipment, can be detrimental to health and can become very costly to the individual and the organization.

because the concepts must be transferred to home and other activities. Training in human safety requires knowledge of work, job tasks, activities of daily living, posture, body mechanics, and biomechanical factors.

Developing corrective measures to improve human safety requires the use of checklists especially constructed to identify the risk factors. Once the risk factors are identified, guidelines can be established and developed. Tables 20–1 through Table 20–4 and Figures 20–3 through 20–12 present examples of ergonomic guidelines specific to enhance human safety in a general workplace, in an office workplace, in a computer workplace, and during laptop computer activities.

Workplace Safety

Workplace safety and human safety are interrelated. The implementation of ergo-nomic guidelines to improve human safety can be far more effective if workplaces are designed with human safety in mind. Numerous ergonomic considerations in equip-ment and tools design have been developed and published in the general literature as well as in industry standards. Practical ergonomic solutions have been demonstrated in workplaces of all sizes across many industries. Many employers have developed effective ergonomic programs and common sense solutions to address workplace injuries. Often these injuries can be prevented by simple and inexpensive changes in the workplace. Adjusting the height of working surfaces, varying tasks for workers, and encouraging short rest breaks can reduce the risks. Reducing the size of items that must be lifted or providing lifting equipment may aid workers.

Many employers have proven that establishing a systematic program to address such issues as repetition, excessive force, awkward postures, and heavy lifting results in fewer injuries to workers. The crucial elements in the development of an effective ergonomic program in the workplace are:

1. Management leadership
2. Employee participation

Text continued on page 572

Table 20–1.
General Ergonomic Guidelines for Human Safety

1. Do not design equipment or environments for an average person. For space requirements, accommodate the large person. For reaches, accommodate the small person.
2. Provide adequate space for body movement.
3. Consider the limits of muscular force and strength.
4. Take note of the visual attributes of the individual.
5. Exercise for stretching and strengthening.
6. Maintain proper posture:
    - Keep joints in the neutral position.
    - Avoid unnatural posture.
    - Provide a wide balanced support on the feet while standing.
    - Avoid prolonged periods of sitting.
    - Stand straight without slumping.
    - Alternate the sides of the body.
    - Support the arms and the back while sitting.
    - Analyze posture to pinpoint cause of pain.
    - Practice perfect posture.
    - Reclined postures are acceptable provided there is good support.
    - Maintain knees at optimal level.
    - Distribute weight uniformly.
    - Evaluate auto driving posture.
7. Use proper body mechanics to lift:
    - Think and plan ahead
    - Size and test the object before handling it.
    - Assume a stable lifting position.
    - Grasp firmly.
    - Choose proper lifting technique.
    - Prepare your muscles for action.
    - Lift smoothly.
    - Move with the object.
    - Ask for help if needed.
8. Use proper body mechanics at all times:
    - Practice good body mechanics.
    - Work within the viewing area.
    - Get as close to the work area as possible.
    - Bring objects close to your focus.
    - Shift weight often.
    - Avoid holding the telephone between the head and the shoulder.
    - Avoid carrying too much in one hand.
    - When pulling, switch hands to avoid straining muscles.
    - Don't hunch your trunk over your desk.
    - Don't slouch when reading in a chair.
    - Avoid prolonged hyperextension and hyperflexion.
    - Avoid twisting and sudden turning.
    - Avoid abrupt reflex movements.
    - Minimize repetitive movements.
    - Avoid working overhead for extended periods of time.
    - Minimize overreaching as well as reaching behind the head.
    - Make use of stronger muscles to perform the same task.
    - Modify sleeping habits or re-evaluate bed and pillows.

Table 20–2.
Ergonomic Guidelines for Desk Activities

1. Keep forearms at or about 90 degrees, parallel to writing surface.
2. When using the phone, rest arm on the desk or support it with the other arm.
3. Don't sustain arms up in the air without any support.
4. Don't cradle the telephone between neck and shoulder.
5. Use a footrest when sitting so that knees are slightly higher than hips.
6. Use the chair's backrest.
7. Avoid pressure on sensitive body tissue (for example, under the thigh while sitting and that at the wrist joint while typing).
8. Distribute body weight evenly under the thighs while sitting.
9. Avoid slouched posture when reading in a chair. Don't hunch shoulders over the desk.
10. Lay out the work area within easy reach (horizontal as well as vertical).
11. Face the work area at all times.
12. Practice pacing. Use reminders to stretch at regular intervals of time.

Table 20–3.
Ergonomic Guidelines for Computer-Related Activities

1. Raise computer monitor so that the top of the monitor is at eyesight level.
2. The relative placement of the source documents, the keyboard, and the monitor should minimize head movement.
3. The keyboard should fall directly below the hands with the elbows at about 90 degrees.
4. Gentle rest of the palms and forearms is recommended for long-term keyboard use to support the weight of the upper extremity and allow shoulder and neck muscles to be relaxed during work.
5. Align yourself with the monitor and the keyboard (especially the part of the keyboard used the most).

Table 20–4.
Ergonomic Guidelines for Laptop Users

1. Use carrying case with a padded shoulder strap and handle. Shift load between hands or shoulders.
2. Consider using a lightweight backpack to spread the weight evenly across your back and shoulders.
3. Make use of wheeled luggage carriers whenever possible.
4. Take "mini-breaks" by focusing on a distant object for a few seconds before continuing work on your screen. Take breaks to stretch.
5. Keep screen clean at all times.
6. Comfortable viewing distance is 18–20 inches.
7. Use indirect, soft light.
8. Keep head in a comfortable position. If light permits, angle the screen so that it is perpendicular to your line-of-sight.
9. Adjust screen brightness and contrast.
10. Increase the font size.
11. Type with a light touch.
12. Keep wrists in a straight, nonrigid position.
13. Hands and wrists should be free to move when typing.
14. Use the wrist-rests to provide support during work and breaks from typing.
15. Keep fingers relaxed and nonrigid.
16. Keep elbow in a relaxed position near the body when possible.
17. If the table and the chair are not adjustable, place a cushion on the chair seat. The extra height helps to eliminate any angling or bending in your wrists.
18. If feet are dangling, use a footrest.
19. If you use the laptop when your car is parked, move to the passenger seat where you will have more room for computing.
20. In airplane: if you have to use the laptop on the plane, try to reserve a bulkhead seat or an exit row in advance of your trip. With a bulkhead seat you will not experience any interference from a seat back reclined in front of you. Exit rows provide more seat-to-seat spacing and allow you to position your arms comfortably while working. Unfortunately the drop-down table on a plane is connected to the person's seat in front of you. If that person reclines while your laptop is open, his or her seat back will hit your screen, forcing you to pull the laptop closer to you.
21. In the airport: Check with airport lounges; most airlines' clubs offer comfortable desks and places to plug in your computer instead of balancing the laptop while waiting at the gate.
22. In bed: Pay close attention to your posture when working in bed. Make sure your lower back is properly supported by pillows. You may want to raise the height of your computer by placing a pillow on your lap. Do not recline too much. Use a pillow to support your head and neck while working.
23. In the office: Using a full-size computer screen and keyboard may be more comfortable. Use your laptop as your central processing unit only, and then you are free to optimize your monitor and keyboard as if you had a regular desktop computer. Docking stations are another useful option. It may be a much better alternative to having both a laptop and a desktop computer.
24. In a meeting/conference room: If you are sitting for a long period of time, try to shift your weight from side to side often and stand regularly to avoid discomfort. Pay close attention to your work-surface height.

Table 20–5.
Ergonomic Guidelines for Workplace Design

1. Design adjustable workstations.
2. Select appropriate seating for the individual and the task.
3. Design tools to facilitate task performance.
4. Keep equipment and supplies for immediate use.
5. Locate control switches within easy reach.
6. Provide good environmental conditions.
7. Choose the right chair:

   - Contoured back and seat supports
   - Upholstered with breathable fabric
   - Flexible tilting
   - Independent adjustment of the seat and the backrest
   - High backrest if needed
   - Angled backrest at about 110 degrees
   - Adjustable seat height and depth
   - Contoured front edge of the seat
   - Width sufficient to allow movement
   - Adjustable armrest
   - Casters, five-spur pedestal, and swivel

8. *Computer workplaces:* Adjust heights such that the top of computer monitor is at eyesight level, keyboard falls directly below the hands, gentle resting of the palms and forearms, a stand for reference material, proper location of the pointing device.
9. *Environment:* Evaluate vibrating tools, slippery floors, sharp objects, protective equipment, glare, heat, dust, noise, chemicals.
10. *Task demand:* Evaluate task demands in terms of strength requirement, endurance requirement, level of concentration, boredom, repetitious, monotonous, requires high level of responsibility, mentally demanding, stressful, etc.
11. *Interaction with work:* Evaluate the operator's level of attentiveness, decision making, speed (work pace), judgment, alertness.

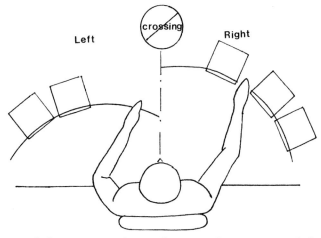

Figure 20–3. Human body joints are not functionally structured to move in straight lines. The layout of work tools must allow natural movements while minimizing repetitive twisting and excessive turning. In this case, work tools should be arranged within the area defined by the "maximum" and "comfortable" reaches of the operator. Excessive "crossing" of the imaginary midline should be minimized, as well as the resulting twisting action.

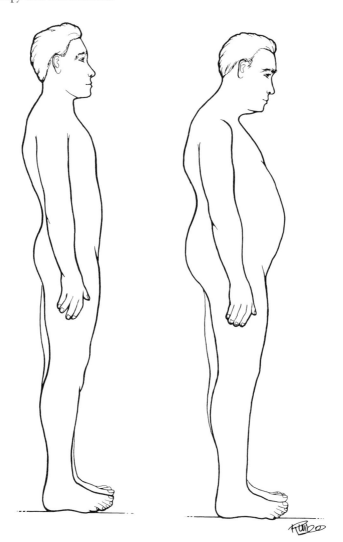

Figure 20–4. Poor posture can be the result of obesity, poor work habits, structural deficiencies, poor self-esteem, muscle weakness, as well as a variety of other factors. Good posture should be consciously practiced and maintained.

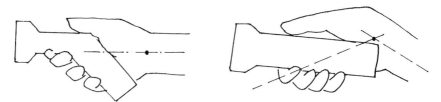

Figure 20–5. In some instances *(right)* the design of tools and equipment does not allow proper natural alignment of body joints, thus placing unnecessary stress on the soft tissue. Whenever possible, better engineering designs *(left)* should be provided. People should be made aware of this type of condition and learn corrective methods.

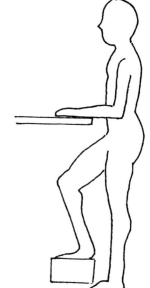

Figure 20–6. By providing a step stool, standing tolerance can be increased. Allowing weight shifting reduces static loading on muscle groups.

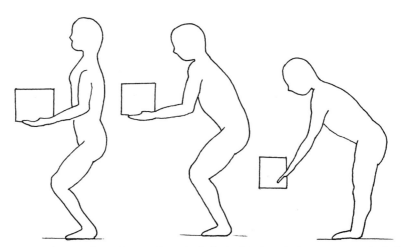

Figure 20–7. Lifting an object far away from the body (*right*) places higher stresses on the body than if the object is held closer to the body's center of gravity (*middle* and *left*). A hot or slippery object, on the other hand, may be difficult to handle while applying proper lifting techniques. In this case, other ergonomic solutions should be investigated.

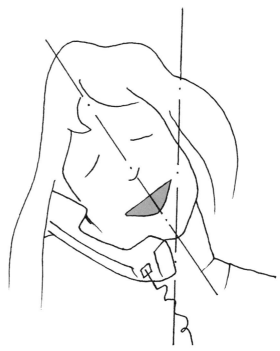

Figure 20–8. A very common, yet incorrect, posture of the head and neck while using the telephone. Such severe deviations from the neutral posture place a significant amount of stress on the neck muscles and can result in myofascial pain. This posture violates the ergonomic principle of "efficiency in muscle use."

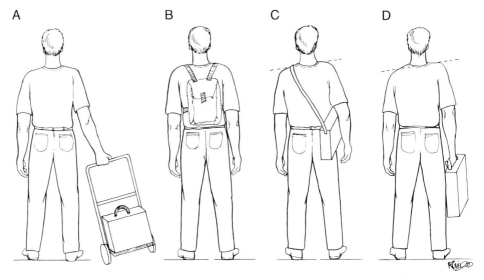

Figure 20–9. There are many ways to perform a single-handed carrying task. Ergonomically, some postures are preferred (A and B) because the resulting biomechanical stresses are lower or are distributed on the body. For some patients who experience recurrent pain on one side, the posture shown in C may be preferred. In this case, weight distribution is shared by the body with some concentration on the nonpainful side. Carrying a heavy load in one hand without alternating sides, as in D, is the least desirable and should be avoided. In all cases, good postural habits should be maintained.

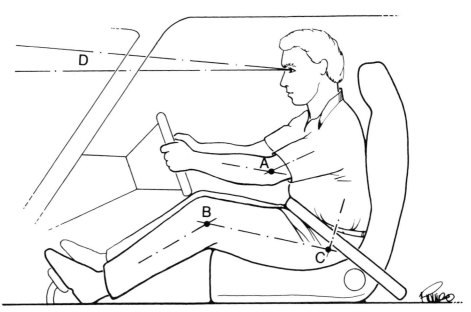

Figure 20–10. Driving postures vary depending on the type of car, the space allowed, and the dimensions of the individual driver. In general, orientation is recommended at the elbows, knees, and hips to allow for comfortable reaching to all controls, sufficient force to apply the brakes safely, and comfortable viewing of the rear-view mirror and the side mirrors.

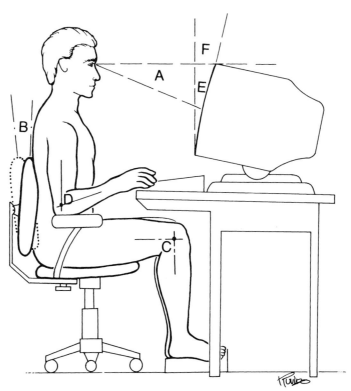

Figure 20–11. The complexity in designing computer workplaces is largely due to the number of variables involved. Recommendations call for a slightly tilted backrest (b), about a 90-degree angle at the elbows (d), knees slightly higher than the hips (c), the video display terminal (VDT) within the viewing area (a), and the VDT screen (e) at an angle that minimizes glare and light reflections (f). The magnitude of these parameters should be individualized for the workplace user.

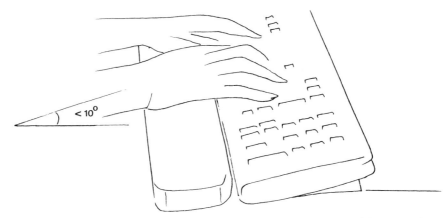

Figure 20–12. With use of a soft support by this computer operator, a comfortable wrist angle can be maintained and shoulder stress resulting from the unsupported weight of the arms can be minimized. Chair arm supports, keyboard holders, and adjusting the chair height may provide a similar effect.

3. Hazard identification and control
4. Employee training
5. Medical management

The keys to success of such efforts are also simple. Ergonomics provides a host of guidelines for designing workplaces in order to control factors such as repeated motions, forceful exertions, poor posture, poor body mechanics, and work-rest schedules. Selected guidelines are presented in Table 20–5 and shown in Figures 20–13 and 20–14.

Manual Lifting and Musculoskeletal Injuries

One risk factor that has been receiving special attention in industrial ergonomics is manual materials handling. Lifting and carrying increase vulnerability to myofascial injuries. There have been attempts to control lifting-related injuries through workers' evaluation, education in proper methods of lifting, and task engineering and design. Various approaches to evaluate the capacity for manual handling tasks have been developed. The most popular of these has been the "psychophysical approach" for determination of lifting capacity in which subjects are allowed to adjust the weight lifted in order to reach what is perceived as the "maximum acceptable weight of lift." Based on this approach, guidelines have been developed for the evaluation and design of tasks involving manual handling of materials. One of the limitations of evaluating lifting tasks is that the amount that a person can lift depends on many variables. Any evaluation aimed at establishing the lifting capacity of an individual should take into consideration[13]:

1. The distance between the person and the load (horizontal distance)
2. The handles (vertical distance, hand spread)
3. Lifting frequency (number of lifts per minute)
4. Load factors (weight distribution, load stability, container's shape and size)
5. Plane of lifting (e.g., in front of the body)
6. Body posture (e.g., twisting, restricted lifting)
7. Pattern of lift (e.g., one-handed vs. two-handed lift; smooth, jerking, style of lifting)
8. Coupling (e.g., handles, floors, and shoes)
9. Ambient environment (space constraints, stairs, altitude)
10. Task variables (e.g., distance that load is to be carried, rest between lifts, time of day, unexpected motions, duration of lift)
11. Human variables (age, gender, fatigue, employee capabilities, employee weight and height, employee skills, past medical history, stress, diet)

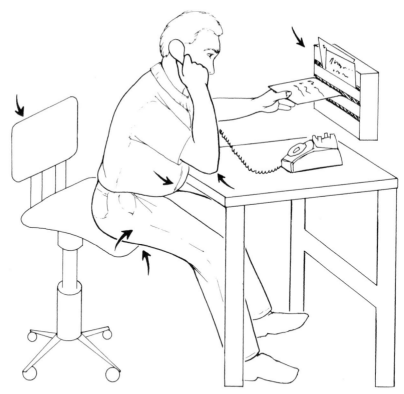

Figure 20–13. It is estimated that more than half of office workers sit either forward or in the middle of the chair. Ergonomics analyzes not only sitting habits but also chair design, individual characteristics, and workplace layout in relation to the task demands.

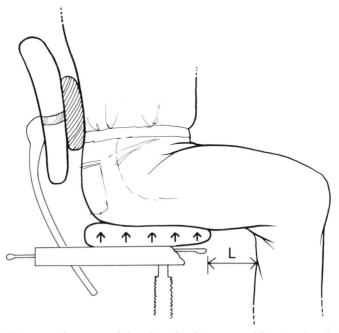

Figure 20–14. Recommending a rounded cushion for this person while using this chair may not be beneficial at all. The added cushion reduces the effective seating area, thus increasing the static pressure under the thighs. The ergonomic approach to this and similar situations relies on fitting equipment to individuals within the constraints of the environment and the requirements of the task.

Current evidence suggests that worker training that emphasizes "lifting technique" only is not very effective in reducing injuries. Often, factors such as task demands, environmental conditions, worker awareness, and fatigue do not permit applying "safe techniques." Programs to teach employees "proper lifting" may not be an effective substitute for a well-engineered workplace and a fit worker. Proper lifting may not be as safe as previously assumed. Loads that can be lifted with the legs can easily exceed the capacity of the low back and can place undue stress on the knees.

Ergonomics in the Rehabilitation Stage (Clinical Ergonomics)

Several medical treatment approaches have been advocated by different care providers to deal with soft tissue injuries and chronic pain problems. The health care professionals that are usually involved in rehabilitation include physicians, physical therapists, occupational therapists, nurses, vocational counselors, psychologists, and psychiatrists. Until the early 1980s, the management of myofascial pain was considered the sole domain of medical professionals. Another profession that has shown to be equally important in a successful rehabilitation effort is ergonomics (Fig. 20–15). In 1982, the concepts of "rehabilitation technology" and "clinical ergonomics" were introduced at the University of Miami Comprehensive Pain and Rehabilitation Center (CPRC). Technology intervention implies the use of ergonomically inspired equipment and techniques to restore performance of patients with chronic injuries to a state of wellness. At the CPRC, ergonomists work jointly with physicians, therapists, and other health care professionals in a rehabilitation environment.[15] This interaction has provided an excellent intervention forum for recognizing and solving many complex problems related to myofascial pain and musculoskeletal injury.

The systematic ergonomic approach to the management of the problem consists of:

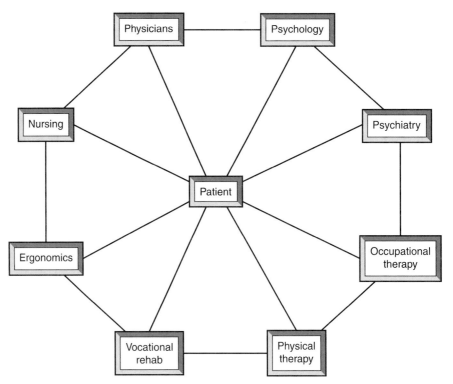

Figure 20–15. At the University of Miami Comprehensive Pain and Rehabilitation Center, ergonomists work jointly with physicians, therapists, and other health care professionals in a multidisciplinary rehabilitation setting to provide the patient with the necessary tools for functional restoration.

1. Evaluating the effect of injury and pain
2. Implementing interventions to deal with the problem and its effects

Patient Evaluation

In postinjury management, a primary goal of ergonomics is quantitative, objective documentation of the effect of pain on the functional abilities of the patient. The evaluation of patients' abilities is an important undertaking in rehabilitation and is accomplished through the establishment of a "performance profile." This profile can then be compared with profiles of healthy persons of equivalent age, sex, and work category in order to determine limitations. Rehabilitation usually involves efforts to restore the patient to the target range of scores for healthy persons. The performance profile can also be used to measure progress and outcome of rehabilitation.

A performance profile can be established through evaluations comprising one or more of the following measures[1]:

1. Measures of *physical* capacities such as static and dynamic strength, flexibility, mobility, posture, sway and balance, psychomotor abilities, and gait
2. Measures of *functional* capacities such as tolerance to sitting, standing, walking, climbing, lifting, carrying, pushing, pulling, driving, stooping, crouching, and squatting
3. Measures of *work* capacities specific to the patient's ability to perform the demands of a job or job category (the Dictionary of Occupational Titles describes 20 physical demands describing every job)[6-9]

The interpretation of findings from the performance profile in pain patients should be based on a clear understanding of the issues surrounding patient evaluation. Among these are:

1. Patient's issues (pain, perceptions, behaviors, motivation, effort, secondary gains, use of medications, prior exposure to similar testing, contraindications, use of assistive devices)[6]
2. Relationship to the Americans with Disabilities Act (ADA), which requires that these evaluations be job specific and task oriented
3. Evaluator's issues (bias, objectivity, training, experience, qualifications)
4. Methodological issues (patient safety, testing equipment, protocols, instructions, sequence of testing)
5. Statistical issues (validity, reliability, sensitivity)
6. Other issues (testing environment, presence of a third party such as the attorneys during testing, method of reporting of results)

By accurately establishing performance parameters of the patients, it is possible to chart their course of treatment, determine their progress, and establish quantitative criteria for return to work.

Engineering Interventions Through Workplace/Task Design

Pain related to work situations is a complex modern problem in industrialized countries. While it is agreed that work may be considered a stress, elements of the work (task, tools, and so on) have been identified as contributors to stress and health problems in the workplace. Meanwhile, the proper design of the same tools and equipment has been linked to good health habits. For example, the shape of a chair is important for good sitting posture. Adjustability, good armrests, good lumbar support, an inclined backrest, and compatibility between the chair and the task have been shown to reduce neck and low back tension significantly. It should, however, be noted that, contrary to common belief, providing patients with ergonomically designed workstations does not necessarily ensure a stress-free situation. It is the combination of good health, good postural habits, and proper body mechanics that augments an ergonomically designed workplace.

Ergonomics can provide engineering solutions that reduce musculoskeletal stresses resulting from the environment, the task, the tools, and the workplace in general.[11] As presented earlier, ergonomics guidelines are numerous and should be interpreted carefully. In order to facilitate the implementation of these guidelines in the design and modification of workplaces, artificial intelligence (known as expert systems) technology has been used to develop software to assist in solving workplace design problems. This SWAD (sitting workplace analysis and design) program combines anthropometric data, workplace information, and recognized principles and considerations to chart an optimal sitting workplace. Using this computer-aided design method, workplaces are designed, analyzed, or modified and proper furniture is determined on an individual basis (Figs. 20–16 and 20–17).

In order to reduce musculoskeletal stresses at work, adjustability has been recommended. Concepts such as tiltable chairs, upwardly slanted desktops, and arm and tool support have been introduced. These features have been shown to induce more mobility, improve posture, facilitate leg movement, and significantly reduce muscle tension. Upwardly inclined desks for reading and writing appear to have a positive effect on posture.

It should be emphasized here that these concepts must not be generalized to all activities or tasks without careful analysis. For example, although a slanted work surface may be preferred for reading tasks, the same surface may not be recommended for writing activities. The same is true for "mobile" chairs where a stationary position is certainly recommended in tasks involving fine motor coordination and activities requiring stability and precision.

The introduction of computers has brought about a new set of health problems. Although computers facilitate work and aid productivity, using computers requires a considerable amount of physical effort, especially of the eyes, head, fingers, and hands. Despite being credited for increased productivity, computers have been accused of causing distress to humans. Eye fatigue and strain, sensitivity to light, blurred vision, changes in color perception, numbness of fingertips, headache, neck strain, back discomfort, skin problems, poor pregnancy outcomes, and stress are but some conditions cited! Some people think that these problems are due to increased repetitive movement, straining of tendons, hyperextension of wrists, and restricted static pos-

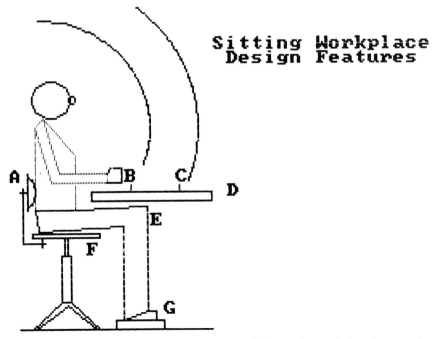

Figure 20–16. Computer printout of SWAD (sitting workplace analysis and design) output showing workplace parameters individualized for its user. The dimensions are produced following automated computerized analysis.

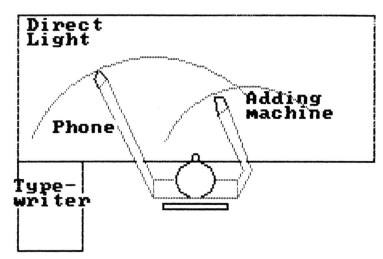

Figure 20–17. SWAD produces a schematic presentation of the recommended layout of the workplace based on inputs to the model combined with rules and principles programmed into the software.

tures, as compared with using a typewriter, which requires manual adjustment of margins and frequent paper changes.

Ergonomics recognizes that computers themselves are a minor contributor to the majority of these symptoms. Many of the reported health problems are a result of improper task and workplace design, poor conditions in the general environment, as well as operators' lack of knowledge of safety issues when dealing with computers. The identification of the origin of the problem is essential for the development of appropriate intervention.

Interventions Through Ergonomic Job/Task Analysis

With ergonomic job analysis, the demands required to perform crucial work tasks are determined through observations, measurement of physical parameters (motion, time, forces, and sensory demands), and interviews with the patient and the employer. The work environment and conditions are assessed for their effect on performance. Information obtained from this analysis is used to determine work duties that an individual can assume, taking into account possible modification or accommodations. This approach is in compliance with the Americans with Disabilities Act (ADA) and its regulations related to employment.

The analysis of work sites can be extremely helpful in preparing an individual to return to work. This approach may require photographing work areas, recording postures and motions, measuring forces and vibration data, and documenting repetitiveness and frequencies of job cycles. These data are then analyzed and examined to determine the risk factors specific to motion economy, postures, and body mechanics. Quantitative data are also analyzed to determine if, for example, forces and vibration data are within exposure ranges. Recommendations are then offered to improve working conditions and/or reduce repetitiveness, vibration, forces, light, and so forth. For example, in order to reduce vibration, the ergonomists may recommend the use of dampen technology, reducing contact surface area, reducing exposure to driving force, isolating vibration, or using material that absorbs vibration.

Another common risk factor that usually requires ergonomic intervention is the task repetitiveness. Common recommendations to reduce the exposure to high-frequency activities can be reducing the number of cycles, augmenting human activities with machines through automation and mechanization (e.g., use of scanners), enlarging jobs (e.g., providing help to workers), and when possible alternating use of extremities. Ergonomic recommendations often include workers' training in proper posture and body mechanics for performing job tasks. Workers are either taught to maintain the neutral postures of their body joints or are provided with technological aids to minimize awkward deviations of body joints.

In order to reduce muscle force, the ergonomists may recommend using machines to replace human effort, improving quality of tools to reduce force, changing tool design to allow use of stronger muscles (e.g., thumb is stronger than any single finger), modifying design to use multiple muscle groups (e.g., group fingers are stronger than a thumb), distributing force over larger area (e.g., using trigger strips), reducing force by having a slip prevention design in hand-held tools, improving tools balance, use of proper gloves (e.g., not too tight at wrist), and utilizing spring action in tools such as scissors and clippers.

A useful tool in data collection is the use of "ergonomic checklists." Although it may be possible to prepare a "generic" checklist, job environments are not alike, thus necessitating customized checklists. An ergonomic checklist should be designed to focus on the human component of the workplace rather than the workplace itself. For example, it should be asked whether a work surface height permits satisfactory postures of the arms rather than simply asking what is a work surface height.

Interventions Through Work Conditioning and Job Simulation

The concepts of job simulation and work conditioning are important to effective return-to-work strategies. The objective here is to improve the physical and functional abilities of an injured individual while he or she is practicing job tasks. It is important to raise the individuals' tolerances to adequate levels in order to maximize their potential of return to work. This is accomplished through exercise, training, work conditioning, and job simulation.

In clinical settings, the ergonomists assist the health care delivery team in developing realistic job simulations within the rehabilitation establishment to permit patients to perform crucial job tasks under medical supervision. Patients are taught to perform their job task properly, which assures them that they are capable of carrying them out in "real life." This also allows the treating physician to certify that the patient has been physically rehabilitated to handle task demands.

During this activity, the ergonomist evaluates posture, body mechanics, motions, time, and forces required to perform the various tasks and relates these demands to the functional abilities of the individual. For this purpose, it is not possible, nor necessary, to *replicate* jobs. It is also not necessary either to simulate a full workday unless a work tolerance evaluation is requested.

Work conditioning programs are highly structured, task focused, goal oriented, individualized, and multidisciplinary/interdisciplinary in nature. The following factors affect the design of a work conditioning program:

1. Intensity (the level of exertion at which patients are expected to perform). The amount of weights to be carried, distances to be covered, and other physical demands are a function not only of the patients' status during treatment but also of their projected goal. The ergonomist seeks input from the rehabilitation team regarding patients' medical status in order to determine work intensity in job simulation.

2. Environment (actual or simulated). In many instances the rehabilitation team may decide that it is necessary to observe patients performing work tasks on the job. This gives an insight into work behaviors and ability to manage stress on the job and helps develop realistic treatment plans and ergonomic recommendations.

3. Personnel involved (medical, ergonomic). In most cases, the ergonomist designs and conducts work conditioning activities with input from the multidisciplinary team. It is not unusual to find a team of the ergonomist, the occupational therapist, physical therapist, the vocational counselor, the biofeedback specialist, and a psychologist working simultaneously with a patient during job simulation. Collectively, these profes-

sionals perform real-time problem-solving to address the physical, functional, biomechanical, and behavioral components of the job. Each professional brings into this process a unique input and perspective and assists in immediate problem-solving. The degree of involvement of each discipline depends on the activities required.

4. Approach (progressive nature of work simulation sessions). A patient who is deconditioned and who must return to a physically demanding job will need a different approach to work conditioning than a patient who will return to a sedentary job. The objective of rehabilitation is to raise the patient's abilities to the maximum attainable physically and functionally. The inclusion of work demands to these abilities will modify the approach to development of the care plan. The care plan also includes essential requirements before work conditioning activities begin. These are:

  a. Increase patients' awareness of posture and body mechanics.
  b. Increase flexibility and mobility.
  c. Increase strength and endurance.
  d. Improve stress management skills.
  e. Improve pain control, safety, and preventive medicine techniques.
  f. Modify behaviors toward work, employment, and return to work.
  g. Involve patient in work conditioning activities early in the treatment program.

The ergonomist provides direct supervision during the work conditioning sessions as well as encouragement, support, and reinforcement to the patient while monitoring behaviors.

Interventions through Patient Education

As discussed earlier, the thrust of the ergonomic approach puts people as the primary element of concern in pain management and functional restoration. Throughout all the interventions described earlier, patients' knowledge and awareness are developed. Patients with pain are taught to recognize their capabilities and limitations and to incorporate and follow ergonomics guidelines when performing virtually any activity. In this process, patients learn not to rely solely on "assistive" devices in order to function. They also learn to realize and identify commercial "gimmicks" directed at their pain and suffering.

Intervention through Postural Correction

The relationship between poor posture and discomfort is well established. Poor, awkward postures cause fatigue, strain, and eventually pain and should be corrected (Figs. 20–18 through 20–25). Poor postures may result in anatomic deformation, pain, many irregularities in the body functions, loss of stability, and falls, slips, and other related accidents. Faulty posture and poor body alignment develop slowly and may not be observed by the individual. Poor posture can develop due to obesity, weakened muscles, osteoporosis, emotional tension, and poor postural habits in the workplace.

Fixed posture is commonly seen in today's offices. It has been indicated that the incidence of pain increases in predominantly sitting work activities as compared with work tasks allowing walking, standing, and sitting.[14] Fixed postures are associated with circulatory disadvantage and diminished blood flow in the muscle, giving rise to pain, reflex muscle contraction, or spasms and eventually tissue damage. A work environment that facilitates movements may reduce the impact of this disadvantage.

It is recognized that postures that place static loading on muscles and place joints in awkward positions are not healthy. Prolonged forward bending of the head and trunk, stooped postures, forced postures, and postures causing constant deviation from neutral alignment are but few examples of poor postures. Many causes of poor postures can be easily identified. Among these are body structural abnormalities such as scoliosis, poor postural habits including slouching when sitting, and poor design of chairs and furniture.

Ergonomics addresses the factors contributing to poor postures from both the physical and the engineering perspective. On the physical level, deficiencies in human

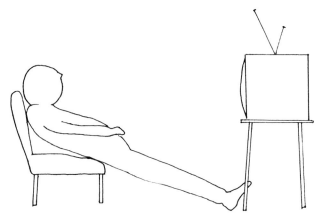

Figure 20–18. Comfortable postures are not necessarily good. Fatigue, pain, and poor habits cause poor postures. Ergonomics education and rationalization are essential in this regard. Principles must be generalized to all activities of daily living.

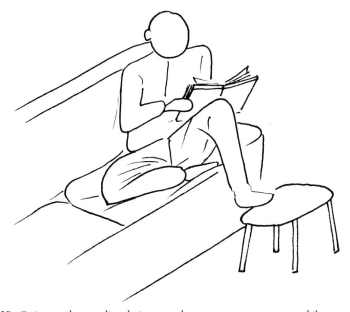

Figure 20–19. Owing to the peculiar design, people assume many postures while on a sofa in their attempt to obtain comfort. Ergonomics can aid in the design and use of sofas as well as in the selection of which activities they should be used for (e.g., reading, watching TV).

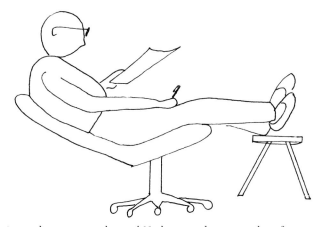

Figure 20–20. An accident waiting to happen! Neck pain and injury resulting from mechanical failure of the chair are possibilities. Ergonomics can intervene for education and task modification to correct this situation.

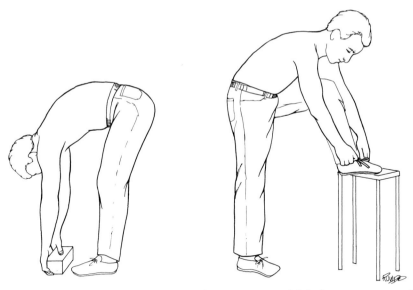

Figure 20–21. Improper body mechanics in performing activities of daily living can cause or lead to injury and pain. Alternative ways should be studied while considering the capabilities and limitations of the individual.

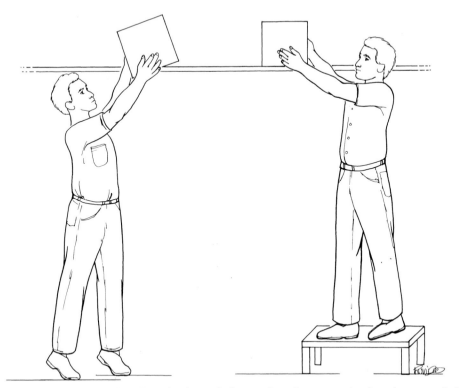

Figure 20–22. The use of mechanical aids can facilitate task performance and reduce the potential of serious injuries.

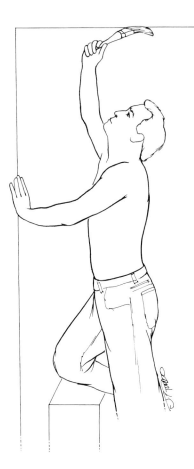

Figure 20–23. Working overhead is one of the most stressful activities involving the shoulder, neck, and arms. Caution must be exercised in such cases and the use of alternative methods must be investigated.

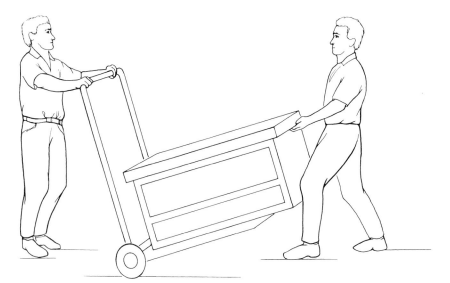

Figure 20–24. The use of mechanical aids and help from coworkers are strongly recommended in tasks involving bulky and heavy objects.

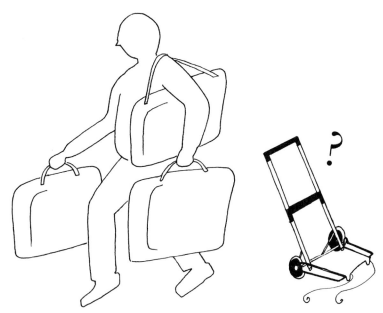

Figure 20–25. Wheeled carts are very useful for daily activities involving handling heavy or bulky objects, provided that there are no stairways or escalators.

structural capabilities can be considered in the design and selection of products and tools. Knowledge and awareness of proper posture can be increased through education and training. Also, products that encourage poor posture must be modified or replaced whenever feasible. Stress and its physiologic consequences can also lead to poor postural habits. People need to be aware of stress as a source of musculoskeletal strain.

In rehabilitation, posture correction is a key element in functional restoration. Patients are taught, through practice and the use of biofeedback, to maintain proper posture, to choose proper equipment, to modify their working environment to encourage good postural habits, and to alternate activities to avoid postural fatigue.

Body Mechanics Interventions

Body mechanics is the manner by which an activity is carried out. Proper body mechanics provides the basis for the safest way to perform daily tasks. Ergonomics intervention in this area consists of education as well as observation during practice. Proper ways to sit, stand, walk, lift, carry, and so forth and their rationale are evaluated and taught to patients. In order to ensure effective implementation, patients must be observed while performing the activity. Feedback can then be offered as patients increase their tolerance to perform the activity. Most often, ergonomics utilizes biofeedback principles to assist patients in learning proper body mechanics and to demonstrate that proper techniques do indeed reduce muscular tension and increase work efficiency.

It is important that body mechanics techniques be taught with sufficient generalization. This will allow patients to accommodate the specific body mechanics technique in the presence of conditions other than pain and as the task demands change. In other words, although it may be advisable to bend the knees and keep the back straight while lifting, this rule may be modified in the presence of knee precautions or as the amount of weight lifted increases beyond a certain value or when the object lifted is of a large size that cannot fit between the legs.

Ergonomics in the Post-rehabilitation Stage

Effective pain management and rehabilitation approaches can succeed in achieving the goal of functional restoration and return to work or a productive lifestyle. However, if no effort is made to ensure that functional gains obtained during rehabilitation are maintained following discharge from treatment, recurrence of pain or disability may result. Also, if efforts are not expended to rectify and correct the cause(s) of pain and injury, reinjury can occur.

In this stage, ergonomics' emphasis is on the re-engineering of the task and the environment to permit a more compatible and safer relationship between the person and his or her working or living environment. During this stage ergonomics contributes by:

1. Designing effective programs for continued health following hospitalization to ensure that the rehabilitated person continues to be active. A properly designed home program (physical, avocational) that incorporates good body mechanics, relaxation, pacing, flare-up management, and so forth should become an integral part of the patient's daily routine indefinitely, even if there is no pain.

2. Re-engineering of the work and home environments. If the patient returns to the same poorly designed environment where, in many cases, he or she sustained the injury, there is a good possibility that reinjury may occur.

Therefore, it becomes a priority to analyze and study the working or living environment (as well as the task) to ensure that the rehabilitated person will be able to perform productively without risk of reinjury. Once again, ergonomically inspired modifications do not necessarily have to be an expensive undertaking.

Managerial and Administrative Interventions

Ergonomics contributions in this area aim at assisting supervisors and employers in facilitating patients' return to work. Among these efforts are:

- Work diversification and variation to allow for changing postures
- Allowing for work breaks and rest pauses
- Periodic work screening to provide better match
- Reducing workload through automation and mechanization
- Enlargement of work team (i.e., getting two people to do the job instead of one)
- Job rotation (allowing the worker to alternate hands, or rotating jobs among workers as an option)
- Providing proper work tools (e.g., sharper knives, thumb or stop triggers, tools with good mechanical balance)
- Changing work methods (e.g., avoiding tight handling of tools, changing grasp, using a power grip instead of the flat palm)
- Considering the use of mechanical restraints for safety
- Rearranging the workplace to preserve neutral postures
- Reducing the amount of force required to perform the task

Ergonomics and the Americans with Disabilities Act

The Americans with Disabilities Act (ADA) is a civil right protection act that provides comprehensive protection to individuals with disabilities. The ADA addresses disability issues in relation to employment, public accommodation, transportation, and telecommunication.

The application of ergonomics methods to individuals with disability necessitates competent knowledge of the ADA and its provisions.[3] A review of the ADA is beyond the scope of this chapter; however, a selected number of relevant issues are discussed here. According to the ADA, an "individual with a disability" is a person who has a physical or mental impairment that substantially limits one or more major life activities, a person who has a record of physical or mental impairment that substantially limits one or more major life activities, or a person who is regarded as having such an impairment.

The ADA prohibits discrimination in all employment practices, including job application procedures, hiring, firing, advancement, compensation, and training. It applies to recruitment, advertising, tenure, layoff, leave, fringe benefits, and all other employment-related activities. An employer may not make a pre-employment inquiry on an application form or in an interview as to whether, or to what extent, an individual is disabled. The employer may ask a job applicant whether he or she can perform particular job functions. If the applicant has a disability known to the employer, the employer may ask how he or she can perform job functions that the employer considers difficult or impossible to perform because of the disability, and whether an accommodation would be needed. A job offer may be conditioned on the results of a medical examination, provided that the examination is required for all entering employees in the same job category regardless of disability, and that information obtained is handled according to confidentiality requirements specified in the act. After an employee enters on duty, all medical examinations and inquiries must be *job related* and necessary for the conduct of the employer's business.

The employment provision of the ADA, therefore, governs the ergonomic approach to assisting an employer in designing job applications, job descriptions, and employment offers. It also affects the approach to functional capacity assessment because evaluations have to be job specific. This, in turn, means that the use of computerized testing equipment for the evaluation of "generic" functional abilities may no longer be valid. Evaluation setting should simulate the work situation. Testing protocols will need to be changed and modified to meet compliance. The ergonomist can also assist the employer in developing practical "post-offer" screening tools in order to test the applicant's ability to perform essential job functions (with or without reasonable accommodations).

The ADA expressly permits employers to establish qualification standards that will exclude individuals who pose a direct threat—i.e., a significant risk—to the health and safety of others, if that risk cannot be lowered to an acceptable level by reasonable accommodation. However, an employer may not simply assume that a threat exists; the employer must establish through objective, medically supportable methods that there is genuine risk that substantial harm could occur in the workplace. By requiring employers to make individualized judgments based on reliable medical evidence rather than on generalizations, ignorance, fear, patronizing attitudes, or stereotypes, the ADA recognizes the need to balance the interests of people with disabilities against the legitimate interests of employers in maintaining a safe workplace. The ergonomist can assist in this area by establishing workplace safety criteria in relation to human factors while taking into account medical information.

Another core issue in the ADA is reasonable accommodation. Reasonable accommodation is any modification or adjustment to a job or the work environment that should be made to enable a qualified applicant or employee with a disability to perform essential job functions. This is another area of primary relevance to ergonomics. Examples of reasonable accommodation include making existing facilities used by employees readily accessible to and usable by an individual with a disability, restructuring a job, modifying work schedules, acquiring or modifying equipment, providing qualified readers or interpreters, and appropriately modifying examinations, training, or other programs. Reasonable accommodation also may include reassigning a current employee to a vacant position for which the individual is qualified if the person becomes disabled and is unable to do the original job. An employer, however, is not required to make an accommodation if it would impose an "undue hardship" on the operation of the employer's business.

Ergonomics and the Performing Artist

Muscial instruments have been termed "instruments of torture." Among the 130,000 individuals in the United States who earn their livelihood playing a musical instrument, 60% to 80% report incidence of overuse syndrome and cumulative trauma disorders.[2] Dancers report injury rates as high as 97%.[10] *Violinists* abrade their chins, *pianists* suffer from arm and fingers pain, and *drummers* suffer trigger fingers and curled-up index finger. It is not uncommon for the performing artist to suffer from swelling, mild to severe discomfort, weakness, soreness, stiffness, cuts and wounds, and sleep disturbance. These disabling symptoms have been attributed to factors such as:

1. Continuous and excessive use of the muscles in performing a certain movement
2. Excessive force to play the instrument
3. Prolonged static pressure to hold the instrument
4. Poor postures while performing
5. Inefficient movements, techniques, and habits
6. Instrument design
7. Duration of activity (including practice, rehearsals, performance)
8. Stress (physical, mental, environmental, performance anxiety)
9. Organization of practice/performance sessions

These stressors manifest themselves in the form of strain, microscopic tears in tendons, ligaments, or muscles, and an added strain upon other tissue due to compensation.

The ergonomic approach to the management of these types of disorders follows the scheme outlined throughout this chapter. Identification of the problem becomes a priority. For example, with the violin, the angle of fingers and elbow position exceeds neutral posture requirement and can cause damage to tendon between index finger and thumb. String and keyboard players have a higher incidence of injury than woodwind, brass, and percussion instrumentalists. Stage chairs are often cited for increased muscle tension and neck and back pain. The handling of instruments before and after performance may also attribute to the cause of injury.

Ergonomic interventions to address these issues require close cooperation with the artist in order to address and solve current problems and avoid future incidence. The performing artist is taught to "do something about the problem!" Only 37% of this group of professionals receive or seek medical care. Others lack proper medical coverage or fear public exposure.[4]

Ergonomically, and depending on the instrument, performers are instructed to adopt preventive measures:

1. Keep hands, arms, and shoulders in proper position.
2. Stay physically fit. Use one of the daily 6 hours of practicing to exercise.
3. Pace yourself. Break up practice time into shorter segments.
4. Change position and posture during the break.
5. Relax when not playing. Take breaks.
6. Pinpoint the cause of the pains and aches.
7. The longer symptoms go unattended, the more complicated and potentially dangerous they become.
8. Stay informed about recent statistics, treatments, and predisposing/preventive factors in music-related injuries.
9. Do not assume that because the instrument has always been played this way, it makes good ergonomic sense.
10. Banjoist—move strap from one shoulder to the other.
11. Pianist—move entire hand to reach the keys rather than poking out with fingers.

Summary

The management of myofascial pain is far from simple. The contributions of ergonomics to the management of myofascial pain are many and should be integrated in all efforts aimed at the prevention and management of the problem. The utilization of ergonomics at the University of Miami CPRC has resulted in valuable approaches that are clinically sound. These approaches originate from actual applications of ergonomics methods with patients presenting with myofascial pain. Not only does ergonomics benefit treatment, its benefits in the prevention of injury (or reinjury) are apparent. Successful ergonomic intervention strategies have demonstrated that pain management should be comprehensive and multidisciplinary. The inclusion of human engineering principles is therefore needed, especially where the objective is functional restoration, reduction of pain, and return to a productive lifestyle.

It is essential that physicians who treat persons of working age, especially worker's compensation patients, be aware of all issues that go beyond the medical findings. They can be confounding and not easily recognized, as medical education does not prepare physicians in these areas. Attention to the vocational, psychosocial, ergonomic, and economic issues are paramount in the assessment and treatment of such patients. Great care should also be taken not to conclude that the pain problem is psychogenic in nature. The physical substrate must be vigorously pursued first along with other issues impacting upon the patient. Prevention and quality of life issues must also be considered.

Many of these patients are desperate and have given up hope. From the standpoint of quality care and compassion, they deserve to be treated holistically in order to achieve the best possible outcome and resumption of a productive and high-quality life. Ergonomics can provide an added dimension in the effort to relieve pain and suffering.

References

1. Abdel-Moty E, Compton R, Steele-Rosomoff R, et al: Process analysis of functional capacity assessment. Journal of Back and Musculoskeletal Rehabilitation 6:223–236, 1996.
2. Amadio PC, Russotti GM: Evaluation and treatment of hand and wrist disorders in musicians. Hand Clin 6:405–416, 1990.
3. Americans with Disabilities Act. Technical Assistance Manual on the Employment Provision (Title) of the ADA. US Equal Employment Opportunities Commission, 1992.
4. Caldron PH, Calabrese L, Clough JD, et al: A survey of musculoskeletal problems encountered in high level musicians. Medical Problems of Performing Artists. 1:136–139, 1986.
5. Fishbain DA, Abdel-Moty E, Cutler R, et al: Detection of a "faked" strength task effort in volunteers using a computerized exercise testing system. Am J Phys Med Rehab 78(3):222–227, 1999.
6. Fishbain DA, Abdel-Moty E, Cutler R, et al: Measuring residual functional capacity in chronic low back pain patients based on the Dictionary of Occupational Titles. Spine 19(8):872–880, 1994.
7. Fishbain DA, Cutler R, Rosomoff H, et al: Movement in work status after pain facility treatment. Spine 22:2662–2669, 1996.
8. Fishbain DA, Cutler R, Rosomoff H, et al: Validity of the Dictionary of Occupational Titles residual functional capacity battery. Clinical J Pain 15(2):102–110, 1999.
9. Fishbain DA, Khalil TM, Abdel-Moty E, et al: Physician limitations when assessing work capacity: a review. Journal of Back and Musculoskeletal Rehabilitation 5:107–113, 1995.
10. Kerr G, Krasnow D, Mainwaring L: The nature of dance injuries. Medical Problems in Performing Artists 7:25–29, 1992.
11. Khalil TM, Abdel-Moty E, Rosomoff RS, Rosomoff HL: Ergonomics in Back Pain: A Guide to Prevention and Rehabilitation. New York, Van Nostrand Reinhold, 1993.
12. Khalil TM, Abdel-Moty E, Rosomoff RS, Rosomoff HL: The role of ergonomics in the prevention and treatment of myofascial pain. In Rachlin E (ed): Myofascial Pain and Fibromyalgia. St. Louis, Mosby-Year Book, 1994, pp 487–523.
13. National Institute for Occupational Safety and Health (NIOSH) 2000. http://www.cdc.gov/niosh/ergopage.html
14. Occupational Safety and Health Administration (OSHA) 2000. http://www.osha-slc.gov/ergonomics-standard/overview.html
15. Rosomoff HL, Rosomoff RS: Comprehensive multidisciplinary pain center approach to the treatment of low back pain. Neurosurgery Clinics of North America 2(4):877–890, 1991.

Index

Note: Page numbers followed by f indicate figures; those followed by t indicate tables.